MANUAL OF
I.V. Therapeutics
Evidence-Based Infusion Therapy

Fifth Edition

MANUAL OF
I.V. Therapeutics

Evidence-Based Infusion Therapy

Fifth Edition

Lynn Dianne Phillips, MSN, RN, CRNI®
Professsor Emeritus
Butte College
Oroville, California
Nursing Education Consultant
President
Infusion Nurses Society 2009–2010

F.A. Davis Company • Philadelphia

F. A. Davis Company
1915 Arch Street
Philadelphia, PA 19103
www.fadavis.com

Printed in the United States of America

Last digit indicates print number: 10 9 8 7 6 5 4 3 2 1

Acquisitions Editor: Thomas A. Ciavarella
Director of Content Development: Darlene D. Pedersen
Sr. Project Editor: Padraic J. Maroney
Project Editor: Christina C. Burns
Art and Design Manager: Carolyn O'Brien

As new scientific information becomes available through basic and clinical research, recommended treatments and drug therapies undergo changes. The author(s) and publisher have done everything possible to make this book accurate, up to date, and in accord with accepted standards at the time of publication. The author(s), editors, and publisher are not responsible for errors or omissions or for consequences from application of the book, and make no warranty, expressed or implied, in regard to the contents of the book. Any practice described in this book should be applied by the reader in accordance with professional standards of care used in regard to the unique circumstances that may apply in each situation. The reader is advised always to check product information (a inserts) for changes and new information regarding dose and contraindications before administering any drug. Caution is especially urged when using new or infrequently ordered drugs.

Library of Congress Cataloging-in-Publication Data

Phillips, Lynn Dianne, 1947-
  Manual of I.V. therapeutics : evidence-based infusion therapy / Lynn Dianne Phillips. — 5th ed.
    p. ; cm.
  Other title: Manual of IV therapeutics
  Includes bibliographical references and index.
  ISBN-13: 978-0-8036-2184-8 (alk. paper)
  ISBN-10: 0-8036-2184-1 (alk. paper)
  1. Intravenous therapy—Handbooks, manuals, etc. I. Title. II. Title: Manual of IV therapeutics.
    [DNLM: 1. Infusions, Intravenous—methods—Examination Questions. 2. Infusions,
  Intravenous—methods—Handbooks. 3. Infusions, Intravenous—nursing—Examination Questions.
  4. Infusions, Intravenous—nursing—Handbooks. WB 39 P561m 2010]
    RM170.P48 2010
    615.5'8—dc22   2010008392

*This book is dedicated to my husband Don,
for all his love and support
My daughter Christa, for her talents and wisdom
And as always
To nursing students—our future*

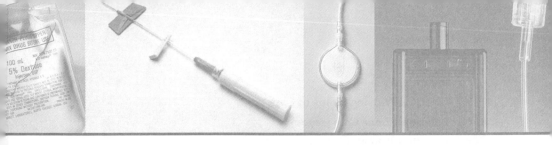

PREFACE

Manual of I.V. Therapeutics: Evidence-Based Infusion Therapy, fifth edition, provides comprehensive information on infusion therapy for the nursing student and practicing nurse. New to this edition is evidence-based nursing practice (EBNP) and evidence-based care (EBC), which is frequently sited as being defined as the conscientious use of current best evidence in making decisions about patient care. Evidence-based nursing practice adds research evidence in the form of systematic reviews and clinical practice guidelines to a clinician's knowledge, judgment, and experience. It de-emphasizes practice based on tradition and ritual. EBNP is important to any nurse performing infusion therapy, due to rapidly expanding dimensions of the nurse's role and the ongoing introduction of new infusion devices and techniques. Also new to this edition is a complete chapter on math calculations for infusion practice. The fifth edition is reorganized to include pediatric and the older adult in a separate section in each chapter. This textbook incorporates Infusion Nurses Society standards of practice and the most current 2008 Centers of Disease Control and Prevention (CDC) guidelines for prevention of intravascular catheter-related infections.

This self-paced, comprehensive text presents information ranging from a simple to complex format, incorporating theory into clinical application. The skills of recall, nursing process, critical thinking, and patient education are covered, along with detailed summaries, providing the foundation one needs to become a knowledgeable practitioner. The psychomotor skills associated with infusion therapy are presented in step-by-step procedures with rationales based on standards of practice at the end of the chapters.

Each chapter has accompanying objectives, defined glossary terms that are bolded within the text, a post-test, chapter highlights summary, and a critical thinking case study. Icons and special boxes are used throughout each chapter to key the reader to web sites, patient education, home care issues, cultural considerations, and standards of practice. SkillChecks, 100 test questions, power point presentations, and math calculations tests are included on the DavisPlus faculty ancillaries which can be used in the educational setting, as well as in agencies, for validating competencies of nurses in infusion skills. **The icons used in this fifth edition are as follows:**

NOTE> Identifies key points of theory content

◖▭▷ **Identifies Nursing Fast Facts** are in italic and shaded within the chapter for important nursing practice information.

EBNP **Identifies Evidence-Based Nursing Practice (EBNP)**

⊕ Identifies Web Sites

⌗ Identifies Nursing Points of Care

▪ Identifies Home Care Issues

● Identifies Patient Education information

◉ Identifies a media link, which refers to the book's accompanying CD–ROM, and is located in the critical thinking case study and post-test sections at the end of each chapter.

INS Standard Identifies Infusion Nurses Society (INS), Standards of Practice

The fifth edition of this textbook is organized from foundations of practice followed by basic practices for all nurses and concludes with specialty infusion practices. The first three foundations chapters are designed to give in-depth information to the reader on nursing practice related to infusion therapy (nursing process applied to infusion therapy, legal and ethical responsibilities, evidence-based practice background, and performance improvement); infection control and risk management practices, and fundamentals of fluid and electrolyte balance.

The subsequent seven chapters provide the essential solid foundation in infusion therapy practices, including parenteral solutions, infusion equipment, peripheral and central line techniques and management, complications, medication infusion modalities and infusion calculations. This fifth edition has incorporated recurring displays for cultural and ethnic related issues. Key concepts for nursing practice are identified as "**Nursing Fast Facts**" and "**>Note**" identifies an important theory concept.

The last two chapters encompass the additional topics of transfusions therapy, nutritional support and phlebotomy.

The CD–ROM accompanying this textbook contains 300 questions based on standards of practice and follows the guidelines of the INS Core Curriculum for certification. The CD–ROM also includes guidelines for discussion and answers to the case studies, and additional math calculations problems and answers. The DavisPlus web site provides the learner with web based ancillaries, additional 50 interactive flash cards for learning terminology, interactive case studies and web links for further research.

The 200 I.V. Flash Cards available from F. A. Davis parallel the terminology in the textbook and provide an additional learning tool for understanding concepts related to infusion practice.

I hope this new edition provides you, whether you are a practicing healthcare professional or student, with valuable insights into the safe practice of infusion therapy and a reference for this rapidly advancing field.

Lynn Phillips

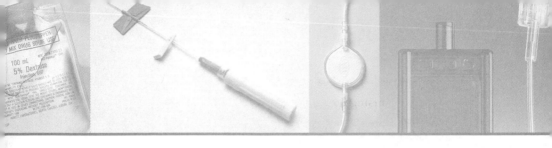

CONTRIBUTORS

CONSULTANTS

Michelle Berreth, RN, CRNI®
Nurse Educator
Infusion Nurses Society
Norwood, Massachusetts

Lynda Cook, MSN, RN, CRNI®
Infusion Nurse Specialist
Greensboro, North Carolina

**Lynn Czaplewski,
MS, APRN, BC, CRNI®, AOCNS**
Clinical Nurse Specialist
Oncology Alliance
Wauwatosa, Wisconsin

Julie Eddins, MSN, RN, CRNI®
Infusion Specialist
Smiths Medical
Fenton, Missouri

***Lisa Gorski,
MS, APRN,B, CRNI®, FAAN**
Clinical Nurse Specialist
Wheaton Franciscan Home Health &
 Hospice
Milwaukee, Wisconsin

Mark Hunter, RN, CRNI®
Clinical Affairs Manager
Global Infusion Systems – Baxter
 Healthcare
Round Lake, Illinois

Brenda Bradley Johansson, MSN, RN
Nursing Instructor
Butte College
Oroville, California

Nancy Moureau, BSN, RN, CRNI®
CEO PICC Excellence
Hartwell, Georgia

***Roxanne Perucca,
MS, APRN, CRNI®**
Director for Magnet/Nursing
 Excellance
University Hospital of Louisville
Louisville, Kentucky

***Cora Vizcarra,
MBA, RN, BSN, CRNI®**
President
MCV Associates Healthcare Inc.
Indianapolis, Indiana

*Mary Walsh, BS, RN, CRNI®
Operations Leader
Hebrew Secret Life
Gloria Adelson Health Care Center
Dedham, Massachusetts

Mary Zugcic, MS, CNS, BC
Clinical Instructor
Wayne State University
Detroit, Michigan

* Past President Infusion Nurses Society

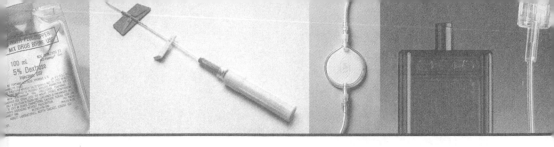

REVIEWERS

Diane Barush, MSN, CRNP
Practical Nursing Faculty
Wilkes-Barre Career and Technical
    Center
Wilkes-Barre, Pennsylvania

Elizabeth Brewington, RN, MSN
ADN Instructor
Saddleback College - Nursing
    Program
Mission Viejo, California

Charlene Gagliardi
BSN Instructor
Mount St. Mary's College
Los Angeles, California

Corrie Hightower
ADN Instructor
Grays Harbor College
Aberdeen, Washington

Cara Leslie, RN, MN
ADN Instructor
South Puget Sound Community
    College
Olympia, Washington

Danny C. Ranchez
ADN Instructor
Glendale Community College
Glendale, California

Rox An Sparks
LPN Instructor
Merced College
Merced, California

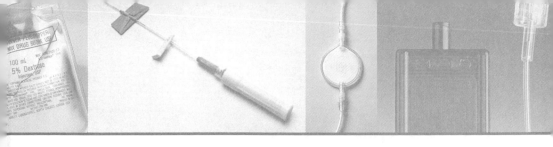

ACKNOWLEDGMENTS

The author would like to acknowledge the following:

The nurses in the specialty practice of infusion therapy

Christa Melton, for her expert organizational skills, and for assisting in acquiring pictures and permissions.

At F. A. Davis:

Tom Ciavarella, Nursing Acquisitions Editor, who assisted in the final development of this manual.

Christina Burns, Project Editor, Nursing, who as project consultant, helped bring this vision to reality.

Padriac J. Maroney, Senior Project Manager.

Sam Rondinelli, Production Manager, for guiding this manuscript through the production process.

Robert G. Martone, Publisher, Nursing, whose foresight brought the project to F. A. Davis

And....

Appreciation is expressed to the following companies who provided product information, pictures and illustrations:

3 M Health Care Division, St. Paul, MN
Bard Access Systems, Inc., Salt Lake City, UT
Bard Access Systems, Inc., Covington, GA
Baxter Healthcare Corporation, Round Lake, IL
B. Braun Medical Inc., Bethlehem, PA
Becton, Dickinson and Company, Sandy, UT
Cardinal Health, San Diego, CA
Enloe Medical Center, Chico, CA
Ethicon, Inc. (J&J Wound Management), Somerville, NJ
Hospira Incorporated, Lake Forest, IL
Infusion Nurses Society, Norwood, MA
I.V. House, Inc., Chesterfield, MO
Lippincott, Williams & Wilkins, Philadelphia, PA
MediVisuals, Inc., Dallas, TX
Norfolk Medical Products, Inc., Skokie, IL
Pall Medical, Ann Arbor, MI
Smiths-Medical Critical Care, Inc., Carlsbad, CA
Teleflex Medical (Arrow), Research Triangle Park, NC
TransLite LLC, Sugar Land, TX
VidaCare, San Antonio, TX

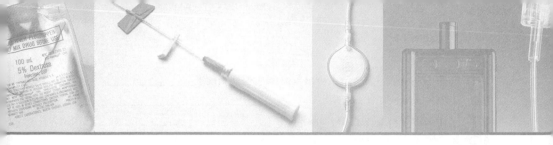

TABLES

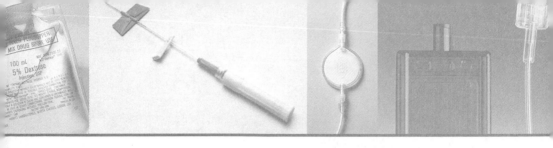

CONTENTS IN BRIEF

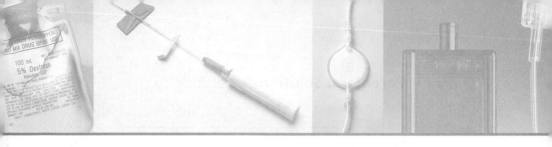

CONTENTS

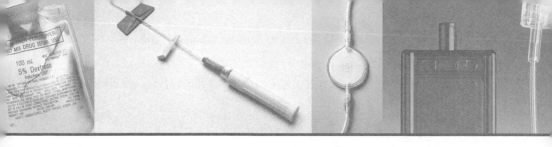

Chapter **1**

Professional Practice Concepts for Infusion Therapy

In dwelling upon the vital importance of sound observation, it must never be lost sight of what observation is for. It is not for the sake of piling up miscellaneous information or curious facts, but for the sake of saving life and increasing health and comfort.

Florence Nightingale, 1873

Chapter Contents

■ LEARNING OBJECTIVES

On completion of this chapter, the reader will be able to:

1. Define the terminology related to infusion-related professional practice.
2. Identify the elements of infusion nurse competency.
3. Discuss the use of competency-based education programs in the practice of infusion therapy.
4. Discuss the value of certification in a specialty practice.
5. Discuss evidence-based practice.
6. Apply the steps needed to incorporate evidence-based health care into nursing practice.
7. Identify the components of the nursing process and how they are applied to infusion practice.
8. Identify the sources of laws.
9. Differentiate between standards of care and standards of practice.
10. Identify the areas of breach of duty for the specialty of infusion nursing.
11. Identify the role of the nurse as an expert witness.
12. Apply quality management strategies to infusion practice.
13. Identify risk management and risk assessment strategies.

⧖ GLOSSARY

Assessment   The systematic and continuous collection, organization, validation, and documentation of data

Audit   A review of care using defined criteria

Bar coding system   Systems that encode data electronically into a format of bars and spaces, scanned by lasers into a computer to identify the object it labels

Benchmarking   Structured, comparative trending of performances that represent "best-known" practices and the identification of goals against which all other levels of performance are measured

Civil law   Laws that affect the legal rights of private persons or corporations

Competency   Integrated behaviors derived from an explicit set of desired outcomes

Criminal law   Offense against the general public; affects welfare of society as a whole

Criteria   Elements necessary to define and measure quality

Data collection   Gathering information through interviewing, observing, and inspecting

Diagnosing   Analysis of assessment data, identification of client strengths and health problems, and formulation of a diagnostic statement

Documentation   A recording, in written or printed form, containing original, official, or legal information

Evaluation   Measuring the degree to which goals/outcomes have been achieved and identifying factors that positively or negatively influence goal achievement.

Evidence-based care   Recognized by nursing, medicine, healthcare institutions, and makers as care based on state-of-the-art science reports

Evidence-based nursing practice (EBNP)   Conscientious, explicit, and judicious use of theory-derived, research-based information in making decisions about care delivery to individuals or groups of individuals

Expert testimony   Witness from the same professional specialty explaining to the court what the standard of care should be in the situation at hand

Goal   Broad statement of a desired outcome

Implementation   Carrying out planned nursing interventions

Liable   Legally responsible for damages, answerable

Malpractice   Negligent conduct of a professional person

Negligence   Not acting in a reasonable or prudent manner

Nursing standard   Specific statement about the quality of a facet of nursing care

Outcome   The result of the performance (or nonperformance) of a function or process(es)

Performance improvement (PI)   The continuous study and adaptation of functions and processes of a healthcare organization to increase the probability of achieving desired outcomes and to better meet the needs of patients and other users of services; the third segment of the performance measurement, assessment, and improvement system

Planning   Determining how to prevent, reduce, or resolve the identified patients problems; how to support client strengths; and how to implement nursing interventions in an organized, individualized, and goal-directed manner

Process   A goal-directed, interrelated series of actions, events, mechanisms, or steps

Quality improvement (QI)   An ongoing process of innovation, prevention of error, and staff development used by an organization that has adopted a quality management philosophy. Used interchangeably with performance improvement

Quality management (QM)   A corporate culture emphasizing customer satisfaction, innovation, and employee involvement in quality improvement activities. Often used interchangeably with total quality management, continuous quality management, quality improvement, and performance improvement.

Risk management   Process that centers on identification, analysis, treatment and evaluation of real and potential hazards

Standard of care   Focuses on the recipient of care consistent with minimum safe professional conduct and describes outcomes of care that patients can expect to receive

Standards of nursing practice   Focuses on the provider and defines competent care along with the activities and behavior needed to achieve positive patient outcomes

Statutes   Written laws enacted by the legislature

Structure   Standard that refers to conditions and mechanisms that provide support for the delivery of care (e.g., policy and resources)

Tort   Private wrong, by act or omission, that can result in a civil action by the harmed person

Total quality management (TQM)   Management system fostering continuously improving performance at every level of every function by focusing on maximization of customer satisfaction; focuses on process

■ Delivery of Quality Care

Clinical Competency

Competency Standards

The Joint Commission for Accreditation of Healthcare Organizations (JCAHO), now called The Joint Commission (TJC, 2007), defines **competency** as "a determination of an individual's capability to perform expectations." Further definition includes documentation in the personnel file that the employee's clinical knowledge, experience, and capabilities are appropriate for assigned duties per the requirements of the minimum data set for competency. Effective January 2008, the Health Care Staffing Services (HCSS) Certification Program Performance Measure Implementation Guide is available from TJC, which presents standardized performance measures. Suggested data sources for documentation of competency include:

1. Clinical skills checklists/competency assessments
2. Continuing education credits

3. Documents that verify training and education
4. References from previous employers (TJC, 2007)

Competency assessment relies on many factors. Competency may be reviewed through information obtained from past and current employers, peer recommendations, validating specialty certifications, testing, ongoing performance data collection, and/or skills observation, either separately on in partnership with customers. The agency customers (clients) need to provide feedback regarding competency assessment to the organization. When the agency chooses to measure competency, it should do so in a thorough and ongoing fashion, including looking at significant, high-risk activities or competencies that are new to the staff member (TJC, 2006).

Based on the National Council of State Boards of Nursing (NCSBN) 2002 job analysis studies, the following are some general patterns of employer expectations. The staff member should:

1. Possess the necessary theoretic background for safe client care and for decision-making.
2. Use the nursing process in a systematic way.
3. Recognize own abilities and limitations.
4. Use communication skills effectively with clients and co-workers.
5. Work effectively with assistive personnel, delegating and supervising nursing care tasks in an appropriate manner.
6. Understand the importance of accurate and complete documentation
7. Possess proficiency in the basic technical nursing skills.
8. Understand and have a commitment to a work ethic.
9. Function with acceptable speed.
(NCSBN, 2003).

A competent nurse in infusion therapy is well qualified by education and capable of performing infusion therapy in an exact and effective manner using the appropriate nursing knowledge, technical expertise, and specialized skills. Within the educational context, competency may be defined as a simultaneous integration of the knowledge, skills, and attitudes required for performance in a designated role and setting.

The practice setting for infusion therapy delivery is as varied as the patient populations served by this specialty practice. In treatment of patients, ranging from hospitalized neonates to elderly persons in extended care facilities or private homes, the competencies of nurses and the combination of knowledge, skills, and abilities necessary to fulfill the role of a nurse administering infusion therapy span all ages and disease processes. Basic competencies are intended to serve as guidelines for practicing nurses and to assist in designing orientation and continuing education programs (Corrigan, 2010).

Infusion nursing is defined as using the nursing process relating to technical and clinical application of fluids, electrolytes, infection control, oncology, pediatrics, pharmacology, quality assurance, technology and clinical applications, parenteral nutrition, and transfusion therapy (Corrigan, 2010). The practice of infusion nursing encompasses the nursing management and coordination of care to the patient in accordance with:

1. State statutes
2. INS Standards of Practice
3. Established institutional policy
4. TJC requirements

Elements

Elements of infusion nursing competency include:

1. Accountability: The role of infusion nurses implies that nurses are astute and knowledgeable enough to adjust their interventions (i.e., interference that may affect outcome) to accomplish short- and long-term care goals.
2. Communication: Exchange of information allows everyone involved in the patient's care to make intelligent decisions based on complete data and professional collaboration.
3. Collaboration: TJC demands multidisciplinary involvement at all levels of patient care. Infusion leaders must develop the skills of collaboration, consultation, and negotiation to achieve positive patient outcomes.
4. Autonomy: Nurses can have increased autonomy by being allowed to make certain decisions independently.

Competency-Based Educational Programs

Competency-based educational programs establish specific goals, accountability, individualization, and behaviors for practitioners by defining clear expectations for levels of performance. The responsibility of ensuring a competent staff often falls to the institution in which a nurse is practicing. A framework for developing staff competencies and ensuring that the institution is delivering safe care includes:

■ Development of standards
■ Development of skills tests
■ Assessment of learning needs
■ Establishment of a plan of educational programs
■ Presentation of educational programs
■ Evaluation of learning outcomes

Competencies should be directed toward essential mandatory aspects of performance, have measurable clinical behaviors, include **evaluation** mechanisms, and test cognitive performance **criteria**. A competency program can consist of self-assessment, skills checklist, self-study modules, written examinations, and program evaluation (Rudzik, 1999).

Three-Part Competency Model

A three-part competency model includes:

1. Competency statement: Statement that reflects a measurable goal
2. Domains of learning criteria: Cognitive criteria (knowledge base) and performance criteria (psychomotor skills: observed behaviors)
3. Evaluation and learning outcomes: Written tests, return demonstrations, and precepted clinical experience

All professional nurses are accountable and responsible for all parts of the tasks associated with infusion therapy and for tasks that are delegated to the licensed practical nurse or technician for care rendered to the patient while under care. The three-part competency model is an effective tool for ensuring competent practice. A competency-based educational model requires developing the three major parts of the model: the competency statement, the performance criteria, and the evaluation and learning options.

INS Standard The nurse providing infusion therapy shall be proficient in its clinical aspects, shall have validated competency in clinical judgment and practice, and shall practice in accordance with the state's Nurse Practice Act, rules and regulations promulgated by the state Board of Nursing, organizational policies and procedures and practice guidelines. (INS, 2006, 5)

Clinical Competency Validation Program

The Infusion Nurses Society has available a clinical competency validation program for infusion therapy published in 2006. The Clinical Competency Validation Program (CCVP) is available for clinicians seeking to validate their infusion-related nursing skills. There are 33 specific nursing competencies in the program, which can be used for procedural validation skills (INS, 2006b). Refer to Table 1-1.

> Table 1-1	ASSESSING COMPETENCY

Acceptable Methods of Assessing Competency

- Direct observation by a supervisor, designated evaluator, instructor, or preceptor while the employee/student demonstrates the skill in the work setting
- Observation by a supervisor, designated evaluator, instructor, or preceptor while the employee/student demonstrates the skills in simulated settings, such as skill laboratories and mock drills.
- Direct observation and return demonstration may be supplemented with other forms of assessment such as tests. The testing should not be the primary means of assessment.

Documentation of Competency
Competency assessments should be documented.
- Competency checklist
- Department job/specific competency

Value of Certification

Professional nursing certification programs have long established their value and importance to healthcare organizations and patients and their families. Certification, as defined by the American Board of Nursing Specialties (ABNS), is the formal recognition of specialized knowledge, skills, and experience demonstrated by achievement of standards identified by a nursing specialty to promote optimal health outcomes (ABNS, 2006).

Basic nursing licensure indicates a minimal professional practice standard; certification denotes a high level of knowledge and practice, with the intent to protect the public (Byrne, Valentine, & Carter, 2004). Certification by credentialing related to the practice of infusion therapy includes the following:

1. Infusion Nurses Certification Corporation: CRNI®. www.ins1.org
2. Oncology Nursing Certification Corporation: OCN®. www.oncc.org
3. Pediatric Nursing Certification Board: CPN®. www.pncb.org
4. American Society for Parenteral and Enteral Nutrition: CNSC. www.nbnsc@nutr.org

The American Board of Nursing Specialties (ABNS) was formed in 1991. Its mission is to "promote the value of specialty nursing certification to all stake holders" (ABNS, 2006). In 2004, the ABNS Research Committee developed a Value of Certification Survey (Evidence-Based Care Box 1-1).

Evidence-Based Care

Evidence-based care (EBC) is clinically competent care based on the best scientific evidence available recognized by nursing, medicine, and healthcare institutions. It incorporates clinical expertise and the patient's preferences.

EVIDENCE-BASED CARE BOX 1-1

Validation of Nurses' Perceptions, Values, and Behaviors Related to Certification

American Board of Nursing Specialties. (2005). A position statement on the value of specialty nursing certification. Retrieved from www.nursingcertification.org (Accessed March 4, 2008).

The American Board of Nursing Specialties (ABNS) Research Committee in 2004 conducted a study of 11,000 nurse respondents, across 20 specialty nursing certification organizations, representing 36 different certification credentials (ABNS, 2005).

Results from the Perceived Value of Certification Tool (PVCT) document a high level of agreement among certified nurses, noncertified nurses, and nurse managers that certification is greatly valued among nurses. This study demonstrates that certification persists as a valuable method for nurses to differentiate themselves in the workplace.

Evidence-based care is a newer term replacing the term evidence-based medicine (EBM), which was coined in 1980s in Canada. Evidence-based care is a process approach to collecting, reviewing, interpreting, critiquing, and evaluating research and other relevant literature for application to patient care (Kelly, 2008).

Evidence-based nursing practice (EBNP) is frequently defined as the conscientious use of current best evidence in making decisions about patient care (Sackett, Straus, Richardson, et al., 2000). The goal of EBNP is to apply valid and reliable research to clinical practice. Evidence-based nursing practice adds research evidence from systematic reviews and clinical practice guidelines to a clinician's knowledge, judgment, and experience. It deemphasizes practice based on tradition and ritual (Valente, 2003). EBNP is important to the infusion nurse owing to rapidly expanding dimensions of the nurse's role and the ongoing introduction of new infusion devices and techniques. Each time a new device or technique is introduced, new practices must be considered. Questions that should be asked when new technology is introduced include: What does science have to say about the change? Does the literature identify differences in practices depending on setting? Between the ongoing safety initiatives being introduced into healthcare setting and the increasing presence of practice guidelines, it is imperative that the infusion nurse use evidence to support infusion practice (Newell-Stokes, 2004).

Research is needed to establish and facilitate consistency in some practice decisions. However, some variations in practice, when they occur, need to be evaluated for appropriateness. Components of EBNP include the following:

- Evidence from research/evidence-based theories, and opinion leaders/expert panels
- Evidence from assessment of patient's history, physical exam, and availability of healthcare resources.
- Clinical expertise
- Information about patient preferences and values (Gorski, 2007).

The use of best evidence in practice is now a measurable goal (Hagle, 2010). The Institute of Medicine (IOM) has set a goal that by 2020, "90% of clinical decisions will be supported by accurate, timely and up-to-date clinical information, and will reflect the best available evidence" (IOM, 2007). EBNP is an international movement, with leadership from nurses in the United Kingdom, the United States, Australia, New Zealand, and Germany.

Using infusion therapy–related research studies to develop changes in procedure or policy, along with published standards such as Infusion Nurses Standards of Practice, is one way to apply evidence-based practice to infusion practice. The application of research to practice is important; however, it requires an investment of attention, methods, and resources to achieve the best outcomes for a specific patient population.

The Institute of Medicine report Health Professions Education: A Bridge to Quality identified five core competencies that all clinicians should possess to improve the quality of health care in the 21st century. The competency of employee evidence-based practice was included, along with providing patient centered care, working in interdisciplinary teams, applying quality improvement, and utilizing informatics (Committee on Health Professions Education, 2003).

Numerous evidence-based models are available; however, all share certain steps as follows:

1. Select a topic.
2. Find and critique the evidence.
3. Adapt the evidence for use in a specific practice environment.
4. Implement the EBP.
5. Evaluate the effect on patient care processes and outcomes (Titler, 2007).

The Agency for Healthcare Research and Quality (AHRQ) has produced a "knowledge transfer framework," which assists in disseminating patient safety research findings (Nieva, 2005). Stetler, Brunell, Giuliano, et al. (1998) developed a strength of evidence of an individual study that reflects basic quality or scientific credibility of a study. There are six levels, with level one the strongest rating. Quality for any level can range from A to D. If the quality is rated as a D it is automatically eliminated from consideration (Alexander, O'Malley, & Androwich, 2008). Refer to Tables 1-2 and 1-3.

> Table 1-2   **STRENGTH OF EVIDENCE OF AN INDIVIDUAL STUDY**

Grade of Research

A.	Strongly recommend; good evidence
B.	Recommend, at least fair evidence
C.	No recommendation for or against; balance of benefits and harms too close to justify a recommendation
D.	Recommend against; fair evidence is ineffective or harm outweighs the benefit
E.	Evidence is insufficient to recommend for or against routinely; evidence is lacking or of poor quality; benefits and harms cannot be determined.

Level and Quality of Evidence	Type of Evidence
Level I (study grade A–D)	Meta-analysis of multiple controlled studies
Level II (study grade A–D)	Individual experimental studies
Level III (study grade A–D)	Quasi-experimental studies such as nonrandomized, controlled single group, time series, or matched case-controlled studies.
Level IV (study grade A–D)	Nonexperimental studies such as comparative and correlational descriptive research qualitative studies
Level V (study grade A–D)	Program evaluation, research utilization, quality improvement projects; or case reports
Level VI (study grade E)	Opinions of respected authorities; or opinions of an expert committee, non-research–based information.

> Table 1-3	SOURCES OF EVIDENCE-BASED RESEARCH

Published research
Published research utilization report
Published quality improvement report
Published meta-analysis
Published systematic or integrative literature review
Published review of the literature
Policies, procedure, protocols
Published guidelines
Practice exemplars, stories, opinions
General or background information/texts/reports
Unpublished research, reviews, poster presentations, or similar materials
Conference proceedings, abstracts, presentations

 Websites

Center for Evidence-Based Nursing: www.york.ac.uk.healthsciences/
centres/evidence/celon.htm
Agency for Healthcare Research and Quality: www.ahrq.gov/downloads/
pub/advances/vol2
Additional websites on Web-based Ancillary—Student/General

NOTE > Throughout this textbook EBNP is threaded within the chapters in
italic type. EBC is presented in boxes, which has a broader application
than only nursing care.

Nursing Process Related to Infusion Therapy

Infusion therapy clinical competencies incorporate the nursing process.
The nursing process provides each nurse with a framework to utilize in
working with the client. For the infusion nurse, the process begins with
good basic assessment skills before beginning infusion therapy and continues until the patient no longer requires assistance of infusion therapy
to meet healthcare maintenance. The accepted standards of nursing care,
as published by the American Nurses Association (ANA) and the Infusion
Nurses Society (INS) Standards of Practice provide a framework for reasonable, prudent nursing care.

The nursing process continues to be a strong expectation for registered nurses. In the 1999 study by National Council of State Boards of
Nursing, newly licensed RNs indicated that they spent 30% of their time
on assessments, 12% on analysis, 14% on planning, 30% implementing
client care, and 14% on evaluation. Seventy-eight percent stated that they
were required to know nursing diagnosis, and 70% used it in their current
position (NCSBN, 2003b).

Assessment

According to INS Standards of Practice (2006a) **assessment** includes the collection of data including related physiologic and psychosocial variables, critical laboratory values, allergies, and environmental issues; and the presence of adverse reactions or complications related to infusion therapy. Assessment is divided into subjective information and objective information. Although not all-inclusive, the following are some key components for the nurse to assess when delivering infusion therapy:

Subjective

- Patient's related fears of infusion therapy
- Patient's experiences with prior infusion therapy
- Patient's needs and stated preferences for venipuncture site, if applicable
- Disclosure of medications including anticoagulants

Objective

- Review of patient's past and present medical history
- Physical assessment including evaluation of periphery for poor vascular return
- Review of laboratory data and radiographic studies
- Assessment of level of growth and development for neonate and pediatric clients.

Diagnosis

The nursing **diagnosis** or problem list is based on the assessment data. The use of nursing diagnosis developed by North American Nursing Diagnosis Association International (NANDA-I, 2007) provides a clear distinction between nursing diagnosis and medical diagnosis. Fifteen new nursing diagnoses recently were approved by NANDA-I, and 25 revisions made by NANDA-I with culturally appropriate nursing interventions were added to care plans (Ackley & Ladwig, 2008). Examples of nursing diagnoses related to infusion therapy are included in each chapter of this textbook. Some that are common for the client receiving infusion therapy include:

1. Fluid volume deficit related to failure of regulatory mechanisms
2. Infection, risk for, related to compromised host defenses
3. Protection ineffective, related to inadequate nutrition

Nursing diagnosis provides a basis for selection of nursing interventions (nursing actions) to achieve outcomes for which the nurse is accountable (Newfield, Hinz, & Tilley, 2007). Collaborative problems are physiologic complications that nurses monitor to detect onset or changes in status.

Nurses manage collaborative problems using physician-prescribed as well as nursing prescribed interventions (Carpenito-Moyet, 2008).

Planning

Planning involves three components: setting priorities, writing expected outcomes and establishing the appropriate interventions. Planning sets the stage for writing nursing actions by establishing the plan of care.

According to INS Standards of Practice (2006a), the outcomes identification includes the establishment of measurable outcomes of care and a time frame for attaining the outcome. Planning also includes development of strategies to attain the outcomes, validation of physician's or authorized prescriber's order(s), coordination and communication with the appropriate ancillary departments, and use of techniques to prevent complications. Outcomes can be developed in one of two ways: using the Nursing Outcomes Classification (NOC) list or developing an appropriate outcome statement. General suggested outcome statement is provided in this textbook (Moorhead, Johnson, & Maas, 2004).

NOTE > In each of the subsequent chapters of this textbook NOC is presented in a table with nursing diagnoses appropriate for the topic and Nursing Intervention Classification (NIC). All care plans must be individualized so the table in the chapters presents suggestion for direction of planning.

The identification of appropriate nursing actions is also called a road map. When determining interventions, evidence-based practice (EBP) should be included. Rationales for practice whenever possible should support appropriate nursing actions (Ackley & Ladwig, 2008).

Implementation of Interventions/Nursing Actions

Implementation is the action plan of nursing process. The interventions are the concepts that link specific nursing activities and actions to expected outcomes.

Nursing actions include both independent and collaborative activities. Independent activities are actions that the nurse performs, using his or her own discretionary judgment. Collaborative activities are actions that involve mutual decision making between two or more healthcare practitioners. Examples of implementation of nursing actions related to infusion may include:

1. Adherence to established infection control practices and maintenance of aseptic techniques
2. Preparation of infusate solutions with medication additives

3. Initiation of appropriate actions in the event of adverse reactions or complications
4. Provision of infusion therapy-related education that is culture and age appropriate
5. Documentation of all care delivered

The Nursing Interventions Classification (NIC) is a comprehensive, standardized classification of treatments that nurses perform. A comprehensive list of NIC interventions is provided in an NIC text by McCloskey, Dochterman, & Bulechek (2004).

NOTE >   In each of the subsequent chapters of this textbook NIC is presented in a table with nursing diagnoses appropriate for the topic and Nursing Outcome Classification (NOC). All care plans must be individualized; therefore the table in the chapters presents suggestions for direction of nursing actions related to the nursing diagnosis.

Evaluation

The evaluation phase of nursing process is the most ignored phase of the nursing process. The evaluation phase is the feedback and control part of the nursing process. **Evaluation** loops back to assessment that was begun in the initial phase. Once new data are collected, a nursing judgment must be made of what modification in the plan of care are needed. Three judgments are possible:

1. The evaluation data indicate that the health-care problem has been resolved.
2. Revise the plan of care.
3. Continue the plan of care based on the conclusion that the outcome has not been met at this time.

■ Legal and Ethical Issues in Infusion Therapy

Sources of Law

In the United States, there are four primary sources of law: (1) constitutional law, (2) statutory law, (3) administrative law, and (4) common law. In addition, law can be divided into two main branches: private law and public law. Constitutional law is a formal set of rules and principles that describe the powers of a government and the right of the people. Rights guaranteed in the Bill of Rights are consistent with the ethical principles of autonomy, confidentiality, respect for persons, and veracity. As participants in the healthcare system, nurses cannot be forced to forfeit any constitutionally guaranteed rights.

Formal laws written and enacted by federal, state, or local legislatures are known as statutory or legislative laws. Only a minimal number of **statutes** dealing with malpractice existed before the malpractice crisis of the mid-1970s. Changes in Medicare and Medicaid laws, statutory recognition of nurses in advanced practice, and proposed healthcare reform legislation are all examples of statutory or legislative law.

Administrative law is a form of law set by administrative agencies, such as the National Labor Relations Board and the Interstate Commerce Commission. State boards of nursing are examples of this type of legislative body. The final source of law is common law, which is court-made law. Most law in the area of malpractice is court-made law. The courts are responsible for interpreting the statutes. Most malpractice law is not addressed by statute but is established by the courts (Burkhardt & Nathaniel, 2008).

Legal Terms

Legal terms that nurses should become familiar with are *criminal law, civil law, tort, malpractice*, and the *rule of personal liability*. **Criminal law** relates to an offense against the general public caused by the potential harmful effect to society as a whole. A government authority prosecutes criminal actions, and punishment includes imprisonment, fine, or both. The administration of I.V. therapy, if performed in an unlawful manner, can involve a nurse in a criminal offense. Violation of the Nurse Practice Act or the Medical Practice Act by an unlicensed person is considered a criminal offense.

Civil law or private law affects the legal rights of private persons and corporations. The branches of private law that are most applicable to nursing practice are contract law and tort law. Noncompliance with private law generally leads to a granting of monetary compensation to the injured party.

A private wrong, by act or omission, is referred to as a **tort**. Most tort law is founded in common law. There are two types of tort: intentional and unintentional. Intentional torts include assault, battery, false imprisonment, restraints as a form of false imprisonment, defamation, and breach of confidentiality (Burkhart & Nathaniel, 2008). When dealing with a rational patient who refuses treatment, it is best to explain the treatment, verbally reassure the patient, and then notify the physician of refusal.

The Joint Commission (2005) defines **negligence** as a "failure to use such care as a reasonably prudent and careful person would use under similar circumstances."

Malpractice is a type or subset of negligence, committed by a person in a professional capacity. Above simple negligence, malpractice is the form of negligence in which any professional misconduct, unreasonable lack of professional skill, or nonadherence to the accepted standard of care causes injury to a patient.

Four components are required to prove liability for malpractice:

1. It must be established that the nurse *had a duty to the patient*.
2. A *breach of standards of care* or failure to carry out that duty must be proven.
3. The patient must *suffer actual harm* or injury.
4. There must be *a causal relationship between the breach of duty and the injury suffered* (Burkhardt & Nathaniel, 2008).

According to the National Practitioner Data Bank created in 1990 under Title V of Public Law 99-660, there are five distinct categories for registered nurses.

1. Nonspecialized RNs
2. Nurse anesthetists
3. Nurse midwives
4. Nurse practitioners
5. Clinical nurse specialists/advance practice nurses (U.S. Department of Health and Human Services [USDHHS], 2004)

Since 1999 studies have shown that nonspecialized RNs were responsible for 62.7% of malpractice payments. Therefore there is an increased liability risk for nonspecialized RNs. Malpractice categories for tracking of infusion-related incidents are listed as I.V. or blood products related or medication related (Diehl-Svrjcek, Dawson, & Duncan, 2007; USDHHS, 2004).

 NURSING FAST FACT!

> *If an act of malpractice does not create harm, legal action cannot be initiated.*
>
> *Coercion of a rational adult patient to place an intravenous catheter constitutes assault and battery.*

The rule of personal liability is "every person is **liable** for his own tortuous conduct" (his own wrongdoing). A physician cannot protect a nurse from an act of negligence by bypassing this rule with verbal assurance. Nurses are liable for their own wrongdoings in carrying out physicians' orders. This rule is relevant to nurses in the areas of medication errors (the most common cause of malpractice claims) and administration of I.V. fluids. Nurses have a legal and professional responsibility to be knowledgeable regarding the I.V. fluids, medications that are administered, and techniques for initiating and maintaining infusion devices.

The terms *assault* and *battery*, although usually used together, have different legal meanings. Both are intentional torts. Assault is defined as the unjustifiable attempt or threat to touch a person without consent that results in fear of immediately harmful or threatening contact. Touching need not actually occur. Battery is the unlawful, harmful, or unwarranted touching of another or the carrying out of threatened physical harm. Regardless of intent or outcome, touching without consent is considered battery. Even when the intention is beneficent and the outcome is positive, if the act is committed without permission, the nurse can be charged with battery.

Standards of Care

The recipient of care, the patient, is the focus of standards of care. The Joint Commission indicates that standards of care must be developed within organizations to measure quality based on expectations (TJC, 2007). Standards of care can be voluntary, such as those promulgated by professional groups, or they may be mandated legislatively. Nursing is regulated by these dual controls, both of which are aimed at providing quality patient care. The legal standards of care for infusion nursing are derived from four sources: federal statutes and regulations, state statutes, professional standards, and institutional standards.

Standards of nursing care reflect the missions, values, and philosophy of the agency. Nursing processes, professional accountability, fiscal responsibility, and other areas of care are included within these standards. **Standards of care** describe the results or outcomes of care and focus on the patient. These are called **performance standards** and should (1) include the minimum acceptable behavior for the nurse congruent with department standards and standards of practice; (2) define performance in observable, measurable behaviors; (3) be specific to the staff nurse role and job description; (4) address all aspects of nurses' roles, including leadership and organizational expectations; and (5) serve as the basis for employee selection decisions and the performance appraisal system.

There are three types of standards in nursing:

1. Standards of structure, which consider the organizational framework
2. Standards of process, which encompass patient procedures in healthcare settings
3. Standards of outcome, which consider the objectives or goals of patient care

For nurses who practice predominantly in the area of infusion therapy, certification is advisable. Certification is the granting of special recognition to nurses who have practiced and pursued an advanced role in a particular area of nursing. A nongovernmental agency or private organization confers certification on nurses who have a higher level of competency than that mandated by state licensure. Membership in the Infusion Nurses Society (INS) and certification (CRNI®) by the Infusion Nurses Certification Corporation (INCC) are options to be considered.

Staying Current with Standards of Care for Infusion Therapy

Whenever nurses administer infusion therapy, they must know and conform to acceptable nursing standards established by the facility as well as state and federal guidelines. The following list presents guidelines for safeguarding practice:

- Apply venous anatomy and physiology to appropriate vein selection sites.
- Use infusion equipment appropriately.
- Clarify unclear orders and refuse to follow orders you know are not within the scope of safe nursing practice.
- Identify adverse responses to medication and special precautions.
- Administer the medications or infusions at the proper or prescribed rate and within the ordered intervals.
- Collect assessment data before beginning infusion therapy.
- Monitor the patient receiving an infusion for complications and implement interventions appropriate for those complications.
- Provide proper patient education.
- Document all aspects of infusion therapy, including patient teaching.
- Follow your institution's policies and procedures.
- Abide by your state's nurse practice act and national standards of I.V. practice, such as the Infusion Nurses Society Standards of Practice and guidelines for the Centers for Disease Control and Prevention and the Occupational Safety and Health Administration.
- Use appropriate evidence-based practice in delivery of infusion therapy.

Standards of Nursing Practice

Standards of practice focus on the provider of care and represent acceptable levels of practice in patient care delivery. Like the standards of care, practice standards address the clinical aspects of patient care services and imply patient outcomes. Standards of nursing practice define nursing accountability and provide a framework for evaluating professional competency. Standards of practice are consistent with research findings, national norms, and legal guidelines, and complement expectations of regulatory agencies. These standards reflect commitment to quality patient care and include generic and specialty standards of practice (Sierchio, 2001).

There are two types of nursing practice: internal and external standards. Internal standards are those developed within the profession of nursing for the purpose of establishing the minimum level of nursing care. These documents guide nursing care and can be used as a yardstick to measure the practice of individual nurses. An example of internal standards is the American Nurses Association (ANA) Standards of Nursing Practice.

ANA Standards of Nursing practice are universal for all types of nursing; specialty standards are applicable to specific areas of practice such as the Infusion Nursing Standards of Practice by the Infusion Nurses Society.

External standards are guides for nursing developed by non-nurses, the government, or institutions. These standards describe the specific expectations of agencies or groups that utilize the services of nurses. Examples of external standards include nurse practice act of each state, guidelines by the Joint Commission and formal policies and procedures for individual agencies (Burkhardt & Nathaniel, 2008).

Legal Causes of Action Related to Professional Practice

There are many causes of action involving nursing practice; however, the two most common are unprofessional practice and professional malpractice. Unprofessional practice or conduct is a departure from, or failure to conform to, the minimal standards of acceptable and prevailing nursing practices. In this case actual injury need not be established (NCSBN, 2003). In the infusion specialty, examples would be breaches in duty to the patient, such as accepting the patient in assignment, and a deficiency in performing that duty, such as failing to perform a venipuncture according to reasonable and prudent standards of care. Unprofessional practice may result in the loss of license to practice.

Breach of Duty

Nurses must be aware at all times that failure to observe, failure to intervene, and verbal rather than written orders are potential risks for all nursing areas. Nurses must assess each patient and formulate a nursing diagnosis to meet the specific patient's needs. At this time, the courts have not extended the concept of nursing diagnosis to the liability of a nurse's practice.

Malpractice cases are most frequently based on negligence in physical care. There are many documented cases of malpractice related to all procedures performed on patients. Sometimes the breach of duty occurs because a nurse fails to perform a procedure according to proper standards of care. A breach of application of standards of care can be the basis for a negligence lawsuit. Always ask what a reasonable and prudent nurse would do. In general, where employers and boards of nursing are concerned, the patient's outcome is a determining factor in deciding whether a nurse breached a standard of nursing practice or violated an employer's policy and therefore may be disciplined by either entity (Higginbotham, 2003). Medication errors are an area in which nurses have faced criminal charges for not following the six rights of medication administration (Institute for Safe Medication Practices [ISMP], 2002).

Because of the risk of malpractice, policy and procedure manuals are vitally important in all aspects of physical nursing care. Practicing and performing specific physical care based on the policies and procedures ensure quality care.

Legal Perils Related to Infusion Therapy Practice

Due to the scope of practice and the required competencies, potential litigation situations exist for nurses involved in infusion therapy. The following are major categories of litigation:

1. Failure to monitor and assess clinical status
2. Failure to prevent infection
3. Failure to use equipment properly
4. Failure to protect the patient from avoidable injury.
   (Diehl-Svrjcek, Dawson, & Duncan, 2007)

 NURSING FAST FACT!

Infusion nurses use multiple types of medical devices on a daily basis. Adherence to the standard of care, scope of practice, necessary competencies and published standards of practice by the infusion nurse is necessary to avoid malpractice.

Monitor and Assess

Patients receiving infusion therapy ongoing assessment should include the catheter/skin junction site and surrounding area, flow rate of medications/infusate, patient response, and potential side effect. Examples of failure to monitor include not assessing the I.V. site with appropriate frequency and not addressing patient complaints about the I.V. site.

Prevent Infections

An infection is the result of an invasion of a pathogen in a host by various modes of transmission. The placement of an infusion device is an invasive process; it is imperative that the infusion nurse follow standard precautions to decrease the possibility of an infection. Other areas that expose the patient to risk of infection and potential malpractice claims include inadequate or ill-timed site care, failure to adhere to aseptic technique, not adhering to rotation of sites, and failure to report clinical manifestations of infection (Diehl-Svrjcek, Dawson, & Duncan, 2007).

Use of Equipment

Failure to use equipment properly may lead to an adverse patient event, specifically the improper use of add-on devices, arm boards, and restraint devices. Incorrect use of filters or electronic infusion devices (EIDs) also has the potential to result in rapid or inadequate rates of infusion. Lack of immediate response to an audible alarm of an EID can compromise patient safety and place the patient at risk.

Protect the Patient from Harm

Failure to protect the patient from avoidable injury is an important practice issue. The Joint Commission via the National Patient Safety Goals emphasizes protection of the patient with adherence to the following 2008 standards:

- Identify the patient correctly.
- Improve staff communication.
- Use medicines safely.
- Prevent infection.
- Check patient medicines.
- Prevent patients from falling.
- Help patients to be involved in their care.
- Identify patient safety risks.
- Watch patients closely for changes in their health status and respond quickly if they need help.
- Prevent errors in surgery.

The Infusion Nurse's Role as Expert Witness

The role of expert witness is relatively new to the nursing profession. The nurse acting as an expert witness strengthens the argument that nursing is an autonomous profession in that no other profession can appropriately judge the practice of nurses.

Serving as an expert witness involves a complex and extensive process of examining evidence, reviewing pertinent nursing literature, giving depositions, and testifying in court (Burkhardt & Nathaniel, 2008). The role of the expert is *NOT* to establish standards of care; rather, the expert's role is to educate the judge and jury regarding the standards already established by the profession. **Expert testimony** increases with the technical complexity of a case. Additional expertise, such as national I.V. certification or research experience, is also important. The Infusion Nursing Standards of Practice (2006a) state "that an expert nurse is certified in I.V. therapy: Certified Registered Nurse Intravenous (CRNI®). An expert nurse gives advice and consultation throughout the litigation process."

Ethical Issues Related to Infusion Therapy

Code of Ethics

A code of ethics acknowledges the acceptance by a profession of the responsibilities and trust that society has conferred and recognizes the duties and obligations inherent in that trust.

The Infusion Nursing Code of Ethics is based on the premise that infusion nurses both individually and collectively practice with awareness, and that there are principles that guide the infusion nurse's actions. It is the purpose of the code to offer the infusion nurse a model for ethical decision-making (INS, 2001). The principles used in ethical and moral decision-making are based on the following:

- Autonomy (right to self-determination, independence)
- Beneficence (doing good for patients)
- Nonmaleficence (doing no harm to patients)
- Veracity (truthfulness)
- Fidelity (obligation to be faithful)
- Justice (obligation to be fair to all people)

The infusion nurse should follow the ethical principles as stated in the Infusion Nursing Code of Ethics and the American Nurses Association Code of Ethics. These codes are designed to serve as a helpful guide to assist the infusion nurse's practice. The codes includes duties to the patient, duties to society, duties to the profession, and limitations of the infusion nurse's duties and obligations, while ensuring compassionate patient care (INS, 2001, 2006a, 7).

HIPAA Privacy Rule

The U.S. Department of Health and Human Services (2003) issued the Standards for Privacy of Individually Identifiable Health Information (the Privacy Rule) under the Health Insurance Portability and Accountability Act of 1996 (HIPAA) to provide the first comprehensive federal protection for the privacy of personal health information. The final rule went into effect in April, 2003. The Privacy Rule requires healthcare providers to take reasonable actions to safeguard protected health information (PHI) and to discipline individuals who violate privacy policies. The Department of Health and Human Services is charged with enforcing the HIPAA legislation. External consequences can mean fines levied on the organization and the individual(s) involved and can include jail time for disclosing PHI maliciously or for personal gain. This rule has affected professional malpractice and has ethical as well as legal ramifications for infusion nurses.

⊕ Websites

U.S. Department of Health and Human Services: www.hhs.gov/ocr/hippa/finalreg.html

■ Quality Patient Management

Quality management is a systematic process to ensure desired patient outcomes. A quality management program includes both risk management and quality assurance and is established to objectively identify, evaluate, and solve problems associated with infusion treatment modalities.

Quality assurance requirements have always been a part of The Joint Commission introduction of the Agenda for Change in 1986, which shifted the emphasis from problem-solving endeavors to continuous improvement of quality. With this shift, TJC initiated the transition from QA to quality improvement (QI). The goal was to create **outcome** monitoring and evaluation processes to assist organizations in improving the quality of care. QA frequently focuses solely on the clinical aspects of care rather than on the interrelated managerial, governance, support, and clinical processes that affect patient care outcomes. Quality cannot be ensured; it can only be assessed.

In 1995 JCAHO changed the wording of continuous quality improvement to **performance improvement (PI).** The goal of improving organization performance is to continuously improve patient health outcomes.

Total Quality Management

Total quality management (TQM) is an outgrowth of several healthcare organizations that have adopted a management system fostering continuous improvement at all levels and for all functions by focusing on maximizing customer satisfaction. This proactive approach emphasizes "doing the right thing" for customers. Total quality management is often interchanged with **quality improvement (QI)** and performance improvement (PI). General principles of quality improvement include the following:

1. The priority is to benefit patients and all other internal and external customers.
2. Quality is achieved through the participation of everyone in the organization.
3. Improvement opportunities are developed by focusing on the work process.
4. Decisions to change or improve a system or process are made based on data.
5. Improvement of the quality of service is a continuous process (McLaughlin & Houston, 2008).

Quality Improvement/Performance Improvement

The use of outcomes and other performance measures complements the application of standards and completes the quality equation. Performance results usually validate the fact that an organization did the right things and provide the baseline stimulus for future quality improvement activities. Performance is what is done and how well it is done to provide health care. Characteristics of what is done and how well it is done are called dimensions of performance.

Doing the right thing includes:

- The *efficacy* of the procedure or treatment in relation to the client's condition
- The *appropriateness* of a specific test, procedure, or service to meet the client's need

Doing the right thing well includes:

- The *availability* of a needed test, procedure, treatment, or service to the client who needs it
- The *timeliness* with which a needed test, procedure, treatment, or service is provided to the client
- The *effectiveness* with which tests, procedures, treatments, and services are provided.
- The *continuity* of the services provided to the client with respect to other services, practitioners, and providers over time
- The *safety* of the client and others to whom the care and services are provided
- The *efficiency* with which care and services are provided (TJC, 2008)
- The *respect and caring* with which care and services are provided

The Joint Commission established standards, scoring, and aggregation rules for improving organization performance that can be downloaded from their website: www.jointcommission.org/standard/Itc-pi.html

The quality improvement process may be performed by using lengthy studies, short-term sampling, or problem solving with documentation and reporting. Three categories are used to create a model for quality management, and each is linked as a measurement of quality patient care. The three categories are structure, process, and outcome.

Structure

Structure consists of the conditions and mechanisms that provide support for the actual provision of care. This is defined as evaluation of resources, both material and human. Material resources are classified as facilities, equipment, mission, philosophy, goals of organization, and financial resources. Human resources include the number and qualifications of nurses performing infusion-related procedures.

Process

Process denotes what is actually done in giving and receiving care. Process is a goal-directed, interrelated series of actions, events, mechanisms, or steps. It includes a patient's activities in seeking care, **data collection**, and a practitioner's activities in making a nursing diagnosis, along with evaluation of actual performance of procedures. This link sets the standards by which evaluation can take place. Process standards focus on job descriptions, performance standards, procedures, and protocols.

Outcome

Outcome denotes the effect of care on the health status of patients. The result of the performance (or nonperformance) of a function or process is the outcome. Improvements in a patient's knowledge and changes in his or her health status are components of outcome criteria. The assessment of outcomes is a method by which quality of care is established. Outcome in the practice of I.V. therapy should reflect final results of the therapy, including patient recovery and rates of complications.

In summary, the goals of PI are to (1) prevent complications, (2) decrease morbidity and mortality, (3) decrease cost, (4) shorten hospital stays, (5) increase patient comfort, and (6) increase patient knowledge.

Strategies to Improve Quality

Audits

An **audit** is a systematic and official examination of a record, process, structure, environment, or account to evaluate performance. The following are used to collect data for audits:

- Retrospective audits: Performed after the patient receives the care
- Concurrent audits: Performed while the patient is receiving the care
- Prospective audits: Attempt to identify how future performance will be affected by current interventions (Marquis & Huston, 2006).

Quality management uses three types of audits: outcome, process, and structure audits.

Outcome Audit

Outcomes are the end result of care as a result of an intervention. Outcome audits determine what results, if any, occurred as a result of specific nursing interventions for a patient. These audits assume that the outcome accurately demonstrates the quality of care delivered. Many experts consider outcome measures to be the most valid indicators of quality, but until this past decade most evaluations of hospital care have focused on structure and process.

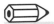 *NURSING FAST FACT!*

> *Joint Commission uses outcome criteria established for 24 hours before discharge when reviewing quality of care. Other postdischarge outcome measures used by TJC include the number of sentinel events, overall error rate, number of reports on possible errors or near misses, hospital readmission rates, and rate of hospital-acquired infections (Bulger, 2003).*

Nursing sensitive outcomes measures for the acute care setting include patient fall rates, nosocomial infection rates, the prevalence of pressure sores, physical restraint use, and patient satisfaction rates.

PROCESS AUDIT

Process audits are used to measure the process of care or how the care was conducted and assume that a relationship exists between the process used by the nurse and the quality of care provided. Process audits tend to be task-oriented (Marquis & Huston, 2006). For example, a process audit might be used to establish whether I.V. catheter sites were rotated every 72 hours.

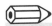 *NURSING FAST FACT!*

> *Standardized clinical guidelines, or critical pathways would be an example of an effort to standardize the process of care. In home care they are addressed as clinical pathways (noncritical).*

STRUCTURE AUDIT

Structure audits assume that a relationship exists between quality of care and appropriate structure. Structural standards, often environmental, are often set by licensing and accrediting bodies; they ensure a safe and effective environment but do not address the actual care delivered. For example, structural audits would include staffing ratios, wait time in clinics or emergency departments, or call lights available to the patient (Marquis & Huston, 2006).

Additional Strategies to Improve Quality

Benchmarking

"**Benchmarking** is continual and collaborative discipline of measuring and comparing the results of keywork processes with those of the best performers" (McLaughlin & Houston, 2008). Consumers are now more aware of healthcare organization quality indicators, such as morbidity and mortality. If an organization cannot demonstrate its own quality care measures, it risks losing patients and managed care contracts. This has propelled benchmarking into the realm of common business practice as a tool to enhance leverage within industry markets (Tran, 2003).

Problem-based benchmarking targets efforts toward improving specific concerns, such as improving medication error rate or decreasing patient waiting times. More recently, facilities are turning to process-based benchmarking, which entails targeting continuous improvement of key processes.

Managers can benchmark to help decide a variety of factors: where to allocate resources more efficiently, when to seek outside assistance, how to quickly improve current operations, and whether customer requirements are being adequately met.

Benchmarking can be used in infusion therapy to validate infusion therapy teams. By monitoring pertinent patient outcomes related to vascular access devices (VADs), facilities that use benchmarking can expect to see fewer problems with VADs, less difficulty starting catheters, less stress for patient and staff, less waiting time for central lines, less interruption of prescribed therapy, a shorter length of hospital stay, and increased patient and staff satisfaction (Galloway, 2002).

Regulatory Requirements

The Joint Commission (TJC) has developed standards to guide critical activities performed by healthcare organizations.

The National Patient Safety Goals (NPSG) for 2008 have a one-year phase in period with full implementation by January of 2009. The 2008 general NPSG goals focus on communication, patient identification, medication safety falls, and medication reconciliation. The new 2008 patient Safety Goals Hospital Program include:

- 3E: Reduce the likelihood of patient harm associated with the use of anticoagulation therapy
- 16: Improve recognition and response to changes in patient's condition
- 16A: The organization selects a suitable method that enables healthcare staff members to directly request additional assistance form a specially trained individual(s) when patient's condition appears to be worsening (TJC, 2008).

Sentinel Event Review

An adverse sentinel event is an unexpected occurrence involving death or serious physical or psychological injury to a patient. Events are called sentinel because they require immediate investigation. An adverse sentinel event presents an opportunity to analyze improving the system. Lending a sentinel event review to the organization's quality improvement system will identify strategies for prevention of future similar events. An example of a sentinel event related to infusion therapy would be a medication delivery error of I.V. potassium resulting in cardiac arrest.

Patient Satisfaction Data

Healthcare facilities receive feedback from patients by having them fill out questionnaires that ask how they feel about their healthcare encounter. If these data can be compared or benchmarked with other organizations' data, they can be helpful in improving quality. Methods of patient data collection include surveys, follow-up phone calls after patient discharge, to obtaining patient satisfaction information via a focus group or postcare interview.

Pay-for-Performance

Pay-for-performance (P4P) sets differing payment levels for providers of care based on their performance on measures of quality and efficiency. Many health plans have been reporting performance using the Health Plan Employer Data Information Set (HEDIS), which measures how well evidence-based medicine is delivered relative to national or regional benchmarks. P4P programs are becoming popular in part because of persistent deficiencies in quality in the U.S. healthcare system. P4P programs reward better performance; 100 P4P programs were operating nationwide as of September 2005. The Centers for Medicare and Medicaid Services (CMS), large employers, business coalitions, health plans, and others have implemented a variety of approaches that seek to reward improvements in quality and high performance by hospitals, physicians, medical groups, and others. An example of CMS plans to tie part of the annual hospital update to actual performance. In 2008, payments to hospitals were reduced for Medicare patients who acquire an infection while in the hospital (Alliance for Health Reform, 2006). Refer to Evidence-Based Care Box 1-2.

■ Risk Management and Risk Assessment

The Infusion Nursing Standards of Practice (INS, 2006) define **risk management** as "a process that centers on identification, analysis, treatment, and evaluation of real and potential hazards." Risk assessment is the scientific process of asking how risky something is. It is a process of collecting and analyzing scientific data "to describe the form, dimension, and characteristics of risk." Risk assessment and risk management are equally important but different processes, with different objectives, information content, and results.

Risk management concepts include the concerns that organizations face with exposure to losses. Organizations handle the chances of losses or risks by financing, purchasing insurance, or practicing loss control. Loss control consists of preventive and protective activities that are performed

---

EVIDENCE-BASED CARE BOX 1-2

Improvement in Outcomes Indicators

Alliance for Health Reform (2006). Pay-for-Performance: A promising start. Brief: Pay-for-performance trends. Retrieved from http://www.allhealth.org (Accessed March 16, 2008).

Early results from demonstration projects by CMS/Premier P4P showed the average improvement across 33 indicators in five clinical areas (acute myocardial infarction; community-acquired pneumonia; hip and knee replacement surgery, coronary artery bypass graft and heart failure) was 6.6% for the more than 260 hospitals participating.

before, during, and after losses are incurred. Risk management involves all medical and facility staff. It provides for the review and analysis of risk and liability sources involving patients, visitors, staff, and facility property. Risk management consists of the following components:

- Identification and management of clinical areas of actual and high risk
- Identification and management of nonclinical (e.g., visitor, staff) areas of actual and high risk
- Identification and management of probable claims events
- Management of property loss occurrences
- Review and analysis of customer surveys and patient complaints
- Review and analysis of risk assessment surveys
- Operational linkages with hospital quality management, safety, and performance improvement programs
- Provision of risk management education
- Compliance with state risk management and applicable federal statutes.

Risk assessment is performed by government agencies such as the U.S. Environmental Protection Agency (EPA). Risk assessment takes different approaches depending on available information. Some assessments look back to try to assess effects after an event. They may also look ahead before a new product is approved for use.

Joint Commission advocates establishing an integrated risk management and quality improvement programs. Risk management strategies combine the elements of both loss reduction and loss prevention. Risk management strategies that may decrease the risk of potential liability are as follows:

- Informed consent
- Unusual occurrence reports
- Sentinel events
- Documentation

Informed Consent

One of the most effective proactive strategies taken in risk management is informed consent. Healthcare professionals have a legal duty to provide a patient with ample information regarding the health treatment or procedure to be performed and obtain an informed consent before proceeding. The purpose of informed consent is to provide patients with enough information to enable them to make a rational decision regarding whether to undergo treatment. The focus is on a patient's understanding the procedure, not just signing consent to have the procedure performed.

The right of self-determination provides the basis for informed consent and is grounded in the bioethical principles of autonomy. A competent adult (competence to consent) is aware of the consequences of a decision and has the ability to make reasonable choices about health care, including the right to refuse health care.

There are categories of necessary elements for informed consent and informed refusal. The first category comprises the information elements. This involves the disclosure of appropriate information. Generally, this disclosure must include benefits and risks of procedure, alternative procedures, benefits and risk of the alternatives, and the qualifications of the provider.

The second category consists of the consent elements. The consent must be voluntary, not coerced. Consent can be manifested by conduct. For example, the infusion specialist states, "I am going to restart your I.V. now," and the patient holds out his or her arm.

There may be limits to consent, such as waiver of consent: the patient must know that options and risks exist even if he or she does not want to know what they are. Other limits to consent include verbal limits; for example, the patient may tell the infusion nurse, "Okay, I will let you try to restart my I.V., but only once."

The duty to obtain informed consent belongs to the person who will perform the procedure, but also may belong to the licensed person who is aware that the patient has not been informed, does not understand, or did not consent. A breach of this duty may result in discipline for unprofessional practice and/or a civil lawsuit for professional malpractice. If the infusion specialist knows that consent does not exist or the patient is not informed and has not waived that right, the infusion specialist must consult with the ordering provider, and go up the chain of command for assistance. Refer to Table 1-4 (Collins, 2001).

> Table 1-4   **ELEMENTS OF INFORMED CONSENT**

Criteria

Patient must be mentally competent.
Patient must be of legal age, or the parent of a minor.
A legally designated healthcare surrogate may act for the patient.
Patient must be able to understand the language.

Information Elements
Clear information about the procedure
Information must include:
    Benefits and risks of the procedure
    Alternative procedures
    Benefits and risks of the alternatives
    Risks of refusing the procedure
    Qualifications of the provider

Consent Elements
Consent form on chart or waiver of consent
Signature on an informed consent is a formality

Adapted from Zonderman (2000); Collins (2001).

INS Standard: The patient or a representative legally authorized to act on the patient's behalf shall be informed of potential complications associated with treatment or therapy. The nurse shall document the information given and patient's or legally authorized representative's response in the patient's medical record. (INS, 2006a, 10)

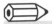 *NURSING FAST FACT!*

> *Informed consents can become invalid if a change in the patient's medical status alters the risks and benefits of treatment.*

Unusual Occurrence Reports

Unusual occurrence reports should be filed every time there is a deviation from the standard. These reports are simple records of an event and are considered an internal reporting mechanism for performance improvement. They should be reported to the superior staff member and the episode must be objectively charted, but reference to the report should not appear in the legal patient record.

The occurrence report should contain the following 10 key points:

1. Patient's admitting diagnosis
2. Date when the incident occurred
3. Patient's room number
4. Age of the patient
5. Location of the incident
6. Type of incident
7. Nature of incident (e.g., medication error, mislabeling, misreading, policy and procedure not followed, overlooked order on chart, patient identification not checked). It should be noted (on the unusual occurrence report) if a physician's order was needed after the occurrence.
8. Factual description of the incident
9. Patient's condition before the incident
10. Results of the incident or injury

 NURSING FAST FACT!

> *Unusual occurrence reports are meant to be nonjudgmental, factual reports of the problem and its consequences.*

Unusual occurrence reports are useful for identification of patterns of infusion medication errors or potentially dangerous situations. Trend analysis monitors patterns of their occurrences. Nursing staff members must feel free to file reports; a report is not an admission of negligence. These reports have the potential to save lives by identifying unsafe practices. More than ever before, risk may be managed by prevention. In 1996, JCAHO implemented five indicators on medication use for its Indicator Measurement System, a performance measurement system intended to help evaluate the performance of healthcare organizations as part of its survey and accreditation process.

INS Standard   An Unusual Occurrence or Sentinel Event report shall document unusual or unanticipated occurrences or variances in practice. The report should be shared with appropriate departments, such as risk management and performance improvement teams. The report should result in specific quality and performance improvement measures as required by organizational policies and procedures. (INS, 2006a, 13)

Sentinel Events

Adverse-event reduction is a key strategy for reducing healthcare mortality and morbidity because patients who suffer adverse events are more likely to die or suffer permanent disability. Nurses have always played a pivotal role in the prevention of adverse events. Adherence to best-practice standards and assurance of quality standards for high-risk/high-volume practices. The Joint Commission calls for voluntary self-reporting of sentinel events by both inpatient institutions and home health agencies (Yoder-Wise, 2007). The most common sentinel events reported in the healthcare arena are listed in Table 1-5.

> Table 1-5	COMMON SENTINEL EVENTS REPORTED IN HEALTHCARE AREAS

Patient suicide
Operative/postoperative complications
Wrong-site surgery
Medication error
Delay in treatment
Patient fall
Patient death/injury in restraints
Assault/rape/homicide
Perinatal death/loss of function
Patient elopement
Infection-related event
Fire
Anesthesia-related event
Maternal death
Ventilator death
Medical equipment related
Infant abduction/wrong family
Utility systems related event

Source: Joint Commission (2005).

Documentation

Documentation provides legal accountability, communicates information to other healthcare workers, provides information for reimbursement, and assists with outcomes monitoring (Moureau & Maney, 2003). **Documentation** should be an accurate, timely, and a complete written account of the care rendered to the patient. The healthcare record charts the patient's history, health status, and goal achievement. It should be objective and completed promptly. Documentation should be legible and include only standard abbreviations. Nurses and other healthcare providers should keep charts free of criticism or complaints. There should be no vacant lines in charts, and every entry should be signed. In an office or home care environment, dates of return visit, canceled or failed appointments, all telephone conversations, and all follow-up instructions should be recorded on the chart.

Since the 1990s, the emphasis has been on quality improvement, with a focus on evaluating organizational and clinical performance outcomes. Documentation is one way of evaluating outcomes. The many formats for charting include the problem-oriented medical record, pie charting, focus charting, narrative charting, and charting by exception. Regardless of the format developed for documenting infusion therapy, basic requirements of the plan of care exist, including goals, actual and potential problems, and nursing interventions and outcomes.

Documentation should include the number of attempts for each procedure, the patient's response to the procedure, adverse events, actions taken in the presence of complications, patient education provided, and descriptive information given for the informed consent and the patient's response (Moureau & Maney, 2003).

The Infusion Nurses Society Standards of Practice (2006a, 14) recommend the following documentation guidelines by the appropriate clinical personnel

- Patient, caregiver, or legally authorized representative's.
- Type, length, and gauge of vascular access device
- Date and time of insertion, number and location of attempts, identification of site, type of dressing, and identification of the person inserting the device.
- Use of visualization and guidance technologies.
- For midline (ML) and peripherally inserted central catheters (PICCs): external catheter length, midarm circumference, effective length of catheter inserted, and radiographic confirmation of the location of catheter tip.
- Site condition and appearance using standardized assessment scales for phlebitis and/or infiltration/extravasation.
- Care of site
- Specific site preparation, infection control, and safety precautions taken.

- Communication among healthcare professionals responsible for patient care and monitoring
- Type of therapy; drug; dose; and rate, time, and method of administration.
- Pertinent diagnosis, assessment, and vital signs
- Patient's symptoms, response to therapy, and/or laboratory test results
- Barriers to care or therapy and/or complications
- Discontinuation of therapy, including catheter length and integrity, site appearance, dressing applied, and patient tolerance.
- When multiple catheter devices or catheter lumens are being used, documentation should clearly indicate what fluids and medications are being infused through each pathway.

INS Standard Documentation shall be legible, accessible to qualified personnel, and readily retrievable. The protocol for documentation should be established in organizational policies and procedures. (INS, 2006a, 14)

Medication Safety

According to The National Coordinating Council for Medication Error and Prevention (2008), the definition of a medication error is "any preventable event that may cause or lead to inappropriate medication use or patient harm, while the medication is in the control of the healthcare professional, patient or consumer. Such events may be related to professional practice, health care products procedures, and systems including: prescribing; order communication; product labeling, packaging and nomenclature; compounding; dispensing; distribution; administration; education; monitoring and use."

 NURSING FAST FACT!

Medication error is the most common type of error affecting patient safety (Bates, Cullen, & Laird, 1997). Preventable adverse drug events (ADEs) are associated with one of every five injuries or deaths occurring in the healthcare system. (Leape, 1995)

Tools have been developed by the American Hospital Association, the Health Research and Education Trust (HRET) and the Institute for Safe Medication Practices (ISMP). The tools are in modular format to be adapted by different organizations and professionals; the three main pathways components help hospital leaders and professionals

- Incorporate medication safety into the organization's strategic plan.
- Identify specific error-prone processes and devise safe alternatives using a process flow diagram, case scenarios, and the ISMP's Ten Key Elements of Medication Use System (ISMP, 2002).

■ Prepare to implement a bedside bar-coding system for administering medications (ISMP, 2002).

Medication use is a complex process that incorporates medication prescribing, order processing, dispensing, administration, and effects monitoring. The key elements that most often affect the medication use process, and the common failures and medication errors associated with them, are the key elements forming the structure within which medications are used.

1. **Patient Information**: Having essential patient information at the time of medication prescribing, dispensing, and administration will result in a significant decrease in preventable adverse drug events.
2. **Drug information:** Drug information needs to be up to date, accurate, and accessible to the staff through a multitude of sources (drug references, pharmacist, formulary, protocols, dosing scales).
3. **Communication of drug information:** Verify drug information and eliminate communication barriers to minimize the amount of medication errors caused by miscommunication.
4. **Drug labeling, packaging, and nomenclature:** Drug names that look alike, sound alike, have confusing drug labeling, and nondistinct drug packaging contribute to medication errors. Use of proper labeling and the use of unit dose systems reduce the incidence of medication errors.
5. **Drug storage, stock, and standardization:** Standardizing drug administration times, drug concentrations, and limiting the dose concentration of drugs available in patient care areas will reduce the risk of medication errors.
6. **Drug device acquisition, use, and monitoring:** Assessment of drug delivery devices should be evaluated before purchase. A system of independent double-checks should be used within the institution to prevent device-related errors such as selecting the wrong drug or drug concentration, setting the rate improperly, or mistaking the infusion line up with another.
7. **Environmental factors:** Environmental factors that contribute to medication errors include poor lighting, noise, interruptions, a significant workload, and chaos of the home environment. Having a well-designed system offers the best chance of preventing errors; however, the environment in which medication is distributed can contribute to medication errors.
8. **Competency and staff education:** Staff education should focus on new medications being used in all practice settings, high-alert medications, medication errors that have occurred both internally and externally, and protocols, policies, and procedures related to medication use.
9. **Patient education:** Patients can play a vital role in preventing medication errors when they have been encouraged by physicians,

pharmacists, and nursing staff to ask questions and seek answers about their medications.

10. **Quality processes and risk management:** The way to prevent errors is to redesign the systems and processes that lead to errors rather than focusing on correcting the individuals who make errors. Effective strategies for reducing errors include making it difficult for staff to make an error and promoting the detection and correction of errors before they reach a patient and cause harm.
(ISMP, 2002)

Characteristics of Medication Errors

The most frequently reported types of errors include: (1) omission errors (failure to administer a prescribed medication; (2) improper dose (medication dose, strength, or quantity different from that prescribed); (3) unauthorized drug errors (the medication dispensed and/or administered was not authorized by the prescriber) (Kleinpell, 2001).

Factors that contribute to IV infusion medical errors include:
- Illegible order
- Incorrect dose prescribed
- Pump programming errors
- RN distracted or fatigued
- Math error converting mcg/kg/min to mL/hr
- Inadequate staffing for time out/double check
- Pharmacy not available 24 hours (Obsheatz, 2004)

Barcoding and Radiofrequency Identification Tags

Barcodes were implemented in 2004 as a response to the alarming number of patient deaths due to medication errors uncovered by the Institute of Medicine. Barcode medication administration (BCMA) technology generates standard reports from recorded errors made, errors prevented, and reasons why nurses overrode warning messages. This quality improvement strategy to prevent medication errors is one step toward performance improvement (Douglas & Larrabee, 2003).

 NURSING FAST FACT!

- *Barcode medication administration (BCMA) technology does not detect or prevent intravenous infusion programming errors.*
- *Integration of BCMA with I.V. medication safety systems can further improve medication administration accuracy and documentation.*
- *Integrating these two systems provides real-time visibility of the status of infusions. (Obsheatz, 2004)*

Radiofrequency identification (RFID) tags were first used in World War II as transponders to prevent American and British warplanes from shooting at each other. The benefits of RFID in health care can be applied from equipment tracking to patient identification. RFID tags contain more embedded data than a bar code, are more durable, have a wider field of readability with a scanner, and are readable through materials such as patient clothing and bed coverings. The disadvantage is that it is expensive. With RFID ease of use, it is a passive way to ensure correct patient information to prevent treatment and medication errors (Roark & Miguel, 2006).

 Home Care Issues

The home infusion nurse must deliver safe, effective quality care in the home. Safe and effective care is ensured when the nurse is educated and competent in infusion therapy, when the patient is assessed for appropriateness of home care, and when the intended infusion therapy is appropriate for home administration. The home care nurse must have a variety of well developed skills, which include the following:
• Excellent assessment skills
• Ability to effectively teach patients and caregivers
• Ability to effectively communicate with patients, caregivers, and other healthcare-related professionals including physicians, pharmacists, insurance case managers, and other members of the agency healthcare team.
• In-depth knowledge of infusion access devices and infusion equipment including
  • Knowledge of community resources and reimbursement
  • Good organizational skills with the ability to function independently (Gorski, 2005)

 NURSING FAST FACT!

The HIPAA privacy act pertains to all healthcare settings; therefore, confidentiality has the same legal boundaries in the home care setting as in the hospital.

A successful home infusion program must ensure patient safety with the following processes and structures in place:
• Written agency policies and procedures for home infusion therapy
• Discharge planning and/or agency intake processes which include evaluation of the patient's status and appropriateness and safety of administering the prescribed infusion drug or fluid in the home.
• Nurses are educated in agency protocols with validated competency in administration of home infusion therapies provided by the agency. Competency is validated.

Home Care Issues—cont'd

- Tools and educational resources are available to support home infusion nurses, patients, and caregivers (Gorski, 2005).

   Healthcare providers deliver a variety of services in the home care setting. The following interventions may be provided:

1. Phlebotomy
2. Routine peripheral chatter site changes
3. Daily peripheral site checks
4. Insertion and maintenance of midline catheters
5. Preparation of selected large-volume parenteral solutions and IV medications
6. Evaluation of infusion therapy-related equipment
7. Central venous catheters
   a. Routine central venous catheter (CVC) dressing changes
   b. Implanted port access
   c. Declotting of CVCs
   d. Insertion and maintenance of PICCs
   e. Blood withdrawal from CVCs
   f. Consultation and teaching for long-term CVCs
8. Administration of intraspinal medications
9. Maintenance of intraspinal catheters
10. Administration of chemotherapy
11. Administration of parenteral nutrition (PN)
12. Data collection for infusion-related statistics

NOTE > Each subsequent chapter addresses home care issues related to the chapter topic.

 Patient Education

Teaching is a major component of clinical infusion practice, and is an independent nursing function. In many states, the requirement to teach is included as part of the Nurse Practice Act. According to the American Nurses Association (ANA) Code of Ethics for Nurses (2001), nurses are responsible for promoting and protecting the health, safety, and rights of patients. The Joint Commission standards require that educators in healthcare organizations consider the literacy, developmental, and physical limitations, financial limitations, language barriers, culture, and religious practices of every client.

Patient Education—cont'd

Teaching must also include any person who will be responsible for client's care (TJC, 2007). The "Patient Care Partnership" (previously the "Patient's Bill of Rights") establishes the right of patients to receive complete and current information regarding diagnosis, treatment, and prognosis in ways they can understand, as well as the right to be informed of hospital/agency policies and practices that relate to them (American Hospital Association [AHA], 2003).

NOTE > Each subsequent chapter will present key patient education points related the content of that chapter.

Chapter Highlights

- Clinical competency is the determination of individual capability to perform expectations. It is evidenced by clinical skills checklists/competency assessments; continuing education; documentation of training and education.
- Evidence-based nursing practice (EBNP) is the conscientious use of current best evidence in making decisions about patient care.
- Components of EBNP include evidence from research/evidence-based theories, and opinions of leaders; evidence from assessment of patient's history, physical exam, and availability of health resources; clinical expertise; and information about patient preferences and values.
- Evidence-based care (EBC) is recognized by nursing, medicine, healthcare institutions, and health policy makers as care based on state-of-the-art science reports. This has replaced evidence-based medicine.
- Clinical competencies incorporate the nursing process. The nursing process includes assessment of the client before beginning infusion therapy; identifying nursing diagnoses that apply to client to deliver safe nursing practice and provide a basis for selection of nursing interventions; planning that incorporates setting priorities, writing expected outcomes, and establishing appropriate interventions; and implementation of the interventions, which is the action plan and evaluation that provides feedback.
- Legal issues for the infusion nurse require that the practitioner be aware of the four primary sources of law and understand legal terms, especially *malpractice* and the *rule of personal liability* and *negligence*. In infusion therapy breaches in duty to the patient would include once a patient assignment is accepted that a deficiency in performing that

duty was incurred; or failing to initiate, care, and maintain infusion therapy according to reasonable and prudent standards of care

- Codes of ethics dictate responsibilities, trust, and the obligations inherent in that trust. The Infusion Code of Ethics and the American Nurses Association Code of Ethics guide the ethical practice of infusion therapy.
- Standards of Care focus on the recipient of care.
- Standards of Practice focus on the provider of care and represent acceptable levels of practice.
- Quality management is a systematic process to ensure desired patient outcomes. The terms quality improvement (QI) and performance improvement (PI) are used interchangeably and focus on "doing the right thing" for customers.
- The quality improvement process has three categories: structure, process, and outcome.
- Strategies to improve quality include audits (retrospective, concurrent, and prospective audits). Benchmarking is the continual and collaborative discipline of measuring and comparing the results of key work processes with those of the best performers. Regulatory requirements, sentinel event review, patient satisfaction data, and pay-for-performance are additional strategies.
- Risk management is a process that centers on identification, analysis, treatment, and evaluation of real and potential hazards.
- Risk management strategies include informed consents, unusual occurrence reports, sentinel events, documentation, medication administration safety, and bar coding.

■■ Thinking Critically: Case Study

You are the supervisor of a home care infusion company. The chief executive officer has requested that you chair a newly established quality management committee because you have had some experiences in your past position of developing audit criteria. A review of the patient population indicates that a high percentage of your clients receive total parenteral nutrition. The committee has decided to review this patient population first. They have chosen to develop a tool for a *prospective audit* that would be appropriate for monitoring the quality of an initial home visit to set up total parenteral nutrition.

What is the goal of quality management?

Identify process criteria for the tool.

Who should be included on this committee?

Design an audit tool that would be appropriate and convenient to use to collect data.

Media Link: Answers to the case study questions and more critical thinking activities are provided on the CD-ROM.

Post-Test

1. The three parts of a competency-based program include:
   a. Competency statement, goal, and return demonstration
   b. Competency statement, criteria for learning, and evaluation
   c. Goal, evaluation, and feedback
   d. Assessment, problem statement, implementation

2. Which of the following describes the benchmarking process?
   a. Comparing your medical unit's data on phlebitis rate with that of the ICU.
   b. Collecting data on all patients with peripheral IVs.
   c. Collecting evidence-based practice to change policy and procedure on care and maintenance of peripheral IV sites.
   d. Comparing your unit's data on phlebitis rates to that of other organizations to identify improvement opportunities.

3. A tool used to report sentinel events would be a:
   a. Performance improvement sheet
   b. Unusual occurrence report
   c. Competency validation tool
   d. Root-cause analysis tool

4. To differentiate between standard of care and standard of practice, the standard of practice would be defined as:
   a. Activities and behaviors of the practitioner needed to achieve patient outcomes
   b. Focuses on the recipient of care and describes outcomes that the patient can expect to receive
   c. An ongoing systematic process for monitoring and problem solving
   d. Conditions and mechanisms that provide support for the delivery of care

5. A nurse walks into a patient's room and finds the I.V. solution container dry. The bag of 1000 mL of 5% dextrose and 0.9% sodium chloride had been hung 1 hour earlier. The nurse informs the charge nurse and the physician that this has occurred. The nurse is instructed to complete an unusual occurrence report. The report allows the analysis of adverse patient events by:
   a. Evaluating quality care and the potential risks for injury to the patient
   b. Determining the effectiveness of nursing interventions
   c. Providing a method of reporting injuries to local, state, and federal agencies
   d. Providing clients with necessary stabilizing treatments

6. Characteristics of performance improvement (doing the right thing well) include which of the following? (*Select all that apply.*)
   a. Availability of a needed test
   b. Documenting the quality of care received
   c. Timeliness with which the test, procedure, and treatment are provided
   d. Continuity of the services provided

7. The definition of a tort is:
   a. A written law enacted by the legislature
   b. A private wrong, by act or omission, that can result in a civil action by the harmed person
   c. An offense against the general public
   d. Being capable or able; knowing how to function

8. The major purpose of evidence-based practice in infusion therapy is:
   a. To increase variability in delivery of nursing care
   b. To determine what medical models can be applied by nursing
   c. To provide clinically competent care
   d. To take the place of quality improvement in nursing care delivery

9. Which of the following organizations develops clinical practice guidelines? (*Select all that apply.*)
   a. The Agency for Healthcare Research and Design
   b. The Joint Commission
   c. Infusion Nurses Society
   d. American Nurses Association

10. The assessment phase of the nursing process related to infusion therapy would include which of the following? (*Select all that apply.*)
   a. Physical assessment
   b. Review of laboratory data
   c. Teaching the patient and family central line care.
   d. Applying a nursing diagnosis of risk of infection related to tunneled catheter placement.

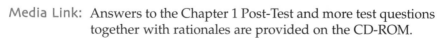 **Media Link:** Answers to the Chapter 1 Post-Test and more test questions together with rationales are provided on the CD-ROM.

■ References

Ackley, B.J., & Ladwig, G.B. (2008). *Nursing diagnosis handbook: An evidence-based guide to planning care.* St. Louis, MO: Mosby Elsevier.

Alexander, R., O'Malley, A.A., & Androwich, I.M. (2008). Evidence-based health care. In: P. Kelly (Ed.), *Nursing leadership and management* (2nd ed., pp. 111–123). Clifton Park, NY: Thomson Delmar Learning.

Alliance for Health Reform (2006). Pay-for-Performance: A promising start. Brief: Pay-for-performance trends. Retrieved from http://www.allhealth.org (Accessed March 16, 2008).

American Board of Nursing Specialties. (2005). A position statement on the value of specialty nursing certification. Retrieved from www.nursingcertification. org (Accessed March 4, 2008).

American Board of Nursing Specialties. (2006). Definition of certification. Retrieved from www.nursingcertification.org (Accessed March 4, 2008).

American Hospital Association (AHA) (2003). *The patient care partnership.* Chicago: Author. Retrieved from http://www.hospitalconnect.com:80/aha/ ptcommunicaiton/partnership/partnership/index.html (Accessed March 16, 2008).

American Nurses Association (2001). *The code for nurses with interpretive statements.* Kansas City, MO: American Nurses Association.

Bates, D.W., Cullen, D.J., & Laiard, N. (1997). The cost of adverse events in hospitalized patients. *JAMA, 227,* 307–311.

Bulger, R.J. (2003). The quest for therapeutic institutions. Washington, DC: Association of Academic Health Centers.

Burkhardt, M.A., & Nathaniel, A. (2008). *Ethics and issues in contemporary nursing* (3rd ed.). Clifton Park, NY: Thomson Delmar Learning.

Byrne, M., Valentine, W., & Carter, S. (2004). The value of certification: A research journey. *AORN J, 79,* 825–835.

Carpenito-Moyet, L.J. (2008). *Nursing diagnosis: Application to clinical practice* (12th ed.). Philadelphia: Lippincott, Williams & Wilkins.

Collins, S.E. (2001). Litigation risks for infusion specialists: Understanding the issues. *Journal of Infusion Therapy, 24*(6), 375–380.

Committee on the Health Professions Education Summit. (2003*). Health professions education: A bridge to quality.* Washington, DC: The National Academies Press. Retrieved from http://www.nap.edu/catalog/10681.html (Accessed February 23, 2008).

Corrigan, A. (2010). Infusion nursing as a specialty. In: M. Alexander, A. Corrigan, L. Gorski, J. Hankins, & R. Perucca (Eds.), *Infusion nursing: An evidence-based approach* (pp. 1–9). St. Louis, MO: Saunders Elsevier.

Diehl-Svrjcek, B.C., Dawson, B., & Duncan, L.L. (2007). Infusion nursing: Aspects of practice liability. *Journal of Infusion Nursing, 30*(5), 274–292.

Douglas, J., & Larrabee, S. (2003). Bring barcoding to the bedside. *Nursing Management, 34*(5), 37–40.

Galloway, M. (2002). Using benchmarking data to determine vascular access device selection. *Journal of Infusion Therapy, 25*(5), 32.

Gorski, L. (2005). *Pocket guide to home infusion therapy.* Sudbury, MA: Jones and Bartlett.

Gorski, L. (2007). Advancing of the science of infusion therapy: Understanding evidence-based practice. *Newsline, 29*(4). Norwood, MA: Infusion Nurses Society.

Hagle, M.E. (2010). Evidence-based practice. In: M. Alexander, A. Corrigan, L. Gorski, J. Hankins, & R. Perucca (Eds.), *Infusion nursing: An evidence-based approach* (p. 10). St. Louis, MO: Saunders Elsevier.

Higginbotham, E. (2003). Does error+injury = negligence? *RN, 66*(5), 67–68.

Infusion Nurses Society (INS). (2001). Infusion Nursing Code of Ethics. *Journal of Infusion Nursing, 24*(4), 242–243.

Infusion Nurses Society (INS). (2006a). Infusion Nursing Standards of Practice, *29*(1S). Norwood, MA: Author.

Infusion Nurses Society (INS). (2006b). *Clinical competency validation program for infusion therapy (CCVP)* (2nd ed.). Norwood, MA: Author.

Institute of Medicine (IOM). (2007). *The learning healthcare system: workshop summary* (p. ix), Washington, DC: The National Academies Press.

Institute for Safe Medication Practices (ISMP). (2002). The ten key elements of medication use system. Retrieved from www.ismp.org/faq.asp (Accessed March 16, 2008).

Kelly, P. (2008). *Nursing leadership and management* (2nd ed). Clifton Park, NY: Thomson Delmar Learning.

Kleinpell, R.M. (2001). Abstracted in *Nursing Spectrum, 2*(2), 39.

Leape, L.L., Bates, D.W., Cullen, K.J., et al. (1995). Systems analysis of adverse drug events. *JAMA, 274*(4), 35–43.

Marquis, B., & Huston, C. (2006). *Leadership roles and management functions in nursing.* Philadelphia: Lippincott Williams & Wilkins.

McCloskey Dochterman, J.C., & Bulechek, G.M. (2004). *Nursing intervention classification* (NIC) (4th ed.). St. Louis, MO: C.V. Mosby.

McLaughlin, M., & Houston, K. (2008). Managing outcomes using organizational quality improvement model. In: P. Kelly (Ed.), *Nursing leadership & management* (2nd ed.). Clifton Park, NY: Thomson Delmar Learning.

Moorhead, S., Johnson, M., & Maas, M. (2004). *Nursing outcomes classification* (NOC) (3rd ed.). St. Louis, MO: C.V. Mosby.

Moureau, N., & Maney, S. (2003). Legal aspects of infusion nursing. *Journal of Vascular Access Devices, 8*(1), 8–12.

NANDA-I (2007). Nursing diagnoses: Definitions and classification, 2007–2008. Philadelphia: Author.

National Council of State Boards of Nursing (NCSBN). (2003). *Report of findings from the 2002 RN practice analysis.* Chicago: National Council of State Boards of Nursing.

Newell-Stokes, G. (2004). Applying evidence-based practice: A place to start. *Journal of Infusion Nursing, 27*(6), 381–385.

Newfield, S.A., Hinz, M.D., Tilley, D.S., et al. (2007). *Cox's clinical applications of nursing diagnosis* (5th ed.). Philadelphia: F.A. Davis.

Nieva, V. (2005). From science to service: A framework for the transfer of patient safety research into practice. In: *Advances in patient safety: From research to implementation* (vol. 2). Rockville, MD: Agency for Healthcare Research and Quality.

Obsheatz, M. (2004). Integrating bar code medication administration and intravenous medication safety systems. Pathways for Medication Safety: Strategies for Leadership. 4th Conference, June 11, 2004, Ohio Valley, PA.

Premier, Inc. (2003). Hospital Quality Incentive Demonstration Project. Retrieved from www.premierinc.com/quality-safety/tools (Accessed March 20, 2008).

Roark, D.C., & Miguel, K. (2006). Bar codings' replacement? *Nursing Management, 37*(2), 29–31.

Rudzik, J. (1999). Establishing and maintaining competency. *Journal of Intravenous Therapy, 22*(2), 69–73.

Sackett, D.L., Straus, S.E., Richardson, W.S., et al. (2000). *Evidence-based medicine: How to practice and teach EBM* (2nd ed.). Edinburgh: Churchill Livingstone.

Sierchio, G.P. (2001). Quality management. In: J. Hankins, R.A. Lonsway, C. Hedrick, & M. Perdue (Eds.), *Infusion Nurses Society: The infusion therapy in clinical practice* (2nd ed., pp. 26–49). St. Louis, MO: W.B. Saunders.

Stetler, D.B., Brunell, M., Giuliano, K.K., et al. (1998). Evidence-based practice and the role of nursing leadership. *Journal of Nursing Administration, 28*(7/8), 45–53.

The Joint Commission (TJC). (2005). *Sentinel event alert.* Oakbrook Terrace, IL: Joint Commission.

The Joint Commission (TJC). (2007). *Comprehensive accreditation manual for hospitals.* Oakbrook Terrace, IL: Joint Commission.

The Joint Commission (TJC). (2008). National Patient Safety Goals. Retrieved from www.jointcommisssion.org/PatientSafety/NationalPatientSafety Goals/08 (Accessed March 8, 2008).

The National Coordinating Council for Medication Error and Prevention (NCCMERP). (2008). *Definition of medication error.* Retrieved from www. nccmerp. about Med errors. (Accessed March 20, 2008).

Titler, M. (2007). Translating research into practice. *American Journal of Nursing, 107*(6 Suppl), 26–33.

Tran, M.N. (2003). Take benchmarking to the next level. *Nursing Management, 34*(1), 19–23.

U.S. Department of Health and Human Services (USDHHS). (2003). The HIPAA Privacy Rule and Research. Retrieved from www.hhs.gov/ocr/hipass/ finalreg.html (Accessed February 19, 2010).

U.S. Department of Health and Human Services (USDHHS). (2004). National practitioner data bank: 2004 report. Retrieved from http://www. npdb-hipdb.com (Accessed March 16, 2008).

Valente, S. (2003). Research dissemination and utilization, improving care at the bedside. *Journal Nurse Care Quality, 18*(2), 114–121

Yoder-Wise, P.S. (2007). *Leading and managing in nursing* (4th ed.). St. Louis, MO: Mosby Elsevier.

Zonderman, A. (2000). An overview of informed consent. *Journal of Vascular Access Device, 5*(3), 20–24.

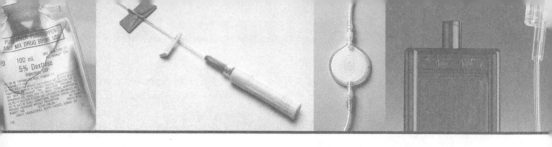

Chapter **2**

Infusion-Related Infection Control and Occupational Risks

It may seem a strange principle to enunciate as the very first requirement in a hospital that it should do the sick no harm. It is quite necessary to lay down such a principle.
Florence Nightingale, 1859

Chapter Contents

▪ LEARNING   *On completion of this chapter, the reader will be able to:*
OBJECTIVES
1. Review the definitions in the glossary of terms.
2. Describe the function of the immune system.
3. Identify the organs involved in the immune system.
4. Identify the factors important for maintaining the well-being of the host.
5. State the four major factors affecting immune dysfunction.
6. Discuss the links in the chain of infection.
7. Identify strategies to prevent infection.
8. State the factors that influence formation of infusion phlebitis.
9. Discuss sources of intravascular cannula-related infections.
10. State the most prevalent microorganisms found in infusion-related infections.
11. Discuss the point of care for infection control practices related to infusion therapy.
12. Identify the three occupational risks for the infusion nurse.

GLOSSARY

Aerobic   Occurring in the presence of oxygen

Airborne Precautions   Techniques used to decrease infection by microorganisms carried by the air. Precautions used in addition to Standard Precautions for illnesses transmitted by airborne droplet nuclei

Anaerobic   Occurring in the absence of oxygen; concerning an organism that lives and reproduces in the absence of oxygen

Antibodies   A substance produced by B lymphocytes in response to a unique antigen. Antibodies neutralize or destroy antigens

Antigens   A protein marker on the surface of cells that identifies the cell as self or nonself; identifies the type of cell and stimulates the production of antibodies

Aseptic technique   A method used by healthcare workers designed to reduce the risk of transmission of pathogenic microorganisms to patients; part of Standard Precautions

Bloodborne pathogens Microorganisms carried in blood and body fluids that are capable of infecting other persons

Bloodstream infection (BSI) An infection that flows through the circulatory system.

Chain of infection The process by which infections spread

Colonization Growth of microorganisms in a host without producing overt clinical symptoms or detected immune reaction

Contact Precautions Techniques used in addition to standard precautions that decrease infection by microorganisms transmitted through direct contact with the patient or patient care items

Contamination Microorganisms present on a body surface without tissue invasion or physiologic reaction

Dissemination Shedding of microorganisms from an individual into the immediate environment or movement of microorganisms from a confined site (skin to the bloodstream to other parts of the body)

Droplet Precautions Infection due to inhalation of respiratory pathogens suspended on liquid particles exhaled from someone already infected

Endogenous Produced within or caused by factors within the organism

Epidemiology Branch of science concerned with the study of the factors determining and influencing the frequency and distribution of disease, injury, and other health-related events and their causes in a defined human population for the purpose of establishing programs to prevent and control their development and spread

Exogenous Originating outside of the organism

Extrinsic contamination Contamination with microorganisms during preparation or administration

Hand hygiene A general term that applies to handwashing, antiseptic handwash, antiseptic hand rub, or surgical hand antisepsis

Healthcare-associated infections (HAIs) Infections that patients acquired during the course of receiving treatment for other conditions or that healthcare workers (HCWs) acquire while performing their duties within a healthcare setting

Hematogenous Produced by or derived from the blood; disseminated through the bloodstream or by the circulation

Host The organism from which a microorganism obtains its nourishment

Immunosuppression Interference with the development of immunologic responses; may be artificially induced by chemical, biologic, or physical agents or may be caused by disease

Intrinsic contamination Contamination during manufacturing

Leukopenia Any condition in which the number of leukocytes in the circulating blood is lower than normal, the lower limit of which is generally regarded as 4000/5000 mm^3

Pathogenicity The state of producing or being able to produce pathological changes and disease

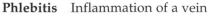

Phlebitis   Inflammation of a vein

Reservoir   Living or nonliving material in or on which an infectious agent multiplies, develops and is dependent on for its survival in nature

Resident flora   Microorganisms that are indigenous to each individual and are present mainly on the skin and in the respiratory, gastrointestinal, and reproductive systems

Septicemia   The presence of pathogenic microorganisms or their toxins in the blood or other tissues; the condition associated with such a presence

Standard Precautions   Guidelines recommended by the Centers for Disease Control and Prevention to reduce the risk of the spread of infection in hospitals. Also referred to as Universal Precautions

Susceptible host   Person with inadequate defenses against an invading pathogen. Host is the organism from which a parasite obtains its nourishment

Transient flora   Microorganisms that are picked up, usually on the skin, that can be removed fairly easily with hand hygiene

Transmission   The movement of an organism from the source to the host

Vector-borne transmission   A carrier, usually an insect or other animal, that transmits the causative organisms of disease from infected to noninfected individuals

Vehicle-borne transmission   Any substance that serves as an intermediate means to transport and introduce an infectious agent into a susceptible host through a suitable portal of entry

Virulence   Relative power and degree of pathogenicity possessed by organisms to produce disease

▪ Introduction to Infusion-Related Infection Control

The intravenous system provides a direct access into the vascular system. Therefore an understanding of basic epidemiology principles and common causative organisms provides a foundation for implementation of standards of care to prevent infusion-related infections. In the United States, the following organizations set standards and guidelines for infection control related to infusion therapy.

- Association of Practitioners in Infection Control and Epidemiology, Inc. (APIC), which emphasizes prevention and promotion of zero tolerance for healthcare-associated infections and adverse events. APIC: www.apic.org
- Centers for Disease Control and Prevention (CDC), which is a division of the U.S. Department of Health and Human Services

and establishes guidelines for infection control practices. CDC: www.cdc.org

■ Centers for Medicare & Medicaid Services (CMS), whose goal is to achieve a transformed and modernized healthcare system. CMS: www.cms.hhs.gov

■ Infusion Nurses Society (INS), which sets standards for practice and provides a framework for the development of infusion policies and procedures in all practice settings. INS: www.ins1.org

■ The Joint Commission (TJC), which oversees and establishes standards of quality and performance measurement in health care. TJC: www.jointcommission.org

■ U.S. Occupational Safety and Health Administration (OSHA), which is the enforcing agency that provides the mandates to protect employees of all fields. OSHA: www.osha.gov

To be a competent practitioner, it is important to have an understanding of the functioning of the immune system, the principles of epidemiology, infectious disease processes, and infections caused by infusion therapy.

■ Immune System Function

The immune system is a dynamic network of immune organs and immune cells that recognizes self from nonself and protects against foreign agents such as microorganisms and abnormal cells that arise within the body (Sommer, 2004). The immune system provides the body with a way of distinguishing itself from foreign invaders. These invaders constantly bombard the body and trigger immune responses. They are termed **antigens** and can include microbes such as viruses, bacteria, and parasites. The appropriate immune response occurs when the immune system recognizes and destroys invading antigens.

The immune system also acts as a "clean-up crew" that disposes of used, mutant, or damaged cells that result from catabolism, growth, and injury (Smeltzer, Bare, Hinkle, & Cheever, 2008).

Organs of the Immune System

The organs and cells involved in the immune system form a complex when antigens and immune system cells are constantly moving through the lymph system, blood circulation, and lymphatic organs. The primary organs of the immune system are the thymus and bone marrow. Secondary organs include lymph nodes, spleen, liver, Peyer's patches, appendix, tonsils and adenoids, and lungs. Table 2-1 shows the locations and functions of these organs.

> Table 2-1   **ORGANS OF THE IMMUNE SYSTEM**

Organs	Location	Function
Primary		
Thymus	Mediastinal cavity	Provides immune function in early years: T-cell development
Bone marrow	Ribs, sternum, long bones	Produces stem cells, which are precursors to leukocytes and lymphocytes
Secondary		
Lymph nodes	Interconnected system of vessels and modes; chains of pathway of lymph drainage	Stores T cells, B cells, macrophages; circulates leukocytes; drains and filters waste products (cellular debris)
Spleen	Left upper abdominal quadrant beneath diaphragm	Stores red cells, leukocytes, platelets, lymphocytes; serves as hematopoietic organ; filters out antigens
Liver	Right upper abdominal quadrant, small intestine	Kupffer cells filter out antigens
Peyer's patches, appendix	Right lower abdominal quadrant	Areas of lymphoid tissue that contain B cells and T cells
Pharynx, tonsils and adenoids	Pharynx	Unknown
Lungs	Thoracic cavity	Filter antigenic material and cellular debris

Mechanisms of Defense

A mutual compatibility exists between a healthy host (human) and environmental microbes. The factors most important in maintaining the well-being of the host are nonspecific responses and specific immune responses. The natural immune response consists of nonspecific defenses present at birth. These mechanisms function without prior exposure to an antigen. Specific immunity is acquired and functions when there has been prior exposure to antigens (Wilkinson & Van Leuven, 2007).

Nonspecific and specific mechanisms include:
- First-line mechanisms
  - Physical: Skin, mucous membranes, epiglottis, respiratory tract cilia, sphincters
  - Chemical: Tears, gastric acidity, vaginal secretions
  - Mechanical: Lacrimation, intestinal peristalsis, urinary flow
- Second-line mechanisms
  - Phagocytosis, complement cascade, inflammation, and fever
- Tertiary mechanisms
  - Specific immunity and lymphocytes

First Line of Defense/Nonspecific or Innate Defenses

Physical nonspecific mechanisms of defense against infections include intact skin, mucosal barriers, the respiratory tree (nares, trachea, and bronchi), gastrointestinal tract and genitourinary tract and are considered to be the first line of defense. The skin forms the first barrier against infection; it is a physical barrier that contains secretions with antibacterial actions. This tight network of cells provides an impenetrable physical barrier against invasion by microbes that reside on the external or internal environment.

Chemical barriers inhibit growth and invasion by environmental microbes. Chemical barriers include acid secretion by mucus, urine acidity, a variety of lipids secreted in the skin, and tears.

There are also physiologic mechanisms. The nares, trachea, and bronchi are covered with mucous membranes that trap pathogens which are then expelled. The nose contains hairs that filter the upper airway, and the nasal passages, sinuses, trachea, and larger bronchi are lined with cilia that sweep microorganisms upward from the lower airways. Coughing and sneezing forcefully expel organisms from the respiratory tract. Through mechanical action, peristalsis in the gastrointestinal (GI) tract and urinary tract expels organisms from the internal environment of the host (Wilkinson & Van Leuven, 2007).

Second Line of Defense/Specific Immune Response

Pathogens that pass the first line of defense release wastes and secretions that activate a set of secondary defenses.

- Phagocytosis: The process by which white blood cells (WBCs) engulf and destroy pathogens directly.
- The complement cascade: A process by which a set of blood proteins called complement triggers the release of chemicals that attack the cell membranes of the pathogens, causing them to rupture. Complement also signals WBCs called basophils to release a chemical called histamine, which prompts inflammation.
- Inflammation: Process that begins when histamine and other chemicals are released directly from damaged cells or from basophils in response to the activation of complement.
- Fever: A rise in core body temperature that increases metabolism, inhibits multiplication of pathogens, and triggers specific immune responses. It is believed that low-grade fevers are a necessary natural defense mechanism (102°F [38.9°C]) (Wilkinson & Van Leuven, 2007).

Tertiary Defenses/Specific Immunity

Acquired or specific host defense mechanisms function most efficiently when there has been prior exposure to invading **antigens**. Passive acquired immunity is transient and develops by passage of immune cells from one person to another or by gamma-globulin infusion. Active acquired immunity develops from direct contact with antigens by disease. The key players in specific immune response are leukocytes, T-cell lymphocytes, B lymphocytes, immunoglobulin, and the complement cascade.

Leukocytes make up one of the most important components of the immune system. A differential white blood cell (WBC) count provides specific information related to infections and disease. **Leukopenia** is defined as a reduction of the number of leukocytes in the blood to a count of less than 5000/mm³. Normal WBC counts range from 5000 to 10,000/mL. Refer to Table 2-2.

Lymphocytes

Other components of the immune system are the B and T lymphocytes, which form the specific immune response system. Lymphocytes have specific antigen recognition and can neutralize toxin and phagocytize invading bacteria and viruses. Lymphocytes recognize a specific antigen because of the presence in the antigens of genes known as human leukocyte antigen (HLA) genes.

Immunoglobulin (Ig) circulates throughout the body, aiding in the destruction of microorganisms and neutralizing toxin. Immunoglobulins are divided into five major classes: IgA, IgD, IgE, IgG, and IgM. The absence of one or more of these substances has been linked to infection or disease processes.

> Table 2-2   **TYPES AND FUNCTIONS OF WHITE BLOOD CELLS**

Type and % of Total WBCs	Function
Granular	
Basophils: 0.5–1%	Release histamine, heparin, and serotonin granules as part of the inflammatory response.
Eosinophils: 1–3%	Destroy helminths; mediate allergic reactions; have limited role in phagocytosis.
Neutrophils: 55–70%	Phagocytize pathogens. Body's first line of defense through phagocytosis.
Agranular	
Lymphocytes: 20–35%	T cells: Responsible for cell-mediated immunity; recognize, attack and destroy antigens
Formed in bone marrow T cells mature in thymus	B cells: Responsible for humoral immunity; produce immunoglobulins and attack and destroy antigens.
Monocytes: 3–8% Similar to lymphocytes Stay in peripheral blood for 70 hours.	Able to phagocytize directly as well as to differentiate into macrophages, which help clean up damaged or injured tissue.

Source: Van Leeuwen, A.M., Kranpitz, T.R., & Smith, L. (2006). Davis's comprehensive handbook of laboratory and diagnostic tests with nursing implications (2nd ed.). Philadelphia: F.A. Davis.

The phagocytic cells provide a first line of defense against invasion by bacteria and selected fungi. These cells circulate in the bloodstream until summoned by chemical mediators to sites of infections. The immune system provides a surveillance network that enables the host to monitor and identify foreign material and generate specific protection against invading pathogens. Immunologic responses are mediated through the production of **antibodies** that circulate in the plasma.

The complement system consists of a complex of about 17 different proteins that are responsible for several steps in the inflammatory process, including summoning phagocytic cells to the site of infection. Complement also attaches to the infectious agent and promotes ingestion by the phagocyte. The complement proteins are numbered C1 through C9 and act in a cascade fashion to initiate action of the next protein. These proteins are part of the nonspecific and specific response systems. As a nonspecific immune response, C3 and C5 increase vascular permeability and chemically attract granulocytes. As part of the specific response, the normally inactive proteins are activated by specific antibodies in two pathways: the classic pathway requires interaction of C1 with the antigen–antibody complex, or the alternative pathway occurs in the absence of a specific antibody (Smeltzer, Bare, Hinkle, & Cheever, 2008).

Impaired Host Resistance

Many factors can result in impaired host defense. Persons who acquire an infection because of a deficiency in any of their multifaceted host defenses are referred to as compromised hosts. Persons with major defects related to specific immune responses are referred to as **immunosuppressed** hosts. These two terms often are used interchangeably.

The following is a general clinical picture of the four major factors affecting immune dysfunction:

1. Infections occur frequently.
2. Infections are more severe than usual.
3. Unusual infecting agents or infections with opportunistic organisms occur.
4. There is an incomplete response to treatment without complete elimination of the infecting agent.

Primary immunodeficiency disorders are congenital or inherited. B-cell immunodeficiencies account for about 50% of primary immunodeficiencies, and T-cell immunodeficiencies account for about 40% (Smeltzer, Bare, Hinkle, & Cheever, 2008).

Secondary immunodeficiencies arise from disease processes or therapies that decrease immune system organ or cell function. These deficiencies are acquired. Causes of secondary immune deficiency are age, stress, trauma, poor nutritional status, and drug therapy. Often these types of immunodeficiencies are transient and respond well to antibody therapy with IgG or a removal of the cause (Swenson, 2000).

Basic Principles of Epidemiology

Epidemiology is the "study of things that happen to people." Historically, it involves the study of epidemics. Epidemiology is the study of determinants, occurrence, and distribution of health and disease in a population (Ostrowsky, 2007).

Colonization

Infection is the replication of organisms in the tissue of a host and development of clinical signs and symptoms. **Colonization** is the presence of a microorganism in or on a host, with growth and multiplication of the microorganisms with no clinical symptoms or detected immune reaction at the time of isolation.

A carrier (or colonized person) is an individual colonized with a specific microorganism and from whom the organism can be recovered but who shows no signs or symptoms of the presence of the microorganism. A carrier may have a history of previous disease. The carrier state may be transient (short term), intermediate (on occasion), or chronic (long term, permanent, or persistent).

Dissemination

Dissemination is the shedding of microorganisms into the immediate environment from a person carrying them. Cultures of air samples, surfaces, and objects reveal dissemination or shedding of microorganisms. Some facilities routinely culture all or selected asymptomatic staff in an attempt to identify carriers of certain organisms; however, such surveys lack practical relevance unless related to a specific outbreak of disease. Usually only a fraction of colonized persons are disseminating; therefore, nondisseminators are not associated with the actual spread of infection.

The risk of dissemination is generally greater from individuals with disease caused by that organism than from individuals with subclinical infection or those who are colonized with the organism.

Chain of Infection

Infections result from interaction between infectious agents and susceptible hosts. This interaction is called **transmission.** The **chain of infection** refers to six links that make up the chain: the causative agent or microorganism;

the place where the organism naturally resides (reservoir); a method (mode) of transmission; a portal of entry into a host; and the susceptibility of the host. To control infection, the chain of infection must be attacked at its weakest link (Fig. 2–1).

First Link: Causative Agent

The first link in the chain of infection is the microbial agent or source, which may be a bacterium, fungus, virus, or parasite. The majority of healthcare-associated infections (HAIs) are caused by bacteria and viruses. The ability of an organism to induce disease is called its **virulence** or invasiveness. The ability of microorganisms to induce disease is referred to as **pathogenicity**, and it may be assessed via disease-colonization ratios.

Second Link: Reservoir

All organisms have a **reservoir**, or source of microorganisms. Common sources include other humans, the client's own microorganisms, plants, animals, or the general environment. People themselves are the most common source of infection for others. The reservoir is the place where the organism maintains its presence, metabolizes, and replicates. Viruses survive better in human reservoirs, whereas the reservoir of gram-negative bacteria may have either a human or an animal reservoir or an inanimate reservoir is usually a human **transmission**.

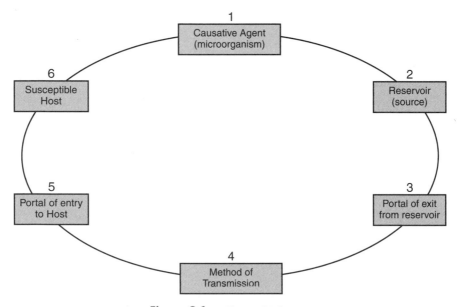

Figure 2-1 ◼ Chain of infection.

Third Link: Portal of Exit from Reservoir

The exit site is important in transmission of infection. Organisms from humans usually have a single portal of exit, but can be multiple. The major portals of exit are the respiratory tract, gastrointestinal (GI) tract, and skin (e.g., in wounds). In addition, blood may be a portal of exit and is a concern for infusion nurses.

Fourth Link: Method (Mode) of Transmission

After a microorganism leaves its source or reservoir, it requires a means of transmission to reach another person or host through a receptive portal of entry. There are five mechanisms of transmission:

1. Contact transmission. Contact transmission can be divided into two subgroups The first, direct transfer of organisms, involves body surface-to-body surface contact and physical transfer of microorganisms between a susceptible host and an infected or colonized person (e.g., turning a patient, or performing other patient-care activities) or through touching, biting, kissing, or sexual intercourse. The second subgroup, indirect-contact transmission, involves contact of a susceptible host with a contaminated intermediate object, usually inanimate (e.g., contaminated instruments, needles, dressing, or hands). Examples of organisms that can be transmitted via contact are *Staphylococcus* and *Enterococcus* (Siegel, Rhinehart, Jackson, & Chiarello, 2007).

2. Droplet transmission. Droplet transmission is a form of contact transmission. The mechanism of transfer of the pathogen to the host is different from contact transmission. Droplet transmission is considered a separate route of transmission. Transmission via large-particle droplets (>5 µm in size) requires close contact between the source and recipient, usually 3 feet. Examples of pathogens transmitted by the droplet route are *Bordetella pertussis* and *Neisseria meningitides* (Siegel, Rhinehart, Jackson, & Chiarello, 2007).

3. Airborne transmission. Airborne transmission occurs by dissemination of either air-borne droplet nuclei (small-particle residues, <5 µm) of evaporated droplets containing microorganisms that remain suspended in the air for long periods of time. Examples of airborne transmission are *Mycobacterium tuberculosis*, rubeola and varicella viruses (Siegel, Rhinehart, Jackson, & Chiarello, 2007).

4. Common vehicle-borne transmission. A vehicle is any substance that serves as an intermediate means to transport and introduce an infectious agent into a susceptible host. Examples are toys, handkerchiefs, soiled linen, or clothes.

5. Vector-borne transmission. A vector is an animal or flying or crawling insect that serves as an intermediate means for transporting an

infectious agent. An example is the mosquito carrying the West Nile virus (Siegel, Rhinehart, Jackson, & Chiarello, 2007).

Fifth Link: Portal of Entry to the Susceptible Host

A person can become infected once the organism enters the body. The skin is a barrier to infectious agents; however, any break in the skin can readily serve as a portal of entry. The mucous membranes and respiratory, gastrointestinal, and urinary tracts are also portals of entry. An organism may colonize one site and cause no disease, but the same organism at another site may result in clinical disease. For example, *Escherichia coli* routinely colonizes the gastrointestinal tract and under normal circumstances does not cause disease; however, the same organism in the urinary tract can cause infection (Ostrowsky, 2007).

Sixth Link: Host Response

A **host** can respond to a microorganism in one of three ways: a subclinical infection, a clinically apparent illness, or the extreme response of death. The same organism infecting different hosts can result in a clinical spectrum of disease that is the same, similar, or different in various individuals. A **susceptible host** is a person with inadequate defenses against the invading organism. Examples include the very young or very old, and those receiving immune suppression treatment for cancer, chronic illness, or following a successful organ transplant.

Classification of Infections

Location

Infections can cause harm in a limited region of the body (e.g., upper respiratory tract or urethra), these infections are considered local. Systemic infections occur when the pathogens invade the blood or lymph and spread through the body. A bacteremia is the clinical presence of bacteria in the blood, whereas **septicemia** is symptomatic systemic infection spread via the blood. The source of the pathogen must be identified.

Endogenous infections are caused by a person's own flora. For endogenous infections, the patient either was admitted to the facility colonized with these microorganisms or became colonized at some point during hospitalization. **Exogenous infections** are from sources outside a person's body. It may not always be possible to determine whether a particular organism isolated from a patient with healthcare-associated infections (HAIs) is exogenous or endogenous. The term autogenous infection indicated that the infection was derived from the flora of the patient, whether or not the infecting organism became part of the patient's flora subsequent to admission (Ostrowsky, 2007).

Stages

Many infections follow a fairly predictable course of events; the duration and intensity of symptoms may vary from one individual to the next.

- Incubation: The stage between successful invasion of the pathogen into the body and the first appearance of symptoms
- Prodromal stage: Characterized by the first appearance of vague symptoms. Not all infections have a prodromal stage.
- Illness: The stage marked by appearance of signs and symptoms characteristic of the disease.

NOTE > If the patient's immune defenses and medical treatment are ineffective, this stage can end in death of the patient.

- Decline: The stage during which the patient's immune defenses, along with any medical therapies, successfully reduce the number of pathogens. Symptoms begin to fade
- Convalescence: Characterized by tissue repair and return to health (Wilkinson & Van Leuven, 2007).

Healthcare-Associated Infections

The terms hospital-acquired or nosocomial infections have been replaced with the term **healthcare-associated infections (HAIs)**. The CDC defines HAIs as infections that patients acquire during the course of receiving treatment for other conditions or that healthcare workers (HCWs) acquire while performing their duties within a healthcare setting (CDC, 2006). The branch of CDC that was formally the Hospital Infections Program broadened its name to the Division of Healthcare Quality Promotion to reflect the expanding epidemiology (CDC, 2006).

In hospitals alone, HAIs account for an estimated 2 million infections, 90,000 deaths, and $4.5 billion in excess healthcare costs annually (CDC, 2006). Factors affecting the challenge of controlling HAIs include:

- Shift in the patient population that healthcare facilities care for to more complicated patients with comorbidities
- Increasing number of patients who are severely immunocompromised
- Use of a larger number of devices and procedures and for longer duration in patients
- Staffing shortages
- Antimicrobial resistant pathogens
- Emerging infectious diseases (Burke, 2003)

A HAI is identified as one that has resulted in a localized or systemic condition that results from adverse reaction or the presence of an infectious agent or agents, or their toxins which were not present or incubating at the time of admission to the hospital or facility. For bacteria HAIs this means that the infection usually occurs 48 hours or longer after admission (Ostrowsky, 2007).

Cannula-related bloodstream infection (CR-BSI) is perhaps the least frequently recognized HAI. The device that poses the greatest risk of iatrogenic BSI is the central venous catheter (CVC) in its numerous forms. It has been estimated that 90% of CR-BSIs originate from CVCs, leading to 55,000 BSIs in U.S. ICUs each year (Mermel, 2000). In the past several years, studies have demonstrated that a zero tolerance for catheter-related infection is needed. From 2001 to 2006 the CDC collected data on implementation of interventions using a "bundle approach" (Maki, Kluger, & Crinch, 2006). More information on the bundle approach is provided in the section "Strategies for Preventing/Treating Infection" in this chapter.

■ Infusion-Related Infections

Epidemiology

Health-care institutions purchase millions of intravascular catheters each year. The incidence of catheter-related bloodstream infections (CRBSI) vary considerably by type of catheter, frequency of catheter manipulation, and patient factors. Peripheral catheters are the devices most frequently used for vascular access. In the United States, more than 5 million central venous devices of various types are inserted annually, with an estimated 15 million CVC days occur in ICUs each year. An estimated 250,000 cases of central line–associated **bloodstream infections** (BSIs) occur annually in hospitals in the United States, with an estimated attributed mortality of 12% to 25% for each infection, with a marginal cost to the health-care system of $25,000-$45,000 per episode (CDC, 2002a; Krywda & Andris, 2005).

A percentage of intravascular devices are colonized by skin organisms at the time of removal, and colonized cannulas are more likely than non-colonized ones to show phlebitis or local inflammation. One of the most serious forms of intravascular device-related infection occurs when intravascular thrombus surrounding the cannula becomes infected. This causes septic thrombophlebitis when associated with peripheral IV cannulas or septic thrombosis of a central vasculature when associated with centrally placed catheters.

Infections related to central venous access device (CVAD) generally are categorized as early and delayed infections. Early infections are those occurring within the first 2 to 3 weeks after CVAD implantation. Early infections generally are caused by bacterial contamination during the initial catheter insertion. These infections are most commonly caused by skin flora.

Delayed infections occur after 3 weeks of catheter insertion because of poor wound care, migration of organisms along the catheter tract, or seeding of the CVAD from a secondary source.

Clinical manifestations of infection are variable and depend on the type of infection present. Local infection may present as cellulitis with erythema, induration, pain, and inflammation. Serosanguineous or purulent discharge may be present from the skin exit site, indicating inflammation around the catheter.

NOTE > "Any patient with an IV catheter who develops high-grade bloodstream infection that persists after an infected cannula has been removed, it is likely the patient has infected thrombus in the recently cannulated vein, and may even have secondary endocarditis or seeding to other distant sites" (Raad & Sabbagh, 1992).

The major sources of cannula-related infections are the skin flora, contamination of the catheter hub, contamination of infusate, and hematogenous colonization of the device. Refer to Figure 2-2.

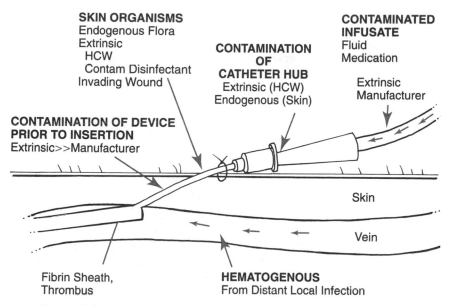

SKIN ORGANISMS
Endogenous Flora
Extrinsic
  HCW
  Contam Disinfectant
Invading Wound

CONTAMINATION OF CATHETER HUB
Extrinsic (HCW)
Endogenous (Skin)

CONTAMINATED INFUSATE
Fluid
Medication

Extrinsic
Manufacturer

CONTAMINATION OF DEVICE PRIOR TO INSERTION
Extrinsic>>Manufacturer

Skin

Vein

Fibrin Sheath,
Thrombus

HEMATOGENOUS
From Distant Local Infection

Figure 2-2 ■ Sources of I.V. cannula-related infections. (From *Bennett & Brachman's hospital infections* [5th ed.]. Lippincott Williams & Wilkins. Used with permission.)

Primary risk factors associated with central infusion line infections include duration of catheterization (number of catheter days), multiple lines, colonization of catheter insertion site by skin organisms, location of catheter subclavian placement, aseptic dressing changes, and aseptic insertion technique. Factors contributing to a lesser degree to central line infections include secondary bacteremia, host defense status, contaminated infusate, and number of catheter lumens (single versus triple lumen).

Factors that predispose patients with CVADs to infection include longer durations of catheter placement, catheters with multiple lumens, catheters made of polyvinyl chloride, catheters that develop fibrin sheaths at the distal catheter tip, port systems that accumulate sludge or blood products within the port reservoir, and a compromised immune status in patients (Ray, 1999). Implantable devices are associated with the lowest rate of infectious complications of all CVAD systems (Maki & Mermel, 2007). Refer to Table 2-3 for management of patient with central venous catheter-related bloodstream infection.

Since 1970, CDC's National Nosocomial Infection Surveillance (NNIS) System, now the National Healthcare Safety Network (NHSN), has been collecting data on the incidence and etiologies of hospital-acquired (healthcare-associated) infections, including catheter related-bloodstream infections (CR-BSIs).

There are three major sources of BSI associated with intravascular devices:

1. Colonization of the cannula wound
2. Colonization of the cannula hub
3. Contamination of the infusate

The forms of device-related inflammation or infection range from infusion phlebitis to asymptomatic colonization of the intravascular device (usually by skin) to overwhelming septic shock originating from an infected thrombus in a cannulated central vein.

Infusion Phlebitis

The presence of **phlebitis** connotes a substantially increased risk of infection and indicates the need for immediate removal of the catheter to reduce the severity of phlebitis, for symptomatic relief, and to prevent catheter colonization from progressing to bloodstream infection. Most researchers have concluded that infusion phlebitis is primarily a physiochemical phenomenon related to many factors. A few of the risk factors for increased phlebitis rates include phlebitis exceeds 50% by the fourth day after catheterization, female gender, and catheter materials. Refer to Table 2-4 for a complete list of risk factors (Maki & Mermel, 2007).

> Table 2-3

MANAGEMENT OF PATIENTS WITH CENTRAL VENOUS CATHETER–RELATED BLOODSTREAM INFECTIONS

Nontunneled CVCs

Complicated		Uncomplicated	
Cause	Treatment	Cause	Treatment
Septic thrombosis or endocarditis	Remove CVC. Treat with systemic antibiotic for 4–6 weeks.	Coagulase-negative *Staphylococcus*	Remove CVC. Treat with systemic antibiotic for 5–7 days. *Staphylococcus aureus*
Osteomyelitis	Remove CVC. Treat with systemic antibiotic for 6–8 weeks.	*Staphylococcus aureus*	Remove CVC. Treat with systemic antibiotic for 14 days.
		Gram-negative bacilli	Remove CVC. Treat with systemic antibiotic for 10–14 days.
		Candida spp.	Remove CVC. Treat with antifungal therapy for 14 days.

Tunneled Catheters and Implanted Devices

Complicated		Uncomplicated	
Cause	Treatment	Cause	Treatment
Tunnel infection Port abscess	Remove CVC/ID. Treat with systemic antibiotic for 10–14 days.	Coagulase-negative *Staphylococcus*	■ May retain CVC/ID. Use systemic antibiotic for 7 days plus antibiotic lock therapy for 10–14 days. ■ Remove CVC/ID if there is clinical deterioration or persisting or relapsing bacteremia.
Septic thrombosis or endocarditis	Remove CVC/ID. Treat with antibiotics for 4–6 weeks	*Staphylococcus aureus*	■ Remove CVC/ID. Treat with systemic antibiotic for 14 days if TEE(–). ■ For CVC/ID salvage therapy, if TEE(–) use systemic and antibiotic lock therapy for 14 days. ■ Remove CVC/ID if there is clinical deterioration or persisting or relapsing bacteremia.
Osteomyelitis	Remove CVC/ID. Treat with systemic antibiotic for 6–8 weeks.	Gram-negative bacilli	■ Remove CVC/ID. Treat with systemic antibiotic for 10–14 days. ■ For CVC/ID salvage, use systemic and antibiotic lock therapy for 14 days. ■ If no response, remove and treat with systemic antibiotic therapy for 10–14 days.
		Candida spp.	■ Remove CVC/ID. Treat with antifungal therapy for 14 days after last positive blood culture.

TEE = Transesophageal echocardiography.
Source: Mermel, L.A., Farr, B., Sherertz, R.J., et al. (2001). Guidelines for the management of intravascular catheter-related infections. Journal of Intravenous Nursing, 24(3), 180–205. Used with permission.

> Table 2-4   RISK FACTORS FOR INFUSION PHLEBITIS

Catheter Material

Polypropylene > Teflon
Silicone elastomer > polyurethane
Teflon > polyetherurethane
Teflon > steel needle

Catheter Size

Large bore > smaller bore
8-inch Teflon > 2-inch Teflon
Insertion in emergency room > inpatient units
Disinfection of skin with antiseptic before catheter insertion

Experience, Skill of Person Inserting Catheter

House officers, nurses > hospital I.V. team
House officers, nurses > decentralized unit I.V. nurse educator
Increasing duration of catheter placement in site
Subsequent catheters beyond the first infusate
Low-pH solutions (e.g., dextrose-containing solutions)
Potassium chloride
Hypertonic glucose, amino acids, lipid for parenteral nutrition
Antibiotics (especially β-lactams, vancomycin, metronidazole)
High rate of flow of I.V. fluid (>90 mL/hr)

Disinfection of Insertion Site Before Catheter Insertion

None > chlorhexidine-alcohol

Frequent I.V. Dressing Changes

Daily > every 48 hours

Catheter-Related Infection

Host factors
"Poor quality" peripheral veins
Insertion site
Upper arm, wrist > hand

Age

Children: Older > younger
Adults: Younger > older

Gender

Female > male

Ethnicity

European American > African American
Underlying medical disease
Individual biologic vulnerability

NOTE: The > symbol denotes a significantly greater risk of phlebitis.
Source: Maki, D.G., & Ringer, M. (1991). Risk factors for infusion-related phlebitis with small peripheral venous catheters. A randomized controlled study. Annals of Internal Medicine, 114, 845–854. Used with permission.

EBNP In a prospective clinical study of 1054 peripheral I.V. catheters, the risk for phlebitis exceeded 50% by the fourth day after catheterization (Maki & Ringer, 1991).

INS Standard The peripheral-short catheter in the adult patient shall be removed every 72 hours and immediately upon suspected contamination, complication, or therapy discontinued. (INS, 2006a, 49)

 NURSING FAST FACT!

The presence of phlebitis connotes a substantially increased risk of infection and indicates the need for immediate removal of the catheter to reduce the severity of phlebitis, for symptomatic relief and to prevent catheter colonization from progressing to BSI (Maki & Mermel, 2007).

Infusate-Related Bloodstream Infections

Contamination of parenteral solutions can occur by **extrinsic contamination**, contamination with microorganisms during preparation or administration; or **intrinsic contamination** (contamination during manufacturing) can occur.

Extrinsic contamination of parenteral fluids can occur during administration of solutions and medications due to the duration of uninterrupted infusion through the same administration set and to the frequency with which the set is manipulated. Microorganisms gain access from air entering bottles, from entry points into the administration set, from the I.V. device through the line, or at the junction between the administration set and the catheter hub.

A meta-analysis of five studies in which more than 9000 infusions in five hospitals were prospectively cultured, with no associated episodes of bacteremia or candidemia identified with an incidence of endemic BSI due to contaminated infusate of less than one episode per 2000 I.V. infusions (Maki, Botticelli, LeRoy, et al., 1987).

NOTE > The I.V. infusate can be identified as the source of BSI only if it is cultured. Most endemic BSIs caused by contaminated fluid go unrecognized or are attributed to the intravascular device (Maki & Mermel, 2007).

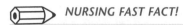

NURSING FAST FACT!

*The most important measures to prevent BSIs from contaminated in-use (extrinsic) infusate are stringent asepsis during the preparation and compounding of admixtures in the hospital central pharmacy or on individual patient-care units. **Aseptic technique** should be followed when infusions are handled during use, during injections of medications, or changing bags or bottles of fluids. Replacing the administration set at periodic intervals can prevent the buildup of dangerous introduced contaminants and further reduce the risk of related BSI. Total replacement of all equipment during the cannula change results in a substantial reduction in epidemic BSIs (Maki & Mermel, 2007).*

INS Standard Primary and secondary continuous administration sets shall be changed no more frequently than every 72 hours and immediately upon suspected contamination or when the integrity of the product or system has been compromised. The primary administration set change shall coincide with peripheral catheter change and with initiation of a new container of solution. (INS, 2006a, 48)

Intrinsic contamination during manufacturing has been reported, with more than 12 epidemics of infusion-related BSI caused by this form of contamination. Intrinsic contamination is rare; however, its potential for producing harm is great because of the large numbers of patients in multiple hospitals who may be affected. The direct contamination of infusate at the manufacturing level gives contaminants time to proliferate to dangerously high concentrations (Maki & Mermel, 2007).

If intrinsic contamination of commercially distributed product is identified or even strongly suspected, the local, state and federal (CDC and the Food and Drug Administration [FDA]) public health authorities must be contacted.

NOTE > Unopened samples of the suspect lot or lots should be quarantined and saved for analysis.

Before use, containers of fluid should be examined against light and dark backgrounds for cracks, defects, turbidity, and particulate matter. Any glass container lacking a vacuum when opened should be considered contaminated. Additional factors that contribute to contamination of infusion-related infection include:

1. *Faulty handling.* Glass containers can become cracked or damaged and plastic bags punctured; bacteria and fungi may invade a hairline crack in an I.V. container.
2. Admixtures. The risk of contamination when admixtures are prepared is decreased when trained personnel prepare mixtures under laminar flow hoods. The use of strict aseptic technique is vital.

3. *Manipulation of in-use I.V. equipment.* Faulty technique in handling equipment can lead to contamination.
4. *Injection ports.* Aseptic technique must be maintained when injection ports are used for "piggyback" or secondary infusions. The injection port located at the distal end of the tubing can expose the patient to excreta and drainage.

INS Standard To prevent the entry of microorganisms into the vascular system, the injection or access port should be aseptically cleansed with an approved antiseptic solution immediately prior to use; antiseptic solution containers in a single-use package should be used. (INS, 2006a, 35)

5. *Three-way stopcocks.* These adjunct devices are potential sources of transmission of bacteria because their ports, unprotected by sterile covering, are open to moisture and contaminants. These devices are usually connected to CVCs and arterial lines and are frequently used for drawing blood. Using aseptic technique is vital.

Refer to Table 2-5 for microorganisms most frequently encountered in catheter-related, central venous catheter–related, infusate-related, and blood product–related infections.

> Table 2-5   **MICROORGANISMS MOST FREQUENTLY ENCOUNTERED**

Source	Pathogens
Catheter Related *Peripheral I.V. Catheter*	Coagulase-negative staphylococci* *Staphylococcus aureus* *Candida* spp.*
Central Venous Catheters	Coagulase-negative staphylococci *Staphylococcus aureus* *Candida* spp. *Corynebacterium* spp. (especially JK-1) *Klebsiella* and *Enterobacter* spp. *Mycobacterium* spp. *Trichophyton beigelii* *Fusarium* spp. *Malassezia furfur**
Contaminated I.V. Infusate	*Tribe Klebsiella* *Enterobacter cloacae* *Enterobacter agglomerans* *Serratia marcescens* *Klebsiella* spp. *Burkholderia cepacia* *Bukrholderia acidovorans, Burkholderia picketti* *Stenotrophomonas maltophilia* *Citrobacter freundii* *Flavobacterium* spp. *Candida tropicalis* *E. cloacae*

> Table 2-5	MICROORGANISMS MOST FREQUENTLY ENCOUNTERED—cont'd	
Source	**Pathogens**	
Contaminated Blood Products	*S. marcescens* *Ochrobactrum anthropi* *Flavobacterium* spp. *Burkholderia* spp. *Yersinia* spp. *Salmonella* spp.	

*Also seen with peripheral I.V. catheters in association with the administration of lipid emulsion for parenteral nutritional support.
Source: Maki, D.G. & Mermel, L.A. (2007). Infections due to infusion therapy. In W. Jarvis (Ed.), Bennett & Brachman's hospital infections (5th ed., p. 620). Philadelphia: Lippincott Williams & Wilkins. Used with permission.

Culturing Techniques

When an infusion-related infection is suspected, obtain cultures from the suspected source of infection. This can include one or all of the following:
- Catheter–skin junction
- Peripheral infusion catheter
- Administration set
- Infusate
- Patient's blood
  (INS, 2006b)

The recommended method for culturing a catheter is the semiquantitative culture technique (Procedures Display 2-1). If culturing at the catheter–skin site do not cleanse the area to be cultured. If culturing the infusion catheter, thoroughly cleanse the area around the insertion site with 70% alcohol and permit the area to air dry. Alcohol is recommended because residual antimicrobial activity of iodine-containing solutions may kill organisms on the catheter when it is removed. If blood culture is required, use venipuncture technique for blood draw using culture tubes.

The following are disadvantages of this semiquantitative method: (1) this method may fail to detect bacteremia of the internal lumens of the catheter tip and (2) the catheter must be removed for culturing and may not actually be the source of infection.

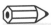 *NURSING FAST FACT!*

> A positive, semiquantitative culture of 15 or more colony-forming units (CFUs) confirms a local cannula infection (Maki & Mermel, 2007).
> Culture any purulent drainage from the site. If the I.V. solution is the suspected source of infection, send the fluid container and tubing to a laboratory for analysis.
> Blood cultures drawn through a peripheral vein and through the I.V. cannula can be a helpful alternative to culturing the cannula. If the results of the catheter blood sample are five times the peripheral blood sample, a catheter-related infection is suspected and the catheter should be removed.

Strategies for Preventing/Treating Infection

Nurses involved in maintaining vascular access devices must have the knowledge base and competency to initiate infusion-related protocols to prevent infection. The principles of infection control provide the foundation for the delivery of infusion therapy. Prevention begins with knowledge regarding the techniques used to prevent infection.

NOTE > Using evidence-based practices and education of personnel in the care of peripheral catheters, using aseptic technique for insertion and care, labeling of insertion sites and all tubing with the date and time of insertion, inspecting every 8 hours for signs of infection, recording, and reporting have shown to reduce catheter-associated bloodstream infection rates (Warren, Cosgrove, Diekema, et al., 2006). Refer to Evidence-Based Care Box 2-1.

---

1. Follow CDC Standard Precautions Guidelines

The Hospital Infection Control Practice Advisory Committee (HICPAC) of the CDC developed new isolation guidelines that better addressed the growing concerns of the transmission of resistant organisms. Standard Precautions and Transmission–Based Precautions are intended to be applied to the care of all patients in all healthcare settings, regardless of the suspected or confirmed presence of infectious agent. The specific elements of Standard and Transmission-Based Precautions are as follows (Siegel, Rhinehart, Jackson, & Chiarello, 2007).

Tier One: Standard Precautions

Standard precautions incorporate the fundamentals of universal precautions (designed to reduce exposure risks to bloodborne pathogens) and

---

EVIDENCE-BASED CARE BOX 2-1

Education-Based Intervention

Warren, D., Cosgrove, S. Diekema D., et al. (2006). A multicenter intervention ot prevent catheter– associated bloodstream infections. Infection Control & Hospital Epidemiology, 27(7), 662–669.

The study was done to assess a multicenter intervention to prevent catheter-associated bloodstream infections. Twelve intensive care units and one bone marrow transplantation unit at six academic medical centers were chosen. Results demonstrated increase in site dressing begin dated from 26% to 34%, and overall rate of CR-BSI decreased from 11% to 8.9% per 1000 catheters.

Results: This study demonstrated than an education-based intervention that uses evidence-based practices can be successfully implemented in a diverse group of medical and surgical units and reduced catheter-associated bloodstream infection rates.

body substance isolation (designed to reduce risk of exposures to pathogens residing in moist body fluids) and require consistent use for all patients regardless of their infection status.

Standard precautions are imposed when (1) there is risk of exposure to blood; (2) there is risk of exposure to all other body fluids, including secretions and excretions (not including sweat), whether or not evidence of blood is present; (3) nonintact skin is present; and (4) there will be contact with any mucous membranes.

Standard Precautions constitutes the primary strategy for the prevention of healthcare-associated transmission of infectious agents among patients and healthcare personnel (Siegel, Rhinehart, Jackson, & Chiarello, 2007).

The new elements of Standard Precautions include three areas of practice:

1. Respiratory Hygiene/Cough Etiquette
2. Safe Injection practices
3. Use of masks for insertion of catheters or injection of material into spinal or epidural spaces via lumbar punctures procedures (Siegel, Rhinehart, Jackson, & Chiarello, 2007).

RESPIRATORY HYGIENE/COUGH ETIQUETTE

The need for vigilance and prompt implementation of infection control measures at the first point of encounter within a healthcare setting (e.g., reception and triage areas, outpatient clinics and physician offices) necessitated the new strategy triaged at patient and accompanying family members with undiagnosed transmissible respiratory infections. The term cough etiquette is derived from recommended source control measures for *Mycobacterium tuberculosis*. The elements include:

- Education of healthcare facility staff, patients, and visitors
- Posted signs in language(s) appropriate to the population served with instructions to patients and accompanying family members or friends
- Source control measures (covering the mouth/nose with a tissue when coughing and prompt disposal of used tissues), using surgical masks on the coughing person when tolerated and appropriate.
- Hand hygiene after contact with respiratory secretions
- Spatial separation, ideally greater than 3 feet of persons with respiratory infections in common waiting areas when possible.

 NURSING FAST FACT!

Healthcare personnel are advised to observe Droplet Precautions (i.e., wear a mask) and hand hygiene when examining and caring for patients with signs and symptoms of respiratory infection (Siegel, Rhinehart, Jackson, & Chiarello, 2007).

SAFE INJECTION PRACTICES

Infection control practices and aseptic technique related to injection practice will be monitored for adherence. Two areas of concern are (1) reinsertion of used needles into a multidose vial or solution container and (2) use of a single needle/syringe to administer intravenous medication to multiple patients. Whenever possible, use of single-dose vials is preferred over multiple-dose vials, especially when medications will be administered to multiple patients. Outbreaks related to unsafe injection practices indicate that some healthcare personnel are unaware of, do not understand, or do not adhere to basic principles of infection control and aseptic technique.

NOTE > A survey of U.S. healthcare workers who provide medication through injection found that 1% to 3% reused the same needle and/or syringe on multiple patients (Williams, Perz, & Bell, 2004).

INS Standard Single use flushing systems shall be used. (INS, 2006a, 50)

INFECTION CONTROL PRACTICES FOR SPECIAL LUMBAR PUNCTURE PROCEDURES

In October 2005, The Healthcare Infection Control Practices Advisory Committee (HICPAC) reviewed evidence related to eight cases of bacterial meningitis by *Streptococcus* species from oropharyngeal flora from HCW post-myelography. The conclusion warranted the additional protection of a face mask for the individual placing a catheter or injecting material into the spinal or epidural spaces.

> **INS Standard** Sterile technique, including mask and gloves, should be used when accessing, caring for, and maintaining an intraspinal access device. (INS, 2006a, 62)

Tier Two: Transmission-Based Precautions

Transmission-based precautions are the second tier of the isolation precautions. These additional precautions are based on the known or suspected infectious state of the patient and the possible routes of transmission. There are three categories of transmission-based precautions:

1. **Airborne precautions**, which require special air handling and ventilation to prevent the spread of these organisms. The infectious agents remain infectious over long instances when suspended in the air, such as those causing tuberculosis, varicella, and measles. The preferred patient placement is in an airborne infection isolation room (AIIR). The AIIR is a single-patient room that is equipped with special air handling and ventilation capacity

that meet the American Institute of Architects/Facility Guidelines Institute standards for AIIRs (i.e., monitored negative pressure relative to the surrounding area, 12 air exchanges per hour for new construction and renovation and 6 air exchanges per hour for existing facilities, air exhausted directly to the outside or recirculated through HEPA filtration before return). Healthcare personnel caring for the patient on Airborne Precautions wear a mask or respirator (HEPA or N95 respirators for patients with tuberculosis) depending on the disease-specific recommendations, which is donned before room entry (Siegel, Rhinehart, Jackson, & Chiarello, 2007).

2. **Droplet precautions**, which require the use of mucous membrane protection (eye protection and masks) to prevent infectious organisms from contacting the conjunctivae or mucous membranes of the nose or mouth. Examples of infections are mumps, rubella, influenza, adenovirus, rhinovirus, and pertussis. The pathogens do not remain infectious over long distances in a healthcare facility; special air handling and ventilation are not required to prevent droplet transmission. A single patient room is preferred. Patients on Droplet Precautions who must be transported outside of the room should wear a mask if tolerated and follow Respiratory Hygiene/Cough Etiquette (Siegel, Rhinehart, Jackson, & Chiarello, 2007).

3. **Contact precautions**, which require the use of gloves and gowns when direct skin-to-skin contact or with contaminated environment is anticipated. Don PPE on room entry and discard before exiting is done to contain pathogens, especially those that have been implicated in transmission through environmental contamination such as vancomycin-resistant *Enterococcus* (VRE), *Clostridium difficile*, noroviruses and other intestinal tract pathogens, and respiratory syncytial virus (RSV) (Siegel, Rhinehart, Jackson, & Chiarello, 2007).

    NURSING FAST FACT!

Implementation of standard precautions has implications for infusion therapy nurses; use of I.V. therapy carts and trays may be limited for patients who are on contact transmission precautions.

2. Follow Hand Hygiene Procedure

Skin Function/Barrier Protection

The primary function of the skin is to reduce water loss, provide protection against abrasive action and microorganisms, and act as a permeability barrier to the environment. Barrier function arises from the dying, degeneration, and compaction of underlying epidermis and from the process of synthesis of the stratum corneum occurring at the same rate as loss. The barrier to percutaneous absorption lies within the stratum corneum, the thinnest and smallest compartment of the skin. The formation of the skin barrier is under homeostatic control, which is illustrated by the epidermal response to barrier disturbance by skin stripping or solvent extraction.

The goal of using specific products for **hand hygiene** is to maintain normal barrier function. The normal barrier function is biphasic: 50% to 60% of barrier recovery typically occurs within 6 hours, but complete normalization of barrier function requires 5 to 6 days (CDC, 2002b).

TRANSMISSION OF PATHOGENS ON HANDS

Transmission of healthcare-associated pathogens from one patient to another via the hands of healthcare workers (HCWs) requires the following sequence of events:

1. Organisms present on the patient's skin or that have been shed onto inanimate objects must be transferred to the hands of HCWs.
2. These organisms must then be capable of surviving for at least several minutes on the hands of personnel.
3. Handwashing or hand antisepsis by the worker was inadequate or omitted entirely, or the agent used for hand hygiene was inappropriate.
4. The contaminated hands of the HCW must come in direct contact with another patient (CDC, 2002b).

 NURSING FAST FACT!

> Studies have documented contamination of HCWs hands with potential healthcare-associated pathogens. Serial cultures revealed that 100% of HCWs carried gram-negative bacilli at least once, and 64% carried Staphylococcus aureus at least once (CDC, 2002b).

PREPARATIONS USED FOR HAND HYGIENE

Alcohol-based products are more effective for standard handwashing or hand antisepsis by HCWs than soap or antimicrobial soaps. Applying friction removes most microbes and should be used when placing invasive devices, when persistent antimicrobial activity is desired, and when it is important to reduce the numbers of **resident skin flora** in addition to transient microorganisms (CDC, 2002b). Alcohols are not appropriate for use when hands are visibly dirty or contaminated.

> EBNP One study demonstrated that by introducing the use of hand rubbing with an alcohol solution, there was significant improved hand-cleansing compliance. When using an alcohol-based hand rub, apply product to palm of one hand and rub hands together, covering all surfaces of hands and fingers, until hands are dry. Note that the volume needed to reduce the number of bacteria on hands varies by product (Girou & Oppein, 2001).

CDC RECOMMENDATIONS FOR HAND HYGIENE IN HEALTHCARE SETTINGS

Indications for handwashing and hand antisepsis:

- When hands are visibly dirty or contaminated with blood or other body fluids, wash hands with either a non-antimicrobial soap or water or an antimicrobial soap and water.
- If hands are not visibly soiled use an alcohol-based hand rub for routinely decontaminating hands in all other clinical situations.
- Decontaminate hands before having direct contact with patients.
- Decontaminate hands before donning sterile gloves when inserting a central intravascular catheter.
- Decontaminate hands before inserting a peripheral vascular catheter.
- Decontaminate hands after contact with patient's intact skin (taking pulse, blood pressure).
- Decontaminate hands after contact with body fluids or excretions, mucous membranes, nonintact skin, and wound dressing if hands are not visibly soiled.
- Decontaminate hands if moving from a contaminated body site to a clean body site during patient care.
- Decontaminate hands after removing gloves.
- Before eating and after using a restroom, wash hands with a non-antimicrobial soap and water or with an antimicrobial soap and water.
- Antimicrobial-impregnated wipes (towelettes) may be considered as an alternative to washing hands with non-antimicrobial soap and water.

> ### NURSING FAST FACT!
>
> - It is recommended that healthcare agencies provide personnel with efficacious hand-hygiene products that have a low irritancy potential, particularly when these products are used multiple times per shift.
> - Using gloves should not replace handwashing and does not provide complete protection.
> - For insertion of peripheral catheters good hand hygiene before catheter insertion or maintenance, combined with proper aseptic technique during catheter manipulation, provides protection against infection. Central venous catheter (CVC) insertion carries a substantially greater risk for infection; therefore, the level of barrier precautions needed to prevent infection during insertion of CVC should be more stringent (CDC, 2002a & b).

ADDITIONAL HAND HYGIENE RECOMMENDATIONS

- Do not wear artificial fingernails or extenders when having direct contact with patients at high risk.
- Keep natural nail tips less than ¼ inch long.
- Wear gloves when in contact with blood or potentially infectious materials, mucous membranes, and nonintact skin.

- Remove gloves after caring for a patient. Do not wear the same pair of gloves for the care of more than one patient, and do not wash gloves between uses with different patients.
- Change gloves during patient care if moving from a contaminated body site to a clean body site.

3. Use Appropriate Skin Antisepsis

The Infusion Nurses Society (2006a, 41) Standards of Practice and Centers for Disease Control and Prevention (CDC) support the use of the following antiseptic solutions to prepare the site before venipuncture:
- Iodophors: Povidone-iodine
- 70% Isopropyl alcohol
- 2% Aqueous chlorhexidine-based solution

Povidone-iodine has been the most widely used antiseptic for cleansing insertion sites; however, recent studies support the use of 2% aqueous chlorhexidine gluconate with alcohol as a superior solution to lower BSI rates. The 2% chlorhexidine-based preparation has also been shown to decrease the skin irritations reported from use of other skin preparation agents (Hibbard, Mulberry, & Brady, 2002; Maki, Alvarado, & Ringer, 1991). Refer to Evidence-Based Practice Box 2-2.

> *EBNP Meticulous care of all invasive sites using chlorhexidine gluconate with alcohol reduced catheter-related bloodstream infections and catheter colonization more than the use of povidone iodine (Chaiyakunapruk, Veenstra, Lipsky, et al., 2002; Young, Commiskey, & Wilson, 2006).*

Practice criteria for insertion of peripheral, midline, arterial, central, and peripherally inserted central catheters (PICCs) include the use of aseptic technique and site preparation with antimicrobial solutions (INS,

---

EVIDENCE-BASED CARE BOX 2-2

Use of Chlorhexidine Gluconate for Vascular Catheter Site Care

Chaiyakunapruk, N., Veenstra, D.L., Lipsky, B.A., et al. (2002). Chlorhexidine compared with povidone-iodine solution for vascular catheter-site care: A meta analysis. Annals of Internal Medicine, 136(11), 792.

Randomized, controlled trials comparing chlorhexidine gluconate with povidone-iodine solutions for catheter-site care. Eight studies involving a total of 4143 catheters met the inclusion criteria.

Results: Suggested that incidence of bloodstream infections is significantly reduced in patients with central vascular lines who receive chlorhexidine gluconate versus povidone–iodine for insertion site skin disinfection.

2006a, 51). In addition, the following guidelines should be used to maintain integrity of the infusion site (INS, 2006a, 41):

- Hand hygiene procedures should be observed
- Protocols for site preparation should be established in organizational policies and procedures and practice guidelines
- The process for applying the chosen antiseptic agent is dependent on and should be consistent with manufacturer's labeled use and directions.
- After initial access site preparation, powder-free gloves (sterile for midline, arterial, central, and peripherally inserted central catheter placement) should be used.
- When necessary, clipping should be performed to remove excess hair at the intended vascular access site
- Antimicrobial solutions in a single-unit use configuration should be used.
- Alcohol should not be applied after the application of povidone-iodine preparation because alcohol negates the effect of povidone-iodine.
- The antimicrobial preparation solution should be allowed to air-dry completely before proceeding with the vascular access device insertion procedure.
- Maximum barrier precautions including sterile gown, gloves, cap, masks, protective eyewear, surgical scrub, and large sterile drapes and towels should be used for midline, arterial, central, and peripherally inserted central catheters or guidewire exchanges.

NOTE > The CDC recommends to observe proper hand-hygiene procedures either by washing hands with conventional antiseptic-containing soap and water or with waterless alcohol-based gels or foams. Use of gloves does not obviate the need for hand hygiene (CDC, 2002b).

4. Use Catheter Site Dressing Regimens

Transparent, semipermeable polyurethane dressing is used in many clinical settings. These dressings reliably secure the infusion device, permit continuous visual inspection of the catheter site, permit patients to bathe and shower without saturating the dressing, and require less frequent changes than do standard gauze and tape dressings. Various studies have been done comparing TSM dressing and gauze dressings on a variety of types of infusion devices that found limited increase in cutaneous colonization under either dressing (Maki & Ringer, 1987).

> *EBNP Data from studies suggest that colonization among catheters dressed with transparent dressings (5.7%) is comparable to that of those dressed with gauze (4.6%) and that no clinically substantial differences exist in the incidences of either catheter colonization or phlebitis (Maki & Ringer, 1987).*

The CDC recommendations include use of sterile gauze or sterile transparent semipermeable dressing to cover the catheter site. If the patient is diaphoretic, or if the site is bleeding or oozing, a gauze dressing may be preferred. The dressing should be replaced if it becomes damp, loosened, or visibly soiled. The CDC also recommends replacing gauze dressings used on short-term CVC sites every 2 days and transparent dressings every 7 days (CDC, 2002a).

INS Standard A sterile dressing shall be applied and maintained on access devices. Gauze dressings that prevent visualization of insertion sites should be changed routinely every 48 hours. A TSM dressing on the peripheral vascular access device should be changed at the time of catheter site rotation and immediately if the integrity of the dressing is compromised. (INS, 2006a, 44)

New Dressing Technology

A chlorhexidine (CHG)-impregnated TSM dressing is now available from 3M Company. The Tegaderm™ CHG dressing cover protects and secures the catheter site while allowing visualization of the insertion site, which has been shown to reduce the risk of site colonization. Refer to Figure 2-3. The CHG-impregnated dressing, at this time, has not been studied in a randomized clinical study as to its effectiveness in preventing CR-BSIs (3M HealthCare Division, 2008).

A chlorhexidine-impregnated urethane sponge composite (Biopatch®, J&J Wound Management) has been shown significantly to reduce CVC-BSIs from 21 to 13 per 1000 catheter days (Keyeserling, Dykes, Newsome, et al., 1994). In a randomized control trial, Maki, Mermel, Klugar, et al. (2000) found that technology using CHG urethane sponge reduced both CR-BSIs and local site infections compared to gauze dressings. Refer to Figure 2-4.

> *EBNP In a multicenter study a chlorhexidine-impregnated sponge (Biopatch®) placed over the site of short-term arterial and CVDs reduced the risk of catheter colonization and catheter-related BSIs. No adverse systemic effects resulted from use of this device (Maki, Mermel, Kluger, et al., 2000).*

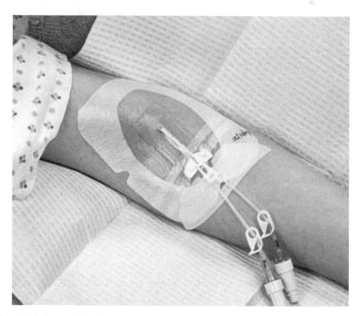

Figure 2-3 ■ Chlorhexidine (CHG) TSM dressing. (Courtesy of 3M Medical Division, St. Paul, MN.)

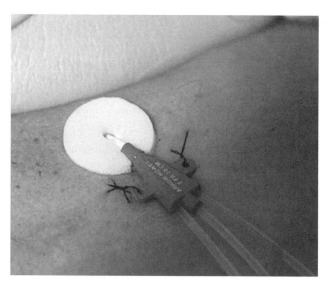

Figure 2-4 ■ Biopatch®. (Courtesy of J&J Wound Management, division of Ethicon, Inc., Somerville, NJ.)

5. Use Catheter Securement Devices

Sutureless devices are available and can be advantageous over sutures in preventing catheter-related BSIs. One study compared sutureless device with sutures for the securement of PICCs; in this study, catheter-related bloodstream infections were reduced in the group of patients receiving the sutureless device (Yamamoto, Solomon, Soulen, et al., 2002). The Statlock® I.V. stabilization device in a study (2006) lowered the rate of total IV complications by 67% and reduced unscheduled IV restarts by 76% (Schears, 2006). This evidence-based stabilization device is one strategy to decrease the risk of infection through migration of the catheter. Refer to Figure 2-5.

> **INS Standard** Catheter stabilization shall be used to preserve the integrity of the access device and to prevent catheter migration and loss of access.
> A catheter that has migrated externally should not be readvanced prior to restabilization. (INS, 2006a, 43)

6. Use Antimicrobial/Antiseptic-Impregnated Catheters and Cuffs

Catheters and cuffs that are coated or impregnated with antimicrobial or antiseptic agents can decrease the risk for catheter-related bloodstream

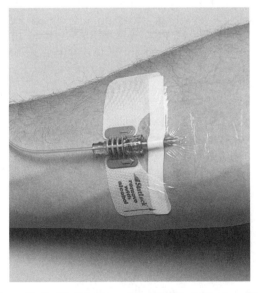

Figure 2-5 ■ Statlock®. (Courtesy of Bard Medical Division, C.R. Bard, Inc., Covington, GA.)

infections. Several different types of materials are used to coat catheters and cuffs. They include:

- Chlorhexidine/silver sulfadiazine: Newest generation available with coating over both the internal and external luminal surfaces. More expensive than standard catheters.
- Minocycline/rifampin: Available impregnated on both the external and internal surfaces. May increase the risk of resistance among pathogens, especially staphylococci.
- Platinum/silver: Ionic metals have a broad antimicrobial activity and are being used in catheters and cuffs.
- Silver cuffs: Ionic silver has been used in subcutaneous collagen cuffs attached to CVCs. Provides antimicrobial activity and cuff provides a mechanical barrier to the migration of microorganisms.

7. Use Anticoagulants

The use of anticoagulants as a routine strategy to reduce CR-BSI is not recommended (Abdelkefi, Torjamn, Ladeb, et al., 2005).

8. Tissue-Interface Barrier

A tissue-interface barrier (VitaCuff®; Vitafore Corp., San Carolos, CA) has been developed that incorporates aspects of the technology of Hickman and Broviac catheters; the device consists of a detachable cuff made of biodegradable collagen to which silver ion is chelated. Refer to Figure 2-6. The cuff can be attached to CVCs immediately before insertion. After insertion, subcutaneous tissue grows into the collagenous matrix, anchoring the catheter and creating a barrier against invasive organisms from the skin (Maki & Mermel, 2007).

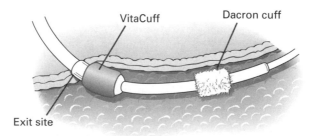

VitaCuff   Dacron cuff

Exit site

Proper VitaCuff positioning

Figure 2-6 ■ VitaCuff®. (Courtesy of Bard Medical Division, C.R. Bard, Inc., Salt Lake City, UT.)

9. Implementation of Central Venous Catheter Bloodstream Infection Prevention Bundle

The 100,000 Lives Campaign

As of June 2006, U.S. hospitals taking part in an unprecedented 18-month effort to prevent 100,000 unnecessary deaths by dramatically improving patient care have exceeded that goal. Hospitals enrolled in the 100,000 Lives Campaign have collectively prevented an estimated 122,300 avoidable deaths (Institute for Health Improvement [IHI], 2006).

As per the statistic at the beginning of this chapter, CVCs account for 15 million CVC-days per year in ICUs. Studies report mortality for infections of these catheters between 5% and 25%. Thus, it is estimated that between 500 and 4000 U.S. patients die annually due to bloodstream infections.

Part of the 100,000 Lives Campaign included prevention of central line infections by implementing a series of scientifically grounded steps called "the Central Line Bundle."

CENTRAL LINE BUNDLES

Care bundles, in general, are groupings of best practices with respect to a disease process that individually improve care, but when applied together result in substantially greater improvement. The central line bundle is a group of evidence-based interventions for patients with intravascular central catheters that, when implemented together, result in better outcomes than when implemented individually.

The basic components of the central line bundle from the Institute for Healthcare Improvement (IHI) include:

- Hand hygiene
- Maximal barrier precautions on insertion
- Chlorhexidine skin antisepsis
- Optimal catheter site selection, with the subclavian vein as the preferred site for nontunneled catheters
- Daily review of line necessity with prompt removal of unnecessary lines.
  (IHI, 2006)

The Central Line Bundle has been expanded to add a few more key evidence-based interventions that have significantly reduced CR-BSIs. Refer to Table 2-6.

New Strategies

Hub Connectors

The membranous septum of needleless Luer-activated connectors can be heavily contaminated, and conventional disinfection with 70% alcohol does not reliably prevent entry of microorganisms. In a study of

> Table 2-6	IMPLEMENTATION OF CENTRAL LINE BUNDLE

Key Components

a. Hand hygiene
b. Maximal Barrier Precautions on insertion (gowns, gloves, mask, cap)
c. Chlorhexidine (with alcohol) skin antisepsis of insertion site
d. Trained catheter inserters
e. Proper selection of type of catheter and insertion site
f. Time out called if proper procedures are not followed (then start again)
g. Use of aseptic technique using catheter manipulation (including hub disinfection)
h. Remove catheters when no longer medically necessary.
i. Optimal catheter site selection, with subclavian vein as the preferred site for non-tunneled catheters
j. Daily review of line necessity with prompt removal of unnecessary lines.

105 commercial, needleless Luer-activated valved connectors demonstrated a high level of protection using a novel chlorhexidine-impregnated barrier cap. Reduction of hub-related BSI using the barrier cap reduced the incidence of BSI fourfold (Menyhay & Maki, 2006).

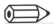 *NURSING FAST FACT!*

> It is important to scrub the hub cap for at least 15 seconds using 70% alcohol or 2% chlorhexidine with friction to ensure that contaminants are removed prior to access (Kaler & Chinn, 2007).

I.V. Fluid and Admixture Antiseptics

Fluid contamination using vancomycin-containing flushes or catheter/valve dwells have been shown to reduce the risk of CR-BSI and to potentially salvage some contaminated CVCs (Safdar & Maki, 2006). In another study, the use of EDTA with minocycline reduced CR-BSIs (Bleyer, Mason, Russel, et al., 2006). These solutions reduced the risk of CR-BSI in high-risk patients.

NURSING POINTS-OF-CARE:
PREVENTION OF INFUSION-RELATED INFECTIONS

Nursing Assessments

History

- History of any exposure to pathogens in the environment, including work, recent travel, contact with people who are ill
- Past and present disease history

- Current level of stress
- Immunization history
- History of risk factors: Fever, diarrhea

Physical Assessment

- Baseline immunologic studies: T-cell count, WBC count, differential. Refer to Table 2-7 for a complete list of laboratory tests
- Vital signs, especially elevated temperature and elevated pulse rate
- Assess for signs of local infection: Redness, inflammation, purulent drainage, tenderness, and warmth of catheter site.
- Assess skin turgor and mucous membranes.

Key Nursing Interventions

1. Reduce exposure to pathogens through the use of aseptic technique.
2. Follow standard precautions (especially hand hygiene)
3. Maintain skin integrity and natural defenses against infection.
4. Recognize that client stress reduction can improve immune system.
5. Promote immune function through collaborative care.
6. Use sterile technique when inserting and removing catheter and when maintaining infusion systems.
7. Ensure complete skin preparation before insertion of catheter using 2% chlorhexidine gluconate and 70% alcohol and allow to dry.
8. Remove the peripheral catheter within 72 hours.
9. Change the insertion site dressing when wet, soiled, or nonocclusive.
10. Secure proximal I.V. connections with a Luer locking set.
11. Monitor for:
    a. Signs and symptoms of sepsis (fever, hypotension, positive blood cultures).
    b. Oxygen saturation with oximetry.
12. Inspect all infusates before administering.
13. Implement central-line bundles.

> Table 2-7	COMMON TESTS FOR EVALUATING THE PRESENCE OF OR RISK OF INFUSION RELATED INFECTIONS

Test	Description
White blood cell count with differential	A breakdown of the types of WBCs; normal WBC count is 5000 to 10,000/mm^3. Constitute the body's primary defense system against foreign organisms, tissues and other substances. Life span of a normal WBC is 13–20 days. Produced in bone marrow Leukocytosis ($\downarrow$WBC), and leukopenia ($\uparrow$WBC). Acute leukocytosis is initially accompanied by changes in WBC count, followed by changes in individual WBCs

Continued

> Table 2-7	COMMON TESTS FOR EVALUATING THE PRESENCE OF OR RISK OF INFUSION RELATED INFECTIONS—cont'd
Test	**Description**
Blood culture	A sample of blood placed on culture media and evaluated for growth of pathogens. Collected whenever bacteremia or septicemia is suspected, determines sepsis.
Panels to evaluate specific disease exposure Immunoglobulin (IgA, IgG, IgM) levels	Blood tests to evaluate exposure to specific diseases (e.g., HIV, hepatitis). Identifies immunocompromised status. Blood tests to evaluate humoral immunity status. Immunoglobulins neutralize toxic substances, support phagocytosis and destroy invading microorganisms. Evaluates humoral immunity status. IgA: evaluate anaphylaxis associated with the transfusion of blood and blood products. IgG: chronic or recurrent infections. IgM: viral infections
C-reactive protein (CRP)	C-reactive protein is a glycoprotein produced by the liver in response to acute inflammation. CRP assay is a nonspecific test that determines the presence (not the cause) of inflammation; it is often ordered in conjunction with erythrocyte sedimentation rate (ESR).
Cold agglutinin titer	Used to diagnose atypical infections by detecting antigens in the blood. Cold agglutinins are antibodies that cause clumping or agglutination of RBCs at cold temperatures in individuals who are infected by a particular organism.
Erythrocyte (red blood cell) sedimentation rate (ESR or sedimentation rate)	Measures rate of sedimentation of red blood cells in an anticoagulated whole blood sample over a specified period of time. The basis of the ESR test is the alteration of blood proteins by inflammatory and necrotic processes. Nonspecific indicator of widespread inflammatory reaction due to infection or autoimmune disorders.

Source: Van Leeuwen, A.M., Kranpitz, T.R., & Smith, L. (2006). Davis's comprehensive handbook of laboratory and diagnostic tests with nursing implications (2nd ed.). Philadelphia: F.A. Davis.

■ Occupational Risks

Two types of occupational hazards are associated with infusion therapy: biologic and physical hazards. Inserting intravenous catheter lines, giving injections, handling and discarding sharps, and assisting with sterile procedures and many other high-risk procedures are an ordinary part of the daily practice regimen for nurses, especially those specializing in infusion therapy.

Biological Hazards

Hazards of bloodborne pathogens must be communicated to infusion nurses during training. Training should include information on bloodborne pathogens, as well as OSHA regulations and employers' exposure control plans. Healthcare employees face a significant risk as the result of occupational exposure to materials that may contain bloodborne pathogens, including hepatitis B virus (HBV), which causes hepatitis B (a serious liver disease), and human immunodeficiency virus (HIV), which causes acquired immunodeficiency syndrome (AIDS).

According to OSHA (2001), percutaneous injury with exposure to HIV- or HBV-infected blood in healthcare workers has accounted for 80% of occupational exposures, with 20% occurring before or during the use of needles and up to 70% after use and before disposal. Most needlestick injuries result from using unsafe needle devices rather than from carelessness by healthcare workers. Safer needle devices have been shown to significantly reduce needlestick injuries and exposures to potentially fatal bloodborne illnesses.

Factors that significantly increase infusion nurses' potential for exposure to HIV, HBV, and hepatitis C virus (HCV) include:

1. Use of hollow-bore catheters (over-the-needle catheters)
2. The increasing use of central line catheters in the hospital and home environment
3. The increasing number of nurses placing peripherally inserted central catheters (PICCs) in various settings
4. The expanding application of implantable vascular access catheters with manipulation of needles to access and de-access these devices (NIOSH, 2000b)

Exposure can be minimized or eliminated using a combination of engineering and work practice controls, personal protective clothing and equipment, training, medical surveillance, hepatitis B vaccination, signs and labels, and other provisions (Siegel, Rhinehart, Jackson, et al., 2007).

Prevention of Exposure to Bloodborne Pathogens

- Follow standards established by OSHA regarding glove wearing and handwashing practices. All bodily secretions, and therefore fluids from patients, are potentially infectious. All personnel who have contact with patients must adhere to strict guidelines.
- Follow CDC Standard and Transmission-Based Precautions.
- Use Needleless systems technology according to the Needlestick Safety and Prevention Act of November 2000.

NOTE > Safety features for needleless and needle protection systems are discussed in detail in Chapter 5.

- Use the Exposure Prevention Information Network (EPINet) to obtain manuals and software, data collection tools, and tracking and reporting systems for surveillance of bloodborne exposures.

Postexposure Prophylaxis

Healthcare organizations should have a plan in place before an exposure occurs. This can be easily derived from the CDC updated guidelines of

September 2005 (Panlilio, Cardo, Grohskopf, et al., 2005). The following are essential elements in responding to an actual event:

1. Refer to the exposure plan for the organization.
2. Wash the wound or flush the mucous membrane with water or saline.
3. Report the exposure to the appropriate department or individual ASAP.
4. Evaluate the risk of exposure.
5. Evaluate the source patient.
6. Evaluate the exposed person.
7. Make a decision about postexposure prophylaxis (PEP).

Persons receiving PEP should complete a full 4-week regimen.

Follow new guidelines from CDC on HIV postexposure prophylaxis: PEP for percutaneous injuries with basic two-drug PEP or expanded to 3-drug PEP when exposure is more severe (Panlilio, Cardo, Grohskopf, et al., 2005).

Website

PEPline at http://www.ucsf.edu/hivcntr/Hotlines/Pepline; 888-448-4911

 NURSING FAST FACT!

The primary barriers to protect healthcare workers from blood and/or body fluid exposures are gloves in conjunction with appropriate hand hygiene practices, eye protection, and mucous membrane protection (i.e., face shield or goggles and mask).

Physical Hazards

Physical hazards associated with infusion therapy include chemical exposure, and latex allergy.

Chemical Exposure

OSHA published guidelines for the management of cytotoxic (antineoplastic) drugs in the workplace in 1986. Since that time, surveys indicated further clarification was needed in management of exposure to chemicals. OSHA revised its recommendations for hazardous drug handling in 1995. To provide recommendations consistent with current scientific knowledge, the information was expanded to cover hazardous drugs, in addition to the cytotoxic. The recommendations apply to all settings in which employees are occupationally exposed to hazardous drugs (OSHA, 1999).

Hazardous drugs (HDs) have demonstrated the ability to cause chromosome breakage in circulating lymphocytes and mutagenic activity in urine, along with causing skin necrosis after surface contacts with abraded skin or damage to normal skin. It is recommended that nurses preparing HDs wear surgical latex gloves (double gloves if these do not interfere with techniques) and wear a protective disposable gown made of lint-free, low-permeability fabrics with closed front, long sleeves, and elastic or knit-closed cuffs when indicated. Because surgical masks do not protect against inhalation of aerosols, a biologic safety cabinet or an air-purifying respirator should be used when preparing HDs. A plastic face shield or splash goggles should be worn if a biologic safety cabinet is not used (OSHA, 1999a).

Latex Allergy

Natural rubber latex (NRL) allergy is a serious medical issue for healthcare workers. Latex allergy develops with exposure to NRL, a plant cytosol that is used extensively to manufacture medical gloves and other medical devices. Allergic reactions to latex range from asthma to anaphylaxis that can result in chronic illness, disability, career loss, and death. There is no treatment for latex allergy except complete avoidance of latex. Patients and healthcare providers must be assured of safety from sensitization and allergic reaction to latex.

The following are defining characteristics of allergic response to latex:

1. Life-threatening reactions occurring less than 1 hour after exposure to latex protein (bronchospasm, cardiac arrest, hypotension, respiratory arrest, wheezing); orofacial symptoms (edema of eyelids, edema of sclera, facial erythema, facial itching, nasal congestion, tearing of the eyes); generalized symptoms (flushing, generalized discomfort, increasing complaint of total body warmth)
2. Type IV reactions occurring more than 1 hour after exposure to latex protein: Discomfort reaction to additives such as thiurams and carbamates; eczema; irritation; redness (Ackley & Ladwig, 2008)

Latex allergy affects between 8% and 12% of workers in all health disciplines who are regularly exposed to latex. In the healthcare industry, workers at risk of latex allergy from ongoing latex exposure include physicians, nurses, aides, dentists, dental hygienists, operating room employees, laboratory technicians, and housekeeping personnel (National Institute for Occupational Safety and Health [NIOSH], 1999).

Latex allergy is a type I immunoglobulin E (IgE)–mediated hypersensitivity reaction that involves systemic antibody formation to proteins in products made of NRL. NRL is harvested commercially from the rubber tree, *Hevea brasiliensis*, and used to manufacture rubber products. NRL contains up to 240 potentially allergenic protein fragments.

Nurses working in infusion therapy are at risk because of the common routes of exposure. The routes of exposure for latex reaction for infusion specialists include aerosol and glove contact. Aerosolized latex exposure may be the greatest danger for those with type I latex allergy caused by respiratory distress (Gritter, 1999). For healthcare workers, the exposure route can be powder released in the air during the removal of powdered latex gloves. Latex proteins are carried on the powder from gloves and latex balloons and can remain airborne for as long as 5 to 12 hours. Frequent use of gloves during the insertion and maintenance of I.V. therapy increases the risk of sensitization. Radioallergosorbent testing (RAST) immunoassay is a blood test that measures the serum level of latex-specific IgE.

INS Standard   Latex exposure should be minimized. Healthcare workers and patients are provided education regarding latex allergy or sensitivity and methods to minimize risk of exposure. Nonlatex personal protective equipment is provided to latex-sensitive individuals. Nonlatex supplies and equipment shall be used on patients who have or may have latex allergy or sensitivity. (INS, 2006a, 28)

Those sensitive to latex should take the following precautions:
- Avoid all contact with latex.
- Carry autoinjectable epinephrine.
- Wear a medical identification bracelet.
- Negotiate with hospitals and providers in advance for latex-safe healthcare delivery (NIOSH, 2000a).

To reduce the risk of an allergic response, avoid using hand lotions or lubricants that contain mineral oil, petroleum salves, and other hydrocarbon-based gels or lotions to prevent the breakdown of the glove material and maintain barrier protection. Do not reuse disposable examination gloves because disinfecting agents can damage the barrier properties of gloves. Following hand hygiene guidelines is recommended after gloves are removed and before a new pair is applied. Gloves should not be stored where they will be subjected to excessive heat, direct ultraviolet or fluorescent light, or ozone (NIOSH, 2000a).

NONLATEX GLOVES

Nonlatex gloves made of alternative materials, with barrier protection equal to or better than that of latex gloves, are available. The protective characteristic of each material must be taken into consideration in relationship to the purpose for which the glove will be used (HealthCare Without Harm, 2008).

NOTE >   Manufacturers of nonlatex and nonchlorine (nonvinyl and nonneoprene) containing gloves are listed on the F.A. Davis Web site, along with additional Web site resources of latex allergy.

New Technology

In April 2008, the FDA cleared gloves made from a new form of NRL, guayule latex. The product, the Yulex Patient Examination Glove, is derived from guayule bush, a desert plant native to Southwestern United States. According to Yulex Corp. (2008), the durability, tensile strength, elasticity, comfort, and barrier protection qualities of Yulex natural rubber are far superior to those of petroleum-derived, synthetic latex products. It has the same chemical structure as other NRL material but without the proteins that cause latex allergy.

Early studies indicated that "gloves made from guayule latex may prove to be safer alternative for some people with sensitivity to traditional latex" (American Latex Allergy Association, 2008).

 ### Website

Further information can be obtained from HealthCare Without Harm: www.noharm.org
Yulex Corporation, Maricopa, Arizona: www.yulex.com

NURSING POINTS-OF-CARE
ALLERGIC RESPONSE TO LATEX

Assessment
- Obtain a history of risk factors (persons with neural tube defects, atopic individuals including those with allergies to food products); those who possess a known or suspected NRL allergy; persons who have had an ongoing occupational exposure to NRL (healthcare workers, rubber industry workers, bakers, laboratory personnel, food handlers, hairdressers, janitors, policemen, and firefighters).
- Take a thorough history of the client at risk.
- Question the client about associated symptoms of itching, swelling, and redness after contact with rubber products such as rubber gloves, balloons, and barrier contraceptives.
- Consider a skin prick test with NRL extracts to identify IgE-mediated immunity.

Key Nursing Interventions
- Treat latex-sensitive clients as if they have NRL allergy.
- Supply materials and items that are latex free.
- Collaborate with pharmacy to have available a list of latex-containing drugs.
- Encourage wearing of Medic-Alert bracelet.
- Encourage importance of carrying an emergency kit.

AGE-RELATED CONSIDERATIONS

The Pediatric Client

The pediatric population is diverse, and the risk of infection varies with age, birthweight, underlying disease, host factors, medications, type of device, and nature of the infusate.

For low birth weight infants use hand hygiene with alcohol hand rub and gloves.

> EBNP *The introduction of the alcohol hand rub and glove protocol was associated with a 2.8-fold reduction in the incidence of late-onset systemic infection and a significant decrease in the incidence of methicillin-resistant Staphylococcus aureus septicemia and necrotizing enterocolitis in very low birth weight infants (Ng, Wong, Lyon, et al., 2004).*

Follow meticulous hand hygiene when working with premature infants.

> EBNP *In a study of neonatal intensive care units (NICUs), transmission of Serratia marcescens was likely to occur through the hands of staff. Cross-transmission through transient hand carriage of a healthcare worker appeared to be the probable route of transmission in NICU (Sarvikivi, Lyytikinen, Salmelinna, et al., 2004; Milisavljevic, Wu, Larson, et al., 2004).*

Avoid prophylactic use of topical cream in premature infants.

> EBNP *Prophylactic application of topical ointment increases the risk of co-agulase staphylococcal infection and any healthcare-associated infection. A trend toward increased risk of any bacterial infection was noted in infants prophylactically treated (Conner, Soll, & Edwards, 2004).*

Treat postoperative fever in pediatric oncology clients promptly.

> EBNP *A postoperative fever in immunocompromised pediatric clients indicates infection and may lead to complications if not treated promptly (Chang, Hendershot, & Colapinto, 2006).*

The Older Adult

Chronically ill older adult clients, particularly those with depression, have an increased susceptibility to infection; practice meticulous care of all invasive sites. Depression has been noted as a risk factor for lethal infectious disease in disabled older adults, with reduced reactivity in humoral and cellular immunity (Shinkawa, Nakayama, Hirari, et al., 2002).

Home Care Issues

It is generally believed that at-home risk factors for developing a catheter-related infection are lower than risk factors in a hospital setting. Although there is a need for further research, available studies show that the risk for IV related infections at home is low.

The Environmental Protection Agency (EPA) has developed many advisory committees regarding infectious waste disposal in the home care setting. The Medical Waste Tracking Act of 1988 mandated to the EPA the investigation and development of guidelines for handling home-generated medical waste. The home care provider should establish policies and procedures for handling waste.

- Sharps containers must be used for all contaminated sharps.
- Infusion pharmacies deliver sharps containers to the patient's home and pick them up when therapy is completed or the container is full.
- There are also "mail back" sharps container programs. The patient is provided with packaging and labeling to mail the container when full.
- Prepackaged kits are available from a number of manufacturers and include sharps disposal systems and the CHemBLOC spill kit.

Each home healthcare nurse or aide needs appropriate equipment and supplies related to infection control. The home health clinician carries needed supplies to the home in the "nursing bag" such as antiseptic hand gel and disinfectants such as alcohol to clean equipment after use (e.g., stethoscope diaphragm), a spill kit in the event of a large amount of blood or body fluid is spilled on the floor or a surface, and appropriate containers for disposal and transport of medical waste and contaminated sharps.

Rubbermaid® tubs with a sealing lid work well for transporting medical waste from homes to the home healthcare agency. Whether in an institutional setting or the home, healthcare workers should use an alcohol-based hand rinse or foam, rubbing vigorously to cover all parts of the hands until dry. If hands are visibly soiled, the nurse may have to go out of the way to find a source of running water because alcohol does not remove soil or organic matter.

 Patient Education

In all healthcare environments, patient education is an important component in preventing catheter-related complications. Education regarding vascular access management is crucial. Information regarding catheter management should be individualized to meet the patient's needs but remain consistent with established policies and procedures for infection control.

Patient Education—cont'd

Education should include:

- Instructions on hand hygiene; aseptic technique; and concept of dirty, clean, and sterile
- Proper methods for handling equipment
- Judicious use of antibiotics, which is a major nursing role to slow an epidemic of drug-resistant infections
- Importance of complying with directions for prescribed antibiotics
- Written information on steps for dressing changes
- Assessment of the site and the key signs and symptoms to report to the home care agency, hospital healthcare worker, or physician
- Information regarding emergency procedures if catheter should break or rupture; ECT to call either 911 or go to emergency room

Allergy
- Provide written information about NRL allergy and sensitivity.
- Instruct the client to carry an emergency kit with a supply of nonlatex gloves, antihistamines, and autoinjectable epinephrine syringe.

■ Nursing Process

The nursing process is a five- or six-step process for problem-solving to guide nursing action. Refer to Chapter 1 for details on the steps of the nursing process related to vascular access. The following table focuses on nursing diagnoses, nursing outcomes classification (NOC), and nursing intervention classification (NIC) for infection control and risk management. Nursing diagnoses should be patient specific and outcomes and interventions individualized. The NOC and NIC presented here are suggested direction for development of outcomes and interventions.

Nursing Diagnoses Related to Infection Control and Safety	NOC: Nursing Outcomes Classification	NIC: Nursing Intervention Classification
Allergic response: latex related to: Hypersensitivity to natural latex rubber protein	Allergic response: Localized or systemic; immune hypersensitivity response	Allergy management
Impaired skin integrity related to: VAD; irritation for IV solution; inflammation; infection	Tissue integrity: Primary intention healing of VAD insertion site	Incision site care, skin surveillance

Continued

Nursing Diagnoses Related to Infection Control and Safety	NOC: Nursing Outcomes Classification	NIC: Nursing Intervention Classification
Infection, risk for, related to: Inadequate acquired immunity; inadequate primary defenses; inadequate secondary defenses; increased environmental exposure to pathogens; immunosuppression; invasive procedures (placement of intravenous catheter)	Infection control, risk control, risk detection	Infection control practices and central line bundle implementation
Protection, ineffective, related to: Abnormal blood profile (leukopenia); drug therapy (antineoplastic); immune disorders; inadequate nutrition.	Health-promoting behavior	Injury protection

Sources: Ackley & Ladwig (2008); McCloskey, Dochterman, & Bulechek (2004); Moorhead, Johnson, & Maas (2004); NANDA-I (2007).

Chapter Highlights

- In the United States, the CDC, a division of the Department of Health and Human Services, is the agency that investigates, develops, recommends, and sets standards for infection control practices.
- The purpose of the immune system is to recognize and destroy invading antigens. Organs include primary (thymus and bone marrow) and secondary (lymph nodes, spleen, liver, Peyer's patches, appendix, tonsils and adenoids, and lungs).
- Impaired host resistance includes:
  - B-cell immunodeficiencies (50% of primary immunodeficiencies)
  - T-cell immunodeficiencies (40% of primary immunodeficiencies)
- The chain of infection includes six links:
  - Causative agent
  - Reservoir
  - Portal of exit
  - Method of transmission
  - Portal of entry
  - Host response
- A healthcare-associated infection (HAI) is an infection that a patient acquires during the course of receiving treatment for other conditions or that a healthcare worker (HCW) acquires while performing their duties within a healthcare setting.
- Infusion-related infections
  - Infusion phlebitis: Primarily a physiochemical phenomenon. Increases risk of infusion related infection
  - Catheter-related infection: CR-BSI related to 12% to 25% mortality rate

- Infusion-related infections: Intrinsic contamination (by manufacturer) and extrinsic contamination (during preparation and maintenance). Extrinsic is the most common contamination.
- Culturing techniques: Semiquantitative method
  Culture one or all of the following depending on symptoms and observation of catheter site.
- Catheter-skin junction: Do not use alcohol to cleanse before culturing
- Peripheral infusion catheter
- Infusate with administration set
- Patient's blood
- Strategies to prevent/treat infection include:
  - Following CDC Standard Precautions guidelines
  - Using the correct hand hygiene procedure
  - Using appropriate skin antisepsis
  - Using catheter site dressing regimens
  - Using catheter securement devices
  - Using antimicrobial/antiseptic-impregnated catheters and cuffs
  - Using anticoagulant flush where appropriate
  - Tissue–interface barrier
  - Implementation of central line bundles
- Occupational risks associated with infusion therapy include:
  - Biologic exposure to bloodborne pathogens
  - Needlestick injuries
  - Chemical exposure
  - Latex allergy

■■ Thinking Critically: Case Study

A patient is admitted with uncontrolled diabetes mellitus. She has a saline lock in place in her left wrist area. A symptomatic drop in blood sugar to 38 mg/dL requires she receive 50 mL of 50% dextrose infused at 3 mL/min via the peripheral infusion site. She responds well, but the next day needs another dose of dextrose via the same infusion site for a second drop in blood sugar. At discharge, she complains of burning and pain at the site. The nurse documents that the catheter is intact on discontinuation of the peripheral catheter, but no assessment data or subjective patient complaints are recorded. The patient is admitted 3 days later with purulent drainage from the left wrist infusion site, temperature of 101°F (38.4°C), and pulse rate of 100 beats per minute.

What is the probable cause of the second admission?

What are contributing factors?

What breach of standards of practice occurred?

What are the legal ramifications of this case?

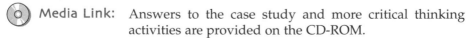 Media Link: Answers to the case study and more critical thinking activities are provided on the CD-ROM.

Post-Test

1. Which of the following constitute the first line of nonspecific defense mechanisms?

   a. Phagocytosis, complement cascade
   b. Leukocytes, proteins
   c. Physical and chemical barriers
   d. Immune system and phagocytes

2. The complement system consists of 17 different:

   a. Glucose molecules
   b. Proteins
   c. Fatty acids
   d. Immune responses

3. The most common immunodeficiency disorders are:

   a. B-cell immunodeficiencies
   b. T-cell immunodeficiencies
   c. Induced by drug therapy
   d. Caused by poor nutritional status

4. The nurse on assessment of a peripheral I.V. site notes the I.V. catheter site is red and swollen with purulent drainage under the TSM dressing. The correct nursing intervention is to:

   a. Culture the catheter and hold catheter restart
   b. Culture the site and reapply the dressing
   c. Culture the site and the catheter, then restart the infusion in a different location.
   d. Cleanse the insertion site with alcohol, remove the catheter, and culture the site.

5. Which of the following describes dissemination?

   a. Shedding of microorganisms into the environment from a person carrying them
   b. Infections that develop within a hospital or are produced by organisms during a patient's hospitalization
   c. Infections caused by a patient's own flora
   d. The first link in the chain of infections

6. Which of the following describe the transmission of organisms from source to host? (*Select all that apply.*)

   a. Contact
   b. Airborne
   c. Vector-borne
   d. Colonized person

7. The most important infection control measure for preventing bacteria transmission during infusion therapy is:

   a. Using non-latex gloves
   b. Using Teflon I.V. catheters
   c. Proper hand hygiene
   d. Use of chlorhexidine skin prep prior to venipuncture

8. Which of the following is included in the central line bundles? (*Select all that apply.*)

   a. Weekly culture of catheter/skin site
   b. Hand hygiene by catheter inserters
   c. Chlorhexidine (with alcohol) skin antisepsis of insertion site
   d. Trained catheter inserters
   e. Proper selection of type of catheter and insertion site.
   f. Time out called if proper procedures are not followed (then start again).

9. Which of the following is the *best* intervention to prevent a central venous catheter bloodstream infection?

   a. Change administration set every 24 hours.
   b. Avoid using the catheter for lab draws.
   c. Change transparent dressing every 72 hours.
   d. Follow standard precautions.

10. Which of the following is the recommended method of culture for purulent drainage?

    a. Agar
    b. Semiquantitative
    c. Semiqualitative
    d. Broth culture

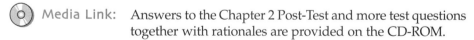 **Media Link:**   Answers to the Chapter 2 Post-Test and more test questions together with rationales are provided on the CD-ROM.

◼ **References**

Abdelkefi, A., Torjman, L., Ladeb, S., et al. (2005). Randomized trial of prevention of catheter-related bloodstream infection by continuous infusion of low-dose unfractionated heparin in patients with hematologic and oncologic disease. *Journal of Clinical Oncology, 23*, 7864–7870.

Ackley, B.J., & Ladwig, G.B. (2008). *Nursing diagnosis handbook: An evidence-based guide to planning care* (8th ed.). St. Louis, MO: Mosby Elsevier.

American Latex Allergy Association. (2008). FDA clears glove made from new type of latex. Retrieved from www.latexallergyresources.org (Accessed June 8, 2008).

Bleyer, A.J., Mason, L., Russel, G., et al. (2006). A randomized, controlled trial of a new vascular catheter flush solution (minocycline-EDTA) in temporary hemodialysis access. *Infection Control & Hospital Epidemiology, 26,* 520–524.

Burke, J.P. (2003). Infection control—a problem for patient safety. *New England Journal of Medicine, 348,* 651–656.

Centers for Disease Control and Prevention (CDC). (2002a). Guidelines for prevention of intravascular catheter related infections. Recommendations of the Hospital Infection Control Practices Advisory Committee (HICPAC), *MMWR Morbidity Mortality Weekly Report,* 51 (RR-10), 1–36.

Centers for Disease Control and Prevention (CDC). (2002b). Guideline for hand hygiene in health-care settings. *MMWR Morbidity Mortality Weekly Report, 51* (RR-16), 1–44.

Centers for Disease Control and Prevention (CDC). (2006). Healthcare-associated infections. Retrieved from www.cdc.gov/ncidod/dhqp/healthDis.html. (Accessed June 6, 2008).

Chaiyakunapruk, N., Veenstra, D.L., Lipsky, B.A., et al. (2002). Chlorhexidine compared with povidone-iodine solution for vascular catheter-site care: A meta analysis. *Annals of Internal Medicine, 136*(11), 792.

Chang, A., Hendershot, E., & Colapinto, K. (2006). Minimizing complications related to fever in the postoperative pediatric oncology patient. *Journal of Pediatric Oncology, 23*(2), 75–81.

Conner, J.M., Soll, R.F., & Edwards, W.H. (2004). Topical ointment for preventing infection in preterm infants. *Cochrane Database System Reviews* (1): CD001150.

Girou, E., & Oppein, F. (2001). Handwashing compliance in a French university hospital: New perspective with the introduction of hand-rubbing with a waterless alcohol-based solution. *Journal of Hospital Infections, 48*(Suppl A), S55.

Gritter, M. (1999). Latex allergy: Prevention is the key. *Journal of Intravenous Nursing, 22*(5), 281–285.

HealthCare Without Harm. (2008). Latex allergy in Health Care Fact Sheet. Washington, DC: HealthCare Without Harm.

Hibbard, J.S., Mulberry, G.K., & Brady, A.R. (2002). A clinical study comparing the skin antisepsis and safety of ChloraPrep, 70% isopropyl alcohol, and 2% aqueous chlorhexidine. *Journal of Infusion Therapy, 25*(4), 244–249.

Infusion Nurses Society (INS). (2006a). Infusion Nursing Standards of Practice. *Journal of Intravenous Nursing, 29*(1S), 1–81.

Infusion Nurses Society (INS). (2006b). *Policies and procedures for infusion nursing* (3rd ed.). Norwood, MA: Author.

Institute for Healthcare Improvement (IHI). (2006). Eliminating central-line related bloodstream infections with bundle compliance. Retrieved from www.ihi.org (Accessed June 8, 2008).

Kaler, W., & Chinn, R. (2007). Successful disinfection of needleless access ports: A matter of time and friction. *JAMA, 12*(3), 140–142.

Keyserling, H., Dykes, F., Newsome, P., et al. (1994). Pilot study of a chlorhexidine disc catheter dressing in a neonatal unit. *NAVAN, 1,* 12–13.

Krywda, E.A., & Andris, D.A. (2005). Twenty-five years of advances in vascular access: Bridging research to clinical practice. *Nutrition in Clinical Practice,* 20(6), 600–606.

Maki, D.G., Botticelli, J.T., LeRoy, M.L., et al. (1987). Prospective study of replacing administration sets for intravenous therapy at 48 vs 72–hour intervals. *JAMA, 258*, 1777–1781.

Maki, D.G., Kluger, D.M., & Crnich, D.J. (2006). The risk for bloodstream infection in adults with different intravascular devices: A systematic review of 200 published prospective studies. *Mayo Clinic Proceedings, 81*, 1159–1171.

Maki, D.G., & Mermel, L.A. (2007). Infection due to infusion therapy. In: W.R. Jarvis (Ed.), *Bennett & Brachman's hospital infections* (5th ed., pp. 611–660). Philadelphia: Lippincott, Williams & Wilkins.

Maki, D.G., Mermel, L.A., Klugar, D., et al. (2000). The efficacy of a chlorhexidine impregnated sponge (Biopatch) for the prevention of intravascular catheter-related infection—a prospective randomized controlled multicenter study (Abstract). Presented at the Interscience Conference on Antimicrobial Agents and Chemotherapy. Toronto, Ontario, Canada. American Society for Microbiology, May.

Maki, D.G., & Ringer, M. (1991). Risk factors for infusion-related phlebitis with small peripheral venous catheters. *Annals of Internal Medicine, 114*, 843–854.

McCloskey-Dochterman, J.C., & Bulechek, G.M. (2004). *Nursing interventions classification (NIC)* (4th ed.). St. Louis, MO: C.V. Mosby.

Menyhay, S.Z., & Maki, D.G. (2006). Disinfection of needleless catheter connectors and access ports with alcohol may not prevent microbial entry: The promise of a novel antiseptic-barrier cap. *Infection Control and Hospital Epidemiology, 27*, 23–27.

Mermel, L.A. (2000). Prevention of intravascular catheter-related infections. *Annals of Internal Medicine, 132*, 391–401.

Mermel, L.A., Farr, B.M., Sherertz, R.J., et al. (2001). Guidelines for the management of intravascular catheter-related infection. *Journal of Intravenous Nursing, 24*(3), 180–205.

Milisavljevic, V., Wu, F., Larson, E., et al. (2004). Molecular epidemiology of *Serratia marcescens* outbreaks in tow neonatal intensive care units. *Infection Control & Hospital Epidemiology, 25*(9), 719–721.

Moorhead, S., Johnson, M., & Maas, M. (2004). *Nursing outcomes classification (NOC)* (3rd ed.). St. Louis, MO: C.V. Mosby.

NANDA-I. (2007). *Nursing diagnoses: Definitions and classification, 2007–2008.* Philadelphia: Author.

National Institute for Occupational Safety and Health (NIOSH) (1999). *Latex allergy: A prevention guide.* Atlanta: CDC Publication 98–113–Latex.

National Institute for Occupational Safety and Health (NIOSH) (2000a). *ALERT: Preventing allergic reactions to natural rubber latex in the workplace.* Publication 97–135. Washington, DC: Author.

National Institute for Occupational Safety and Health (NIOSH) (2000b). *ALERT: Preventing needlestick injuries in health care settings.* U.S. Department of Health and Human Services. Publication No. 2000–108.

Ng, P.C., Wong, H.L., Lyon, D.J., et al. (2004). Combined use of alcohol hand rub and gloves reduces the incidence of late onset infection in very low birth weight infants. *Archives of Diseases in Childhood Fetal and Neonatal Edition, 89*(4), 335–340.

Occupational Safety and Health Administration (OSHA). (1999a). *OSHA technical manual controlling occupational exposure to hazardous drugs.* U.S. Department of Labor Occupational Safety & Health Administration. Section VI: Chapter 2.

Occupational Safety & Health Administration (OSHA). (1999b). Technical Information Bulletin: Potential for allergy to natural rubber latex gloves and other natural rubber products. Washington, DC: U.S. Department of Labor.

Occupational Safety and Health Administration (OSHA). (2001). Occupational exposure to blood borne pathogens; needlesticks and other sharps injuries; final rule. *Federal Register, 66,* 5317–5325.

Ostrowsky, B. (2007). Epidemiology of healthcare-associated infections. In: W. Jarvis (Ed.), *Bennett & Bachman's hospital infections* (5th ed.). Philadelphia: Lippincott Williams & Wilkins.

Panlilio, A.L., Cardo, D.M., Grohskopf, L.A., et al. (2005). Updated U.S. public health service guidelines for the management of occupational exposures to HIV and recommendations for postexposure prophylaxis. *MMWR Morbidity Mortality Weekly Report, 54* (RR09), 1–17.

Radd, I.I., & Sabbah, M.F. (1992). Optimal duration of therapy for catheter-related *Staphylococcus aureus* bacteremia: A study of 55 cases and review. *Clinical Infectious Diseases, 14,* 75–82.

Ray, C.E. (1999). Infection control principles and practices in the care and management of central venous access devices. *Journal of Intravenous Therapy, 22*(6S), S18–25.

Safdar, N., & Maki, D.G. (2006). Use of vancomycin-containing lock or flush solutions for prevention of bloodstream infection associated with central venous access devices: A meta-analysis of prospective randomized trials. *Clinical Infectious Diseases, 43,* 474–484.

Sarvikivi, E., Lyytikinen, O., Salmenlinna, S., et al. (2004). Clustering of *Serratia marcescens* infections in a neonatal intensive care unit. *Infection Control & Hospital Epidemiology, 25*(9), 723–729.

Schears, G.J. (2006). Summary of product trials for 10,164 patients comparing an intravenous stabilizing device to tape. *Journal of Infusion Nursing, 30*(4), 225–231.

Shinkawa, M., Nakayama, K., Hirai, H., et al. (2002). Depression and immunoreactivity in disabled older adults. *Journal of the American Geriatric Society, 50,* 198.

Siegel, J.D., Rhinehart, E., Jackson, M., Chiarello, L., & the Healthcare Infection Control Practices Advisory Committee. (2007). 2007 Guidelines for isolation precautions: Preventing transmission of infectious agents in healthcare settings. Retrieved from Centers for Disease Control and Prevention. www.cdc.gov/ncidod/dhq/pdf/isolation2007.pdf (Accessed August 6, 2008).

Smeltzer, S.C., Bare, B.G., Hinkle, J.L. & Cheever, K.H. (2008). *Brunner & Suddarth's textbook of medical–surgical nursing* (11th ed., pp. 1522–1535). Philadelphia: Lippincott Williams & Wilkins.

Sommer, C. (2004). Immunity and inflammation. In: C. Porth (Ed.), *Pathophysiology: Concepts of altered health states* (7th ed.). Philadelphia: Lippincott Williams & Wilkins.

Swenson, M.R. (2000). Autoimmunity and immunotherapy. *Journal of Intravenous Nursing, 23*(5S), S8–S13.

Van Leeuwen, A.M., Kranpitz, T.R., & Smith, L. (2006). *Davis's comprehensive handbook of laboratory and diagnostic tests with nursing implications* (2nd ed.). Philadelphia: F.A. Davis.

Warren, D., Cosgrove, S., Diekema, D., et al. (2006). A multicenter intervention to prevent catheter-associated bloodstream infections. *Infection Control & Hospital Epidemiology, 27*(7), 662–669.

Wilkinson, J.M., & Van Leuven, K. (2007). *Fundamentals of nursing: Theory, concepts and applications.* Philadelphia: F.A. Davis.

Williams, I.T., Perz, J.F., & Bell, B.P. (2004). Viral hepatitis transmission in ambulatory health care settings. *Clinical Infectious Diseases, 38*(11), 1592.

Yamamoto, A.J., Solomon, J.A., Soulen, M.C., et al. (2002). Sutureless securement device reduces complications of peripherally inserted central venous catheters. *Journal of Vascular Intervention Radiology, 29*(2), 10–14.

Young, E., Commiskey, M., & Wilson, S.J. (2006). Translating evidence into practice to prevent central venous catheter-associated bloodstream infections: A systems-based interventions. *American Journal of Infection Control, 34*(8), 503–506.

Yulex Corporation (2008). Yulex natural rubber. Retrieved from www.yulex.com/med/products (Accessed August 6, 2008).

PROCEDURES DISPLAY 2-1

Steps in Culturing Catheter–Skin Junction, Catheter, Infusate, and Blood

Equipment needed:
Sterile scissors
Sterile gloves
Barrier field:
70% Alcohol swab
Sterile specimen container
Label
Delegation:
This procedure should not be delegated. It is a registered nurse responsibility to assess and apply critical thinking skills to obtain the necessary cultures.

Procedure	Rationale
1. Check the authorized prescriber's order.	1. An authorized order is needed for laborabory analysis
2. Introduce yourself to the patient.	2. Establish nurse-patient relationship
3. Check patient ID using two forms (check ID bracelet and ask patient to state name).	3. The Joint Commission (2003) safety goal recommendation
4. Wash hands using friction for 15–20 seconds.	4. Good hand hygiene is the single most important means of preventing the spread of infection.

PROCEDURES DISPLAY 2-1

Steps in Culturing Catheter–Skin Junction, Catheter, Infusate, and Blood—cont'd

Procedure	Rationale
5. Inform patient of purpose of culture and that there is no discomfort or pain associated with this procedure.	5. Patient education begins prior to the procedure and patient cooperation implies consent for culture.
6. Place the patient in a comfortable position.	

Catheter-skin junction culture (a)

Procedure	Rationale
7a. Don clean gloves.	7. Follow Standard Precautions
8a. Remove dressing over I.V. site and place in biohazard bag.	8. Soiled dressings contain contaminants and should be treated as biohazardous waste.
9a. Don another pair of clean gloves.	9. Prevent contamination.
10a. If purulent drainage is present, culture of drainage should be taken first.	10. Removes purulent drainage from the catheter-skin junction.
11a. *Do not* cleanse area to be cultured	11. Removes bacteria needing to be cultured.
12a. Swab purulent drainage with a sterile swab.	12. To obtain bacteria present at catheter skin junction. Swab cultures collect surface bacteria.
13a. Uncap the culture tube.	
14a. Drop swab into culture tube using aseptic technqiue; crush the ampule of culture medium at the bottom of the tube.	13. Allow for transfer of swab into tube without contamination.
	14. The ampule contains medium for growth of the organism.
15a. Recap the culture tube and label the culturette tube with the patient's name, date and time, and source of culture.	15. Ensures obtaining the results from the correct patient.

Continued

PROCEDURES DISPLAY 2-1

Steps in Culturing Catheter–Skin Junction, Catheter, Infusate, and Blood—cont'd

Procedure	Rationale
Infusion Catheter (b)	
Follow steps 1–6, 7a–8a.	
9b. Disinfect venipuncture site with alcohol and allow to air dry.	**9.** Prevents transfer of skin pathogens onto catheter.
10b. Don sterile gloves and place sterile towel in close proximity to catheter-skin junction.	**10.** Provide a sterile barrier.
11b. Remove catheter avoiding contact with surrounding skin.	**11.** Prevent transfer of skin pathogens.
12b. Uncap the culture tube	**12.** Allow for transfer of catheter into culturette.
13b. For peripheral-short, cut entire length of catheter from catheter hub using sterile scissors.	**13.** Use sterile scissors to prevent contamination.
14b. For longer catheters, cut a 2-inch segment from the catheter tip with sterile scissors.	
15b. Drop the catheter into the culture tube; crush the ampule of culture medium at the bottom of the tube.	**15.** The ampule contains medium for growth of the organism.
16b. Recap the culture tube and label the culturette tube with patient's name, date and time, and specimen type.	**16.** Ensures obtaining the results from the correct patient.
17b. Apply pressure to the catheter exit site with sterile gauge and secure with tape.	**17.** Prevent hematoma formation.
Infusate (Infusion Solution) (c)	
Follow steps 1–6 and 7a.	
8c. Disinfect injection port of infusate container with alcohol for 15 seconds using a twisting motion.	**8.** Prevent cross-contamination from port site.

PROCEDURES DISPLAY 2-1

Steps in Culturing Catheter–Skin Junction, Catheter, Infusate, and Blood—cont'd

Procedure	Rationale
9c. Insert sterile needleless syringe into injection port of infusate bag.	**9.** To obtain sterile sample of infusate
10c. Withdraw approximately 5 mL of infusate into syringe.	**10.** Amount needed for culture
11c. Remove the syringe from the infusate container.	
12c. Uncap the culture tube.	
13c. Inject the syringe's contents into culture tube and crush the ampule of culture medium at the bottom of the tube.	**13.** The ampule contains medium for growth of the organism.
14c. Recap culture tube and label the culturette tube with patient's name, date and time and specimen type.	**14.** Ensures obtaining the results from the correct patient.
15c. Discard syringe in appropriate container.	**15.** Syringe is considered contaminated and should be treated as biohazardous waste.
16c. Send infusate with administration set intact to microbiology laboratory.	**16.** Cultures can be obtained from administration set, bag, and infusate.

Blood culture: Peripheral site (d)
Follow steps 1–6

7d. Blood cultures are collected in sets of two and use special tubes or bottles, one aerobic (with air) and one anaerobic (without air).

8d. Carefully disinfect the venipuncture site. Chlorhexidine gluconate is the recommended blood culture site disinfectant.

Continued

PROCEDURES DISPLAY 2-1

Steps in Culturing Catheter–Skin Junction, Catheter, Infusate, and Blood—cont'd

Procedure	Rationale
9d. Collect 10–20 mL for adult patients or 1–5 mL for pediatric of whole blood.	
10d. Follow laboratory guidelines for obtaining blood culture (Chapter 7).	

Blood culture: Central line
Follow steps 1–6
Do not discard first draw.
Follow steps in obtaining blood specimen from central line (Chapter 8).
Fill culture tubes with blood.

Post-Procedure All	**17, 18.** Follow Standard Precautions
17. Remove gloves	
18. Wash hands	**19.** To maintain proper docu- mentation and communicate that a culture has been obtained. To maintain legal record.
19. Document all relevant information:	
■ Record on the patient's chart the taking of the specimen and source.	
■ Include the date and time; the appearance of the exudate; the color, consistency, amount, and odor of any drainage; and any discomfort experienced by the patient.	

Sources: Infusion Nurses Society (2006). Policies and procedures for infusion nursing (3rd ed.). Norwood MA: Infusion Nurses Society; Van Leeuwen, A.M., Kranpitz, T.R., & Smith, L. (2006). Davis's comprehensive handbook of laboratory and diagnostic tests with nursing implications (2nd ed.). Philadelphia: F.A. Davis.

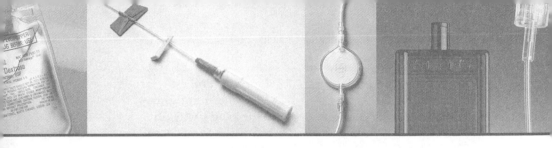

Chapter **3**

Fundamentals of Fluid and Electrolyte Balance

Chinese say that water is the most powerful element, because it is perfectly nonresistant. It can wear away rock and sweep all before it.
—*Florence Scovel Shinn*

■ **LEARNING**
OBJECTIVES

On completion of this chapter, the reader will be able to:

1. Define terminology related to fluids and electrolytes.
2. Identify the three fluid compartments within the body.
3. State the functions of body fluids.
4. Differentiate between active and passive transport.
5. Define the concept of osmosis and give examples of this concept.
6. Describe the homeostatic mechanisms.
7. Compare and contrast the movement of water in hypotonic, hypertonic, and isotonic solutions.
8. Compare and contrast fluid volume deficit and fluid volume excess.
9. List the six major body systems assessed for fluid balance disturbances.
10. State the seven major electrolytes within the body fluids.
11. Differentiate between cations and anions.
12. Contrast each of the seven electrolytes and their major roles in body fluids.
13. Identify signs and symptoms of deficits of sodium, potassium, calcium, magnesium, chloride, and phosphate.
14. Identify signs and symptoms of excesses of sodium, potassium, calcium, magnesium, chloride, and phosphate.
15. Discuss patients at risk for electrolyte imbalances.
16. State the normal pH range of body fluids.
17. Identify regulatory organs of acid–base balance.
18. Compare clinical manifestations of metabolic acidosis and alkalosis.
19. Compare clinical manifestations of respiratory acidosis and alkalosis.
20. Identify nursing diagnoses and interventions related to fluid and electrolyte balance.

GLOSSARY OF TERMS

Acidosis   An actual or relative increase in the acidity of blood due to an accumulation of acids or an excessive loss of bicarbonate. Blood pH below normal (less than 7.35)

Active transport   The process by which a cell membrane moves molecules against a concentration or electrochemical gradient. Metabolic work is required.

Alkalosis   An actual or relative increase in blood alkalinity due to an accumulation of alkalies or reduction of acids in the blood. Blood pH above normal (greater than 7.45)

Anion   Negatively charged electrolyte

Antidiuretic hormone (ADH)   A hormone secreted from the pituitary mechanism that causes the kidney to conserve water; sometimes referred to as the "water-conserving hormone"

Atrial natriuretic peptide (ANP)   ANP is a cardiac hormone found in the atria of the heart that is released when atria are stretched by high blood volume.

Body fluid   Body water in which electrolytes are dissolved

Cation   Positively charged electrolyte

Chvostek's sign   A sign elicited by tapping the facial nerve about 2 cm anterior to the earlobe, just below the zygomatic process; the response is a spasm of the muscles supplied by the facial nerve

Diffusion   The movement of a substance from a region of high concentration to one of lower concentration

Extracellular fluid (ECF)   Body fluid located outside the cells.

Filtration   The process of passing fluid through a filter using pressure

Fingerprinting edema   A condition in which imprints are made on the hands, sternum, or forehead when pressed firmly by the fingers

Fluid volume deficit (FVD)   A fluid deficiency. Hypovolemia. An equal proportion of loss of water and electrolytes from the body.

Fluid volume excess (FVE)   The state of exceeding normal fluid levels. Hypervolemia. Retention of both water and sodium in similar proportions to normal ECF

Homeostasis   The state of dynamic equilibrium of the internal environment of the body that is maintained by the ever-changing processes of feedback and regulation in response to external or internal changes.

Hypertonic   Solutions that have a higher osmolality than body fluids—above 375 mOsm

Hypotonic   Solutions that have a lower osmolality than body fluids—below 250 mOsm

Insensible loss   Fluid loss that is not perceptible to the individual; nonvisible form of water loss that is difficult to measure, for example, perspiration

Interstitial fluid   Body fluid between the cells

Intracellular fluid (ICF)   Body fluid inside the cells

Intravascular fluid   The fluid portion of blood plasma

Isotonic   Having an osmotic pressure equal to that of blood; equivalent osmotic pressure; between 250 and 375 mOsm

Oncotic pressure   The osmotic pressure exerted by colloids (proteins), as when albumin exerts oncotic pressure within the blood vessels and helps to hold the water content of the blood in the intravascular compartment

Osmolarity   A measure of solute concentration; the concentration of a solution in terms of osmoles of solutes per liter of solution

Osmosis   The movement of water from a lower concentration to a higher concentration across a semipermeable membrane

pH   A measure of hydrogen ion (H^+) concentration.

Sensible loss   Output that is measurable, for example, urine

Solute   The substance that is dissolved in a liquid to form a solution

Syndrome of inappropriate antidiuretic hormone (SIADH) secretion   A condition in which excessive ADH is secreted, resulting in hyponatremia

Tetany   Continuous tonic spasm of a muscle

Trousseau's sign   A spasm of the hand elicited when the blood supply to the hand is decreased or the nerves of the hand are stimulated by pressure; elicited within several minutes by applying a blood pressure cuff inflated above systolic pressure

Body Fluid Composition

Body fluid is body water in which electrolytes are dissolved. Water is the largest single constituent of the body. Body water, the medium in which cellular reactions take place, constitutes approximately 60% of total body weight (TBW) in young men and 50% to 55% in women. Table 3-1 provides percentages of total body fluids in relation to age and gender. Fat tissue contains little water, and the percentage of total body water varies considerably based on the amount of body fat present. In addition, total body water progressively decreases with age, making up about 50% of body weight in elderly people (Metheny, 2000).

CULTURAL AND ETHNIC CONSIDERATIONS

A person's age, gender, ethnic origin, and weight can influence the amount and distribution of body fluid. For example, African Americans often have larger numbers of fat cells compared with other groups and therefore have less body water (Giger & Davidhizar, 2004).

> Table 3-1	PERCENTAGES OF TOTAL BODY FLUID IN RELATION TO AGE AND GENDER
Age	**Total Body Fluid (% of Body Weight)**
Full-term newborn	70–80
1-year-old	64
Puberty to 39 years	Men: 60 Women: 55
40–60 years	Men: 55 Women: 47
Older than 60 years	Men: 52 Women: 46

Source: Metheny, N.M. (2000). Fluid and electrolyte balance. In: N.M. Metheny (Ed.). Nursing considerations (4th ed). Philadelphia: Lippincott Williams & Wilkins. Copyright 2000 by Lippincott Williams & Wilkins. Reprinted with permission.

■ Fluid Distribution

Homeostasis is dependent on fluid and electrolyte intake, physiologic factors (e.g., organ function, hormones, age, gender), disease state factors (e.g., respiratory, renal, or metabolic disorders), external environmental factors (e.g., temperature, humidity), and pharmacologic interventions.

Water is a neutral polar molecule in which one part is negative and one part is positive. Body water is distributed within cells and outside cells. The body water within the cells is referred to as **intracellular fluid** (ICF); fluid outside the cells is referred to as **extracellular fluid** (ECF) and consists of two compartments, interstitial and intravascular. Approximately 40% of the TBW is composed of the fluid inside the cell (ICF). Another 20% is fluid outside the cell (ECF) and is divided between interstitial and intravascular spaces, with 15% in the tissue (interstitial) space and only 5% represented in the plasma (intravascular) space. The interstitial fluid lies outside of the blood vessels in the interstitial spaces between the body cells. Lymph and cerebrospinal fluids, although highly specialized, are usually regarded as interstitial fluid. Figure 3-1 gives a representation of body water distribution.

An exchange of fluid occurs continuously among the intracellular, plasma, and interstitial compartments. Of these three spaces, the intake or elimination of fluid from the body directly influences only the plasma. Changes in the intracellular and interstitial fluid compartments occur in response to changes in the volume or concentration of the plasma.

The internal environment needs to remain in homeostasis; therefore, the intake and output of fluid must be relatively equal, as in healthy individuals. In those who are ill, this balance is frequently upset, and intake of fluid may become diminished or even cease. Output may vary with the influences of increased temperature, increased respiration, draining wounds, or gastric suction.

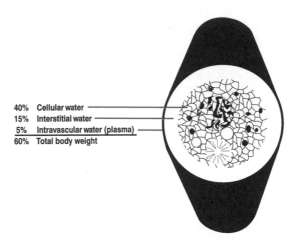

40% Cellular water
15% Interstitial water
5% Intravascular water (plasma)
60% Total body weight

Figure 3-1 ■ Percentages of body fluid.

Normal sources of water per day include liquids, water-containing foods, and metabolic activity. In healthy adults, the intake of fluids varies from 1000 to 3000 mL/day, and 200 to 300 mL is produced from oxidation.

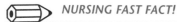 NURSING FAST FACT!

Normally intake and output will approximately balance only every 72 hours; thus, an appropriate target date for fluid rehydration would be 3 days (Newfield, Hinz, Tilley, et al., 2007).

The elimination of fluid is considered either **sensible** (measurable) loss or **insensible** (not measurable) loss. Water is eliminated from the body by the skin, kidneys, bowels, and lungs. Approximately 300 to 500 mL of water are eliminated through the lungs every 24 hours, and the skin eliminates about 500 mL/day of water in the form of perspiration. The amount of insensible loss in an adult is considered to be approximately 500 to 1000 mL/day. Losses through the gastrointestinal (GI) tract are only about 100 to 200 mL per day because of the reabsorption of most of the fluid in the small intestines. Increased losses of GI fluids can occur from diarrhea or intestinal fistulas (Metheny, 2000).

The metabolic rate increases with fever; it rises approximately 12% for every 1°C (7% for every 1°F increase in body temperature). Significant sweat losses occur if a patient's body temperature exceeds 101°F (38.3°C) or if the room temperature exceeds 90°F. Fever also increases the respiratory rate, resulting in additional loss of water vapor through the lungs (Porth & Martin, 2008). Insensible loss is also increased if respirations are increased to more than 20 per minute.

■ Fluid Function

Fluids within the body have several important functions. The ECF transports nutrients to the cells and carries waste products away from the cells by means of the capillary bed. Body fluids are in constant motion, maintaining living conditions for body cells (Metheny, 2000). The fluid within the body also has the following functions:

1. Maintains blood volume.
2. Regulates body temperature.
3. Transports material to and from cells.
4. Serves as an aqueous medium for cellular metabolism.
5. Assists digestion of food through hydrolysis.
6. Acts as a solvent in which solutes are available for cell function.
7. Serves as a medium for the excretion of waste.

Fluid Transport

Body fluids are in constant motion, maintaining healthy living conditions for body cells. The ECF interfaces with the outside world and is modified by it, but the ICF remains stable. Nutrients are transported by the ECF to the cells and wastes are carried away from the cells by means of the capillary bed (Metheny, 2000).

Movement of particles through the cell membrane occurs through four transport mechanisms: passive transport consisting of diffusion, osmosis, and filtration; and active transport. Materials are transported between the ICF and the extracellular compartment by these four mechanisms.

Passive Transport

Passive transport is also referred to as non–carrier-mediated transport. It is the movement of solutes through membranes without the expenditure of energy. It includes passive diffusion, osmosis, and filtration.

Passive Diffusion

Passive diffusion is the passive movement of water, ions, and lipid-soluble molecules randomly in all directions from a region of high concentration to an area of low concentration. Diffusion occurs through semipermeable membranes by the substance either passing through pores, if small enough, or dissolving in the lipid matrix of the membrane wall. If there is no force opposing diffusion, particles distribute themselves evenly. Many substances can diffuse through the cell membrane, and these substances diffuse in both directions. Influencing factors in the diffusion process are concentration differences, electrical potential, and pressure differences across the pores. The greater the concentration, the greater the rate of diffusion. An increase in the pressure on one side of the membrane increases the molecular forces striking the pores, thus creating a pressure gradient. Other factors that increase diffusion include:

- Increased temperature
- Increased concentration of particles
- Decreased size or molecular weight of particles
- Increased surface area available for diffusion
- Decreased distance across which the particle mass must diffuse

Filtration

Filtration is the transfer of water and a dissolved substance from a region of high pressure to a region of low pressure; the force behind it is hydrostatic pressure (i.e., the pressure of water at rest). The pumping heart provides hydrostatic pressure in the movement of water and electrolytes from the arterial capillary bed to the interstitial fluid. Diffusion moves in either direction across a membrane; filtration moves in one direction only because of the hydrostatic, osmotic, and interstitial fluid pressure. Filtration is likened to pouring a solution through a sieve: the size of the opening in the sieve determines the size of the particle to be filtered.

The plasma compartment contains more protein than the other compartments. Plasma protein, composed of albumin, globulin, and fibrinogen, creates an osmotic pressure at the capillary membrane, preventing fluid from the plasma from leaking into the interstitial spaces. Osmotic pressure created within the plasma by the presence of protein (mainly albumin) keeps the water in the vascular system.

Starling's Law of the Capillaries (1896) maintains that under normal circumstances, fluid filtered out of the arterial end of a capillary bed and reabsorbed at the venous end is exactly the same, creating a state of near-equilibrium. However, it is not exactly the same because of the difference in hydrostatic pressure between the arterial and venous capillary beds. The pressure that moves fluid out of the arterial end of the network amounts to a total of 28.3 mm Hg. The pressure that moves fluid back into circulation at the venous capillary bed is 28 mm Hg. The small amount of excess remaining in the interstitial compartment is returned to the circulation by way of the lymphatic system (Craven & Hirnlel, 2003).

Active Transport

Active transport is similar to diffusion except that it acts against a concentration gradient. Active transport occurs when it is necessary for ions (electrolytes) to move from an area of low concentration to an area of high concentration. By definition, active transport implies that energy expenditure must take place for the movement to occur against a concentration gradient. Adenosine triphosphate (ATP) is released from the cell to enable certain substances to acquire the energy needed to pass through the cell membrane. For example, sodium concentration is greater in ECF; therefore, sodium tends to enter by diffusion into the intracellular compartment. This tendency is offset by the sodium–potassium pump, which is located on the cell membrane. In the presence of ATP, the sodium–potassium pump actively moves sodium from the cell into the ECF. Active transport is vital for maintaining the unique composition of both the extracellular and intracellular compartments (Metheny, 2000).

Osmosis

Osmosis is the passage of water from an area of lower particle concentration toward one with a higher particle concentration across a semipermeable membrane. For a membrane to be semipermeable, it has to be more permeable to water than to solutes. This process tends to equalize the concentration of two solutions.

Osmosis governs the movement of body fluids between the intracellular and ECF compartments, therefore influencing the volumes of fluid within each. Through the process of osmosis, water flows through semipermeable membranes toward the side with the higher concentration of particles (thus from lower to higher).

OSMOTIC PRESSURE GRADIENTS

Osmotic pressure develops as solute particles collide against each other. Osmotic pressure is the amount of hydrostatic pressure needed to draw a solvent (water) across a membrane and develops as a result of a high concentration of particles colliding with one another. As the number of solutes increases, there is less space for them to move; therefore, they come in contact with one another more frequently. This results in increased osmotic pressure, which causes the movement of fluid. The osmotic pressure differs at the cell membrane and capillary membrane. At the capillary membrane, the terminology is referred to as osmotic pressure (Hankins, 2006). The colloid osmotic pressure is influenced by proteins, due to the proteins being the only dissolved substances in the plasma and interstitial fluid that do not diffuse readily through capillary membranes. The concentration of protein in plasma is two to three times greater than that of the proteins found in the interstitial fluid. Only the substances that do not pass through the semipermeable membrane exert osmotic pressure. Therefore, proteins in the extracellular fluid (ECF) spaces are responsible for the osmotic pressure at the capillary membrane. Osmotic pressure is measured in milliosmoles (mOsm).

OSMOLARITY VERSUS OSMOLALITY

The osmotic activity of a solution may be expressed in terms of either its osmolarity or osmolality. Osmolarity refers to the osmolar concentration in 1 liter (L) of solution and osmolality is the osmolar concentration of 1 kilogram (kg) of water. Osmolarity is usually used when referring to fluids outside the body and osmolality for describing fluids inside the body. Because 1 L of water weighs 1 kg, the terms osmolarity and osmolality are often used interchangeably (Porth & Martin, 2008).

Tonicity of Solutions

A change in water content causes cells to either swell or shrink. The term tonicity refers to the tension or effect that the effective osmotic pressure of a solution with impermeable solutes exerts on the cell size because of water movement across a cell membrane. Tonicity is determined solely by effective solutes such as glucose that cannot penetrate the cell membrane, thereby producing an osmotic force that pulls water into or out of the cell and causing it to change size. Solutions to which body cells are exposed can be classified as isotonic, hypotonic, or hypertonic depending on whether they cause cells to swell or shrink. Cells placed in an isotonic solution, which has the same effective osmolality as intracellular fluids, neither shrink or swell (Porth & Martin, 2008).

When cells are placed in a hypotonic solution, which has a lower effective osmolality than intracellular fluids, they swell as water moves into the cell. When they are placed in a hypertonic solution, which has a greater effective osmolality than intracellular fluids, they shrink as water is pushed out of the cell.

Figure 3-2 shows the movement of water by osmosis in hypotonic, isotonic, and hypertonic solutions.

Isotonic solutions, such as 0.9% sodium chloride (NaCl) and 5% dextrose in water, have the same osmolarity as that of normal body fluids. Solutions that have an osmolarity of 250 to 375 mOsm/L are considered isotonic solutions and have no effect on the volume of fluid within the cell; the solution remains within the ECF space. Isotonic solutions are used to expand the ECF compartment.

Hypotonic solutions contain less salt than the intracellular space, and when infused, have an osmolarity below 250 mOsm/L, and move water into the cell, causing the cell to swell and possibly burst. By lowering the serum osmolarity, the body fluids shift out of the blood vessels into the interstitial tissue and cells. Hypotonic solutions hydrate cells and can deplete the circulatory system. An example of a hypotonic solution is 2.5% dextrose in water.

Hypertonic solutions, conversely, cause the water from within a cell to move to the ECF compartment, where the concentration of salt is greater, causing the cell to shrink. Hypertonic solutions have an osmolarity of 375 mOsm/L and above. These solutions are used to replace electrolytes. When hypertonic dextrose solutions are used alone, they also are used to shift ECF from interstitial tissue to plasma. Examples of hypertonic solutions are 5% dextrose and 0.9% NaCl, or 5% dextrose and lactated Ringer's solution. Figure 3-3 illustrates tonicity (osmolarity) ranges.

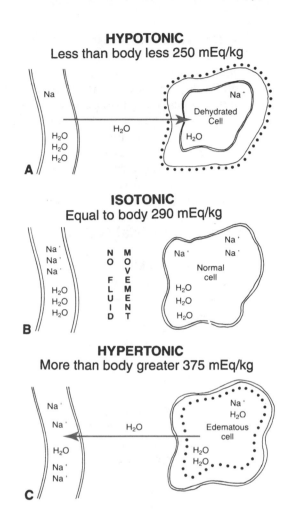

HYPOTONIC
Less than body less 250 mEq/kg

ISOTONIC
Equal to body 290 mEq/kg

HYPERTONIC
More than body greater 375 mEq/kg

Figure 3-2 ■ Effects of fluid shifts in (*A*), hypotonic, (*B*), isotonic, and (*C*), hypertonic states. (From Kuhn, M. [1998]. *Pharmacotherapeutics: A nursing process approach* [4th ed., p. 128]. Philadelphia: F.A. Davis, with permission.)

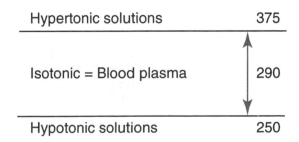

Hypertonic solutions	375
Isotonic = Blood plasma	290
Hypotonic solutions	250

Figure 3–3 ■ Tonicity osmolarity ranges of solutions.

Fluid and Electrolyte Homeostatic Mechanisms

Regulation of body water is maintained through exogenous sources, such as the intake of food and fluids, and endogenous sources that are produced within the body through chemical oxidation process. Several homeostatic mechanisms are responsible for the balance of fluid and electrolytes within the body. When homeostasis is compromised and imbalance occurs, the nurse is responsible for managing the exogenous source of fluid replacement via the intravenous route. The endogenous sources of balancing fluid and electrolytes are through various body systems such as the cardiovascular, lymphatic, renal, respiratory, nervous, and endocrine systems.

Cardiovascular System and Atrial Natriuretic Factor

The pumping action of the heart provides circulation of blood through the kidneys under pressure, which allows urine to form. Renal perfusion makes renal function possible. Blood vessels provide plasma to reach the kidneys in sufficient volume (20% of circulating blood volume) to permit regulation of water and electrolytes. Baroreceptors located in the carotid sinus and aortic arch respond to the degree of stretch of the vessel wall, which has been generated by the body's reaction to hypovolemia. The response is to stimulate fluid retention.

Atrial natriuretic factor (ANFs) are produced by the cardiac atria, ventricles, and other vessels in response to changes in ECF volume. When atrial pressure is increased, ANF released by the atrial and ventricular myocytes acts on the nephron to increase sodium excretion. Additionally, ANF is a direct vasodilator, lowering systemic blood pressure (Metheny, 2000).

Lymphatic System

The lymphatic system serves as an adjunct to the cardiovascular system by removing excess interstitial fluid (in the form of lymph) and returning it to the circulatory system. Fluid overload in the interstitial compartment would result if it were not for the lymphatic system. The lymphatic system carries the excess fluid, proteins, and large particulate matter that cannot be reabsorbed by the venous capillary bed out of interstitial compartment. This minute excess (0.3 mm Hg) accounts for 1.7 mm/min of fluid. If the lymphatic system were not continually removing this small amount of fluid, there would be a buildup of 2448 mL in the interstitial compartment over a 24-hour period of time (Porth & Martin, 2008).

Kidneys

The kidneys are vital to the regulation of fluid and electrolyte balance. The kidney is the main regulator of sodium. The kidney monitors arterial pressure and retains sodium when arterial pressure is decreased and eliminates it when arterial pressure is increased (Porth & Martin, 2008). The kidneys normally filter 170 L of plasma per day in the adult, and excrete only 1.5 L of urine (Metheny, 2000). They act in response to bloodborne messengers such as aldosterone and antidiuretic hormone (ADH). Renal failure can result in multiple fluid and electrolyte imbalances.

Functions of the kidneys in fluid balance are:

- Regulation of fluid volume and osmolarity by selective retention and excretion of body fluids
- Regulation of electrolyte levels by selective retention of needed substances and excretion of unneeded substances
- Regulation of pH of ECF by excretion or retention of hydrogen ions (H^+)
- Excretion of metabolic wastes (primarily acids) and toxic substances (Metheny, 2000).

Renin–Angiotensin–Aldosterone Mechanism

The renin–angiotensin–aldosterone system exerts its action through angiotensin II and aldosterone. Renin is a small enzyme protein that is released by the kidney in response to changes in arterial pressure, the glomerular filtration rate, and the amount of sodium in the tubular fluid. Aldosterone acts at the level of the cortical collecting tubules of the kidneys to increase sodium reabsorption while increasing potassium elimination (Porth & Martin, 2008).

Respiratory System

The lungs are vital for maintaining homeostasis and constitute one of the main regulatory organs of fluid and acid–base balance. The lungs regulate acid–base balance by regulation of the hydrogen ion (H^+) concentration. Alveolar ventilation is responsible for the daily elimination of approximately 13,000 mEq of H^+ ions. The kidneys excrete only 40 to 80 mEq of hydrogen daily. Under influence from the medulla, the lungs act promptly to correct metabolic acid–base disturbances by regulating the level of carbon dioxide (a potential acid) in the ECF. Functions of the lungs in body fluid balance are:

- Regulation of metabolic alkalosis by compensatory hypoventilation, resulting in carbon dioxide (CO_2) retention and increased acidity of the ECF
- Regulation of metabolic acidosis by causing compensatory hyperventilation, resulting in CO_2 excretion and thus decreased acidity of the ECF
- Removal of 300 to 500 mL of water daily through exhalation (i.e., insensible water loss)

Endocrine System

The glands responsible for aiding in homeostasis are the adrenal, pituitary, and parathyroid glands. The endocrine system responds selectively to the regulation and maintenance of fluid and electrolyte balance through hormonal production.

Water

Holliday and Segar (1957) established that regardless of age, all healthy persons require approximately 100 milliliters (mL) of water per 100 calories metabolized, for dissolving and eliminating metabolic wastes. That means a person who expends 1800 calories of energy requires approximately 1800 mL of water for metabolic purposes. Two main physiologic mechanisms assist in regulating body water: thirst and antidiuretic hormone (ADH). Both mechanisms respond to changes in extracellular osmolality and volume.

Thirst

Thirst is controlled by the thirst center in the hypothalamus. There are two stimuli for true thirst based on water need: cellular dehydration caused by an increase in extracellular osmolality and a decrease in blood volume, which may or may not be associated with a decrease in serum osmolality. Thirst develops when there is as little as 1% to 2% change in serum osmolality (Ayus & Arieff, 1996).

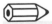 *NURSING FAST FACT!*

Thirst is one of the earliest symptoms of hemorrhage and is often present before other signs of blood loss appear.

Antidiuretic Hormone

The pituitary hormone influencing water balance is antidiuretic hormone (ADH) also called vasopressin. This hormone, which affects renal reabsorption of water, is also referred to as the "water-conserving" hormone. Functions of ADH are to maintain osmotic pressure of the cells by controlling renal water retention or excretion and control of blood volume. Excessive secretion of ADH results in the syndrome of inappropriate antidiuretic hormone secretion (SIADH).

As with thirst, ADH levels are controlled by extracellular volume and osmolality. A small increase in serum osmolality is sufficient to cause ADH release. A blood volume decrease of 5% to 10% produces a maximal increase in ADH levels. As with many other homeostatic mechanisms, acute conditions produce changes in ADH levels (Berne & Levy, 2000).

Numerous drugs (e.g., alcohol, narcotic antagonists) can block ADH activity or reduce tubular responsiveness to ADH (e.g., lithium, demeclocycline), which results in increased water loss, causing dehydration and hypernatremia. Increased ADH secretion may be the result of disease (hormone-secreting tumor, head injury) or may be related to administration of drugs such as chlorpropamide, Vinca alkaloids, carbamazepine, cyclophosphamide, tricyclic antidepressants, and narcotics (Metheny, 2000; Porth & Martin, 2008).

Factors that affect ADH production include pathologic changes such as head trauma and tumors of the brain or lung, anesthesia and surgery in general, and certain drugs (e.g., barbiturates, antineoplastics, and nonsteroidal anti-inflammatory agents).

Parathyroid Hormone

The parathyroid gland is embedded in the corners of the thyroid gland and regulates calcium and phosphate balance. The parathyroid gland influences fluid and electrolytes, increases serum calcium levels, and lowers serum phosphate levels. A reciprocal relationship exists between extracellular calcium and phosphate levels. When the serum calcium level is low, the parathyroid gland secretes more parathyroid hormone. The parathyroid hormone can increase the serum calcium level by promoting calcium release from the bone as needed. Calcitonin from the thyroid gland increases calcium return to the bone, thus decreasing the serum calcium level.

Aldosterone

The adrenal cortex is important in fluid and electrolyte homeostasis. The primary adrenocortical hormone influencing the balance of fluid is aldosterone. Aldosterone is responsible for the renal reabsorption of sodium, which results in the retention of chloride and water and the excretion of potassium. Aldosterone also regulates blood volume by regulating sodium retention.

Epinephrine

Epinephrine, another adrenal hormone, increases blood pressure, enhances pulmonary ventilation, dilates blood vessels needed for emergencies, and constricts unnecessary vessels.

Cortisol

When produced in large quantities, the adrenocortical hormone cortisol can produce sodium and fluid retention and potassium deficit. Table 3-2 summarizes the regulators of fluid and electrolyte balance.

> Table 3-2   **REGULATORS OF FLUID BALANCE**

Homeostatic Mechanism	Action
Cardiovascular	Baroreceptor in carotid sinus and aortic arch responds to hypovolemia. ANF is a direct vasodilator-lowering BP.
Lungs	Lungs excrete 400–500 mL of water daily through normal breathing
Kidneys	Kidneys excrete 1000–1500 mL of body water daily. Water excretion may vary according to the balance between fluid intake and fluid loss.
Lymphatics	Plasma protein that shifts to the tissue spaces cannot be reabsorbed into the blood vessels. Lymphatic system promotes the return of water and protein from the interstitial spaces to the vascular spaces.
Skin	Skin excretes 300–500 mL of water daily through normal perspiration
Electrolyte	Sodium promotes water retention. With a water deficit, less sodium is excreted via kidneys; thus more water is retained
Nonelectrolytes	Protein and albumin promote body fluid retention. These nondiffusible substances increase the colloid osmotic (oncotic) pressure in favor of fluid retention.
Hormones	
Antidiuretic hormone (ADH)	ADH is produced by the hypothalamus and stored in the posterior pituitary gland. ADH is secreted when there is an ECF volume deficit or an increased osmolality. ADH promotes water reabsorption from the distal tubules of the kidneys.
Aldosterone	Aldosterone is secreted from the adrenal cortex. It promotes sodium, chloride, and water reabsorption from the renal tubules.
Renin	Decreased renal blood flow increases the release of renin, an enzyme, from the juxtaglomerular cells of the kidneys. Renin promotes peripheral vasoconstriction and the release of aldosterone (sodium and water retention).

■ Physical Assessment of Fluid and Electrolyte Needs

A body systems approach is the best method for assessing fluid and electrolyte imbalances related to infusion therapy. The nurse should begin by obtaining a history, assessing vital signs, performing a focused physical assessment, monitoring pertinent laboratory tests, and evaluating intake and output. The purpose of this data gathering is to identify clients at risk for or already experiencing alterations in fluid and electrolyte balance.

Nursing history related to fluid and electrolyte balance includes questions about past medical history, current health concerns, food and fluid intake, fluid elimination, medications, and lifestyle. The physical assessment correlates data with the nursing history validating subjective information. Focused assessment includes, but is not limited to, neurological evaluation of level of consciousness (LOC), cardiovascular system, respiratory system, skin, special senses, and weight. Laboratory data should be reviewed in a comprehensive review of patient fluid and electrolyte needs.

Neurologic System/Focus on LOC

Changes in level of consciousness occur with changes in serum osmolality or changes in serum sodium, and can also occur with acute acid–base imbalances. Fluid volume changes, along with serum sodium levels, affect the central nervous system (CNS) cells, resulting in irritability, lethargy, confusion, seizures, or coma. CNS cells shrink in sodium excess and expand when serum sodium levels decrease (Metheny, 2000). Sensation of thirst depends on excitation of the cortical centers of consciousness (Heitz & Horne, 2005). The use of antianxiety agents, sedatives, or hypnotic agents can lead to confusion and disorientation, causing the patient to forget to drink fluid.

Assessment of neuromuscular irritability is particularly important when imbalances in calcium, magnesium, sodium, and potassium are suspected. Electrolyte imbalances can cause neurologic system signs and symptoms. Abnormal reflexes occur with calcium and magnesium imbalances including Trousseau's and Chvostek's signs. Hyperkalemia (increase in potassium level) can cause flaccid paralysis. Paraesthesia may occur in acid–base imbalances (Heitz & Horne, 2005).

There is a progressive loss of CNS cells with advancing age, along with decreases in the sense of smell and tactile sense. The thirst mechanism in elderly people may be diminished and is a poor guide for fluid needs in older patients. An ill patient may not be able to verbalize thirst or to reach for a glass of water.

Cardiovascular System

The quality and rate of the pulse are indicators of how the patient is tolerating the ECF volume. The peripheral veins in the extremities provide a way of evaluating plasma volume. Examination of hand veins can evaluate the plasma volume. Peripheral veins empty in 3 to 5 seconds when the hand is elevated and fill in the same amount of time when the hand is lowered to a dependent position. Peripheral vein filling takes longer than 3 to 5 seconds in patients with sodium depletion and extracellular dehydration (Metheny, 2000). Slow emptying of the peripheral veins indicates overhydration and excessive blood volume (Fig. 3-4).

A 20-mm Hg fall in systolic blood pressure when shifting from the lying to the standing position (postural hypotension) usually indicates fluid volume deficit. The jugular vein provides a built-in manometer for evaluation

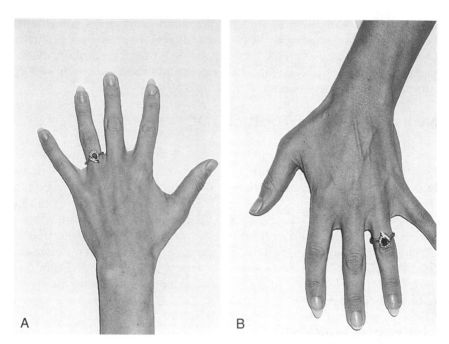

A　　　　　　　　　　　B

Figure 3-4 ■ Hand vein assessment. Peripheral vein takes longer than 3 to 5 seconds in patients with sodium depletion and dehydration. Slow emptying of hand veins indicates overhydration and excessive blood volume.

of central venous pressure (CVP). Changes in fluid volume are reflected by changes in neck vein filling.

The external jugular veins, with the patient supine, fill to the anterior border of the sternocleidomastoid muscle. Flat neck veins in the supine position indicate a decreased plasma volume. When the patient is in a 45-degree position, the external jugular vein distends no higher than 2 cm above the sternal angle. Neck veins distending from the top portion of the sternum to the angle of the jaw indicate elevated venous pressure (Fig. 3-5).

Edema indicates expansion of interstitial volume. Edema can be localized (usually caused by inflammation) or generalized (usually related to capillary hemodynamics). Edema should be assessed over bony surfaces of the tibia or sacrum and rated according to severity from 1+ to 4+ (Fig. 3-6). The presence of periorbital edema suggests significant fluid retention.

EBNP Dependent edema was found to demonstrate the greatest sensitivity as a defining characteristic for excess fluid volume (Rios, Delaney, & Kruckeberg, 1991).

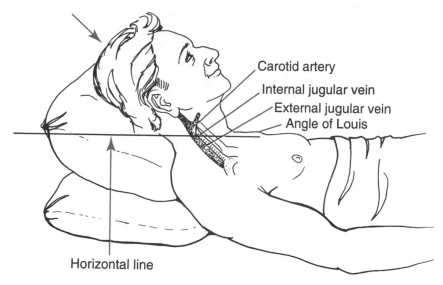

Carotid artery
Internal jugular vein
External jugular vein
Angle of Louis

Horizontal line

Figure 3-5 ■ Jugular venous distention.

Respiratory System

A key to the assessment of circulatory overload is an assessment of the lung fields. Changes in respiratory rate and depth may be a compensatory mechanism for acid–base imbalance. Tachypnea (greater than 20 respirations/min) and dyspnea indicate fluid volume excess (FVE). Moist crackles in the absence of cardiopulmonary disease indicate fluid volume excess. Shallow, slow breathing may indicate metabolic alkalosis or respiratory acidosis. Deep, rapid breathing may indicate respiratory alkalosis or metabolic acidosis.

Skin Appearance and Temperature

Assessments of temperature and skin surface are key in determining fluid volume changes. Pinching the area over the hand, inner thigh, sternum, or forehead can assess skin turgor. In a well-hydrated person, the pinched skin immediately falls back to its normal position when released. This

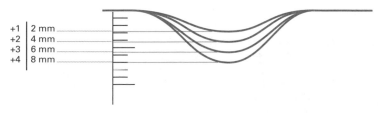

+1	2 mm
+2	4 mm
+3	6 mm
+4	8 mm

Figure 3-6 ■ Edema.

elastic property, referred to as turgor, is partially dependent on interstitial fluid volume. In a person with a fluid volume deficit, the skin may remain slightly elevated for many seconds. In persons older than age 55 years, skin turgor is generally reduced because of loss of elasticity, particularly in areas that have been exposed to the sun. A more accurate assessment can be made on the skin over the sternum. A condition in which placement of fingers firmly on the patient's skin leaves finger imprints is called fingerprinting and is associated with fluid volume excess. Fingerprint edema is demonstrated by pressing a finger firmly over the sternum or other body surface for a period of 15 to 30 seconds. On removal of the finger, a positive sign is a visible fingerprint similar to that seen when a fingerprint is made on paper with ink.

Special Senses

The eyes, mouth, lips, and tongue are also key indicators of fluid volume imbalances. The absence of tearing and salivation in a child is a sign of fluid volume deficit. In a healthy person, the tongue has one longitudinal furrow. In the person with fluid volume deficit, the tongue has additional longitudinal furrows and is smaller because of fluid loss (Metheny, 2000).

Mucous membranes often show the first sign of dehydration; as fluid volume decreases, the mouth becomes dry and sticky and the lips dry and cracked. In fluid volume deficit, the patient's eyes tend to appear sunken; in significant fluid volume excess, periorbital edema is present.

 NURSING FAST FACT!

Good oral hygiene is imperative with mouth-breathing patients. If the patient is receiving good oral care and the crusted, dry, furrowed tongue does not improve, fluid volume deficit must be restored to aid in solving this problem.

Body Weight

Taking daily weights of patients with potential fluid imbalances is an important clinical tool. Accurate body weight measurement is a better indicator of gains or losses than intake and output records. A loss or gain of 1 kg (2.2 lb.) reflects a loss or gain of 1 L of body fluid. Generally, fluid volume deficit or excess is considered severe when body weight fluctuates 15% higher or lower than the person's normal body weight.

EBNP A study by Armstrong (2005) found that asystematic review demonstrated measurement of weight is a safe technique to assess hydration status, especially for dehydration that occurs over a period of 1 to 4 hours; less frequent measurement may reflect changes in respiratory water loss or gain or loss of adipose tissue; thus weight changes may be a less accurate indicator of hydration status.

Table 3-2 summarizes the regulators of fluid balance.

> *EBNP Urine color significantly correlates with urine osmolality, serum sodium, and blood urea nitrogen (BUN)/creatinine ratios. In a hydrated person urine should be light yellow—the color of lemonade, with the color of apple juice indicating slight dehydration (Wakefield, Mentes, & Diggelmann, 2002).*

Refer to Evidence-Based Care Box 3-1.

EVIDENCE-BASED CARE BOX 3-1

Correlation of Urine Color to Hydration State

Wakefield, B., Mentes, J., & Diggelmann, L. (2002). Monitoring hydration status in elderly veterans. Western Journal of Nursing Research, 24 (2), 132.

A study of 89 veterans from two Veteran's Affairs facilities over a 10 hour period. Urine color was compared to the criterion standard of urine specific gravity and osmolality. Urine color was graded on an eight–level color chart. Significant positive associations existed between urine color and both urine specific gravity and urine osmolality. Potential for color chart as a low-cost technology to monitor dehydration status.

Laboratory Values

The review and interpretation of a patient's laboratory findings are important objective data for analysis of alterations in fluid balance and for the major electrolyte imbalances. The blood gas analysis is a key indicator, along with physical assessment, of acid–base imbalances. Tests that reflect the proper function of the heart and kidneys are of particular importance and require close scrutiny for early detection of fluid imbalances. Table 3-3 summarizes laboratory findings for monitoring fluid and electrolyte imbalances.

Disorders of Fluid Balance

Fluid volume imbalances may reflect an increase or a decrease in total body fluid or an altered distribution of body fluids. There are two major alterations in ECF balance: fluid volume deficit (FVD) and fluid volume excess (FVE).

Fluid Volume Deficit (Hypovolemia)

Extracellular fluid volume deficit (hypovolemia) reflects a contracted vascular compartment caused either by a significant ECF loss or by an accumulation of fluid in the interstitial space. ECF deficit is also referred to

> Table 3-3   **SUMMARY OF LABORATORY EVALUATION FOR FLUID AND ELECTROLYTE IMBALANCES**

Test	Clinical Considerations
Kidneys	
BUN	Assess nutritional support; evaluate hydration, and renal function.
Creatinine	Evaluate for renal impairment. Assess known or suspected disorder involving muscles in the absence of renal disease.
Specific gravity	Urine concentration reflects fluid volume concentrations and hydration status.
Urine osmolarity	Monitor for fluid imbalances.
Blood Chemistry	
Calcium, ionized	Identify individuals with hypocalcemia, monitor patients with renal failure in whom secondary hyper parathyroidism may occur. Monitor patient with sepsis or magnesium deficiency.
Chloride, blood	Assist in confirming diagnosis of disorder associated with abnormal chloride values in acid-base and fluid volume imbalances. Differentiate between types of acidosis.
Magnesium, blood	Determine electrolyte balance in renal failure and chronic alcoholism. Evaluate cardiac dysrhythmias.
Potassium, blood	Assess known or suspected disorder associated with renal disease, glucose metabolism, trauma, or burns. Evaluate electrolyte imbalances (especially elderly). Evaluate cardiac dysrhythmias especially during digitalis therapy. Monitor acidosis (potassium moves from RBCs into extracellular fluid in acidotic states).
Sodium, blood	Determine whole body stores of sodium. Monitor the effectiveness of drug therapy, especially diuretics on serum sodium levels. Determine hydration status.
Complete blood count (CBC)	Complete blood count screening for hemoglobin, hematocrit, red blood cell, white blood cell and platelets prior to replacement of these components or when expanding ECF
Blood Gases	Evaluation of acid–base status
pH, Hydrogen ion	The pH, negative logarithm of the hydrogen ion concentration, determines the acidity or alkalinity of body fluids.
Bicarbonate (HCO_3^-)	Alkaline substance that is over half of the total buffer base in the blood. Role in maintaining a pH of 7.35–7.45.
Partial pressure of oxygen (Pa_{CO_2})	Determines the amount of oxygen available to bind with hemoglobin. The PaO_2 is decreased in respiratory diseases.
Partial pressure of carbon dioxide (Pa_{CO_2})	Partial pressure of carbon dioxide reflects the adequacy of alveolar ventilation. The pH affects the combining power of oxygen and hemoglobin.
Miscellaneous	
Serum glucose	Monitor osmotic diuresis.

Source: Van Leeuwen, A., Kranpitz, T.R., & Smith, L. (2006). Laboratory and diagnostic tests with nursing implicaitons (2nd ed.). Philadelphia: F.A. Davis.

as dehydration. It may be caused by an actual decrease in body water; excessive fluid loss or inadequate fluid intake; or a relative decrease in which fluid (plasma) shifts from the intravascular compartment to the interstitial space, a process called "third spacing" (Metheny, 2000). Depending on the type of fluid lost, hypovolemia may be accompanied by acid–base, osmolar, or electrolyte imbalances. Prolonged hypovolemia may lead to the development of acute renal failure (Heitz & Horne, 2005).

Etiology

Fluid volume deficit occurs when there is either an excessive loss of body water or an inadequate compensatory intake. The ECF consists predominantly of the electrolytes sodium and chloride, both of which tend to attract water; loss of these electrolytes also leads to loss of water. Gastrointestinal dysfunction is the most common cause of ECF deficit. Other common causes include overzealous use of diuretics and diaphoresis.

Fluid volume deficit also occurs in third spacing, which is caused by peritonitis, intestinal obstruction, postoperative conditions, thrombophlebitis, acute pancreatitis, ascites, fistula drainage, and burns. Third spaces are extracellular body spaces in which fluid is not normally present in large amounts, but in which fluid can accumulate. Fluid that accumulates in third spaces is physiologically useless because it is not available for use. Common sites for collection of third space fluid include tissue spaces, abdomen, pleural spaces, and pericardial space (Hogan & Wane, 2003).

COMMON CAUSES OF ISOTONIC DEHYDRATION

- Hemorrhage resulting in loss of fluid, electrolytes, proteins, and blood cells in proportional amounts, resulting in inadequate vascular volume
- Gastrointestinal losses: Vomiting, diarrhea, nasogastric suction, drainage from fistulas and tubes. Tend to be lost in proportional amounts.
- Fever, environmental heat, and diaphoresis result in profuse sweating, causing water and sodium loss.
- Burns initially damage skin and capillary membranes allow fluid, electrolytes, and proteins to escape into the burned tissue, resulting in inadequate vascular volume.
- Diuretics cause excessive loss of fluid and electrolytes in proportional amounts.
- Third space fluid shifts occur when fluid moves from the vascular space into physiologically useless extracellular spaces.

COMMON CAUSES OF HYPERTONIC FLUID DEHYDRATION

- Inadequate fluid intake: Patients who are unable to respond to thirst independently (bedridden, infants, elderly who have nausea, and anorexia, those who are NPO without adequate fluid replacement)

- Decreased water intake results in ECF solute concentration and leads to cellular dehydration (Hogan & Wane, 2003).

Clinical Manifestations

Clinically, ECF deficit is characterized by acute weight loss, altered cardiovascular function that reflects the underlying ECF volume deficit, and complaints of nausea and vomiting. The cardiovascular assessment is the most important part of the process to determine plasma volume changes. In a patient who is hypovolemic, the heart rate increases, the blood pressure decreases, and the peripheral pulses are weak. Symptoms reflect a dehydrated state with sunken eyeballs, poor skin turgor, and oliguria commonly seen.

Laboratory Findings

- Hemoconcentration with the serum hemoglobin, hematocrit, and proteins increased
- Blood urea nitrogen (BUN) is elevated above 20 mg/100 mL
- Urine specific gravity reflects high solute concentration of more than 1.030

NURSING POINTS-OF-CARE
HYPOVOLEMIA (FVD)

Nursing Assessments
1. Complete a client history identifying factors that may cause a fluid volume deficit such as vomiting, diarrhea, limited fluid intake, diabetes mellitus, large draining wound, or diuretic therapy.
2. Assess skin turgor, mucous membranes, cracked lips, and furrows on the tongue.
3. Check vital signs: heart rate increases with blood volume decrease. Check for narrow pulse pressure.
4. Assess urine output for volume and concentration.
5. Assess recent weight loss by percentage.
6. Assess hand or neck vein filling.
7. Review laboratory findings such as BUN, hematocrit, and hemoglobin.

Nursing Interventions
1. Monitor vital signs every 1–4 hours depending upon severity of fluid loss.
2. Provide fluid intake hourly orally or by I.V. replacement.
3. Monitor skin turgor, mucous membranes.
4. Monitor I.V. fluid replacement to ensure infusion rate.

Media Link: Use Web-based interactive for case study with care plans.

Treatment

Treatment for patients with an ECF volume deficit entails fluid replacement (orally or intravenously) until the oliguria is relieved and the cardiovascular and neurologic systems stabilize. Isotonic electrolyte solutions such as 0.9% NaCl or lactated Ringer's solution are used to treat hypotensive patients with a fluid volume deficit. A hypotonic electrolyte solution (0.45% NaCl) is often used to provide electrolyte and free water for renal excretion of metabolic wastes (Metheny, 2000).

 NURSING FAST FACT!

> Extreme caution must be exercised in fluid replacement therapy to avoid fluid overload.

Fluid Volume Excess (Hypervolemia)

ECF volume excess causes an expansion of the ECF compartment. The primary cause of ECF excess is cardiovascular dysfunction. Fluid volume excess is always secondary to an increase in total body sodium content, which causes total body water increase. Normally, the posterior pituitary decreases secretion of the ADH when excess water moves into the cells. This causes the kidney to eliminate excess fluid. However, if a patient has an excessive secretion of ADH, the water will be retained, placing the patient at risk for fluid volume excess. Excessive secretion of ADH can be caused by fear, pain, and postoperative reaction 12 to 24 hours after surgery, along with acute infections.

Etiology

Conditions that cause overhydration include excessive administration of oral or I.V. fluids containing sodium, excessive irrigation of body cavities or organs, and use of hypotonic fluids to replace isotonic fluid loss. When sodium and water are retained in the same proportion, iso-osmolar fluid volume excess occurs. Edema is commonly associated with excess extracellular body fluid or excess fluid due to I.V. overhydration. Physiologic factors leading to edema may be caused by various clinical conditions such as heart failure, kidney failure, cirrhosis of the liver, steroid excess, and retention of sodium (Kee, Paulanka, & Purnell, 2004).

COMMON CAUSES OF ISOTONIC OVERHYDRATION

- Renal failure leading to decreased excretion of water and sodium
- Heart failure leading to stasis of blood in the circulation and venous congestion
- Excess fluid intake of isotonic I.V. solutions

- High corticosteroid levels due to therapy, stress response, or disease resulting in sodium and water retention
- High aldosterone levels (stress response to adrenal dysfunction, liver damage, or metabolic problems)

COMMON CAUSES OF HYPOTONIC OVERHYDRATION (WATER INTOXICATION)

- More fluid is gained than solute.
- Serum osmolality falls, causing cells to swell (cerebral cells most sensitive).
- Repeated plain water enemas.
- Overuse of hypotonic I.V. fluids
- In young children or infants, ingestion of inappropriately prepared formula and/or excess water (use of water bottle as pacifier)
- SIADH causes kidneys to retain large amounts of water without sodium.

Clinical Manifestations

Clinically, ECF volume excess has distinct signs and symptoms, the most prominent being weight gain. A constant irritating nonproductive cough is frequently the first clinical symptom of hypervolemia. It is caused by excess fluid "backed up" into the lungs.

Edema is usually not apparent until 2 to 4 kg of fluid has been retained. Alterations in respiratory and cardiovascular function are present and include hypertension and tachycardia. Moist crackles in the lung usually indicate that the lungs are congested with fluid. Cyanosis is a late symptom of pulmonary edema due to hypervolemia. In addition to common assessment findings, some patients also experience confusion, altered levels of consciousness, skeletal muscle weakness, and increased bowel sounds.

Peripheral edema present in the morning may result from inadequate heart, liver, or kidney function. Peripheral edema in the evening may be due to fluid stasis, dependent edema. An increase in vascular volume may be evidenced by distended neck veins, slow-emptying peripheral veins, a full and bounding pulse, and an increase in central venous pressure.

 NURSING FAST FACT!

Peripheral edema should be assessed in the morning before the patient gets out of bed. A weight gain of 2.2 pounds is equivalent to the retention of 1 liter of body water.

Laboratory Findings

Laboratory findings are variable and usually nonspecific.

- BUN, serum protein, albumin, hemoglobin, and hematocrit may be decreased as a result of hemodilution.
- The serum osmolality will be decreased below 280 mOsm/kg.

- B-type natriuretic peptide (BNP) increased to greater than 100 pg/mL in congestive heart failure
- Serum sodium is decreased if hypervolemia occurs as a result of excessive water retention.
- Urine specific gravity decreased if kidney is attempting to excrete excess volume.

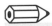 *NURSING FAST FACT!*

> *Severe or prolonged isotonic fluid volume excess in a person with a healthy heart and kidneys is usually compensated through increasing urinary output.*

NURSING POINTS-OF-CARE
HYPERVOLEMIA (FVE)

Nursing Assessments
- Complete a client history to identify underlying health problems that may have contributed to FVE.
- Obtain dietary history that emphasizes sodium, protein, and water intake.
- Assess vital signs; focus on the presence of a bounding pulse.
- Assess for constant irritating cough, difficulty in breathing, neck and hand vein engorgement, and lung crackles.
- Assess extremities for peripheral edema.
- Assess urine output.

Key Nursing Interventions
1. Monitor vital signs; report elevated blood pressure or bounding pulse.
2. Monitor weight daily. Check weight every morning before breakfast.
3. Observe for the presence of edema daily. Check for pitting edema in the extremities every morning.
4. Monitor diet, and teach appropriate food selections to avoid excess salt.
5. Encourage rest periods to support diuresis.

Treatment

Treatment of ECF volume excess is directed toward sodium and fluid restriction, administration of diuretics, and the treatment of the underlying cause (Porth & Martin, 2008). The treatment of FVE focuses on providing a balance between sodium and water intake and output. Diuretic therapy is commonly used to increase sodium elimination. Table 3-4 summarizes the fluid imbalances of hypovolemia and hypervolemia.

> Table 3-4   **QUICK ASSESSMENT GUIDE FOR FLUID IMBALANCES**

Area of Clinical Assessment	Signs and Symptoms of Fluid Volume Deficit (Hypovolemia)	Signs and Symptoms of Fluid Volume Excess (Hypervolemia)
Neurologic	Irritability, restlessness, lethargy, and confusion (seizures and coma) Thirst	Confusion
Cardiovascular	Frank or postural hypotension Tachycardia Weak, thready pulses Decreased pulse volume Cool extremities with delayed capillary refill Flat neck veins Poor peripheral vein filling CVP <4 cm	Galloping heart rhythm (heart S_3 sound) in adults Distended neck veins Slow emptying hand veins CVP >11 cm Bounding full pulse Peripheral edema
Respiratory	Lungs clear Respirations may be rapid and shallow	Tachypnea (>20) and dyspnea Irritated cough Hacking cough – becoming moist and productive Labored breathing Wet lung sounds (moist crackles) Decreased O_2 saturation Cyanosis
Skin Appearance and Temperature	Low-grade fever Dry skin "tenting" Sunken or depressed fontanels in infants	Bulging fontanels in children under 18 months Edematous skin (1+ to 4+)
Eyes	Decreased tearing and dry conjunctiva Sunken eyeballs	Periorbital edema
Lips	Dry lips, cracked	No change
Oral Cavity	Dry Increased tongue furrows, tongue coated Sticky mucous membranes	No change
Urine Volume and Concentration	Concentrated urine and low volume <30 mL/hr Specific gravity high: >1.035	Polyuria Specific gravity <1.005
Body Weight	Weight loss 5%: Mild deficit 5–10%: Moderate deficit >15%: Severe deficit (especially important in children)	Weight gain (acute and rapid) 5%: Mild excess 5–10%: Moderate excess >15%: Severe excess

> Table 3-4	QUICK ASSESSMENT GUIDE FOR FLUID IMBALANCES—cont'd	
Area of Clinical Assessment	Signs and Symptoms of Fluid Volume Deficit (Hypovolemia)	Signs and Symptoms of Fluid Volume Excess (Hypervolemia)
Diagnostic Laboratory Findings	Normal or high hematocrit and BUN Serum osmolarity elevated: >300 Serum sodium >150 mEq Serum glucose elevated >120 mg/dL	Hematocrit and BUN decreased Serum osmolality is low <275 Serum sodium low <125 mEq

Sources: Hogan & Wane (2003); Metheny (2000); Porth & Martin (2008).

▪ Basic Principles of Electrolyte Balance

Chemical compounds in solution behave in one of two ways: they separate and combine with other compounds, or they remain intact. One group of compounds remains intact; these are called nonelectrolytes (e.g., urea, dextrose, and creatinine). These compounds do not separate from their complex form when added to a solution. The second group of compounds, electrolytes, dissociates or separates in solution. These compounds break up into separate particles known as ions in a process called ionization. The major electrolytes in body fluids are sodium, potassium, calcium, magnesium, chloride, phosphorus, and bicarbonate.

Ions, which are the dissociated particles of an electrolyte, each carry an electrical charge, either positive or negative. Negative ions are called **anions** and positive ions are called **cations.**

Electrolytes are active chemicals that unite. The ions are expressed in terms of milliequivalents (mEq) per liter rather than milligrams. A milliequivalent measures chemical activity or combining power rather than weight. For example, when a hostess creates a guest list for a party, she does not invite 1000 pounds of boys per 1000 pounds of girls; rather, she invites the same number of boys and girls. In total, the milliequivalents of cations in a given compartment is equal to the milliequivalents of anions. There are 154 mEq of anions and 154 mEq of cations in the plasma. Each water compartment of the body contains electrolytes. The concentration and composition of electrolytes vary from compartment to compartment. See Table 3-5 for a diagrammatic comparison of electrolyte composition in the fluid compartments.

Most of the electrolytes have more than one physiologic role; often several electrolytes work together to mediate chemical events. The physiologic roles of electrolytes include:

- Maintaining electroneutrality in fluid compartments
- Mediating enzyme reactions
- Altering cell membrane permeability

> Table 3-5	COMPARISON OF ELECTROLYTE COMPOSITION IN FLUID COMPARTMENTS				

Intracellular Water (approx. mEq/L)		Extracellular Water (approx. mEq/L)			
		Plasma	*m*	*Interstitial Fluid*	
Cations	Anions	Cations	Anions	Cations	Anions
205 mEq	205 mEq	154 mEq	154 mEq	154 mEq	154 mEq

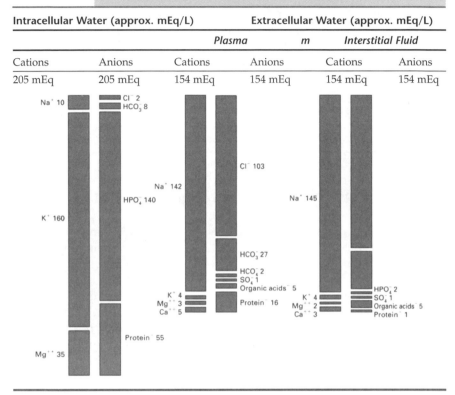

- Regulating muscle contraction and relaxation
- Regulating nerve impulse transmission
- Influencing blood clotting time

The electrolyte content of intracellular fluid (ICF) differs from that of extracellular fluid (ECF). Usually only ECF plasma electrolytes are measured because of the special techniques required to measure the concentration of electrolytes in ICF. The serum plasma levels of electrolytes are important in the assessment and management of patients with electrolyte imbalances.

Nursing Diagnosis and Electrolyte Imbalances

According to Carpenito-Moyet (2008), certain physiologic complications that nurses monitor to detect onset or changes in status are considered collaborative problems. Nurses manage collaborative problems using physician-prescribed and nursing-prescribed interventions to minimize the complications of the events. Electrolyte imbalances are collaborative problems and for collaborative problems nursing focuses on monitoring for onset of change in status of physiologic complications.

General Diagnostic Statement

Potential Complication Metabolic related to electrolyte imbalance. Electrolyte imbalances describes a person experiencing or at risk to experience a deficit or excess of one or more electrolytes.

Nursing goal: The nurse will manage and minimize episodes of electrolyte imbalances using laboratory values and monitor for signs and symptoms of specific electrolyte imbalance.

NOTE > For each of the following electrolytes, the Nursing Points-of-Care focuses on assessments and nursing interventions that support collection of data for monitoring for changes in status.

Sodium (Na⁺)

Normal Reference Value: 135 to 145 mEq/L

Physiologic Role

The physiologic role of sodium includes:
- Neuromuscular: Transmission and conduction of nerve impulses (sodium pump)
- Body Fluids: Responsible for the osmolality of vascular fluids.
- Cellular: Maintain water balance. Sodium shifts into cells as potassium shifts out of cells—depolarization (cell activity). When sodium shifts out of cells, potassium shift back into cell—repolarization (enzyme activity)
- Acid–base: Sodium combines with chloride or bicarbonate to regulate acid–base balance (Kee, Paulanka, & Purnell, 2004).

 NURSING FAST FACT!

Doubling the serum sodium level gives the approximate serum osmolality.

The major function of sodium is to maintain ECF volume. Extracellular sodium level has an effect on the cellular fluid volume based on the principle of osmosis. Sodium represents about 90% of all the extracellular cations. Sodium does not easily cross the cell wall membrane and is therefore the most abundant cation of ECF.

A low serum sodium level results in dilute ECF, therefore allowing water to be drawn into the cells (lower to higher concentration). Conversely if the serum sodium is high, water is drawn out of the cells, leading to cellular dehydration. Figure 3-7 shows the relationship between sodium and cellular fluid. The normal daily requirement for sodium in adults is approximately 100 mEq.

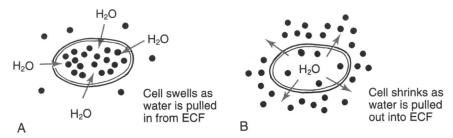

Figure 3-7 ■ Sodium and cellular fluid relationship. *(A)* Hyponatremia. The cell swells as water is pulled in from the extracellular fluid. *(B)* Hypernatremia. The cell shrinks as water is pulled out into the extracellular fluid.

The kidneys are extremely important in the regulation of sodium. This regulation is primarily accomplished through the action of the hormone aldosterone. Hyponatremia is a common complication of adrenal insufficiency because of aldosterone and cortisol deficiencies. Elderly persons have a slower rate of aldosterone secretion, which places them at risk for sodium imbalances.

 NURSING FAST FACT!

The cerebral cells are very sensitive to changes in serum sodium levels and exhibit adaptive changes to sodium imbalances (Hogan & Wane, 2003).

Three factors can create a sodium imbalance:

1. Change in the sodium content of the ECF such as a deficit caused by excessive vomiting
2. Change in the chloride content, which can affect both the sodium concentration and the amount of water in the ECF; when the ratio of chloride to sodium deviates from normal, it is reflected as an acid–base imbalance
3. Change in the quantity of water in the ECF

Serum Sodium Deficit: Hyponatremia

Hyponatremia is a condition in which the sodium level is below normal (less than 135 mEq/L). A low sodium level can be the result of an excessive loss of sodium or an excessive gain of water; in either event, hyponatremia is caused by a relatively greater concentration of water than of sodium. Sodium deficit is usually associated with hypervolemia states.

ETIOLOGY

The pathophysiology that contributes to sodium deficit (hyponatremia) is often a sign of a serious underlying disease; there are also many causes of hyponatremia.

All gastrointestinal (GI) secretions contain sodium; therefore, any abnormal loss of GI secretions can cause a sodium deficit. GI disorders such as vomiting, diarrhea, drainage from suction or fistulas, and excessive tap water enemas may also cause hyponatremia.

Other causes of hyponatremia are losses from skin in excessive sweating, combined with excessive water consumption and the use of thiazide diuretics (especially dangerous with low-salt diets). In addition, excessive parenteral hypo-osmolar fluids such as dextrose in water solutions can cause hyponatremia.

Hormonal factors such as labor induction with oxytocin and the syndrome of inappropriate antidiuretic syndrome (SIADH) cause the amount of sodium per volume to be reduced, in turn causing a dilutional hyponatremia. Oxytocin has been shown to have an intrinsic antidiuretic hormone effect, acting to increase water reabsorption from the glomerular filtrate. Cerebral intracellular fluid excess (hyponatremic encephalopathy) includes the risk of seizures, coma, and death, which can occur when water shifts into the brain cells (Kee, Paulanka, & Purnell, 2004; Metheny, 1997). Researchers (Ayus, Varon, & Arieff, 2000) believe that physiologic responses in premenopausal women place them at higher risk than men for hyponatremic encephalopathy because estrogen stimulates ADH release and antagonizes the brain's ability to adapt to swelling. In men, androgens suppress ADH release and enhance the brain's ability to adapt to swelling. Young women account for most of the reported cases of fatalities secondary to hyponatremia. Marathon runners have been shown to develop hyponatremic encephalopathy related to dilutional hyponatremia. See Evidence-Based Care Box 3-2 for evidence-based practice changes in treating dilutional hyponatremic encephalopathy (Siegel, 2007).

 NURSING FAST FACT!

SIADH has progressed from a rare occurrence to the most common cause of hyponatremia seen in general hospitals. It occurs in patients with inflammatory disorders such as pneumonia; tuberculosis; abscess; oat cell cancer of the lung; and central nervous system (CNS) disorders such as meningitis, trauma, stroke, and degenerative diseases (Metheny, 2000).

EVIDENCE-BASED CARE BOX 3-2

Treatment of Dilutional Hyponatremia

Hew-Butler, T., Almond, C., Ayus, J.C. et al. (2005). Consensus statement of the 1st international exercise-associated hyponatremia development conference. Cape Town, South Africa. Clinical Journal of Sports Medicine, 15:208-13.

An evidence-based consensus statement concluded that both excessive fluid consumption and a decrease in urine formation contribute to dilutional effect in hyponatremia that can lead to life-threatening and fatal cases of pulmonary and cerebral edema. Strategies for prevention and treatment including intravenous hypertonic solutions (such as 3% sodium chloride) to reverse the symptoms related to moderate and life threatening hypotonic encephalopathy.

Chemical agents may also impair renal water excretion, leading to sodium deficit. Pharmacologic agents that contribute to sodium deficit include nicotine, chlorpropamide (Diabinese), cyclophosphamide (Cytoxan), morphine, barbiturates, and acetaminophen.

CLINICAL MANIFESTATIONS

Hyponatremia affects cells of the CNS. Patients with chronic hyponatremia may experience impaired sensation of taste, anorexia, muscle cramps, feelings of exhaustion, apprehension, feelings of impending doom (Na$^+$ less than 115), and focal weaknesses (e.g., hemiparesis, ataxia). Patients with acute hyponatremia caused by water overload experience the same symptoms as well as fingerprint edema (sign of intracellular water excess). Patients undergoing operative procedures involving irrigations may develop hyponatremia (such as transurethral resection of prostate [TURP] and endometrial ablation).

LABORATORY FINDINGS

- Serum sodium: Less than 135 mEq/L
- Serum osmolarity: Less than 280 mOsm/L
- Urine specific gravity: Less than 1.010 (except in SIADH)
- Urine sodium: Decreased (usually less than 20 mEq/L)
- Hematocrit: Above normal when fluid volume deficit (FVD) exists
- Decreased blood urea nitrogen (BUN)

TREATMENT/COLLABORATIVE MANAGEMENT

Treatment of patients with hyponatremia aims to provide sodium by the dietary, enteral, or parenteral route. Patients able to eat and drink can easily replace sodium by ingesting a normal diet. Those unable to take sodium orally must take the electrolyte by the parenteral route. An isotonic saline or Ringer's solution may be ordered, such as 0.9% sodium chloride (NaCl), or lactated Ringer's solution. The immediate goal of therapy is the correction of acute symptoms, the gradual return of sodium to normal level, and if necessary, the restoration of normal ECF volume.

Acute symptomatic hyponatremia requires more aggressive treatment. Treatment must be individualized. Too rapid correction of chronic hyponatremia (lasting greater than 24–48 hours) may result in irreversible neurologic damage and death as a result of osmotic demyelination (Heitz & Horne, 2005).

General treatment guidelines for patients with hyponatremia are:

1. Replace sodium and fluid losses through diet or parenteral fluids.
2. Restore normal ECF volume.
3. Correct any other electrolyte losses such as potassium or bicarbonate.

Treatment of hyponatremia with fluid volume overload includes:

1. Removal or treatment of underlying cause such as SIADH
2. Administering loop diuretic (thiazide diuretics should be avoided)
3. Water restriction to 1000 mL/day establishes negative water balance and increases plasma sodium levels in most adults.

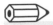 NURSING FAST FACT!

When the primary problem is water retention, it is safer to restrict water than to administer sodium. An I.V. solution that can contribute to hyponatremia is excessive administration of 5% dextrose in water.

 NURSING FAST FACT!

Permanent neurologic damage may occur in patient with acute symptomatic hyponatremia as a result of failure to adequately treat hyponatremic encephalopathy. The replacement of sodium chloride solution by infusion pump should be at a rate calculated to elevate the plasma sodium level about 1 mEq/L/hr. Too rapid elevation of sodium (more than 25 mEq/L in the first 48 hours can cause brain damage (Metheny, 1997).

NURSING POINTS-OF-CARE
HYPONATREMIA

Nursing Assessments
- Obtain a patient history of high-risk factors for hyponatremia (vomiting, diarrhea, eating disorders, low-sodium diet).
- Obtain a history of medications with emphasis on those predisposing patients to hyponatremia (i.e., diuretics).
- Assess for signs and symptoms of hyponatremia.
- Obtain baseline laboratory tests (e.g., serum sodium, serum osmolarity, serum potassium, serum chloride, and urinary specific gravity).

Key Nursing Interventions
1. Monitor laboratory tests with emphasis on serum sodium
2. Monitor GI losses.
3. Monitor for signs and symptoms of hyponatremia: CNS changes (coma, headache), weakness, nausea, muscle cramps, vomiting, diarrhea, and apprehension
4. Monitor for changes in central venous system symptoms.
5. Monitor intake, output, and daily weight.
6. Restrict water when hyponatremia is due to hypervolemia.

Serum Sodium Excess: Hypernatremia

The serum level of sodium is elevated to above 145 mEq/L in hypernatremia. This elevation can be caused by a gain of sodium without water or a loss of water without loss of sodium. There are two primary defenses against hypernatremia: (1) thirst respose, (2) excretion of maximally concentrated urine through increased production of ADH. Sodium is the major determinant of ECF osmolality; therefore hypernatremia causes hypertonicity. Hypertonicity causes a shift of water of the cells, which leads to cellular dehydration. Dehydration of the cerebral cells results in the development of the CNS symptoms (Heitz & Horne, 2005).

ETIOLOGY

Increased levels of serum sodium can occur with water loss or deprivation of water, occurring when a person cannot respond to thirst; during hypertonic tube feeding with inadequate water supplements. Sodium gain can occur with excessive parenteral administration of sodium-containing solutions; and in near drowning in salt water. Sodium is lost with watery diarrhea (a particular problem in infants), increased insensible loss, ingestion of sodium in unusual amounts, profuse sweating, heat stroke, and diabetes insipidus when water intake is inadequate (Hogan & Wane, 2003).

CLINICAL MANIFESTATIONS

Patients with hypernatremia may experience marked thirst; elevated body temperature; swollen tongue; red, dry, sticky mucous membranes; and tachycardia. In severe hypernatremia, disorientation and irritability or hyperactivity when physically stimulated can occur.

LABORATORY FINDINGS

- Serum sodium: Greater than 145 mEq/L
- Chloride may be elevated.
- Serum osmolarity: Greater than 295 mOsm/kg
- Urine specific gravity: Greater than 1.015 (except for those with diabetes insipidus)
- Dehydration test: Water is withheld for 16 to 18 hours; serum and urine osmolarity are checked 1 hour after administration of antidiuretic hormone (ADH); this test is used to identify the cause of polyuric syndromes (central versus nephrogenic diabetes insipidus).

> EBNP Ferry (2005) found that because the aging process causes a decrease in thirst, once a geriatric client experiences thirst, he or she may have a severe water deficit and sodium excess.

TREATMENT/COLLABORATIVE MANAGEMENT

The goal of treatment of patients with hypernatremia is to gradually lower the serum sodium level (usually over 48 hours), infusing a hypotonic

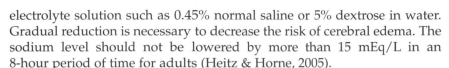

electrolyte solution such as 0.45% normal saline or 5% dextrose in water. Gradual reduction is necessary to decrease the risk of cerebral edema. The sodium level should not be lowered by more than 15 mEq/L in an 8-hour period of time for adults (Heitz & Horne, 2005).

Generally, treatment guidelines for hypernatremia are:

1. Infusion of hypotonic electrolyte solution (0.45% NaCl or 5% dextrose in water). If the sodium level is more than 160 mEq/L, 5% dextrose in water is indicated.
2. Sodium levels can also be decreased by use of diuretics, which induce excretion of water and sodium.
3. Administration of desmopressin acetate (DDAVP) can be given to treat central diabetes insipidus. Treating the underlying cause such as treating fever or diarrhea minimizes abnormal fluid loss.
4. Removal of cause of hypernatremia such as discontinuing medications that cause increase sodium levels (lithium), or correcting electrolyte imbalances such as hypokalemia and hypercalcemia.

NURSING POINTS-OF-CARE
HYPERNATREMIA

Nursing Assessments
- Obtain a patient history of high-risk factors for hypernatremia (e.g., increased sodium intake, water deprivation, increased adrenocortical hormone production, use of sodium-retaining drugs).
- Assess for signs and symptoms of hypernatremia.
- Obtain baseline values of laboratory tests, especially serum sodium.

Key Nursing Interventions
1. Monitor laboratory test results with emphasis on serum sodium and serum osmolarity.
2. Monitor fluid intake, output, and daily weight.
3. Monitor for signs and symptoms of fluid overload including thirst, CNS effects (agitation to convulsions), weight gain and edema, elevated blood pressure, and tachycardia.
4. Monitor for signs of pulmonary edema when the patient is receiving large amounts of parenteral sodium chloride.
5. Promote increased mobility if appropriate.
6. Monitor for seizures.

Potassium (K⁺)

Normal Reference Value: 3.5 to 5.5 mEq/L

Physiologic Role

The physiologic role of potassium includes:
- Regulation of fluid volume within the cell
- Promotion of nerve impulse transmission
- Contraction of skeletal, smooth, and cardiac muscle
- Control of hydrogen ion (H⁺) concentration, acid–base balance; when potassium moves out of the cell, hydrogen ions move in, and vice versa
- Role in enzyme action for cellular energy production.

Potassium is an intracellular electrolyte with 98% in the ICF and 2% in the ECF. Potassium is a dynamic electrolyte. Cellular potassium replaces ECF potassium if it becomes depleted. Potassium is acquired through diet and must be ingested daily because the body has no effective method of storage. The daily requirement is 40 mEq. Potassium influences both skeletal and cardiac muscle activity. Alterations in the concentration of plasma potassium change myocardial irritability and rhythm. Potassium moves easily into the intracellular space when the body is metabolizing glucose. It moves out of the cells during strenuous exercise, when cellular metabolism is impaired, or when the cell dies. Potassium, along with sodium, is responsible for transmission of nerve impulses. During nerve cell innervation, these ions exchange places, creating an electrical current (Metheny, 2000).

There is a relationship between acid–base imbalances and potassium balance. Hypokalemia can cause alkalosis, which in turn can further decrease serum potassium. Hyperkalemia can cause acidosis, which in turn can further increase serum potassium.

The regulation of potassium is related to several other processes, including:
- Sodium level: Enough sodium must be available for exchange with potassium.
- Hydrogen ion excretion: When there is an increase in hydrogen ion excretion, there is a decrease in potassium excretion.
- Aldosterone level: An increased level of aldosterone stimulates and increases excretion of potassium.
- Potassium imbalances are common in clinical practice because of their association with underlying disease, injury, or ingestion of certain medications.

Serum Potassium Deficit: Hypokalemia

Hypokalemia is a serum potassium level below 3.5 mEq/L. It usually reflects a real deficit in total potassium stores; however, it may occur in patients with normal potassium stores when alkalosis is present. Hypokalemia is a common disturbance; many factors are associated with this deficit, and many clinical conditions contribute to it.

ETIOLOGY

Many conditions can lead to potassium deficit, including GI and renal loss, increased use of increased perspiration, shifting of extracellular potassium into the cells, and poor dietary intake. Gastrointestinal loss includes diarrhea or laxative overuse, prolonged gastric suction, and protracted vomiting. Renal loss includes potassium-wasting diuretic therapy; excessive use of glucocorticoids; ingestion of drugs such as sodium penicillin, carbenicillin, or amphotericin B; excessive ingestion of European licorice (which mimics the action of aldosterone); and excessive steroid administration.

Sweat loss includes heavy perspiration in persons acclimated to the heat. Shifting into the cells can occur with total parenteral nutrition therapy without adequate potassium supplementation, alkalosis, and excessive administration of insulin. Poor dietary intake can occur with anorexia nervosa, bulimia, and alcoholism.

CLINICAL MANIFESTATIONS

Patients with hypokalemia may experience neuromuscular changes such as fatigue, muscle weakness, diminished deep tendon reflexes, and flaccid paralysis (late). Other symptoms include anorexia, nausea, vomiting, irritability (early), increased sensitivity to digitalis, electrocardiographic (ECG) changes, and death (in those with severe hypokalemia) caused by cardiac arrest.

LABORATORY AND ECG FINDINGS

- Serum potassium: Less than 3.5 mEq/L
- Arterial blood gas (ABG): May show metabolic alkalosis (increased pH and bicarbonate ion).
- Elevated serum glucose levels (increased insulin secretion and increased osmotic pressure)
- ECG: ST-segment depression, flattened T wave, presence of U wave, and ventricular dysrhythmias. The ECG tracing in Figure 3-8 reflects changes when potassium is below normal.

 NURSING FAST FACT!

Clinical signs and symptoms rarely occur before the serum potassium level has fallen below 3 mEq/L.

Potassium replacement must take place slowly to prevent hyperkalemia. Extreme caution should be used when potassium chloride replacement exceeds 120 mEq in 24 hours. The patient must be monitored for dysrhythmias.

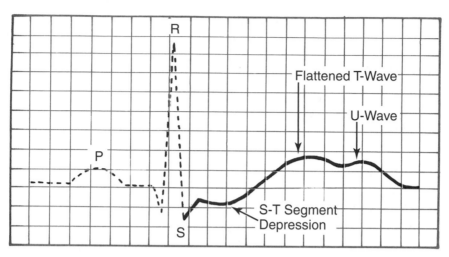

Figure 3-8 ■ Sample ECG tracing: Hypokalemia. The ECG tracing for hypokalemia has ST-segment depression, flattened T wave, and the presence of a U wave.

Treatment/Collaborative Management

Replacement of potassium is the key concept in treating patients with potassium deficit. Replacement of potassium either by mouth or intravenously. The usual oral dose is 40 to 80 mEq/day in divided doses. I.V. potassium is necessary if hypokalemia is severe or if the patient is unable to tolerate oral potassium. I.V. potassium is irritating to the vessels and the rate must be adjusted to prevent phlebitis. Potassium is usually replaced in combination with chloride or phosphate. Hypokalemia is frequently associated with ECF volume deficit and chloride loss; potassium chloride is usually ordered. Hypokalemia associated with metabolic acidosis may be treated with potassium bicarbonate or citrate (Heitz & Horne, 2005).

General treatment guidelines include:

1. Mild hypokalemia is usually treated with dietary increases of potassium or oral supplements.
2. Salt substitutes (e.g., Morton Salt Substitute, Co-Salt, Adolph's Salt Substitute) contain potassium and can be used to supplement potassium intake.
3. If the serum potassium is below 2 mEq/L, monitor the patient's ECG and administer potassium by means of a secondary piggyback set in a volume of 100 mL (Metheny, 2000).

NOTE > Never give potassium I.V. push/bolus.

Table 3-6 gives critical guidelines for nursing in I.V. administration of potassium.

> Table 3-6	CRITICAL GUIDELINES FOR ADMINISTRATION OF POTASSIUM

Never give a potassium I.V. push.
Potassium chloride (KCl) should be added to a nondextrose solution such as isotonic saline to treat severe hypokalemia because administration of KCl in a dextrose solution may cause a small reduction in the serum potassium level.
Never administer concentrated potassium solutions without first diluting them as directed.
KCl preparations greater than 60 mEq/L **should not** be given in a peripheral vein. Concentrations greater than 8 mEq/100 mL can cause pain and irritation of peripheral veins and lead to postinfusion phlebitis.
When adding KCl to infusion solutions, especially plastic systems, make sure the KCl mixes with the solution thoroughly. Invert and agitate the container to ensure mixing.
Do not add KCl to a hanging container!
For patients with any degree of renal insufficiency or heart block, reduce the infusion by 50%. For example, 5–10 mEq/hr rather than 10–20 mEq/hr.
Administer potassium at a rate not to exceed 10 mEq/hr through peripheral veins.
For patients with extreme hypokalemia, rates should be no more than 40 mEq/hr while ECG is constantly monitored.
If KCl is administered into the subcutaneous tissue (infiltration), it is extremely irritating and can cause serious tissue loss. Use extravasation protocol in this situation.

Sources: Gahart & Nazareno (2008); Metheny (2000).

NURSING POINTS-OF-CARE
HYPOKALEMIA

Nursing Assessments
- Obtain history of high-risk factors for hypokalemia such as vomiting, renal disease, and diuretic use.
- Assess for signs of hypokalemia.
- Obtain baseline laboratory test values such as ECG reading, serum potassium, and serum osmolarity.

Key Nursing Interventions
1. Monitor the laboratory test results, especially serum potassium
2. Monitor for signs and symptoms of hypokalemia.
3. Keep accurate intake and output records.
4. Monitor for changes in cardiac response.
5. Monitor for signs of phlebitis (potassium irritates veins) when given by I.V. route
6. When administering potassium by I.V. always dilute and do not exceed 10 mEq/hr in adults. **Never give by IV push.**

Serum Potassium Excess: Hyperkalemia

Hyperkalemia occurs less frequently than hypokalemia, but it can be more dangerous. It seldom occurs in patients who have normal renal function. Hyperkalemia is defined as a serum plasma level of potassium above 5.5 mEq/L. The main causes of hyperkalemia are (1) increased intake of potassium (oral or parenteral), (2) decreased urinary excretion of potassium, and (3) movement of potassium out of the cells and into the extracellular space.

ETIOLOGY

High levels of serum potassium can be caused by either a gain of potassium body or shift of potassium from the ICF to the ECF. Hyperkalemia can be caused by excessive administration of potassium parentally or orally; severe renal failure resulting in reduced potassium excretion; release of potassium from altered cellular function, such as with burns or crush injuries; and acidosis.

Drugs that can cause a predisposition to hyperkalemias include potassium penicillin, indomethacin, amphetamines, nonsteroidal antiinflammatory drugs, alpha agonists, beta blockers, succinylcholine, cyclophosphamide, and potassium-sparing diuretics. Pseudohyperkalemia can occur with prolonged tourniquet application during blood withdrawal (Metheny, 2000).

CLINICAL MANIFESTATIONS

Patients with hyperkalemia may experience changes shown on ECGs, irregular pulse, vague muscle weakness, flaccid paralysis, anxiety, nausea, abdominal cramping, and diarrhea.

LABORATORY AND ECG FINDINGS

- Serum potassium: Greater than 5.5 mEq/L
- ABG values: Metabolic acidosis (decreased pH and bicarbonate ion)
- ECG: Widened QRS, prolonged PR, and ventricular dysrhythmias (Fig. 3–9)
- If dehydration is causing hyperkalemia, then hematocrit, hemoglobin, and sodium and chloride levels should be drawn.
- If associated with renal failure, creatinine and BUN levels should be drawn.

TREATMENT/COLLABORATIVE MANAGEMENT

The goal is to treat the underlying cause and return the serum potassium to a safe level. In acute hyperkalemia, the administration of I.V. calcium gluconate, glucose and insulin, beta$_2$ agonists, or sodium bicarbonate are temporary. It is usually necessary to follow these medications with a therapy that removes potassium from the body (Heitz & Horne, 2005).

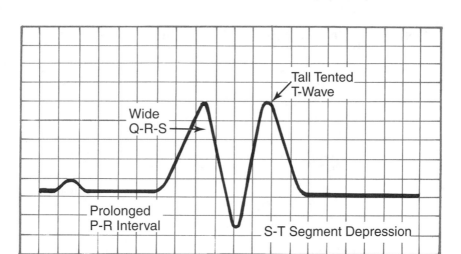

Figure 3-9 ■ Sample ECG tracing: Hyperkalemia. The ECG tracing for hyperkalemia shows progressive changes; tall, thin T waves; prolonged PR intervals; ST-segment depression; widened QRS; and loss of P wave.

The following are guidelines for the treatment of patients with hyperkalemia:

1. The goal is to treat the underlying cause and return the serum potassium level to normal.
2. Restrict dietary potassium in mild cases.
3. Discontinue supplements of potassium.
4. Cation-exchange resins (Kayexalate) may be given PO, NG, or via retention enema to exchange sodium for potassium in the bowel.
5. Administer I.V. calcium gluconate if necessary for cardiac symptoms. Administer I.V. sodium bicarbonate, which alkalinizes the plasma and causes a temporary shift of potassium into the cells.
6. Administer regular insulin (10–25 U) and hypertonic dextrose (10%), which causes a shift of potassium into the cells.
7. Peritoneal dialysis or hemodialysis may be ordered.
8. A $beta_2$ agonist (albuterol or salbutamol), may be ordered by nasal inhalation or I.V. to shift potassium into the cells

Table 3-7 provides critical guidelines for nursing in treatment of patients with potassium excess.

> Table 3-7 | **CRITICAL GUIDELINES FOR REMOVAL OF POTASSIUM**

Treatment Guidelines

■ **Sodium polystyrene sulfonate** is a cation exchange resin that removes potassium from the body by exchanging sodium for potassium in the intestinal tract. This method should not be the sole treatment for severe hyperkalemia because of its slow onset. Oral sodium polystyrene sulfonate (15–30 g); may repeat every 4–6 hours as needed; it removes potassium in 1–2 hours.
Rectal sodium polystyrene sulfonate (50 g) as retention enema; when administered, use an inflated rectal catheter to ensure retention of the dissolved resin for 30–60 minutes; it removes potassium in 30–60 minutes; each enema can lower the plasma potassium concentration by 0.5–1.0 mEq/L

■ **Dialysis** is used when more aggressive methods are needed. Peritoneal dialysis is not as effective as hemodialysis. Whereas peritoneal dialysis can remove approx. 10–15 mEq/hr, hemodialysis can remove 25–35 mEq/hr.

■ **Glucose and insulin**
Insulin facilitates potassium movement into the cells, reducing the plasma potassium level. Glucose administration in nondiabetic patients may cause a marked increase in insulin release from the pancreas, producing desired plasma potassium-lowering effects. 250–500 mL of 10% dextrose with 10–15 units of regular insulin over 1 hour: The potassium-lowering effects are delayed about 30 minutes but are effective for 4–6 hours.

■ **Emergency measures**
Calcium gluconate: 10 mL of 10% calcium gluconate administered slowly over 2–3 minutes. Administer only to patients who need immediate myocardial protection against toxic effects of severe hyperkalemia. Protective effect begins within 1–2 minutes and lasts only 30–60 minutes.
Sodium bicarbonate: 45 mEq (1 ampule of 7.5% sodium bicarbonate) infused slowly over 5 minutes. This temporarily shifts potassium into the cells and is helpful in patients with metabolic acidosis.

Sources: Gahart & Nazareno (2008); Heitz & Horne (2005).

NURSING POINTS-OF-CARE
HYPERKALEMIA

Nursing Assessments
- Obtain client history relative to high-risk factors for hyperkalemia (renal disease, potassium-sparing diuretics, excessive salt substitute use).
- Assess for signs of hyperkalemia.
- Obtain baseline ECG; assess for altered T waves.
- Obtain baseline serum potassium.

Key Nursing Interventions
1. Monitor the laboratory test results, especially serum potassium.
2. Keep accurate intake and output records.
3. Monitor for changes in cardiac response.
4. Monitor vital signs, with special attention to tachycardia and bradycardia.

Calcium (Ca^{2+})

Normal Reference Value: 8.5 to 10.5 mg/dL

Physiologic Role

The physiologic role of calcium includes:

- Maintaining skeletal elements; calcium is needed for strong, durable bones and teeth
- Regulating neuromuscular activity
- Influencing enzyme activity
- Converting prothrombin to thrombin, a necessary part of the material that holds cells together

The calcium ion is most abundant in the skeletal system, with 99% residing in the bones and teeth. Only 1% is available for rapid exchange in the circulating blood bound to protein. The parathyroid hormone (PTH) is responsible for transfer of calcium from the bone to plasma. PTH also augments the intestinal absorption of calcium and enhances net renal calcium reabsorption. Calcium is acquired through dietary intake. Adults require approximately 1 g of calcium daily, along with vitamin D and protein, which are required for absorption and utilization of this electrolyte.

Calcium is instrumental in activating enzymes and stimulating essential chemical reactions. It plays an important role in maintaining the normal transmission of nerve impulses and has a sedative effect on nerve cells. Calcium plays its most important role in the conversion of prothrombin to thrombin, a necessary sequence in the formation of a clot.

Calcium and phosphate have a reciprocal relationship; that is, an increase in calcium level causes a drop in the serum phosphorus concentration, and a drop in calcium causes an increase in phosphorus level.

Calcium is present in three different forms in the plasma: (1) ionized (50% of total calcium); (2) bound (less than 50% of total calcium); and (3) complexed (small percentage that combines with phosphate). Only ionized calcium (i.e., calcium affected by plasma pH, phosphorus, and albumin levels) is physiologically important. A relationship between ionized calcium and plasma pH is reciprocal; an increase in pH decreases the percentage of calcium that is ionized. The relationship between plasma phosphorus and ionized calcium is also reciprocal. Albumin does not affect ionized calcium, but it does affect the amount of calcium bound to proteins.

Serum Calcium Deficit: Hypocalcemia

A reduction of total body calcium levels or a reduction of the percentage of ionized calcium causes hypocalcemia. Total calcium levels may be decreased as a result of increased calcium loss, or altered regulation (hypoparathyroidism). The most common cause of low total calcium level is hypoalbuminemia.

Etiology

Total calcium levels may be decreased because of increased calcium loss, reduced intake secondary to altered intestinal absorption, and altered regulation, as in those with hypoparathyroidism.

The most common cause of hypocalcemia is inadequate secretion of PTH caused by primary hypoparathyroidism or surgically induced hypoparathyroidism. It can also result from calcium loss through diarrhea and wound exudate, acute pancreatitis, hyperphosphatemia usually associated with renal failure, inadequate intake of vitamin D or minimal sun exposure, prolonged nasogastric tube suctioning resulting in metabolic alkalosis, and infusion of citrated blood (citrate–phosphate–dextrose).

Many drugs can lead to the development of hypocalcemia, including potent loop diuretics dioxin, Dilantin, and phenobarbital, antineoplastic drugs, some radiographic contrast media, large doses of corticosteroids, heparin, and antacids (Hogan & Wane, 2003).

Clinical Manifestations

Patients with hypocalcemia may experience neuromuscular symptoms such as numbness of the fingers, cramps in the muscles (especially the extremities), hyperactive deep tendon reflexes, and a positive **Trousseau's sign** (Fig. 3-10) and **Chvostek's sign** (Fig. 3-11).

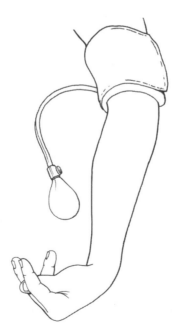

Figure 3-10 ■ Positive Trousseau's sign. Carpopedal attitude of the hand when blood pressure cuff is placed on the arm and inflated above systolic pressure for 3 minutes. A positive reaction is the development of carpal spasm.

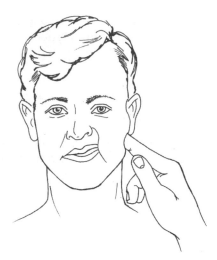

Figure 3-11 ■ Positive Chvostek's sign, which occurs after tapping the facial nerve approximately 2 cm anterior to the earlobe. Unilateral twitching of the facial muscle occurs in some patients with hypocalcemia.

Other symptoms include irritability, memory impairment, delusions, seizures (late), prolonged QT interval, and altered cardiovascular hemodynamics that may precipitate congestive heart failure. In patients with hypocalcemia caused by citrated blood transfusion, the cardiac index, stroke volume, and left ventricular stroke work values have been found to be lower.

The most dangerous symptom associated with hypocalcemia is the development of laryngospasm and tetany-like contractions. A low magnesium level and a high potassium level potentiate the cardiac and neuromuscular irritability produced by a low calcium level. However, a low potassium level can protect patients from hypocalcemic tetany.

LABORATORY AND RADIOGRAPHIC FINDINGS

- Total serum calcium less than 8.5 mg/dL
- Ionized calcium level less than 4.0 mg/dL
- Radiographic films detect bone fractures and thinning
- Bone mass density tests for signs of osteoporosis
- Potential for hypomagnesemia (1 mg/dL)
- Potential for hypokalemia (less than 3.5 mEq/mL)
- Hyperphosphatemia (greater than 2.6 mEq/mL)
- Potential for elevated creatinine from renal insufficiency

TREATMENT/COLLABORATIVE MANAGEMENT

The goal of treatment is to alleviate the underlying cause. Treatment of patients with hypocalcemia consists of:

1. Administration of calcium gluconate, orally (preferred) with calcium supplements, 1000 mg/day, to raise the total serum calcium level by 1 mg/dL.

2. Patients with symptomatic hypocalcemia less than 7.5 mg/dL usually require parenteral calcium. Hypocalcemia in adults is treated with 5 to 20 mL (2.3–9.3 mEq) of a 10% solution by I.V. injection slowly.
Or
Diluted in 1000 mL of 0.9% sodium chloride over 12 to 24 hours. Do not exceed 200 mg/min (Gahart & Nazareno, 2008).

NOTE > Follow current rate administration guidelines for safe I.V. administration of medications.

NURSING POINTS-OF-CARE
HYPOCALCEMIA

Nursing Assessments
- Obtain history relative to potential causes of hypocalcemia, such as low-calcium diet, lack of vitamin D, low-protein diet, chronic diarrhea, or hormonal disorders.
- Obtain history of drugs that could predispose the patient to hypocalcemia, such as furosemide (Lasix) or cortisone.
- Assess for signs of hypocalcemia.
- Obtain baseline values for serum calcium, ionized calcium serum albumin, and acid–base status.

Key Nursing Interventions
1. Observe safety precautions and prepare to adopt seizure precautions if hypocalcemia is severe
2. Monitor laboratory test results with emphasis on serum and ionized calcium.
3. Monitor ECGs for changes in pattern.
4. Monitor for irritation of subcutaneous tissue and tissue sloughing when calcium is given parenterally.
5. Monitor for signs of cardiac arrhythmias in patients receiving digitalis and calcium supplements.
6. Monitor for hypocalcemia in patients receiving massive transfusion of citrated blood.

Serum Calcium Excess: Hypercalcemia

Hypercalcemia is caused by excessive release of calcium from bone, almost always from malignancy, hyperparathyroidism, thiazide-diuretic use, or excessive calcium intake.

ETIOLOGY

Most symptoms of hypercalcemia are present only when the serum calcium level is greater than 12 mg/dL and tend to be more severe if hypercalcemia develops quickly. Causes of hypercalcemia include hyperparathyroidism, Paget's disease, multiple fractures, and overuse of calcium-containing antacids. Patients with solid tumors that have metastasized, such as breast, prostate, and malignant melanomas, and hematologic tumors, such as lymphomas, acute leukemia, and myelomas, are also at risk for developing hypercalcemia.

Drugs that predispose an individual to hypercalcemia include calcium salts, megadoses of vitamin A or D, thiazide diuretics (potentiate the action of PTH), androgens or estrogen for breast cancer therapy, I.V. lipids, lithium, and tamoxifen.

CLINICAL MANIFESTATIONS

Patients with hypercalcemia may experience neuromuscular symptoms such as muscle weakness, incoordination, lethargy, deep bone pain, flank pain, and pathologic fractures (caused by bone weakening). Other symptoms include constipation, anorexia, nausea, vomiting, polyuria or polydipsia leading to uremia if not treated, and renal colic caused by stone formation. Patients taking digitalis must take calcium with extreme care because it can precipitate severe dysrhythmias.

LABORATORY AND RADIOGRAPHIC FINDINGS

- Total serum calcium: May be more than 10.5 mg/dL.
- Serum ionized calcium: Greater than 5.5 mg/dL
- Serum parathyroid hormone: Increased levels in primary or secondary hyperparathyroidism
- Radiography: May reveal osteoporosis, bone cavitations, or urinary calculi.

TREATMENT/COLLABORATIVE MANAGEMENT

Hypercalcemia should be treated according to the following guidelines:

1. Treat the patient's underlying disease.
2. Administer saline diuresis. Fluids should be forced to help eliminate the source of the hypercalcemia. A solution of 0.45% NaCl or 0.9% NaCl I.V. dilutes the serum calcium level. Rehydration is important to dilute the Ca^{2+} ion and promote renal excretion.
3. Give inorganic phosphate salts orally (Neutra-Phos) or rectally (Fleet Enema).
4. Provide hemodialysis or peritoneal dialysis to reduce serum calcium levels in life-threatening situations.
5. Use furosemide, 20 to 40 mg every 2 hours, to prevent volume overloading during saline administration.

6. Administer calcitonin, 4 to 8 U/kg intramuscularly or subcutaneously every 6 to 12 hours. This will temporarily lower the serum calcium level by 1 to 3 mg/100 mL.
7. Give bisphosphonates to inhibit bone reabsorption. Pamidronate is effective, 60 to 90 mg in 1 L of 0.9% NaCl or 5% dextrose in water infused over 24 hours.

NURSING POINTS-OF-CARE
HYPERCALCEMIA

Nursing Assessments
- Obtain a patient history of probable cause of hypercalcemia, such as cancer; excessive use of calcium supplements, antacids, or thiazide diuretics; or steroid therapy.
- Assess for signs of hypercalcemia.
- Obtain baseline values for serum calcium and serum phosphate.
- Obtain baseline ECG.
- Assess client's fluid volume status and mental alertness.

Key Nursing Interventions
1. Monitor changes in vital signs and laboratory tests.
2. Encourage the patient to drink 3 to 4 L of fluid per day.
3. Encourage the patient to consume fluids (e.g., cranberry or prune juice) that promote urine acidity to help prevent formation of renal calculi.
4. Keep accurate fluid intake and output records.
5. Monitor for digitalis toxicity (toxic level greater than 2 ng/mL)
6. Handle the patient gently to prevent fractures.
7. Encourage the patient to avoid high-calcium foods.

Magnesium (Mg^{2+})

Normal Reference Value: 1.5 to 2.5 mEq/L

Physiologic Role
The physiologic role of magnesium includes:
- Enzyme action
- Regulation of neuromuscular activity (similar to calcium)
- Regulation of electrolyte balance, including facilitating transport of sodium and potassium across cell membranes, influencing the utilization of calcium, potassium, and protein

Magnesium is a major intracellular electrolyte. The normal diet supplies approximately 25 mEq of magnesium. Approximately one third of serum magnesium is bound to protein; the remaining two thirds exists as free cations. The same factors that regulate calcium balance have an influence on magnesium balance. Magnesium balance is also affected by many of the same agents that decrease or influence potassium balance.

Magnesium acts directly on the myoneural junction and affects neuromuscular irritability and contractility, possibly exerting a sedative effect. Magnesium acts as an activator for many enzymes and plays a role in both carbohydrate and protein metabolism. Magnesium affects the cardiovascular system, acting peripherally to produce vasodilation. Imbalances in magnesium predispose the heart to ventricular dysrhythmias (Metheny, 2000).

Serum Magnesium Deficit: Hypomagnesemia

Hypomagnesemia is often overlooked in critically ill patients. This imbalance is considered to be one of the most underdiagnosed electrolyte deficiencies (Metheny, 2000). Symptoms of hypomagnesemia tend to occur when the serum level drops below 1.0 mEq/L.

Etiology

Hypomagnesemia can result from chronic alcoholism; malabsorption syndrome, especially if the small bowel is affected; prolonged malnutrition or starvation; prolonged diarrhea; acute pancreatitis; administration of magnesium-free solutions for more than one week; and prolonged nasogastric tube suctioning.

Drugs that predispose an individual to hypomagnesemia include aminoglycosides, diuretics, cortisone, amphotericin, digitalis, cisplatin, and cyclosporine. Infusion of collected blood preserved with citrate can also cause hypomagnesemia (Heitz & Horne, 2005).

Clinical Manifestations

Patients with hypomagnesemia often experience neuromuscular symptoms, such as hyperactive reflexes, coarse tremors, muscle cramps, positive Chvostek's and Trousseau's signs (see Figs. 3-4 and 3-5), seizures, paresthesia of the feet and legs, and painfully cold hands and feet. Other symptoms include disorientation, dysrhythmias, tachycardia, and increased potential for digitalis toxicity.

Laboratory And ECG Findings

- Serum magnesium: Less than 1.5 mEq/L
- Urine magnesium: Helps to identify renal causes of magnesium depletion.

- Serum albumin: A decrease may cause a decreased magnesium level resulting from the reduction in protein-bound magnesium.
- Serum potassium: Decreased because of failure of the cellular sodium–potassium pump to move potassium into the cell and because of the accompanying loss of potassium in the urine
- Serum calcium: May be reduced because of a reduction in the release and action of PTH.
- ECG: Findings of tachydysrhythmia, prolonged PR and QT intervals, widening of the QRS, ST segment depression, and flattened T waves. A form of ventricular tachycardia (i.e., torsades de pointes) associated with all three electrolyte imbalances (i.e., magnesium, calcium, and potassium) may develop.

TREATMENT/COLLABORATIVE MANAGEMENT

Treatment of patients with hypomagnesemia includes identification and removal of the cause.

1. Administering oral magnesium salts: Magnesium oxide (Mag-Ox) or magnesium chloride (Slow-Mag). Magnesium containing antacids may also be used.
2. Administering 4 g diluted in 250 mL of 5% dextrose in water at 3 mL/min.
3. Administering 1 to 2 g (2–4 mL of a 50% solution) diluted in 10 mL of 5% dextrose in water by direct I.V. push at a rate of 1.5 mL/min (Gahart & Navarone, 2008).

NOTE > Follow current rate administration guidelines for safe I.V. administration of medications.

Table 3-8 provides critical guidelines for nurses who are administering magnesium.

> Table 3-8	**CRITICAL GUIDELINES FOR ADMINISTRATION OF MAGNESIUM**

- Double-check the order for magnesium administration to ensure that it stipulates the concentration of the solution to be used. Do not accept orders for "amps" or "vials" without further clarification.
- Use caution in patients with impaired renal function; watch urine output.
- Reduce other CNS depressants when given concurrently with magnesium preparations.
- Therapeutic doses of magnesium can produce flushing and sweating, which occur most often if the administration rate is too fast.
- Closely assess patients receiving magnesium.

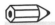

> *NURSING FAST FACT!*
>
> *Be aware that other CNS depressants could cause further depressed sensorium when magnesium sulfate is being administered. Therefore, be prepared to deal with respiratory arrest if hypermagnesemia inadvertently occurs during administration of magnesium sulfate.*

NURSING POINTS-OF-CARE
HYPOMAGNESEMIA

Nursing Assessments
- Obtain a patient history, being alert to factors that predispose to hypomagnesemia such as alcoholism, laxative abuse, total parenteral nutrition (TPN), and potassium-wasting diuretic use.
- Assess for signs and symptoms of hypomagnesemia.
- Obtain baseline values for laboratory tests, serum magnesium, serum calcium, and serum potassium.
- Obtain baseline ECG.

Key Nursing Interventions
1. Monitor vital signs.
2. Monitor for dysphagia, nausea, and anorexia.
3. Monitor for muscle weakness and athetoid movements (slow, involuntary twisting movements).
4. Monitor closely for digitalis toxicity (toxic level >2 ng/mL)
5. Keep accurate intake and output records.
6. Initiate seizure precautions if necessary to protect from injury.

Serum Magnesium Excess: Hypermagnesemia

Hypermagnesemia occurs when a person's serum level is greater than 2.5 mEq/L. The most common cause of hypermagnesemia is renal failure in patients who have an increased intake of magnesium.

ETIOLOGY

Renal factors that lead to hypermagnesemia include renal failure, Addison's disease, and inadequate excretion of magnesium by kidneys.

Other causes include hyperparathyroidism; hyperthyroidism; and iatrogenic causes such as excessive magnesium administration during treatment of patients with eclampsia, hemodialysis with excessively hard water with a dialysate inadvertently high in magnesium, or ingestion of medications high in magnesium, such as antacids and laxatives.

CLINICAL MANIFESTATIONS

The major symptoms of hypermagnesemia are the result of depressed peripheral and central neuromuscular transmissions. Patients with hypermagnesemia may experience neuromuscular symptoms such as flushing and sense of skin warmth, lethargy, sedation, hypoactive deep tendon reflexes, depressed respirations, and weak or absent cry in newborn. Other symptoms include hypotension, sinus bradycardia, heart block, and cardiac arrest (serum level greater than 15 mEq/L) and increased susceptibility to digitalis toxicity, nausea, vomiting, and seizures. Most common cause of hypermagnesemia is individuals with renal failure who have an increased intake of magnesium (Heitz & Horne, 2005).

LABORATORY AND ECG FINDINGS

- Serum magnesium: Greater than 2.5 mEq/L
- ECG: Findings of QT interval and atrioventricular block may occur (at levels greater than 2.5 mEq/L).

TREATMENT/COLLABORATIVE MANAGEMENT

The goal of treatment is to remove cause of hypermagnesemia such as discontinuing or avoiding use of magnesium containing medications, especially in clients with decreased renal function. Guidelines for treatment of patients with hypermagnesemia are:

1. Decrease oral magnesium intake.
2. Administer diuretics and 0.45% sodium chloride solution to enhance magnesium excretion in clients with adequate renal function.
3. Administer I.V. calcium gluconate (10 mL of 10% solution) to antagonize the neuromuscular effects of magnesium for patients with lethal hypermagnesemia.
4. Support respiratory function.
5. Administer peritoneal or hemodialysis in severe cases of hypermagnesemia.

NURSING POINTS-OF-CARE
HYPERMAGNESEMIA

Nursing Assessments
- Evaluate possible causes of hypermagnesemia, including renal insufficiency and chronic laxative use.
- Assess for signs of hypermagnesemia.
- Obtain baseline values for serum magnesium and serum calcium.
- Obtain baseline ECG.

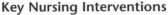

Key Nursing Interventions
1. Monitor vital signs for decreased blood pressure, pulse, and respirations.
2. Observe for flushing of the skin.
3. Monitor laboratory test values (hypochloremia).
4. Monitor for ECG changes.
5. Encourage fluid intake if not contraindicated.
6. Provide ventilatory assistance or resuscitation if necessary.

Phosphate (HPO_4-)

Normal Reference Value: 3.0 to 4.5 mg/dL

Physiologic Role

The physiologic role of phosphorus is:
- Phosphorus is essential to all cells.
- Role in metabolism of proteins, carbohydrates, and fats
- Essential to energy, necessary in the formation of high-energy compounds adenosine triphosphate (ATP) and adenosine diphosphate (ADP)
- As a cellular building block, it is the backbone of nucleic acids and is essential to cell membrane formation.
- Delivery of oxygen; functions in formation of red blood cell enzyme.

Approximately 80% of phosphorus in the body is contained in the bones and teeth, and 20% is abundant in the ICF. PTH plays a major role in homeostasis of phosphate because of its ability to vary phosphate reabsorption in the proximal tubule of the kidney. PTH also allows for the shift of phosphate from bone to plasma.

Phosphorus plays an important role in delivery of oxygen to tissues by regulating the level of 2,3-diphosphoglycerate (2,3-DPG), a substance in red blood cells that decreases the affinity of hemoglobin for oxygen.

 NURSING FAST FACT!

Phosphorus and calcium have a reciprocal relationship: an increase in the phosphorus level frequently causes hypocalcemia.

Serum Phosphate Deficit: Hypophosphatemia

Phosphorus is a critical constituent of all the body's tissues. Hypophosphatemia occurs when the serum level is below the lower limit of normal (less than 2.5 mg/dL). This imbalance may occur in the presence of total body phosphate deficit or may merely reflect a temporary shift of phosphorus into the cells.

Etiology

Hypophosphatemia can result from overzealous refeeding, total parenteral nutrition administered without adequate phosphorus, malabsorption syndromes, or alcohol withdrawal. GI losses include vomiting, chronic diarrhea, and malabsorption syndromes.

Hormonal influences such as hyperparathyroidism enhance renal phosphate excretion. Drugs that predispose an individual to hypophosphatemia include aluminum-containing antacids (which bind phosphorus, thereby lowering serum levels), diuretics, androgens, corticosteroids, glucagon, epinephrine, gastrin, and mannitol. Other causes include treatment of patients with diabetic ketoacidosis (dextrose with insulin causes a shift of phosphorus into cells). In hypophosphatemia the oxygen-carrying capacity of the blood decreases due to decreased 2,3-DPG and gas exchange. With decreased 2,3-DPG levels, the oxyhemoglobin dissociation curve shifts to the right, that is, at a given oxygen tension of arterial blood (PaO_2) level, more oxygen is bound to hemoglobin and less is available to the tissues (Heitz & Horne, 2005).

Clinical Manifestations

Hypophosphatemia can affect the CNS, neuromuscular and cardiac status, and the blood. An affected patient may experience disorientation, confusion, seizures, paresthesia (early), profound muscle weakness, tremor, ataxia, incoordination, dysarthria, dysphagia, and congestive cardiomyopathy. Hypophosphatemia affects all blood cells, especially red cells. It causes a decline in 2,3-DPG levels in erythrocytes. 2,3-DPG in red cells normally interacts with hemoglobin to promote the release of oxygen.

Laboratory and Radiographic Findings

- Serum phosphorus: Less than 2.5 mg/dL (1.7 mEq/L)
- Serum PTH: Elevated
- Serum magnesium: Decreased because of increased urinary excretion of magnesium
- Serum alkaline phosphatase: Increased with increased osteoblastic activity
- Radiography: Skeletal changes of osteomalacia or rickets

Treatment/Collaborative Management

Treatment should focus on identification and elimination of the cause such as avoiding use of phosphorus-binding antacids. Treatment can also include:

1. For mild to moderate deficiency, oral phosphate supplements, such as Neutra-Phos or Phospho-Soda, can be administered.
2. For severe hypophosphatemia, administer I.V. sodium phosphorus or potassium phosphorus solutions.

NURSING POINTS-OF-CARE
HYPOPHOSPHATEMIA

Nursing Assessments
- Obtain a patient history with focus on factors that put patients at high risk for hypophosphatemia, such as alcoholism, use of TPN, and diabetic ketoacidosis.
- Assess for signs of hypophosphatemia.
- Obtain baseline laboratory values of serum phosphate and serum calcium.

Key Nursing Interventions
1. Monitor for cardiac, GI, and neurologic abnormalities.
2. Monitor for changes in laboratory test values.
3. Keep accurate intake and output records.
4. Use safety precautions when a patient is confused.
5. Monitor for refeeding syndrome once oral feeding is restarted after prolonged starvation.
6. Monitor for other electrolyte complications of phosphorus administration (hypocalcemia, hyperphosphatemia).

Serum Phosphate Excess: Hyperphosphatemia

ETIOLOGY

Hyperphosphatemia can result from renal insufficiency, hypoparathyroidism, or increased **catabolism**. It is also seen in patients with cancer states such as myelogenous leukemia and lymphoma.

Drugs that can predispose an individual to hyperphosphatemia include oral phosphates, I.V. phosphates; phosphate laxatives; and excessive vitamin D, tetracyclines, and methicillin. Other causes include massive blood transfusions caused by phosphate leaking from the blood cells.

CLINICAL MANIFESTATIONS

Patients with hyperphosphatemia may experience many symptoms, including hypocalcemia; tetany (short-term); soft tissue calcification (long-term); mental changes, such as apprehension, confusion, and coma; and increased 2,3-DPG levels in red blood cells.

LABORATORY AND RADIOGRAPHIC FINDINGS

- Serum phosphorus: Greater than 4.5 mg/dL (2.6 mEq/L)
- Serum calcium: Useful in assessing potential consequences of treatment
- Serum PTH: Decreased in those with hypoparathyroidism

- BUN: To assess renal function
- Radiography: Skeletal changes of osteodystrophy

TREATMENT/COLLABORATIVE MANAGEMENT

Treatment should include the following regimen:

1. Identify the underlying cause of hyperphosphatemia.
2. Restrict dietary intake.
3. Administer the intake of phosphate-binding gels (e.g., Amphojel, Basaljel, and Dialume).

NURSING POINTS-OF-CARE
HYPERPHOSPHATEMIA

Nursing Assessments
- Obtain a patient history for factors that place patients at high risk for hyperphosphatemia, including renal insufficiency and laxative use.
- Assess for signs and symptoms of hyperphosphatemia.
- Obtain baseline laboratory values for serum phosphate.
- Assess 24-hour urinary output; less than 600 mL/day increases serum phosphate levels.

Key Nursing Interventions
1. Monitor for cardiac, GI, and neuromuscular abnormalities.
2. Monitor changes in laboratory test values.
3. Keep accurate intake and output records.
4. Observe the patient for signs and symptoms of hypocalcemia; when phosphate levels increase, calcium levels decrease.

Table 3-9 summarizes clinical problems associated with electrolyte imbalances.

Chloride (Cl⁻)

Normal Reference Value: 95 to 108 mEq/L

Physiologic Role

The physiologic role of chloride is:
- Regulation of serum osmolarity
- Regulation of fluid balance; when sodium is retained chloride is also retained, causing water retention and increased fluid volume.
- Control of acidity of gastric juice

- Regulation of acid–base balance
- Role in oxygen–carbon dioxide exchange (chloride shift)

Chloride is the major anion in the ECF. Changes in serum chloride concentration are usually secondary to changes in one or more of the

> Table 3-9	CLINICAL PROBLEMS ASSOCIATED WITH ELECTROLYTE IMBALANCES			
Clinical Problem	Sodium (Na⁺)	Potassium (K⁺)	Calcium (Ca²⁺)	Magnesium (Mg²⁺)
Cardiovascular				
Myocardial infarction	Na⁺↓ (hypervolemia)	K⁺↓	—	Mg²⁺↓
Heart failure (HF)	Na⁺↑	K⁺/N	—	Mg2⁺↓/N
Gastrointestinal				
Vomiting and diarrhea	Na⁺↓	K⁺↓	Ca²⁺↓	Mg²⁺↓
Malnutrition	Na⁺↓	K⁺↓	Ca²⁺↓	Mg²⁺↓
Anorexia	Na⁺↓	K⁺↓	Ca²⁺↓	Mg²⁺↓
Intestinal fistula	Na⁺↓	K⁺↓		Mg²⁺↓
GI surgery	Na⁺↓	K⁺↓		Mg²⁺↓
Chronic alcoholism	Na⁺↓	K⁺↓	Ca²⁺↓	Mg²⁺↓
Hyperphosphatemia			Ca²⁺↓	
Transfused citrated blood			Ca²⁺↓	
Endocrine				
Cushing's syndrome	Na⁺↑	K⁺↓		Mg²⁺↓
Addison's disease	Na⁺↓	K⁺↑		Mg²⁺↓
Diabetic ketoacidosis	Na⁺↑	K⁺↑ Diuresis K⁺↓	Ca²⁺↓ ↓ionized	Mg²⁺↓ Diuresis Mg²⁺↓
Parathyroidism (Hypo)			Ca²⁺↓	
Parathyroidism (Hyper)			Ca²⁺↑	
Renal				
Acute renal failure	Na⁺↑	Oliguria K⁺↑ Diuresis K⁺↓		Mg²⁺↑
Chronic renal failure	Na⁺↑		Ca²⁺↑/↓	Mg²⁺↑
Miscellaneous				
Cancer	Na⁺↓	K⁺↓/↑	Ca²⁺↑	Mg²⁺↓
Burns	Na⁺↓	K⁺↓/↑	Ca²⁺↓	Mg²⁺↓
Acute pancreatitis			Ca²⁺↓	
Syndrome of inappropriate antidiuretic hormone (SIADH)	Na⁺↓			
Metabolic acidosis		K⁺↓	Ca²⁺↓	
Metabolic alkalosis		K⁺↓		

N = normal.

other electrolytes. Chloride has a reciprocal relationship with bicarbonate (HCO_3^-). For example, a decrease in HCO_3^- concentrations results in a reciprocal rise in chloride level; when chloride level decreases, HCO_3^- level increases in compensation. Chloride exists primarily combined as sodium chloride or hydrochloric acid. Measurement of serum chloride is most frequently done for its inferential value.

Reabsorption of chloride by the renal tubules is one of the major regulatory functions of the kidneys. As sodium chloride is reabsorbed, water follows through osmosis. It is through this function that vascular blood volume is maintained.

Chloride plays its most important role in acid–base balance. Its role in the pH balance of the ECF is referred to as the "chloride shift." The chloride shift is an ionic exchange that occurs within red blood cells. This shift preserves the electrical neutrality of the red blood cells and maintains a 1:20 ratio of carbonic acid and HCO_3^- that is essential for pH balance of the plasma.

NOTE > Chloride is discussed further under acid–base balance, and imbalances in chloride are reflected in metabolic alkalosis and metabolic acidosis.

▪ Acid–Base Balance

The regulation of the hydrogen ion concentration of body fluids is actually the key component of acid–base balance. The pH of a fluid reflects the hydrogen ion concentration of that fluid. The normal pH of arterial blood ranges from 7.35 to 7.45. A solution is either basic or acidic on the basis of the concentration of hydrogen ions in the solution, and the pH scale is used to describe the hydrogen ion concentration. The pH scale is a logarithmic scale with values from 0.00 to 14.00. A neutral solution (i.e., neither acidic nor basic) has a pH of 7.00 (Porth & Martin, 2008).

The inverse proportion of the pH to the concentration of hydrogen ions is reflected in the concept that the higher the pH value, the lower the hydrogen ion concentration. Conversely, the lower the pH value, the higher the hydrogen ion concentration. Therefore, a pH below 7.35 reflects an acidic state, but a pH greater than 7.45 indicates alkalosis and a lower hydrogen ion concentration. A variation from 7.35 to 7.45 of 0.4 in either direction can be fatal. Figure 3-12 shows the pH scale.

Three mechanisms operate to maintain the appropriate pH of the blood:

1. Chemical buffer systems in the ECF and within the cells
2. Removal of carbon dioxide by the lungs
3. Renal regulation of the hydrogen ion concentration

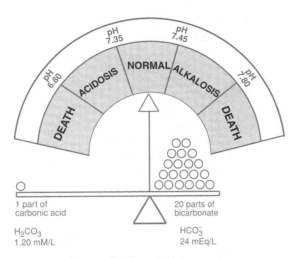

Figure 3-12 ■ Acid–base scale.

Chemical Buffer Systems

The buffer systems are fast-acting defenses that provide immediate protection against changes in the hydrogen ion concentration of the ECF. The buffers also serve as transport mechanisms that carry excess hydrogen ions to the lungs.

A buffer is a substance that reacts to minimize **pH** changes when either acid or base is released into the system. There are three primary buffer systems in the ECF: the hemoglobin system, the plasma protein system, and the bicarbonate system. The capacity of a buffer is limited; therefore, after the components of a buffer system have reacted, they must be replenished before the body can respond to further stress.

The hemoglobin and deoxyhemoglobin found in red blood cells, together with their potassium salts, act as buffer pairs. The electrolyte chloride shifts in and out of the red blood cells according to the level of oxygen in the blood plasma. For each chloride ion that leaves a red blood cell, a bicarbonate ion enters the cell; for each chloride ion that enters a red blood cell, a bicarbonate ion is released.

Plasma proteins are large molecules that contain the acid (or base) and salt form of a buffer. Proteins then have the ability to bind or release hydrogen ions.

The bicarbonate buffer system maintains the blood's pH in the range of 7.35 to 7.45 with a ratio of 20 parts bicarbonate to 1 part carbonic acid by a process that is called hydration of carbon dioxide and is a means of buffering the excess acid in the blood. If a strong acid is added to the body, the ratio is upset. In this acid imbalance, the largest amount of carbon dioxide diffuses in the plasma to the red blood cells; carbon dioxide then combines with plasma protein. Carbon dioxide that is dissolved in the blood combines with water to form carbonic acid (Smeltzer, Bare, Hinkle, & Cheever, 2008).

Respiratory Regulation

In healthy individuals, the lungs form a second line of defense in maintaining the acid–base balance. When carbon dioxide combines with water, H_2CO_3 is formed. Therefore, an increase in the acid carbon dioxide lowers the pH of blood, creating an acidotic state; a decrease in the carbon dioxide level increases the pH, causing the blood to become more alkaline. After H_2CO_3 is formed, it dissociates into carbon dioxide and water. The carbon dioxide is transferred to the lungs, where it diffuses into the alveoli and is eliminated through exhalation. Therefore, the rate of respiration affects the hydrogen ion concentration. An increase in respiratory rate causes carbon dioxide to be blown off by the lungs, resulting in an increase in pH. Conversely, a decrease in respiratory rate causes retention of carbon dioxide and thus a decrease in pH. This means that the lungs can either hold the hydrogen ions until the deficit is corrected or inactivate the hydrogen ions into water molecules to be exhaled with the carbon dioxide as vapor, thereby correcting the excess. It takes from 10 to 30 minutes for the lungs to inactivate the hydrogen molecules by converting them to water molecules (Smeltzer, Bare, Hinkle, & Cheever, 2008).

Renal Regulation

The kidneys regulate the hydrogen ion concentration by increasing or decreasing the HCO_3^- ion concentration in the body fluid by a series of complex chemical reactions that occur in the renal tubules. The regulation of acid–base balance by the kidneys occurs chiefly by increasing or decreasing the HCO_3^- ion concentration in body fluids. Hydrogen is secreted into the tubules of the kidney, where it is eliminated in the urine. At the same time, sodium is reabsorbed from the tubular fluid into the ECF in exchange for hydrogen and combines with HCO_3^- ions to form the buffer, $NaHCO_3$.

The kidneys help to regulate the extracellular concentration of HCO_3^-. Two buffer systems help the kidney to eliminate excess hydrogen in the urine: the phosphate buffer system and the ammonia buffer system. With each of these, an excess of hydrogen is secreted and HCO_3^- ions are formed; sodium is reabsorbed, thus forming $NaHCO_3$. The time it takes for a change to occur in the acid–base balance can range from a fraction of a second to more than 24 hours. Although the kidneys are the most powerful regulating mechanism, they are slow to make major changes in the acid–base balance (Metheny, 2000).

Major Acid–Base Imbalances

There are two types of acid–base imbalances: (1) metabolic (base bicarbonate deficit and excess) **acidosis** and **alkalosis** and (2) respiratory (carbonic acid deficit and excess) acidosis and alkalosis. The balanced pH of the arterial blood is 7.4, and only small variations of up to 0.05 can exist without causing ill effects. Deviations of more than five times the normal concentration of H+ in the ECF are potentially fatal (Horne & Derrico, 1999).

Metabolic Acid–Base Imbalances

Normal Reference Value: 22 to 26 mEq/L

Metabolic Acidosis: Base Bicarbonate Deficit

Metabolic acidosis (HCO_3^- deficit) is a clinical disturbance characterized by a low pH and low plasma HCO_3^- level. This condition can occur by a gain of hydrogen ion (H^+) or a loss of HCO_3^-.

Etiology

Metabolic acidosis occurs with loss of HCO_3^- from diarrhea, draining fistulas, and administration of TPN. Diabetes mellitus, alcoholism, and starvation cause ketoacidosis. Respiratory or circulatory failure, ingestion of certain drugs or toxins (e.g., salicylates, ethylene glycol, or methyl alcohol), some hereditary disorders, and septic shock cause lactic acidosis. It can also result when renal failure results in excessive retention of hydrogen ions.

 NURSING FAST FACT!

Hyperkalemia is usually present in clinical cases of acidosis (Metheny, 2000).

Clinical Manifestations

Patients with metabolic acidosis may experience CNS-related symptoms such as headache, confusion, drowsiness, increased respiratory rate, and Kussmaul respirations. Other symptoms include nausea, vomiting, decreased cardiac output, and bradycardia (when serum pH is less than 7.0).

Laboratory and ECG Findings

- ABG values: pH less than 7.35, HCO_3^- less than 22 mEq/L
- $PaCO_2$: Less than 38 mm Hg
- Serum HCO_3^-: Less than 22 mEq/L
- Serum electrolytes: Elevated potassium possible, because of exchange of intracellular potassium for hydrogen ions in the body's attempt to normalize acid–base environment
- ECG: Dysrhythmias caused by hyperkalemia

COMMON CAUSES OF METABOLIC ACIDOSIS

- Gastrointestinal abnormalities: Starvation, severe malnutrition or chronic diarrhea
- Renal abnormalities: Kidney failure
- Hormonal influences: Diabetic ketoacidosis, hyperthyroidism, thyrotoxicosis

Others: Trauma, shock, excess exercise, severe infection, fever

TREATMENT/COLLABORATIVE MANAGEMENT

Patients with metabolic acidosis are treated by

1. Reversing the underlying cause (e.g., diabetic ketoacidosis, alcoholism related to ketoacidosis, diarrhea, acute renal failure, renal tubular acidosis, poisoning, or lactic acidosis)
2. Eliminating the source (if the cause is excessive administration of sodium chloride)
3. Administering $NaHCO_3$ (7.5% 44.4 mEq/50 mL or 8.4% 50 mEq/50 mL I.V. when pH is equal to or less than 7.2). Concentration depends on severity of acidosis and presence of any serum sodium disorders.
4. Potassium replacement: Hyperkalemia is usually present, but potassium deficit can occur. If a deficit of less than 3.5 mEq/L is present, the potassium deficit must be corrected before $NaHCO_3$ is administered because the potassium shifts back into the ICF when the acidosis is correct.

 NURSING FAST FACT!

> Give $NaHCO_3$ cautiously to avoid patients' developing metabolic alkalosis and pulmonary edema secondary to sodium overload.

NURSING POINTS-OF-CARE
METABOLIC ACIDOSIS

Nursing Assessments
- Obtain a patient history of health problems that relate to metabolic acidosis such as diabetes or renal disease.
- Obtain baseline vital signs with focus on the respiration and cardiac functioning.
- Assess for symptoms of metabolic acidosis.
- Obtain baseline values for arterial blood gases (ABGs) and laboratory tests. Note the serum electrolytes, serum CO_2 content, HCO_3^-, and blood sugar level.

Key Nursing Interventions
1. Provide safety precautions when a patient is confused.
2. Monitor for signs and symptoms of metabolic acidosis.
3. Monitor the patient's dietary and fluid intake and output record.
4. Monitor laboratory results for changes.
5. Monitor the patient for changes in vital signs, especially changes in respiration, cardiac function, and CNS signs.

Metabolic Alkalosis: Base Bicarbonate Excess

Metabolic alkalosis (i.e., HCO_3^- excess) is a clinical disturbance characterized by a high pH and a high plasma HCO_3^- concentration and can be produced by a gain of HCO_3^- or a loss of hydrogen ion.

Etiology

Metabolic alkalosis occurs with GI loss of hydrogen ions from gastric suctioning and vomiting. Renal loss of hydrogen ions occurs from potassium-losing diuretics, excess of mineralocorticoid, hypercalcemia, and hypoparathyroidism. In patients with hypokalemia and carbohydrate refeeding after starvation, hydrogen ions shift from ECF into the cells, depleting serum levels. This also occurs when excessive ingestion of alkalis (e.g., antacids such as Alka-Seltzer), parenteral administration of $NaHCO_3$ during cardiopulmonary resuscitation, and massive blood transfusions increase serum levels of HCO_3^-.

Clinical Manifestations

Patients with metabolic alkalosis may experience dizziness and depressed respirations in addition to impaired mentation, tingling of fingers and toes, circumoral paresthesia, and hypertonic reflexes. Other symptoms include hypotension, cardiac dysrhythmias, hyperventilation, hypokalemia, and decreased ionized calcium (i.e., carpopedal spasm).

Laboratory and ECG Findings

- ABG values: pH greater than 7.45; HCO_3^- greater than 26 mEq/L
- $PaCO_2$: Greater than 42 mm Hg
- Serum HCO_3^-: Greater than 26 mEq/L
- Serum electrolytes: Low serum potassium (less than 4 mEq/L) and low serum chloride
- ECG: Assess for dysrhythmias (Heitz & Horne, 2005).

Common Causes of Metabolic Alkalosis

- Chloride depletion: Loss of gastric secretions, vomiting, NG drainage, diarrhea
- Potassium depletion: Primary aldosteronism, mineral corticoid excess, laxative abuse

- Hypercalcemic states: Hypercalcemia of malignancy, acute milk alkali syndrome
- Miscellaneous: Medication (bicarbonate ingestion, carbenicillin, ampicillin)

Refeeding syndrome, hypoproteinemia.

 NURSING FAST FACT!

Hypokalemia is often present in patients with alkalosis.

TREATMENT/COLLABORATIVE MANAGEMENT

Patients with metabolic alkalosis are treated by

1. Reversing the underlying cause
2. Administration of sufficient chloride for the kidney to excrete the excess HCO_3^- usually isotonic sodium chloride infusion may correct deficit.
3. Replace potassium if K^+ is low, usually potassium chloride is preferred because chloride losses can be replaced simultaneously (Heitz & Horne, 2005).
4. Carbonic anhydrase inhibitors: Acetazolamide (Diamox) is useful for correcting metabolic alkalosis for patients who cannot tolerate rapid volume expansion. Acetazolamide causes a large increase in renal secretion of HCO_3^- and K^+ so may be necessary to supplement potassium prior to administration of medication.
5. Administration of acidifying agents such as diluted HCl, ammonium chloride (NH_4Cl). There are serious side effects therefore this solution is not commonly used (Heitz & Horne, 2005).

NURSING POINTS-OF-CARE
METABOLIC ALKALOSIS

Nursing Assessments
- Obtain history of health problems related to metabolic alkalosis (e.g., peptic ulcer, vomiting, adrenocortical hormone abnormalities).
- Obtain baseline vital signs.
- Assess for signs and symptoms of metabolic alkalosis.
- Obtain baseline values for ABGs and serum electrolyte, serum CO_2 content, and HCO_3^-

Key Nursing Interventions
1. Use safety precautions for hyperexcitability states.
2. Monitor the patient's fluid intake and output.
3. Monitor renal and hepatic function.
4. Monitor laboratory results for changes (ABGs, potassium, and chlroide).
5. Monitor the patient for changes in vital signs, with particular attention to respirations and CNS.
6. Monitor for changes in cardiac rhythm, especially in patients taking cardiac glycosides

Respiratory Acid–Base Imbalances

Normal Reference Value: Partial pressure of carbon dioxide ($Paco_2$): 38 to 42 mm Hg.

Respiratory Acidosis: Carbonic Acid Excess

Respiratory acidosis is caused by inadequate excretion of carbon dioxide and inadequate ventilation, resulting in an increase of serum levels or carbon dioxide and H_2CO_3. Acute respiratory acidosis is usually associated with emergency situations.

ETIOLOGY

Acute respiratory acidosis can result from pulmonary, neurologic, and cardiac causes, such as pulmonary edema; aspiration of a foreign body; pneumothorax; severe pneumonia; severe, prolonged exacerbation of acute asthma; overdose of sedatives; cardiac arrest; and massive pulmonary embolism.

Chronic respiratory acidosis results from emphysema, bronchial asthma, bronchiectasis, postoperative pain, obesity, and tight abdominal binders.

CLINICAL MANIFESTATIONS

Acute signs and symptoms include tachypnea; dyspnea; dizziness; seizures; warm, flushed skin, and ventricular fibrillation. Chronic signs and symptoms occur if $Paco_2$ exceeds the body's ability to compensate, and include respiratory symptoms.

LABORATORY AND RADIOGRAPHIC FINDINGS

- ABG values: *Acute:* pH less than 7.35, $Paco_2$ greater than 42 mm Hg, HCO_3^- greater than 26 mEq/L. *Chronic:* pH less than 7.35, $Paco_2$ greater than 42 mm Hg, HCO_3^- normal or slight increase
- Serum HCO_3^-: Reflects acid–base balance; initial values normal unless mixed disorder is present.
- Serum electrolytes: Usually not altered

- Chest radiography: Determines the presence of underlying pulmonary disease.
- Drug screen: Determines the quantity of drug if patient is suspected of taking an overdose.

Common Causes of Respiratory Acidosis

Acute:

- Pulmonary/thoracic disorders: Severe pneumonia, acute respiratory distress syndrome (ARDS), flail chest, pneumothorax, smoke inhalation
- Increased resistance to air flow: Upper airway obstruction, aspiration, laryngospasm, severe bronchospasm
- CNS depression: Sedative overdose, anesthesia

Chronic:

- Obstructive diseases: Emphysema, chronic bronchitis, cystic fibrosis, obstructive sleep apnea.
- Restriction of ventilation: Kyphoscoliosis, hydrothorax, severe chronic pneumonitis, obesity–hypoventilation (pickwickian syndrome)
- Neuromuscular abnormalities: Spinal cord injuries, poliomyelitis, muscular dystrophy, multiple sclerosis
- Depression of respiratory center: Brain tumor, chronic sedative overdose

Treatment/Collaborative Management

The goal is to treat the underlying cause.
Respiratory acidosis is treated by carrying out the following:

1. Restore normal acid–base balance: Support respiratory function
2. Administer bronchodilators or antibiotics for respiratory infections as indicated.
3. Administer oxygen as indicated.
4. Administer adequate fluids (2–3 L/day) to keep mucous membranes moist and help remove secretions.

NURSING POINTS-OF-CARE
RESPIRATORY ACIDOSIS

Nursing Assessments
- Obtain history of pneumonia, chronic obstructive pulmonary disease (COPD), narcotic use, or emphysema.
- Obtain baseline vital signs.
- Assess for signs and symptoms of respiratory acidosis.
- Obtain baseline values for laboratory tests, especially $Paco_2$.

Key Nursing Interventions
1. Provide safety precautions when a patient is confused.
2. Monitor laboratory results for changes, especially pH and $Paco_2$.
3. Monitor for changes in vital signs.
4. Monitor oxygen and mechanical ventilator when in use.
5. Elevate the head of the patient's bed.
6. Encourage the patient to perform deep-breathing exercise.
7. Perform chest percussions to break up mucus when appropriate.

Respiratory Alkalosis: Carbonic Acid Deficit

Respiratory alkalosis is usually caused by hyperventilation, which causes "blowing off" of carbon dioxide and a decrease in H_2CO_3 content. Respiratory alkalosis can be acute or chronic.

ETIOLOGY

Acute respiratory alkalosis results from pulmonary disorders that produce hypoxemia or stimulation of the respiratory centers. Underlying causes of hypoxemia include high fever, pneumonia, congestive heart failure, pulmonary emboli, hypotension, asthma, and inhalation of irritants. Causes of stimulation of respiratory centers include anxiety (most common), excessive mechanical ventilation, CNS lesions involving the respiratory center, and salicylate overdose (an early sign).

CLINICAL MANIFESTATIONS

Respiratory alkalosis causes light-headedness, the inability to concentrate, numbness and tingling of the extremities (circumoral paresthesia), tinnitus, palpitations, epigastric pain, blurred vision, precordial pain (tightness), sweating, dry mouth, tremulousness, seizures, and loss of consciousness.

LABORATORY AND ECG FINDINGS

- ABG values: pH greater than 7.45, $Paco_2$ less than 38 mm Hg, HCO_3^- less than 22 mEq/L
- Serum electrolytes: Presence of metabolic acid–base disorders
- Serum phosphate: May fall to less than 0.5 mg/dL.
- ECG: Determines cardiac dysrhythmias

COMMON CAUSES OF RESPIRATORY ALKALOSIS

- Hypoxemia: Pneumonia, hypotension, severe anemia, congestive heart failure
- Stimulation of pulmonary or pleural receptors: Pulmonary emboli, pulmonary edema, asthma, inhalation of irritants

- Central stimulation of respiratory center: Anxiety, pain, intracerebral trauma
- Hyperventilation, mechanical: Fever, sepsis (gram negative), hepatic disease

TREATMENT/COLLABORATIVE MANAGEMENT

In respiratory alkalosis, the underlying disorder must be treated.

Treatment of patients with respiratory alkalosis consists of the following:

1. Treat the source of anxiety (instruct patient to breathe slowly into a paper bag).
2. Administer a sedative as indicated.
3. Oxygen therapy if hypoxemia is causative factor.
4. Adjustments to mechanical ventilators: Settings checked and adjustments made to ventilatory parameters in response to ABG results.

NURSING POINTS-OF-CARE
RESPIRATORY ALKALOSIS

Nursing Assessments
- Obtain a patient history of hysteria, fever, or severe infection.
- Check for signs and symptoms of respiratory alkalosis.
- Obtain baseline vital signs.
- Obtain ABG and electrolyte values.

Key Nursing Interventions
1. Encourage the patient who is hyperventilating to breathe slowly.
2. Have the patient rebreathe expired air by breathing into a paper bag.
3. Administer a sedative as directed.
4. Listen to the patient who is in emotional distress.
5. Monitor for respiratory alkalosis.
6. Determine the cause of hyperventilation.
7. Monitor ABG values and electrolyte levels (potassium, calcium).

Table 3-10 presents a summary of acute acid–base imbalances.

> Table 3-10 **SUMMARY OF ACUTE ACID–BASE IMBALANCES**

The Body's Reaction to Acid–Base Imbalance

Condition	pH	$Paco_2$	HCO_3^-	How the Body Compensates
Respiratory acidosis	↓	↑	Normal	
With compensation	↓	↑	↑	Kidneys conserve HCO_3^- and eliminate H^+ to increase pH
Respiratory alkalosis	↑	↓	Normal	
With compensation	Slightly ↓ or normal	↓	↓	Kidneys eliminate HCO_3^- and conserve H^+ to decrease pH
Metabolic acidosis	↓	Normal	↓	
With compensation	↓	↓	↓	Hyperventilation to blow off excess CO_2 and conserve HCO_3^-
Metabolic alkalosis	↑	Normal	↑	
With compensation	Slightly ↓ or normal	↑	↑	Hypoventilation to ↑ CO_2; kidneys keep H^+ and excrete HCO_3^-

Common Causes of Acid–Base Imbalance

Respiratory acidosis	Asphyxis, respiratory depression, CNS depression
Respiratory alkalosis	Hyperventilation, anxiety, PE (causing hyperventilation)
Metabolic acidosis	Diarrhea, renal failure, salicylate overdose such as ASA (aspirin)
Metabolic alkalosis	Hypercalcemia, overdose on an alkaline substance such as antacid

AGE-RELATED CONSIDERATIONS

The Pediatric Client

Infants have proportionately more body fluid (70–80% of body weight) than any other age group. Infants are at higher risk for fluid volume deficit during times of increased external temperatures. In infants (children younger than 18 months of age) sunken or depressed fontanels can indicate fluid volume deficit (FVD) and bulging fontanels can indicate FVE. In addition, in children, skin turgor begins to diminish after 3% to 5% of body weight is lost.

Assess FVD in children focus on capillary refill time, skin turgor and respiratory pattern because these factors are more significant in identifying dehydration, but imprecise and still difficult to determine the exact degree of dehydration (Steiner, DeWalt, & Byerley, 2004).

> *EBNP Recommendations by Aker (2002) for pediatric NPO times have been revised to allow clear liquids up to 2 hours preoperatively for pediatric clients less than 6 months of age and up to 3 hours preoperatively for pediatric clients 6 months and older to fluid deficit id decreased (Aker, 2002).*

There are two types of hypocalcemia in newborn infants. The first occurs early after birth during the first 3 days of life; this is attributed to parathyroid immaturity or maternal hyperparathyroidism. This resolves within the first week of life (Metheny, 2000). The second type of neonatal hypocalcemia occurs about 1 week after birth and is associated with hyperphosphatemia and hypomagnesemia. Providing milk with a high phosphorus level can lead to hyperphosphatemia and then hypocalcemia (Narins, 1994).

The Older Adult

Fluid balance in elderly persons is affected by physiologic changes associated with aging. Older people do not possess the fluid reserves of younger individuals or the ability to adapt readily to rapid changes. Alterations in fluid and electrolyte balance frequently accompany illness. The total body water in the elderly is reduced by 6%, which creates a potential for fluid volume deficit. In an elderly person, the thirst mechanism is less effective than it is in a younger person. Older persons are more prone to dehydration. Cardiovascular and respiratory changes in the elderly combine to contribute to a slower response to the stress of blood loss, fluid depletion, shock and acid–base imbalances (Metheny, 2000).

The elderly client has a decreased ability to adapt to rapid increases in intravascular volume and can quickly develop fluid overload. Sodium and fluid overload is common in hospitalized elderly clients and can result in increased morbidity and mortality in surgical clients (Allison & Lobo, 2004).

Dehydration and chronic hyponatremia can lead to confusional states that interfere with fluid intake in elderly people, who are very susceptible to dehydration.

> *EBNP Dehydrated older adults have significantly lower systolic and diastolic blood pressures and significantly higher BUN levels but similar creatinine levels compared with nondehydrated adults (Bennett, Thomas, & Riegel, 2004).*

Home Care Issues

- Consider home health care for patients with diabetes mellitus, cardiovascular disorders, and severe GI disorders.
- Consider home health care for patients taking drug therapy (diuretics) for edema.
- Consider home health care for dietary follow up, and instructions on use of pressure stockings.
- Assess patient taking oral electrolyte supplements for adherence

Patient Education

- Teach patient risk factors for development of FVD or FVE.
- Explain to client and family the reasons for intake and output records.
- Teach the client to keep track of oral liquids consumed.
- Assess the patient's understanding of the type of fluid loss being experienced.
- Give verbal and written instructions for fluid replacement (drink at least 3 quarts of liquid).
- Teach the patient to increase the fluid intake during hot days, in the presence of fever or infection and to decrease activity during extreme weather.
- Teach how to observe for dehydration (especially in infants).
- Instruct the patient to seek medical consultation for continued dehydration.
- Teach appropriate use of laxatives, enemas, and diuretics.
- Inform the patient to notify the physician if he or she has excessive edema or weight gain (more than 2 lbs) or increased shortness of breath.
- Provide literature concerning low-salt diets; consult with dietitian if necessary.
- Provide dietary education on sodium and potassium and teach to avoid adding salt while cooking, and in addition information on salt substitutes
- Teach to avoid caffeine because it acts as a mild diuretic.
- Provide written material and verbal instructions regarding any medications.
- Provide information on predisposing factors associated with specific electrolyte imbalances.

Patient Education—cont'd

■ Review indicators of digitalis toxicity, if appropriate.
■ Provide information on dietary sources of electrolytes in deficit situations when appropriate.
■ Provide information on over-the-counter medications (e.g., magnesium and aluminum hydroxide, antacids and phosphorus-binding antacids, laxatives, multivitamin and mineral supplements) when appropriate.
■ Educate the patient with cancer about symptoms of hypercalcemia.
■ Educate the patient on the high phosphorus content of processed foods, carbonated beverages, and over-the-counter medications when appropriate.

■ Nursing Process

The nursing process is a five- or six-step process for problem-solving to guide nursing action. Refer to Chapter 1 for details on the steps of the nursing process related to vascular access. The following tables focus on nursing diagnoses and nursing outcomes for patients with fluid, electrolyte, and acid–base imbalances. Nursing diagnoses should be patient specific and outcomes and interventions individualized. The NOC and NIC presented here are suggested direction for development of outcomes and interventions.

Nursing diagnoses and interventions are specific to the underlying pathophysiologic process. In addition, these may be considered.

Nursing Diagnoses to Fluid and Related Imbalance Electrolyte	NOC: Nursing Outcomes Classification	NIC: Nursing Intervention Classification
Activity intolerance risk for: risk factor: Muscle weakness or neuromuscular irritability secondary to electrolyte imbalance	Activity tolerance, energy conservation	Energy management
Cardiac output decreased related to: Negative inotropic changes associated with reduced myocardial functioning from severe phosphorus depletion Electrical alterations associated with tachydysrhythmias or digitalis toxicity; possible dysrhythmia from electrolyte imbalance	Cardiac pump effectiveness, circulation status, tissue perfusion, vital signs	Cardiac care

Nursing Diagnoses to Fluid and Related Imbalance Electrolyte	NOC: Nursing Outcomes Classification	NIC: Nursing Intervention Classification
Fluid volume deficit or excess related to: Failure of regulatory mechanisms; active fluid volume loss or gain	Electrolyte and acid–base balance, fluid balance, hydration	Fluid management, hypovolemia management, shock management: volume, fluid monitoring
Injury risk for related to: neurosensory alterations: Altered mental functioning, drowsiness and weakness; sensory or neuromuscular dysfunction from hypophosphatemia-induced central nervous system disturbances Altered sensorium from primary hypernatremia or cerebral edema occurring with too-rapid correction of hypernatremia Tetany—precipitation of calcium phosphate in the soft tissue and periarticular region of the large joints sensory or neuromuscular dysfunction as a result of hypomagnesemia Tetany and seizures related to neurosensory alterations from severe hypocalcemia	Personal safety; risk control; safe home environment. Remain free of injury.	Health education; environmental modification
Knowledge deficit related to: The purpose of phosphate binders and the importance of reducing GI absorption of phosphorus Importance of avoiding excessive or inappropriate use of magnesium-containing medications for client with chronic renal failure	Knowledge of diet, disease process, health behavior, health resources, medication, and treatment regimen	Teaching: disease process, learning facilitation
Nutrition altered: more than body requirements related to: Excessive intake in relation to metabolic needs: excess intake of phosphate containing compounds; oral and I.V. magnesium supplements and chronic use of drugs containing magnesium	Nutritional status, nutrient intake	Nutrition management
Nutrition altered: less than body requirements, related to: Inadequate nutritional intake, chronic alcoholism, intravenous fluid (including TPN) with lack of phosphate additive, magnesium related to history of poor intake, anorexia, or alcoholism Effects of vitamin D deficiency, renal failure, malabsorption, laxative use	Nutritional status; food and fluid intake, nutrient intake	Feeding, nutrition management
Tissue perfusion, ineffective (peripheral perfusion) related to: Hypervolemia; hypovolemia	Fluid balance	Circulatory care and monitoring

Sources: Ackley & Ladwig (2008); Carpenito-Moyet (2008); McCloskey, Dochterman, & Bulechek (2004); Moorhead, Johnson, & Maas (2004); NANDA-I (2007); Newfield, Hinz, & Tilley (2007).

Nursing Diagnoses Related to Acid–Base Balance	NOC: Nursing Outcomes Classification	NIC: Nursing Intervention Classification
Airway clearance ineffective related to: Physiological factors or obstructed airway	Aspiration prevention; respiratory status: airway patency, gas exchange, ventilation	Airway management, airway suctioning, cough enhancement
Gas exchange, impaired related to: Alveolar-capillary membrane changes; ventilation-perfusion imbalance secondary to hypercapnia; hypercarbia; hypoxemia; hypoxia	Respiratory status: gas exchange	Acid–base management, airway management
Injury risk for related to: Internal: abnormal blood profile; tissue hypoxia	Personal safety behavior; risk control	Education to prevent iatrogenic harm.
Tissue perfusion, ineffective related to: Decreased hemoglobin concentration in blood; hypoventilation; impaired transport of oxygen; mismatch ventilation with blood flow	Tissue perfusion: cardiac, cerebral, peripheral	Circulatory care: arterial insufficiency

Sources: Ackley & Ladwig (2008); Carpenito-Moyet (2008); McCloskey, Dochterman, & Bulechek (2004); Moorhead, Johnson, & Maas (2004); NANDA-I (2007); Newfield, Hinz, & Tilley (2007).

Chapter Highlights

- Fluid is distributed in three compartments: Intracellular (40%), intravascular (5%), and interstitial (15%); total body weight in water is 60% for an average adult.
- Fluid is transported passively by filtration, diffusion, and osmosis.
- Electrolytes are actively transported by ATP on cell membranes and the sodium–potassium pump.
- Osmosis is the movement of water from a lower concentration to a higher concentration across a semipermeable membrane.
- The osmolarity of I.V. solutions has the following ranges:
  - Isotonic solutions: 250 to 375 mOsm/L
  - Hypotonic solutions: Less than 250 mOsm/L
  - Hypertonic solutions: Greater than 375 mOsm/L
- The homeostatic organs that regulate fluid and electrolyte balance include the kidneys; heart and blood vessels; lungs; and adrenal, parathyroid, and pituitary glands.
- There are six areas to assess for fluid balance: Neurologic status, cardiovascular, respiratory, integumentary, special senses, and body weight.
- Fluid imbalances fall into two categories:
  - Fluid volume deficit caused primarily by disorders of the GI system; signs and symptoms reflect a dehydrated individual. Treatment is aimed at rehydration with isotonic sodium chloride.

- Fluid volume excess caused primarily by cardiovascular dysfunction, renal or endocrine dysfunction, and too-rapid administration of I.V. fluids; signs and symptoms reflect fluid overload. Treatment is aimed at decreasing the sodium level, using diuretics to increase the excretion of fluids, and treating the underlying cause.
- The seven major electrolytes and their symbols are:
  - *Cations:* Sodium: Na^+, Potassium: K^+, Calcium: Ca^{2+}, Magnesium: Mg^{2+}
  - *Anions:* Chloride: Cl^-, Phosphate: HPO_4^-, Bicarbonate: HCO_3^-
- The prefix hypo-: Deficit in an electrolyte
- The prefix hyper-: Excess in an electrolyte
- Key nursing interventions for electrolyte imbalances reflect collaborative practice and are specific to the imbalance.
- Key laboratory values that the nurse must recognize:
  - Potassium (K^+): 3.5 to 5.5 mEq/L
  - Calcium (Na^+): 135 to 145 mEq/L
  - Magnesium (Mg^{2+}): 1.5 to 2.5 mEq/L
  - Phosphate (HPO_4^-): 3.0 to 4.5 mg/dL
  - Chloride (Cl^+): 95 to 108 mEq/L
- Critical guidelines for infusion potassium include:
  - Never give potassium I.V. push.
  - Concentrations of potassium greater than 60 mEq should not be given in a peripheral vein.
  - Concentrations greater than 8 mEq/100 mL can cause pain and irritation of peripheral veins, leading to phlebitis.
  - Do not add potassium to a hanging container.
  - Administer potassium at a rate not exceeding 10 mEq/hr through peripheral veins.
- Calcium and phosphate have a reciprocal relationship: When one is elevated, the other is decreased.
- Patients with calcium imbalances may need seizure precautions. The most dangerous symptom of hypocalcemia is laryngospasm.
- The four major acid–base imbalances in the body are respiratory acidosis (carbonic acid excess), respiratory alkalosis (carbonic acid deficit), metabolic acidosis (base bicarbonate deficit), and metabolic alkalosis (bicarbonate excess).
- Acid–base balance is maintained through three major reaction-specific buffer systems that regulate hydrogen ion concentration: the carbonic acid–bicarbonate system, the phosphate buffer system, and the protein buffer system.

▄▄ Thinking Critically: Case Study 1

A 60-year-old man admitted to the hospital ED with a history of diarrhea (average 8 watery stools per day) over a period of several weeks, he stated he was able to eat some and tried to increase fluids. He admitted increased stress at home and in his job. The following laboratory data was obtained:

Sodium = 135 mEq/L
Potassium = 3.0 mEq/L
Chloride = 111 mEq/L
Arterial pH = 7.25
$Paco_2$ = 28 mm Hg
HCO_3^- = 12 mEq/L

What is the focus of your assessment? What nursing diagnoses can be made from these data?

What collaborative diagnosis can be made? What interventions would you anticipate?

■■ Thinking Critically: Case Study 2

A 28-year-old woman was admitted to the hospital after 3 days of severe diarrhea and poor intake. She weighs 120 lbs (54.5 kg) on admission, pre-illness weight, 132 lbs (60 kg). Her BUN was 40 mg/dL and serum creatinine was 1.3 mg/dL, potassium was 3.2 mEq/mL, sodium 133 mEq/mL. Skin turgor was poor and urine output was 15 mL/hr (specific gravity 1.030). Blood pressure was 120/80 mm Hg recumbent and fell to 98/60 mm Hg when erect. Pulse was 110, weak and regular.

What percentage of body weight did she lose?
What concerns would the nurse have regarding her laboratory work?
What nursing diagnoses would apply to this woman?
What nursing interventions would be implemented?
What collaborative orders would you anticipate?

 Media Link: Answers to the case study questions and more critical thinking activities are provided on the CD–ROM.

Post-Test

1. The nurse administering 0.45% sodium chloride in 5% dextrose in water understands that this solution will hydrate the intravascular and intracellular spaces based on which of the following transport mechanisms?

   a. Diffusion
   b. Osmosis
   c. Filtration
   d. Sodium–potassium pump

2. You have just completed a physical assessment of a 68-year-old man. He knows who he is but is unsure of where he is (previous orientation normal). His eyes are sunken, his mouth is coated with an extra longitudinal furrow, and his lips are cracked. Hand vein filling takes more than 5 seconds, and tenting of the skin appears over the sternum. His vital signs are blood pressure of 128/60 mm Hg, pulse

of 78, and respiratory rate of 16 (previously 150/78, 76, 16, respectively). Your assessment would lead you to suspect:

a. Fluid volume deficit
b. Hyponatremia
c. Fluid volume excess
d. Hypernatremia

3. If the external temperature is 101°F (38.4°C), which of the following age groups is at highest risk for fluid volume deficit?

a. Infants
b. School-age children
c. Adolescents
d. Middle-aged adults

4. Which of the following could be the etiology for a nursing diagnosis of fluid volume excess? (*Select all that apply.*)

a. Excessive infusion of 0.9% sodium chloride solution
b. Use of diuretics
c. SIADH
d. Congestive heart failure

5. Which of the following laboratory values are consistent with fluid volume deficit?

a. Urine specific gravity 1.005
b. Blood urea nitrogen 6 mg/100 mL
c. Hematocrit 52%
d. Serum osmolarity 305 mOsm/kg

6. Match the following signs and symptoms in Column I to the clinical manifestation in Column II.

Column I	Column II
a. Flushing, lethargy, hypoactive deep tendon reflexes, depressed respirations	1. Hypokalemia
b. Weakness, deep bone pain, pathologic fractures	2. Hypermagnesemia
c. Fatigue, headache, apprehension, serum Na^+ 115 mEq/L	3. Hypocalcemia
d. ECG with flat or inverted T wave, depressed ST segment	4. Hypercalcemia
e. ECG with peaked, narrow T wave, shortened QT interval, prolonged PR interval followed by disappearance of P wave.	5. Hypernatremia

f. Marked thirst, dry sticky mucous membranes, disorientation, chloride may be elevated.

6. Hyponatremia

g. Positive Trousseau's sign and Chvostek's sign, numbness of fingers

7. Hyperkalemia

7. Treatment for a patient with metabolic alkalosis includes which of the following? (*Select all that apply.*)
   a. Removal of underlying cause
   b. I.V. fluid administration with NaCl
   c. Replacement of potassium deficit
   d. Administer I.V. solution with sodium bicarbonate

8. To correct metabolic acidosis, the parenteral fluid of choice is:
   a. $NaHCO_3$
   b. NaCl
   c. Albumin
   d. 5% dextrose in water

9. A nursing diagnosis that would be appropriate for the patient with calcium deficit would be:
   a. Ineffective breathing pattern related to biochemical imbalances
   b. Altered comfort related to injuring agent
   c. Risk for protection ineffective: Risk of tetany and seizures related to neurosensory alterations from severe hypocalcemia.
   d. Altered urinary elimination pattern related to changes in renal function.

10. An 80-year-old frail man has had nausea, vomiting, and diarrhea for several days. When he becomes weak and confused he is admitted to the hospital. The best indicator of the client's rehydration status, the nurse should assess the client's:
    a. Mucous membranes
    b. Weight gain of 2.2 lbs
    c. Urinary output
    d. Skin turgor

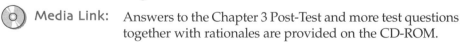

Media Link: Answers to the Chapter 3 Post-Test and more test questions together with rationales are provided on the CD-ROM.

▪ References

Ackley, B.J., & Ladwig, G.B. (2008). *Nursing diagnosis handbook: An evidence-based guide to planning care.* St. Louis: Mosby Elsevier.

Aker, J. (2002). Pediatric fluid management. *Current Review of Pain, 24*(7), 73–84.

Allison, S.P., & Lobo, D.N. (2004). Fluid and electrolytes in the elderly. *Current Opinion in Clinical Nutrition and Metabolic Care, 7*(1), 27.

Armstrong, L.E. (2005). Hydration assessment technqiues. *Nutrition Reviews, 63*(6Pt2), S40–S54.

Ayus, J.C., & Arieff, A.L (1999). Symptomatic hyponatremia: Making the diagnosis rapidly. *Journal of Critical Care, 5*(8), 846–856.

Ayus, J.C., & Arieff, A.L. (1996). Abnormalities of water metabolism in the elderly. *Seminars in Nephrology, 16*(4), 277–288.

Ayus, J.C., Varon, J., & Arieff, A.I. (2000). Hyponatremia, cerebral edema, and noncardiogenic pulmonary edema in marathon runners. *Annals of Internal Medicine, 32,* 711–714.

Bennett, J.A., Thomas V., & Riegel, B. (2004). Unrecognized chronic dehydration in older adults: Examining prevalence rate and risk factors. *Journal of Gerontology Nursing, 30*(11), 22–28.

Berne R.M., & Levy, M. (2000). *Principles of physiology* (3rd ed., p. 438). St. Louis, MO: C.V. Mosby.

Carpenito-Moyet, L.J. (2008). *Nursing diagnosis: Application to clinical practice* (12th ed.). Philadelphia: Lippincott, Williams & Wilkins

Craven, R.F., & Hirnle, C.J. (2003). *Fundamentals of nursing: Human health and function* (4th ed.). Philadelphia: Lippincott, Williams & Wilkins.

Gahart, L., & Nazareno, A.R. (2008). 2008 *Intravenous medications* (24th ed.). St. Louis, MO: Mosby Elsevier.

Giger, J.N., & Davidhizar, R.E. (2004). *Transcultural nursing: Assessment and intervention* (4th ed.). St. Louis, MO: C.V. Mosby.

Hankins, J. (2006). The role of albumin in fluid and electrolyte balance. *Journal of Infusion Nursing, 29*(5), 260–265.

Heitz, Y., & Horne, M.M. (2005). *Pocket guide to fluid, electrolyte and acid-base balance* (5th ed.). St. Louis, MO: C.V. Mosby.

Hew-Butler, T., Almond C., Ayus, J.C., et al. (2005). *Consensus statement of the 1st international exercise-associated hyponatremia development conference.* Cape Town, South Africa. *Clinical Journal of Sports Medicine, 15,* 208–213.

Hogan, M.A., & Wane, D. (2003). *Fluids, electrolytes, and acid–base balance: Reviews and rationales* (pp. 17–27). Upper Saddle River, NJ: Prentice-Hall.

Holliday, M.A., & Segar, W.E. (1957). The maintenance need for water in parenteral fluid therapy. *Pediatrics, 19,* 823–832.

Horne, C., & Derrico, D. (1999). Mastering ABGs. *American Journal of Nursing, 99*(8), 26–33.

Kee, J.L., Paulanka, B.J., & Purnell, L.D. (2004). *Fluids and electrolytes with clinical applications a programmed approach* (7th ed.). Clifton Park, NY: Thomson Delmar Learning

McCloskey-Dochterman, J.C., & Bulechek, G.M. (2004). *Nursing interventions classification (NIC)* (4th ed.). St. Louis, MO: C.V. Mosby.

Metheny, N.M. (1997). Focusing on the dangers of D5W. *Nursing 97, 10*, 55–59.

Metheny, N.M. (2000). Fluid and electrolyte balance. *Nursing considerations* (4th ed.). Philadelphia: Lippincott Williams & Wilkins.

Moorhead, S., Johnson, M., & Maas, M. (2004). *Nursing outcomes classification (NOC)* (3rd ed.). St. Louis, MO: C.V. Mosby.

NANDA-I (2007). *Nursing diagnoses: Definitions and classification, 2007–2008.* Philadelphia: Author

Newfield, S., Hinz, M., Tilley, D.S., et al. (2007). *Cox's clinical applications of nursing diagnosis.* Philadelphia: F. A. Davis.

Porth, C.M., & Martin, G. (2008). *Pathophysiology concepts of altered health states* (8th ed.). Philadelphia: Lippincott Williams & Wilkins

Rios, H., Delaney, C., & Kruckeberg, T. (1991). Validation of defining characteristics of four nursing diagnoses using a computerized data base. *Journal of Professional Nursing, 7*, 293.

Siegel, A.J. (2007). Hypertonic (3%) sodium chloride for emergent treatment of exercise-associated hypotonic encephalopathy. Conference paper. *Sports Medicine, 37*, 94–95, 459–462.

Smeltzer, S.C., Bare, B.G., Hinkle, J.L., & Cheever, K.H. (2008). *Brunner & Suddarth's textbook of medical-surgical nursing* (7th ed.). Philadelphia: Lippincott, Williams & Wilkins

Starling, E.H. (1896). On the absorption of fluids from connective tissues spaces. *Journal of Physiology, 19*(3), 12–26.

Steiner, M.J., DeWalt, D.A., & Byerley, J.S. (2004). Is this child dehydrated? *JAMA, 291*(22), 2764.

Wakefield, B., Mentes, J., & Diggelmann, L. (2002). Monitoring hydration status in elderly veterans. *Western Journal of Nursing Research, 24*(2), 132.

Wilkinson, J.M., & Van Leuven, K. (2007). *Fundamentals of nursing: Theory, concepts, and applications.* Philadelphia: F.A. Davis.

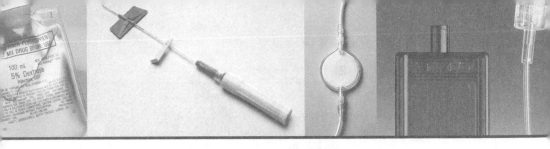

Chapter **4**

Parenteral Solutions

Let the patient's taste decide. You will say that, in cases of great thirst, the patient's craving decides that it will drink a great deal of tea, and that you cannot help it. But in these cases be sure that the patient requires diluents for quite other purposes than quenching the thirst; he wants a great deal of some drink, not only of tea, and the doctor will order what he is to have, barley water or lemonade, or soda water and milk, as the case may be.
—*Florence Nightingale, 1859*

Chapter Contents

■ LEARNING OBJECTIVES	*On completion of this chapter, the reader will be able to:*

1. Define terminology related to parenteral solutions.
2. Identify the three objectives of parenteral therapy.
3. List the key elements in intravenous (I.V.) solutions.
4. List the uses of maintenance fluids.
5. List the four functions of glucose as a necessary nutrient when administered parenterally.
6. Explain the roles of vitamin C and vitamin B complex in maintenance therapy.
7. Describe the uses of hypotonic, isotonic, and hypertonic fluids.
8. Identify the major groupings of I.V. solutions.
9. Compare the advantages and disadvantages of dextrose, sodium chloride, hydrating fluids, and balanced electrolyte fluids.
10. Identify the main role of hydrating fluids.
11. Identify the use of alkalinizing and acidifying fluids.
12. State the most commonly used isotonic multiple electrolyte solution.
13. Compare and contrast the use of colloid volume expanders (albumin, hetastarch, dextran, and gelatin).
14. Identify the formulas available for calculating the fluid needs of pediatric clients.

▧ GLOSSARY

Balanced solution   Parenteral solution that contains electrolytes in proportions similar to those in plasma; also contains bicarbonate or acetate ion

Body surface area   Surface area of the body determined through use of a nomogram.

Caloric method   Calculation of metabolic expenditure of energy, used in pediatric fluid maintenance and replacement.

Catabolism   The breakdown of chemical compounds by the body; an energy-producing metabolic process

Colloid   A substance (e.g., blood, plasma, albumin, dextran) that does not dissolve into a true solution and is not capable of passing through a semipermeable membrane

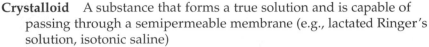

Crystalloid   A substance that forms a true solution and is capable of passing through a semipermeable membrane (e.g., lactated Ringer's solution, isotonic saline)

Dehydration   A deficit of body water; can involve one fluid compartment or all three

Hydrating solution   A solution of water, carbohydrate, sodium, and chloride used to determine adequacy of renal function

Hypertonic solution   A solution with an osmolarity higher than that of plasma, above 375 mOsm

Hypotonic solution   A solution with an osmolarity lower than that of plasma, usually below 250 mOsm

Isotonic solution   A solution with the same osmolarity as plasma, usually 250–375 mOsm

Maintenance therapy   Fluids that provide all nutrients necessary to meet daily patient requirements; usually water, glucose, sodium, and potassium

Meter square method   Formula using a nomogram to determine surface areas of a pediatric client for maintenance of fluid needs

Normal saline   Solution of salt (0.9% sodium chloride)

Oncotic pressure   The osmotic pressure exerted by colloids (proteins), as when albumin exerts oncotic pressure within the blood vessels and helps to hold the water content of the blood in the intravascular compartment

Parenteral therapy   Introduction of substances other than through the gastrointestinal tract; particularly to the introduction of substances into an organism by intravenous route, or subcutaneous, intramuscular, or intramedullary injection

Plasma volume expander   A high molecular weight compound in a solution suitable for intravenous use

Replacement therapy   Replenishment of losses when maintenance cannot be met and when patient is in a deficit state

Restoration therapy   Reconstruction of fluid and electrolyte needs on a continuing basis until homeostasis returns

Weight method   Formula based on weight in kilograms to estimate the fluid needs of the pediatric client

▪ Rationales and Objectives of Parenteral Therapy

Objectives of Delivery of Infusion Therapy

The nurse has the main responsibility of delivery of **parenteral fluid therapy**. The nurse initiates the written parenteral therapy order, monitors for patient response, and must be knowledgeable about the contents of parenteral fluids, their purposes, action on the body and the complications that may occur once delivered to the patient. The complex subject of fluids and electrolytes is covered in Chapter 3, which provides the requisite background knowledge for this chapter on parenteral therapy. To understand the use of parenteral solutions the nurse must understand two important concepts: (1) the reason or objective for the authorized physician prescriber's order of infusion therapy and (2) the type of solution ordered, together with the composition and clinical use of that solution. The goals for administration of parenteral therapy fall into three broad categories:

1. Maintenance therapy for daily body fluid requirements
2. Replacement therapy for present losses
3. Providing fluids and electrolytes necessary to replace ongoing losses (restoring homeostasis)

These three objectives differ with regard to the time necessary to complete the therapy, the purpose of the I.V. fluid, and the type of patient who is to receive the I.V. solution. Factors affecting the choice of objective in prescribing parenteral fluid and the rate of administration by the physician are the patient's renal function, daily maintenance requirements, existing fluid and electrolyte imbalance, clinical status, and disturbances in homeostasis as a result of parenteral therapy (Metheny, 2000).

Maintenance Therapy

Maintenance therapy provides nutrients that meet the daily needs of a patient for water, electrolytes, and dextrose. Water has priority. Water is also an important dilutor for waste products excreted by the kidneys. Approximately 30 mL of fluid is needed per kilogram of body weight (i.e., 15 mL/kg) for maintenance needs (Metheny, 2000). The typical patient profile for maintenance therapy is an individual who is allowed nothing by mouth (NPO) or whose oral intake is restricted for any reason. Remember that insensible loss is approximately 500 to 1000 mL every 24 hours. Maintenance therapy should be 1500 mL per square meter (m^2) of body surface over 24 hours (Metheny, 2000). For example, a man weighing 85 kg (187 lbs.) has a body surface area of 2 (m^2); 1500 times 2 equals 3000; therefore, he needs 3000 mL of fluids for maintenance therapy.

Solutions for maintenance therapy include water, daily needs of sodium and potassium, and glucose. Glucose, a necessary component in maintenance therapy, is converted to glycogen by the liver. It has four main uses in maintenance parenteral therapy:

1. Improves hepatic function.
2. Supplies necessary calories for energy.
3. Spares body protein.
4. Minimizes ketosis.

NURSING FAST FACT!

> *The basic caloric requirement for an adult is 1600 calories/day for a 70-kg adult at rest. Approximately 100–150 g of carbohydrates are needed daily to minimize protein catabolism and prevent starvation. One liter of 5% dextrose in water contains 50 g of dextrose (Metheny, 2000).*

Replacement Therapy

Replacement therapy is necessary to take care of the fluid, electrolyte, or blood product deficits of patients in acute distress; this type of therapy is supplied over a 48-hour period. Examples of conditions of patients needing replacement infusion therapy (and their replacement requirements) are:

- Hemorrhage (for replacement of cells and plasma)
- Low platelet count (for replacement of clotting factors)
- Vomiting and diarrhea (for replacement of losses of electrolytes and water)
- Starvation (for replacement of losses of water and electrolytes)

When the maintenance requirements of the body cannot be met, the physician should institute **replacement therapy**. The physician must figure the losses and calculate replacement over a 48-hour period. Kidney function is the first thing that should be checked before replacement therapy is begun. Patients requiring replacement therapy, except those in shock, require potassium. Patients under stress from tissue injury, wound infection, or gastric or bowel surgery also require potassium.

Most hospitalized patients receiving additional saline or glucose infusions are prone to developing potassium deficiency. In addition, hospitalized patients are usually under physiologic stress. Excretion of potassium in their urine can increase to 60 to 120 mEq/day even with limited intake. Tissue injury significantly increases the loss of potassium. Normal dietary intake of potassium is 80 to 200 mEq/day. Potassium is often included as part of replacement therapy (Metheny, 2000).

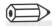 *NURSING FAST FACT!*

> *Never give more than 120 mEq of potassium in a 24-hour period unless cardiac status is monitored continuously, because it can create a life-threatening situation. Key nursing assessment: Check kidney function before administering potassium in replacement therapy.*

Carefully monitor replacement solutions with potassium for the following patients:

1. Those with dysfunction of the:
   - Renal system
   - Cardiovascular system

- Adrenal glands
- Pituitary gland
- Parathyroid gland
2. Those with deficits of:
   - Sodium
   - Calcium
   - Base bicarbonate
   - Blood volume (hypovolemic)
3. Those with excess of:
   - Base bicarbonate
   - Extracellular potassium
   - Extracellular calcium

Vitamins are necessary for utilization of the nutrients and are often added to postoperative replacement therapy. Vitamin C and vitamin B complex are used frequently in postoperative parenteral therapy, to assist in replacement, and to promote wound healing. Vitamin B complex has a role in metabolism of carbohydrates and maintenance of gastrointestinal (GI) function.

Restoration: Providing Fluids and Electrolytes to Restore Ongoing Losses

When maintenance and replacement therapy do not meet the needs of the patient, fluid and electrolyte management is accomplished with restoration therapy. With restoring ongoing losses (e.g., nasogastric tubes to suction, bleeding) critical evaluation of the source of the loss is done at least every 24 hours. Accurate documentation of intake and output is extremely important in this type of management of fluid and electrolyte therapy. Restoration of homeostasis depends on the nursing assessment of intake of I.V. fluids as well as on the documentation of all body fluid losses. The types of clinical patients who require 24-hour evaluation are those with draining fistulas, abscesses, nasogastric tubes, burns, and abdominal wounds. With these types of patients, you will see frequent changes in the types of solutions ordered, in the amounts of electrolytes ordered based on laboratory values ordered, and in the rate of infusion.

Third-space shifts such as in peritonitis, bowel obstruction, burns, ascites, some cancers, major surgery involving extensive tissue trauma, and sepsis are considered ongoing losses that must have special consideration when determining fluid needs (Heitz & Horne, 2005). Third-spacing refers to a shift of fluid from the vascular space into a portion of the body from which it is not easily exchanged with the rest of the extracellular fluid (ECF). The trapped fluid is sequestered and not available for functional use. Fluid can be sequestered from the intravascular space into body spaces (pleural or peritoneal) or it can become trapped in the bowel by obstruction or in the interstitial space as edema after burns (Metheny, 2000).

Major considerations in differentiating the fluid volume deficit associated with third-spacing from that associated with fluid lost through vomiting or diarrhea are that measurable fluid can be replaced using replacement therapy which third-space fluid cannot; in addition, decreased body weight does not occur in third spacing. Accurate dosing of fluid therapy requires monitoring, and treatment is directed at correcting the cause of the third-space shift of body fluids and be tailored to the patient's response.

Parkland Formula: Burn Resuscitation

Fluid resuscitation is complicated. The Parkland formula is often used to calculate fluid resuscitation. This formula also states that one half of the amount is given over the first 8 hours, one fourth is administered in the second 8 hours, and one fourth of the total in the third 8–hour period after the burn. Lactated Ringer's solution at 4 mL/kg/%TBSA burned. The second 24 hours the solution of choice is 25% albumin plus 5% dextrose in water with volume to maintain desired urine output.

> **Example:** A child who weighs 10 kg sustains an estimated total body surface area (TBSA) burn of 50% from a house fire. The Parkland formula of fluid resuscitation is used to determine the amount of fluid that this child requires. According to this formula, a nurse should intravenously administer _____ mL of fluid to the child in the first 8 hours from the time of the injury. Fill in the blank.
>
> **Ans:** 1000
>
> **Rationale:** The Parkland formula is:
> 4 mL of lactate solution × kg of body weight × % of TBSA burned
> 4 mL × 10 kg × 50% = 2000 mL

■ Key Elements in Parenteral Solutions

The key elements that make up crystalloid parenteral fluids include water, carbohydrates (glucose), protein, vitamins, and electrolytes. The pH of crystalloid solutions can affect the initial response to crystalloid administration and must be considered by nurses providing the infusion.

Water

There are two main physiologic mechanisms that assist in regulating body water: thirst and antidiuretic hormone (ADH). Thirst is primarily a regulator of water intake and ADH a regulator of water output. Both mechanisms respond to changes in extracellular osmolality and volume (Porth & Martin, 2008). The human body is a contained fluid environment of water and electrolytes. Holliday and Segar (1957) established that regardless of age, all healthy persons require approximately 100 milliliters (mL) of water per 100 calories metabolized, for dissolving and eliminating metabolic wastes. This means that a person who expends 1800 calories of energy requires approximately 1800 mL of water for metabolic purposes. These water needs are increased in patients with sensible water losses such as respiratory rate above 20 breaths/min, fever, and diaphoresis, as well as in low–humidity environments; in patients with decreased renal concentration ability; and in elderly people. The average adult loses 500 to 1000 mL in the form of insensible water every 24 hours. Water must be provided for adequate kidney function.

Carbohydrates (Glucose)

Glucose, a nutrient included in maintenance, restoration, and replacement therapies, is converted into glycogen by the liver, which improves hepatic function. By supplying calories for energy, it spares body protein. Sources of carbohydrates include dextrose (glucose) and fructose. When glucose is supplied by infusion, all the parenteral glucose is bioavailable. The addition of 100 g of glucose per day minimizes starvation. Every 2 L of 5% dextrose in water contains 100 g of glucose.

Amino Acids

Amino acids (protein) are the body-building nutrients whose major functions are contributing to tissue growth and repair, replacing body cells, healing wounds, and synthesizing vitamins and enzymes. Amino acids are the basic units of protein. The parenteral proteins currently used are elemental, provided as synthetic crystalline amino acids. These proteins are available in concentrations of 3.5 to 15% and are used in total parenteral nutrition (TPN) centrally or peripherally. When administered by infusion, protein bypasses the GI and portal circulation (Metheny, 2000). The usual daily requirement is 1 g of protein/kg of body weight. For example, a 54-kg woman needs 54 g of protein per day.

Vitamins

Vitamins are added to restorative and replacement therapies. Certain vitamins (i.e., the fat-soluble A, D, E, and K and water-soluble B and C vitamins) are necessary for growth and act as catalysts for metabolic processes. Some disease conditions alter vitamin requirements (Metheny, 2000). Vitamins B and C are the most frequently used in parenteral therapy. Vitamin B complex is important in the metabolism of carbohydrates and the maintenance of GI function, which is especially important in postoperative patients. Vitamin C promotes wound healing.

Electrolytes

Electrolytes are the major additives to replacement and restorative therapies. Correction of electrolyte imbalances is important in the prevention of serious complications associated with excess or deficit of electrolytes. There are seven major electrolytes in normal body fluids and the same seven major elements are supplied in manufactured I.V. solutions. (Chapter 3 reviews these electrolyte functions.) The electrolytes of major importance in parenteral therapy are potassium, sodium, chloride, magnesium, phosphorus, calcium, and bicarbonate or acetate ion (important for acid–base balance).

pH

The pH reflects the degree of acidity or alkalinity of a solution. Blood pH is not a significant problem for routine parenteral therapy. Normal kidneys can achieve an acid–base balance as long as enough water is supplied. The USP standards require that solution pH must be slightly acidic (a pH of between 3.5 and 6.2). Many solutions have a pH of 5. The acidity of solutions allows them to have a longer shelf life.

 NURSING FAST FACT!

> As the acidity of a solution increases, the solution's ability to irritate vein walls increases.

◾ Osmolality and Osmolarity of Parenteral Solutions

The osmotic activity of a solution may be expressed in terms of either its osmolarity or osmolality. Osmolarity refers to the osmolar concentration in 1 liter (L) of solution (mOsm/L) and osmolality is the osmolar concentration 1 kilogram (kg) of water (mOsm/kg of H_2O). Osmolarity is usually used when referring to fluids outside the body and osmolality for describing fluids inside the body. Because 1 L of water weighs 1 kg the terms osmolarity and osmolality are often used interchangeably (Porth & Martin, 2008).

Extracellular osmolality is primarily determined by the sodium level because it is the main solute found in extracellular fluid. A rough estimation of extracellular osmolality can be made by multiplying the plasma sodium concentration by 2 (Porth & Martin, 2008).

The term *tonicity* refers to the tension or effect that the effective osmotic pressure of a solution with impermeable solutes exerts on cell size because of water movement across the cell membrane. Tonicity is determined solely by effective solutes such as glucose that cannot penetrate the cell membrane, thereby producing an osmotic force that pulls water into or out of the cell and causing it to change size.

Solutions to which body cells are exposed can be classified as isotonic, hypotonic or hypertonic depending on whether they cause cells to swell or shrink. Cells placed in an isotonic solution, which has the same effective osmolality as intracellular fluids (ICFs; 280–295 mOsm/L), neither shrink or swell. When cells are placed in hypotonic solution, which has a lower effective osmolality than ICFs, they swell as water moves into the cell, and when they are placed in a hypertonic solution, which has a greater effective osmolality than ICF, they shrink as water is pulled out of the cell. Administration of intravenous fluids is guided by the tonicity of the solution and falls into three categories: isotonic or isosmolar, hypotonic, and hypertonic (Kraft, 2000). The effect of I.V. fluid on the body fluid compartments depends on how its osmolarity compares with the patient's serum osmolarity. Intravenous fluids can change the fluid compartment in one of three ways:

1. Expand the intravascular compartment
2. Expand the intravascular compartment and deplete the intracellular and interstitial compartments.
3. Expand the intracellular compartment and deplete the intravascular compartment

---

NOTE > Review Chapter 3 for further information on osmolarity and diagrams of fluid shifts.

Isotonic or Iso-osmolar Fluids

Isotonic solutions have an osmolarity of 250 to 375 mOsm/L. Blood and normal body fluids have an osmolarity of 285 to 295 mOsm/kg. These fluids are used to expand the ECF compartment. No net fluid shifts occur between isotonic solutions because the osmotic pressure gradient is the same inside and outside the cells. Many isotonic solutions are available. Examples include 0.9% sodium chloride, 5% dextrose in water, and lactated Ringer's solution.

Isotonic solutions are commonly used to treat fluid loss, dehydration, and hypernatremia (sodium excess). Five percent dextrose solution is used for dehydration because it replaces fluid volume without disrupting the interstitial and intracellular environment. However, this solution becomes hypotonic when dextrose is metabolized; the solution should be used cautiously in patients with renal and cardiac disease because of the increased risk of fluid overload (Kraft, 2000). This solution also does not provide enough daily calories and can lead to protein breakdown if used for extended periods of time.

Caution: The danger with the use of isotonic solutions is circulatory overload. These solutions do not cause fluid shifts into other compartments. The problem with overexpanding the vascular compartment is that the fluid dilutes the concentration of hemoglobin and lowers hematocrit levels.

Hypotonic Fluids

Hypotonic fluids have an osmolarity lower than 250 mOsm/L. By lowering serum osmolarity, the body fluids shift out of blood vessels into cells and interstitial spaces. The resulting osmotic pressure gradient draws water into the cells from the ECF, causing the cells to swell. Hypotonic solutions are used for patients who have hypertonic dehydration, water replacement, and diabetic ketoacidosis after initial sodium chloride replacement (Kraft, 2000). Examples of hypotonic solutions include 0.45% sodium chloride (half-strength saline), 0.33% sodium chloride, and 2.5% dextrose in water.

Hypotonic solutions hydrate cells and can deplete the circulatory system. Water moves from the vascular space to the intracellular space when hypotonic fluids are infused.

Caution: Do not give hypotonic solutions to patients with low blood pressure because it will further a hypotensive state.

Hypertonic Fluids

Hypertonic fluids have an osmolarity of 375 mOsm/L or higher. The resulting osmotic pressure gradient draws water from the intracellular space increasing extracellular volume and causing cells to shrink. Examples of hypertonic fluids include 5% dextrose in 0.45% sodium chloride, 5% dextrose in 0.9% sodium chloride, 5% dextrose in lactated Ringer's, 10% dextrose in water, and colloids (albumin 25%, plasma protein fraction, dextran, and hetastarch).

These fluids are used to replace electrolytes, to treat hypotonic dehydration, and in temporary treatment of circulatory insufficiency and shock. When hypertonic dextrose solutions are used alone, they also are used to shift ECF from the interstitial fluid to the plasma.

Caution: Hypertonic solutions are irritating to vein walls and may cause hypertonic circulatory overload. Some hypertonic solutions are contraindicated in patients with cardiac or renal disease because of the increased risk of congestive heart failure and pulmonary edema. Give hypertonic solutions slowly to prevent circulatory overload.

■ Types of Parenteral Solutions

Crystalloid Solutions

Crystalloids are materials capable of crystallization (i.e., have the ability to form crystals). **Crystalloids** are solutes that, when placed in a solution, mix with and dissolve into a solution and cannot be distinguished from the resultant solution. Because of this, crystalloid solutions are considered true solutions that are capable of diffusing through membranes. The vascular fluid is 25% of the ECF, and 25% of any crystalloid administered remains in the vascular space. Crystalloids must be given in three to four times the volume to expand the vascular space to a degree equal to that brought about by a colloid solution. Types of crystalloid solutions include dextrose solutions, sodium chloride solutions, balanced electrolyte solutions, and alkalizing and acidifying solutions.

Crystalloid Physiologic Initial and Therapeutic Responses

INITIAL RESPONSE EFFECT ON THE VEIN INTIMA AND RBCs

Crystalloid administration can be divided into two phases: the initial response and the therapeutic response. The initial response is the immediate reaction that occurs when the I.V. solution is introduced into the circulation (Cook, 2003). As the solution enters the blood stream, it comes into immediate contact with red blood cells (RBCs) and the cells of the vein intima. The initial response of crystalloid therapy to the vein intima may be dramatic but is not life-threatening. The intima, at the point of fluid injection, will be repeatedly subjected to the fluid. Hypotonic and hypertonic solutions change the immediate surroundings of the cell. Isotonic solutions do not alter the tonicity of the ECF; therefore the RBCs are not initially affected (Cook, 2003).

Hypotonic fluids will cause the endothelial cells to swell as water is absorbed and hypertonic solutions to draw fluid from the endothelial cells. The rate of swelling and the risk of lysis increase as the tonicity of the fluid decreases. The cells will return to their normal shape as they move into a more isotonic environment (Hill, 2004; Metheny, 2000).

Hypertonic solutions draw fluid from the endothelial cells, causing shrinkage of the RBCs. The risk of cellular dehydration increases as the tonicity of fluid increases. As red cells move toward a more isotonic environment, they regain their original shape (Hill, 2004). The administration of hypertonic saline or dextrose preparations greater than 10% through small veins is associated with phlebitis, as a result of this cellular dehydration (Cook, 2003).

THERAPEUTIC RESPONSE/SYSTEMIC EFFECTS

The therapeutic response of crystalloid administration occurs as the fluid disperse through the ECF and ICF. The therapeutic response is predictable and is the reason one fluid is chosen over another. The therapeutic response to isotonic solutions when administered by the intravenous route result in the tonicity of the plasma to remain unchanged. The solutions 0.9% sodium chloride and lactated Ringer's solutions remain isotonic even after they disperse into the interstitial spaces; therefore, the tonicity of the interstitial space is unchanged. The interstitial space is three times as large as the intravascular space; 75% of the fluid will be dispersed interstitially and 25% will remain in the plasma (Jordan, 2000).

The solution of 5% dextrose in water is considered isotonic in the initial response but the mechanics are different than with isotonic electrolyte solutions. Dextrose in water is an electrolyte-free solution. As the fluid disperses throughout ECF, the dextrose is absorbed into the cells to be used for energy. What is left is free water that dilutes the osmolality of the ECF (Porth & Martin, 2008). The cells are suddenly suspended in a hypotonic environment and, osmosis will occur, with the cells absorbing the fluid until the two compartments are isotonic. The intracellular compartment is two thirds the size of the ECF; 67% of the water will enter the cells and 33% will remain in the ECF. The dispersion of 1 liter of 5% dextrose in water will divide the 1000 mL into 667 intracellular and approximately 250 mL into the interstitial space, and 83 mL into plasma.

Many crystalloid solutions are made up of a combination of dextrose and electrolyte solutions, most of which are hypertonic initially. The therapeutic response to these fluids can be predicted based on the tonicity of the solution. Once the cells use the dextrose, the remaining sodium chloride and electrolytes will be dispersed as isotonic electrolyte solution, hydrating only the ECF. The dispersion of the solution to ECF and ICF will be dependent on the osmolarity of the solution. Remember that 5% dextrose when added to other solutions rapidly is absorbed into the cells to be used for energy (Popcock & Richards, 2000). The remaining electrolyte solution is dispersed between the ECF and ICF. The only true hypertonic crystalloid solutions are 3% and 5% sodium chloride. These remain consistently hypertonic and can cause severe cellular dehydration (Jordan, 2000).

Dextrose Solutions

Carbohydrates can be administered by the parenteral route as dextrose, fructose, or invert sugar. Dextrose is the most commonly administered carbohydrate. The percentage solutions express the number of grams of solute per 100 g of solvent. Thus a 5% dextrose in water (D5W) infusion contains 5 g of dextrose in 100 mL of water.

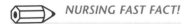 *NURSING FAST FACT!*

One milliliter of water weighs 1 g, and 1 mL is 1% of 100 mL. Milliliters, grams, and percentages can be used interchangeably when calculating solution strength. Thus, 5% dextrose in water equals 5 g of dextrose in 100 mL, and 1 L of 5% dextrose in water contains 50 g of dextrose. (Example: 250 mL of 20% dextrose in water solution contains 50 g of dextrose.)

When carbohydrate needs are inadequate, the body will use its own fat to supply calories. Dextrose fluids are used to provide calories for energy, reduce catabolism of protein, and reduce protein breakdown of glucose to help prevent a negative nitrogen balance.

The monohydrate form of dextrose used in parenteral solutions provides 3.4 kcal/g. It is difficult to administer enough calories by I.V. infusion, especially with 5% dextrose in water, which provides only 170 calories per liter. One would have to administer 9 L to meet calorie requirements, and most patients cannot tolerate 9000 mL of fluid in 24 hours. Concentrated solutions of carbohydrates in 20% to 70% dextrose are useful for supplying calories. These solutions containing high percentages of dextrose must be administered slowly for adequate absorption and utilization by the cells (Metheny, 2000).

Dextrose is a nonelectrolyte, and the total number of particles in a dextrose solution does not depend on ionization. Dextrose is thought to be the closest to the ideal carbohydrate available because it is well metabolized by all tissues. The tonicity of dextrose solutions depends on the particles of sugar in the solution. Dextrose 5% is rapidly metabolized and has no osmotically active particles after it is in the plasma. The osmolarity of a dextrose solution is determined differently from that of an electrolyte solution. Dextrose is distributed inside and outside the cells, with 8% remaining in the circulation to increase blood volume. The USP pH requirements for dextrose is 3.5 to 6.5 (Metheny, 2000).

Dextrose in water is available in various concentrations including 2.5%, 5%, 10%, 20%, 30%, 40%, 50%, and 70%. Dextrose is also available in combination with other types of solutions. The 5% and 10% concentrations can be given peripherally. Concentrations higher than 10% are given through central veins. A general exception is the administration of limited amounts of 50% dextrose given slowly through a peripheral vein for emergency treatment of hypoglycemia (usually 3 mL/min; Gahart & Nazareno, 2008).

ADVANTAGES

■ Acts as a vehicle for administration of medications.
■ Provides nutrition.

- Can be used as treatment for hyperkalemia (using high concentrations of dextrose).
- Can be used in treatment of patients with dehydration.
- Provides free water.

DISADVANTAGES

- The main disadvantage of dextrose solutions intravenously is vein irritation, which is caused by the slightly acidic pH of the solution. Vein irritation, vein damage, and thrombosis may result when hypertonic dextrose solutions are administered in a peripheral vein.
- Hyponatremic encephalopathy can develop rapidly in postoperative patients who receive excessive infusion of 5% dextrose in water. Postoperative hyponatremia can affect any patient but is much more serious in women of childbearing age. Premenopausal women who develop hyponatremic encephalopathy are 25 times more likely to have permanent brain damage or die, compared to men (Metheny, 1997).

> EBNP Siegel (2007) discusses research presented on treating acute onset of
> hyponatremia with a sodium concentration of <135 mEq/L with 3% sodium
> chloride for emergent treatment of moderate and life-threatening symptoms.

Refer to Evidence-Based Care Box 4-1.
- Solutions of 20% to 70% dextrose when infused rapidly, act as an osmotic diuretic and can pull interstitial fluid into plasma, causing severe cellular **dehydration**. Any solution of dextrose infused rapidly can place the patient at risk for dehydration. To prevent this adverse reaction, infuse the dextrose solution at the prescribed rate.
- Rapid infusion of 20% to 70% dextrose can also lead to transient hyperinsulin reaction, in which the pancreas secretes extra insulin to metabolize the infused dextrose. Sudden discontinuation of any hypertonic dextrose solution may leave a temporary excess of insulin. To prevent hyperinsulinism, infuse an isotonic dextrose solution (5–10%) to wean the patient off hypertonic dextrose. The infusion rate should be gradually decreased over 48 hours. When administering dextrose solutions, remember that they do not provide any electrolytes.
- Dextrose solutions cannot replace or correct electrolyte deficits, and continuous infusion of 5% dextrose in water places patients at risk for deficits in sodium, potassium, and chloride. In addition, dextrose cannot be mixed with blood components because it causes hemolysis (i.e., agglomeration) of the cells.

NOTE > Before any medication is added to a dextrose solution, compatibility information should be checked. Dextrose may also affect the stability of admixtures.

EVIDENCE-BASED CARE BOX 4-1

Use of 3% Sodium Chloride to Treat Hypotonic Encephalopathy

Hew-Butler, T., Almond, C., Ayus, J.C., et al. (2005). Consensus statement of the 1st international exercise-associated hyponatremia consensus development conference. Cape Town, South Africa. Clinical Journal of Sports Medicine, 15, 208–213.

A recent evidence-based consensus statement concluded that both excessive fluid consumption and a decrease in urine formation contribute to dilutional effect in hyponatremia that can lead to life-threatening and fatal cases of pulmonary and cerebral edema. Strategies for prevention and treatment including intravenous hypertonic solutions, such as 3% sodium chloride to reverse the symptoms related to moderate and life-threatening hypotonic encephalopathy. Further studies are needed to investigate dilutional hyponatremia.

▷ *NURSING FAST FACT!*

Do not play "catch up" if the solution infusion is behind schedule. Make sure the I.V. solution does not "run away" and that it does not infuse rapidly into the patient.

All dextrose solutions are acidic (pH 3.5–5.0) and may cause thrombophlebitis. Assess the I.V. site frequently.

EBNP A study by van Wissen and Breton (2004) concluded that intraoperative fluid replacement should not contain glucose because plasma cortisol increases during surgery, which in turn causes hyperglycemia.

Refer to Table 4-1 for summary of dextrose solution osmolarity, pH and electrolyte content; refer to Table 4-2 for indications and precautions.

Sodium Chloride Solutions

Sodium chloride solutions are available in 0.25%, 0.45%, 0.9%, 3%, and 5% concentrations. Sodium chloride 0.9% solution, often referred to as normal saline, has 154 mEq of both sodium and chloride, or about 9% higher than normal plasma levels of sodium and chloride ions without other plasma electrolytes. The term *normal saline* is therefore misleading.

There are many clinical uses of sodium chloride solutions, including treatment of shock, hyponatremia, use with blood transfusions, resuscitation in trauma situations, fluid challenges, metabolic alkalosis

Text continued on page 207

> Table 4-1   CONTENTS OF AVAILABLE INTRAVENOUS FLUIDS

Solution	Osmolarity	Dextrose, g/100 mL	pH	Cal/100 mL	Na^+	Cl^-	K^+	Ca^+	Mg^{++}	Acetate	Lactate
				Dextrose in Water (D/W)							
5% D/W	Isotonic—252	5	4.8	17							
10% D/W	Hypertonic—505	10	4.7	34							
20% D/W	Hypertonic—1010	20	4.8	68							
50% D/W	Hypertonic—2526	50	4.6	170							
70% D/W	Hypertonic—3532	70	4.6	237							
				Sodium Chloride (NaCl)							
0.225% NaCl (¼ strength)	Hypotonic—77		4.5		34	34					
0.33% NaCl	Hypotonic—115		4.5		51	51					
0.45% NaCl (½ strength)	Hypotonic—154		5.6		77	77					
0.9% NaCl (full strength)	Isotonic—308		6.0		154	154					
3% NaCl	Hypertonic—1027		6.0		513	513					
5% NaCl	Hypertonic—1711		6.0		855	855					
0.25% D and 0.9% NaCl	Isotonic—321	2.5	4.5	8	154	154					

Continued

> Table 4-1   CONTENTS OF AVAILABLE INTRAVENOUS FLUIDS—cont'd

Solution	Osmolarity	Dextrose, g/100 mL	pH	Cal/100 mL	Na+	Cl-	K+	Ca+	Mg++	Acetate	Lactate
Dextrose and Sodium Chloride (D/NaCl)											
5% D and 0.225% NaCl	Isotonic—321	5	4.6	17	34	34					
5% D and 0.45% NaCl	Hypertonic—406	5	4.6	17	77	77					
5% D and 0.9% NaCl	Hypertonic—560	5	4.4	17	154	154					
Balanced Electrolyte Solutions											
Lactated Ringer's solution	Isotonic—273		6.5		130	109	4	3			28
Ringer's injection	Isotonic—309		5.5		147	156	4	4			
Normosol-R*	Isotonic—295		7.4		140	98	5		3	27	
D5 and Normosol-M*	Isotonic—363		5.0	17	40	98	40		3	27	16
Speciality Solutions											
⅙ M Sodium lactate	Isotonic—335		6.5		167						167
10% Mannitol	Hypertonic—549		5.7								
20% Mannitol	Hypertonic—1098		5.7								
NaHCO₃	Isotonic—333		8.0		595						595

Ca = calcium; Cal = calories; Cl = chloride; K = potassium; Mg = magnesium; Na = sodium; NaCl = sodium chloride.
*Hospira Pharmaceuticals.

> Table 4-2	QUICK-GLANCE CHART OF COMMON I.V. FLUIDS	
Solutions	**Indications**	**Precautions**
	Dextrose Solutions	

5% Dextrose
10% Dextrose
20% Dextrose
50% Dextrose
70% Dextrose
	Spares body protein.
	Provides nutrition.
	Provides calories.
	Provides free water.
	Acts as a diluent for I.V. drugs.
	Treats dehydration.
	Treats hyperkalemia.
		Possible compromise of glucose
		  tolerance by stress, sepsis, hepatic
		  and renal failure, corticosteroids,
		  and diuretics
		Does not provide any electrolytes.
		May cause vein irritation,
		Possible agglomeration of RBCs.
		Use cautiously in the early
		  postoperative period to prevent
		  water intoxication
		ADH secretions as a stress response
		  to surgery
		Use with caution in patients with
		  known subclinical or overt
		  diabetes mellitus.
		Hypertonic fluids may cause
		  hyperglycemia, osmotic
		  diuresis, hyperosmolar coma, or
		  hyperinsulinism.

	Sodium Chloride (NaCl) Solutions	

0.225% NaCl
0.45% NaCl
0.9% NaCl
3% NaCl
5% NaCl
	Replaces ECF and electrolytes.
	Replaces sodium and chloride.
	Treats hyperosmolar diabetes.
	Acts as diluent for I.V. drug
	  administration.
	Used for initiation and discon-
	  tinuation of blood products.
	Replaces severe sodium and
	  chloride deficit.
	Helps to correct water overload.
	Acts as an irrigant for
	  intravascular devices.
		Fluid and/or solute overload, with
		  potential congested states or
		  pulmonary edema
		Calorie depletion
		Hypernatremia or hyperchloremia
		Deficit of other electrolytes
		Can induce hyperchloremic acidosis
		  because of a loss of bicarbonate
		  ions.
		Does not provide free water or
		  calories.
		Use with caution in older adults.

	Combination Dextrose and Sodium Chloride Solutions	

5D/0.225% NaCl
  (hydration
  solution)
5D/0.45% NaCl
  (hydration
  solution)
5D/0.9% NaCl
	Assesses kidney function.
	Hydrates cells.
	Promotes diuresis.
	For temporary treatment of
	  circulatory insufficiency
	  hydrating fluids.
	Replaces nutrients and
	  electrolytes.
	Supplies some calories.
	Reduces nitrogen depletion.
	Used in place of plasma
	  expanders.
		Use with caution in patients with
		  edema and those with cardiac,
		  renal, or liver disease.
		Do not use in patients in diabetic
		  coma.
		Do not use in patients who are
		  allergic to corn.

Continued

> Table 4-2   **QUICK-GLANCE CHART OF COMMON I.V. FLUIDS—cont'd**

Solutions	Indications	Precautions
Balanced Electrolyte Solutions		
Normosol M – and Dextrose 5% Balanced maintenance solution	Parenteral maintenance of routine fluid and electrolyte requirements with minimal carbohydrate calories. Magnesium help prevent iatrogenic Mg^{2+} deficiency. Provide free water, calories, and electrolytes. Provides routine maintenance Relieves physiologic stress leading to inappropriate release or ADH.	**Fluid or solute overload – overhydration with congested states or pulmonary edema** Dilution of serum electrolyte concentrations Use with care in patients with congestive heart failure, and severe renal insufficiency. Solutions with dextrose should be used with caution in patient with known subclinical or overt diabetes mellitus.
Normosol R – Balanced solution for replacement of acute losses of extracellular fluid in surgery, trauma, burns or shock	Provide calories and electrolytes. Provides fluid and electrolyte replacement. Provides calories. Spares protein. Replaces ECF losses and electrolytes Sodium acetate provides an alternate source of bicarbonate by metabolic conversion in the liver.	Use with care in patients with congestive heart failure, severe renal insufficincy and in clinical states of sodium retentnion. Hyerkalemia Use with caution in patients with metabolic or respiratory alkalosis. **Fluid or solute overloading, overhydration and congested states or pulmonary edema.** *Elderly have increased risk of developing fluid overload and dilutional hyponatremia.*
5% D in Ringer's injection	Provides calories Spares body protein Replaces ECF losses and electrolytes Composition similar to plasma	Contraindicated in patients with renal failure Use with caution in patients with congestive heart failure Tolerated well in pateints with liver disease.
5% Dextrose and lactated Ringer's solutions (Ionic composition similar to plasma)	Treats mild metabolic acidosis Replace fluid losses from burns and trauma Contains bicarbonate precursor Replaces fluid losses from alimentary tract Rehydrates in all types of dehydration Ionic composition similar to plasma	Contraindicated in patients with lactic acidosis Circulatory overload May cause metabolic acidosis Hypernatremia Fluid overload Contraindicated in patients with renal failure Use with caution in patients with congestive heart failure Composition similar to plasma Tolerated well in patients with liver disease Contraindicated in patients with lactic acidosis Circulatory overload May cause metabolic acidosis. Ionic composition similar to plasma Contains bicarbonate precursor

Bold type indicates the most common precaution or risk.

hypercalcemia, and fluid replacement in diabetic ketoacidosis, to list a few. Sodium chloride solutions should be used cautiously in patients with congestive heart failure, edema, or hypernatremia because it replaces ECF and can lead to fluid overload.

ADVANTAGES

- Provides ECF replacement when chloride loss is greater than or equal to sodium losses (e.g., a patient undergoing nasogastric suctioning).
- Treats patients with metabolic alkalosis in the presence of fluid loss (the 154 mEq of chloride helps compensate for the increase in bicarbonate ions).
- Treats patients with sodium depletion.
- Initiates or terminates a blood transfusion (the saline solutions are the only solutions to be used with any blood product; Gahart & Nazareno, 2008).

DISADVANTAGES

- Provides more sodium and chloride than patients need, causing hypernatremia. The adult dietary sodium requirements are 90 to 250 mEq daily. Three liters of sodium chloride (0.9%) provides a patient with 462 mEq of sodium, a level that exceeds normal tolerance. To prevent this overload of electrolytes, assess for signs and symptoms of sodium retention.
- Can cause acidosis in patients receiving continuous infusions of 0.9% sodium chloride because sodium chloride provides one third more chloride than is present in ECF. The excess chloride leads to loss of bicarbonate ions, leading to an imbalance of acid.
- May cause low potassium levels (i.e., hypokalemia) because of the lack of the other important electrolytes over a period of time.
- Can lead to circulatory overload. Isotonic fluids expand the ECF compartment, which can lead to overload of the cardiovascular compartments.

 NURSING FAST FACT!

During stress, the body retains sodium, adding to hypernatremia.

Hypotonic saline (0.45%) can be used to supply normal daily salt and water requirements safely. Hypertonic saline solution (3–5%) is used only to correct severe sodium depletion and water overload.

Hyperosmolar saline (3% or 5% NaCl) can be dangerous when administered incorrectly. Nurses should follow these steps to ensure safe administration of hyperosmolar sodium chloride (3% and 5%).

- Check serum sodium level before and during administration.
- Administer only in intensive care settings.
- Monitor aggressively for signs of pulmonary edema.
- Only small volumes of hyperosmolar fluids are usually administered.
- Use a volume-controlled device or electronic infusion pump.

Refer to Table 4-1 for sodium chloride solution osmolarity, pH and electrolyte content; refer to Table 4-2 for indications and precautions.

Dextrose Combined with Sodium Chloride

When sodium chloride is infused, the addition of 100 g dextrose prevents formation of ketone bodies. Dextrose prevents **catabolism,** which is the breakdown of chemical compounds by the body. Consequently, there is a loss of potassium and intracellular water.

Carbohydrates and sodium chloride fluid combinations are best used when there has been an excessive loss of fluid through sweating, vomiting, or gastric suctioning. Refer to Table 4-1 for available dextrose and sodium chloride solution osmolarity, pH and electrolyte content; refer to Table 4-2 for indications and precautions.

ADVANTAGES

- Temporarily treats patients with circulatory insufficiency and shock caused by hypovolemia in the immediate absence of a plasma expander.
- Provides early treatment of burns, along with plasma or albumin.
- Replaces nutrients and electrolytes.
- Acts as a **hydrating solution** to assist in checking kidney function before replacement of potassium.

DISADVANTAGE

- Same as for sodium chloride solutions (see earlier section): hypernatremia, acidosis, and circulatory overload.

Hydrating Solutions (Combinations of Dextrose and Hypotonic Sodium Chloride)

Solutions that contain dextrose and hypotonic saline provide more water than is required for excretion of salt and are useful as hydrating fluids. Hydrating fluids are used to assess the status of the kidneys. The administration of a hydrating solution at a rate of 8 mL/m² of body surface per minute for 45 minutes is called a fluid challenge. When urinary flow is established, it indicates that the kidneys have begun to function; the hydrating solution may then be replaced with a specific electrolyte solution. If the urinary flow is not restored after 45 minutes, the rate of infusion should be reduced and monitoring of the patient should continue without administration of electrolyte additives, especially potassium (Metheny, 2000). Carbohydrates in hydrating solutions reduce the depletion of nitrogen and liver glycogen and are also useful in rehydrating cells.

Hydrating solutions are potassium free. Potassium is essential to the body but can be toxic if the kidneys are not functioning effectively and are therefore unable to excrete the extra potassium. See Table 4-1 for types of hydrating fluids.

Combination solutions can be used via hypodermoclysis or subcutaneous route for hydration in clients with poor venous access. The use of 5% dextrose in 0.45% sodium chloride for rehydration using hypodermoclysis or subcutaneous infusion was found in two randomized controlled studies to be comparably safe and effective as intravenous delivery of the solutions for rehydration in this client population (Turner & Cassano, 2004).

Refer to Evidence-Based Care Box 4-2.

ADVANTAGES

- Help assess the status of the kidneys before replacement therapy is started.
- Hydrate patients in dehydrated states.
- Promote diuresis in dehydrated patients.

EVIDENCE-BASED CARE BOX 4-2

Use of Hypodermoclysis/Subcutaneous Route for Administration of Combination (Dextrose and Sodium Chloride) Solutions for Rehydration

1. Slesak, G., Schnurle, J.W., Kinzel, E., et al. (2003). Comparison of subcutaneous and intravneous rehydration in geriatric patients: a randomized trial. Journal of the American Geriatric Society, 51, 155–160.

A study of 96 elderly patients (mean age 85.3) with signs of mild to moderate dehydration needing parenteral fluid replacement over a 20-month period. Participants were block randomized to either subcutaneous infusion or I.V. infusion of 5% D/0.45% NaCl. The authors concluded that rehydration by S.C. and I.V. infusion were equally well accepted with comparable safe and effective outcomes.

2. O'Keeffe, S.T., & Lavan, J.N. (1996). Subcutaneous fluid in elderly hospital patient with cognitive impairment. Gerontology, 42, 36–39.

In this study the 60 participants (mean age 80) were cognitively impaired admitted to an acute geriatric unit who required parenteral fluids for at least 48 hours due to mild dehydration. The participants were randomly allocated to S.C. infusion or I.V. infusion. In both treatment groups, patients received either 0.9% or 0.45% sodium chloride and 5% D. The authors concluded that study demonstrated the advantages of S.C. infusion in elderly due to less interference with S.C. infusion.

DISADVANTAGE

- Require cautious administration in edematous patients (e.g., patients with cardiac, renal, or liver disease).

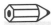 *NURSING FAST FACT!*

Do not give potassium to any patient unless kidney function has been established. Use hydrating fluid to check kidney function.

Balanced Electrolyte Solutions

A variety of balanced electrolyte fluids are available commercially. Balanced fluids are available as hypotonic or isotonic maintenance and replacement solutions. Maintenance fluids approximate normal body electrolyte needs; replacement fluids contain one or more electrolytes in amounts higher than those found in normal body fluids. Balanced fluids also may contain lactate or acetate (yielding bicarbonate), which helps to combat acidosis and provide a truly "balanced solution."

See Table 4-1 for balanced electrolyte solution osmolarity, pH and electrolyte content; refer to Table 4-2 for indications and precautions.

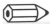 *NURSING FAST FACT!*

Multiple electrolyte fluids are recommended for use in patients with trauma, alimentary tract fluid losses, dehydration, sodium depletion, acidosis, and burns.
Do not use gastric replacement fluid in patients with hepatic insufficiency or renal failure.

Many types of balanced electrolyte replacement fluids are available. Special fluids are available from each manufacturer for gastric replacement, which provide the typical electrolytes lost by vomiting or gastric suction. These isotonic fluids usually contain ammonium ions, which are metabolized in the liver to hydrogen ions and urea, replacing hydrogen ions lost in gastric juices. Lactated Ringer's injection is considered an isotonic multiple electrolyte solution.

Hypertonic multiple electrolyte solutions are also used as replacement fluids. Usually 5% dextrose has been added, which raises the osmolarity of the solution.

Ringer's Solution and Lactated Ringer's

The Ringer's solutions (i.e., Ringer's injection and lactated Ringer's injection) are classified as balanced or isotonic solutions because their fluid and electrolyte contents are similar to those of plasma. They are used to replace electrolytes at physiologic levels in the ECF compartment.

Ringer's Solution (Injection)

Ringer's injection is a fluid and electrolyte replenisher, which is used rather than 0.9% sodium chloride for treating patients with dehydration after reduced water intake or water loss. Ringer's solution (injection) is similar to **normal saline** (i.e., 0.9% sodium chloride) with the substitution of potassium and calcium for some of the sodium ions in concentrations equal to those in the plasma. Ringer's injection, however, is superior to 0.9% sodium chloride as a fluid and electrolyte replenisher and it is preferred to normal saline for treating patients with dehydration after drastically reduced water intake or water loss (e.g., with vomiting, diarrhea, or fistula drainage). This solution has some incompatibilities with medications, so it is necessary to check drug compatibility literature for guidelines.

 NURSING FAST FACT!

> *Ringer's injection does not contain enough potassium or calcium to be used as a maintenance fluid or to correct a deficit of these electrolytes.*

Ringer's injection is used for the following:
- Treatment of any type of dehydration
- Restoration of fluid balance before and after surgery
- Replacement of fluids resulting from dehydration, GI losses, and fistula drainage

Use this solution instead of lactated Ringer's when the patient has liver disease and is unable to metabolize lactate.

Advantages

- Tolerated well in patients who have liver disease.
- May be used as blood replacement for a short period of time.

Disadvantages

- Provides no calories.
- May exacerbate sodium retention, congestive heart failure, and renal insufficiency.
- Contraindicated in renal failure.

Lactated Ringer's Solution

This solution is also called Hartmann's solution. Lactated Ringer's is the most commonly prescribed solution, with an electrolyte concentration closely resembling that of the ECF compartment. This solution is commonly used to replace fluid loss resulting from burns, bile, and diarrhea.

Lactated Ringer's is used for the following:
- Rehydration in all types of dehydration
- Restoration of fluid volume deficits
- Replacement of fluid lost as a result of burns
- Treatment of mild metabolic acidosis
- Treatment of salicylate overdose

 NURSING FAST FACT!

Lactated Ringer's solution has some incompatibilities with medications, so it is necessary to check drug compatibility literature for guidelines.

ADVANTAGES

- Contains the bicarbonate precursor to assist in acidosis.
- Most similar to body's extracellular electrolyte content.

DISADVANTAGES

- Three liters of lactated Ringer's solution contains about 390 mEq of sodium, which can quickly elevate the sodium level in a patient who does not have a sodium deficit.
- Lactated Ringer's solution should not be used in patients with impaired lactate metabolism, such as those with liver disease, Addison's disease, severe metabolic acidosis or alkalosis, profound hypovolemia, or profound shock or cardiac failure.
- In the above conditions, serum lactate levels may already be elevated.

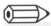 *NURSING FAST FACT!*

At present isotonic sodium chloride is recommended as the first line fluid in resuscitation of hypovolemic trauma patients (Revell, Porter, & Greaves, 2002).

Alkalizing and Acidifying Infusion Fluids

ALKALIZING FLUIDS

Metabolic acidosis can occur in clinical situations in which dehydration, shock, liver disease, starvation, or diabetes causes retention of chlorides, ketone bodies, or organic salts or when too large an amount of bicarbonate is lost. Treatment consists of infusion of an alkalizing fluid. Two I.V. fluids are available when there are excessive bicarbonate losses and metabolic acidosis occurs: $\frac{1}{6}$ molar isotonic sodium lactate and 5% sodium bicarbonate injection. The lactate ion must be oxidized in the body to carbon dioxide before it can affect the acid–base balance. Sodium lactate to bicarbonate requires 1 to 2 hours. Oxygen is needed to increase bicarbonate concentrations. The isotonic solution sodium bicarbonate injection provides bicarbonate ions in clinical situations in which there are excessive bicarbonate losses.

Alkalizing fluids are used in treating vomiting, starvation, uncontrolled diabetes mellitus, acute infections, renal failure, and severe acidosis with severe hyperpnea (sodium bicarbonate injection).

The ⅙ molar sodium lactate solution is useful whenever acidosis has resulted from sodium deficiency; however, it is contraindicated in patients suffering from lack of oxygen and in those with liver disease. Patients receiving this fluid should be watched for signs of hypocalcemic tetany.

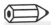 **NURSING FAST FACT!**

Sodium bicarbonate injection is used to relieve dyspnea and hyperpnea; the bicarbonate ion is released in the form of carbon dioxide through the lungs, leaving behind an excess of sodium.

ACIDIFYING FLUIDS

Metabolic alkalosis is a condition associated with an excess of bicarbonate and deficit of chloride. Isotonic sodium chloride (0.9%) provides conservative treatment of metabolic alkalosis. Ammonium chloride is the solution used to treat metabolic alkalosis. Acidifying fluids are used for severe metabolic alkalosis caused by a loss of gastric secretions or pyloric stenosis.

An advantage is that the ammonium ion is converted by the liver to hydrogen ion and to ammonia, which is excreted as urea. However, a disadvantage is that ammonium chloride must be infused at a slow rate to enable the liver to metabolize the ammonium ion. In fact, rapid infusion can result in toxicity, causing irregular breathing and bradycardia.

NURSING FAST FACT!

Ammonium chloride must be used with caution in patients with severe hepatic disease or renal failure and is contraindicated in any condition in which a high ammonium level is present.

NURSING POINTS-OF-CARE
CRYSTALLOID ADMINISTRATION

Nursing Assessments
- History of present illness of fluid loss
- Observe ability to ingest and retain fluids.
- Obtain vital signs
- Obtain weight
- Initial physical assessment for signs and symptoms of fluid imblance.
- Review prescriber's order for accuracy and match the solution to the order.

Nursing Management
1. Administer I.V. fluids at room temperature.
2. Administer I.V. medications at prescribed rate and monitor for results.
3. Use open containers immediately.
4. Monitor I.V. site during infusion.
5. Monitor for
   a. signs and symptoms of fluid overload
   b. urine output and specific gravity
   c. trending of pertinent laboratory values (electrolytes, prothrombin time (PT), partial thromboplastin time (PTT), serum amylase)
   d. complications associated with infusion therapy (phlebitis, erratic flow rates, infiltration).
6. Monitor for I.V. patency before administering I.V. medications.
7. Replace I.V. cannula and apparatus every 72 hours.
8. Replace fluid containers at least every 24 hours.
9. Flush peripheral I.V. catheters between administration of incompatible solutions with sodium chloride
10. Record intake and output.
11. Provide information outlining current I.V. therapy.
12. Maintain standard precautions.

Colloid Solutions

Patients with fluid and electrolyte disturbances occasionally require treatment with colloids. Colloid solutions contain protein or starch molecules that remain distributed in the extracellular space and do not form a "true" solution. Colloid solutions are referred to as **plasma volume expanders**. When colloid molecules are administered, they remain in the vascular space for several days in patients with normal capillary endothelia. These fluids increase the osmotic pressure within the plasma space, drawing fluid to increase intravascular volume. Colloid solutions do not dissolve and do not flow freely between fluid compartments. Infusion of a colloid solution increases intravascular colloid osmotic pressure (pressure of plasma proteins). The most common colloid volume expanders are dextran, albumin, hetastarch, mannitol and gelatin.

Ideal colloid solutions would include the following advantages:
■ Distributed to intravascular compartment only
■ Readily available
■ Long shelf life
■ Inexpensive
■ No special storage or infusion requirements
■ No special limitations on volume that can be infused
■ No interference with blood grouping or cross matching
■ Acceptable to all patients and no religious objections.

Albumin

Albumin is a natural plasma protein prepared from donor plasma. Albumin is the predominant plasma protein and remains the standard against which other colloids are compared (Roberts & Bratton, 1998). The colloid osmotic pressure is influenced by proteins. The concentration of protein in plasma is 2 to 3 times greater than proteins found in the interstitial fluid (i.e., plasma, 7.3 g/dL; and interstitial fluid, 2 to 3 g/dL) (Hankins, 2006). This colloid is available as a 5%, 20%, or 25% solution. Five (5) percent albumin is osmotically and oncotically equivalent to plasma. The 5% is usually indicated in hypovolemic patients and cardiopulmonary bypass. The initial dose is 5%, which is available in 50-mL, 250-mL, 500-mL, and 1000-mL containers, 12.5 to 25 g. The 5% solution is isotonic.

The 25% solution is equivalent to 500 mL of plasma or two units of whole blood. It is indicated for patients whose fluid and sodium intake should be minimized. The 25% solution (25 g/100 mL) is available in 20-mL, 50-mL, or 100-mL vials. The 20% solution is available in 100-mL vials from one manufacturer. The 25% solution is used in hypoproteinemia, hypovolemia and burns, acute nephrosis, hemodialysis, red blood cell resuspension, and cardiopulmonary bypass (Gahart & Nazareno, 2008). The 20% and 25% solutions are hypertonic. In well hydrated patients, each volume of the 25% solution draws about 300 to 500 mL in intravascular volume for every 100 mL infused (McEvoy, 2007).

NOTE > These products are subject to an extended heating period during preparation and therefore do not transmit viral disease.

ADVANTAGES

■ Free of danger of serum hepatitis
■ Expands blood volume proportionately to amount of circulating blood
■ Improves cardiac output
■ Prevents marked hemoconcentration
■ Aids in reduction of edema, raises serum protein levels
■ Maintains electrolyte balance and promote diuresis in presence of edema
■ Acts as a transport protein that binds both endogenous and exogenous substances, including bilirubin and certain drugs

DISADVANTAGES

■ May precipitate allergic reactions (e.g., urticaria, flushing, chills, fever, or headache)
■ May cause circulatory overload (greatest risk with 25% albumin)
■ May cause pulmonary edema
■ May alter laboratory findings

> *EBNP In 2004, a prospective, multicenter, double-blind controlled trial published in the New England Journal of Medicine looked at albumin versus saline in critically ill patient. Refer to Evidence-Based Care Box 4-3.*

Refer to Table 4-3 for summary of albumin osmolarity, expansion and side effects.

EVIDENCE-BASED CARE BOX 4-3

Saline versus Albumin Fluid Evaluation (SAFE) Study

Finfer, S., Bellomo, R., Boyce, N., et al. (2004). A comparison of albumin and saline for fluid resuscitation in the intensive care unit. New England Journal of Medicine, 350, 2247–2256.

One of the largest prospective clinical studies to date, the SAFE (Saline versus Albumin Fluid Evaluation) trial randomized a heterogeneous group of 7000 critically ill patients requiring fluid resuscitation to receive iso-oncotic albumin or isotonic crystalloid. Overall, 28-day mortality was 21% and did not differ according to treatment assignment.

Dextran

Dextran fluids are polysaccharides that behave as colloids that are **plasma volume expanders**. They are available as low molecular weight dextran (dextran 40) and high molecular weight dextran (dextran 70). Low molecular weight dextran (Dextran 40) is a rapid, but short-acting plasma volume expander. It increases plasma volume by once or twice its own volume. Improves microcirculatory flow and prevents sludging in venous

> Table 4-3   COMMON COLLOID VOLUME EXPANDERS

Solution	Molecular Wt.	Osmolality	Max Volume* Expansion (%)	Duration of Expansion	Side Effects
Albumin 4%, 5%	69	290	70–100	12–24 hours	Allergic reactions
Albumin 20%, 25%	69	310	300–500	12–24 hours	Allergic reactions
Starches Hetastarch 3%, 6%, 10%	450	300–310	100–200	8–36 hours	Renal dysfunction
Starches Pentastarch 10%	280	326	100–200	12–24 hours	Renal dysfunction
Dextrans 10% 10 % Dextran 40	40	280–324	100–200	1–2 hours	Anaphylactoid reactions
3% Dextran–60 6% Dextran–70	70	280–324	80–140	<8–24 hours	Anaphylactoid reactions
Gelatins Succinylated and cross–linked: 2.5%, 3%, 4% Urea–linked: 3.5%	30–35	300–350	70–80	<4–6 hours	High calcium content (urea–linked forms)

*Max volume expansion % is expressed as a percentage of administered volume.
Adapted from Martin, G.S., & Matthay, M.A. (2004). Evidence-based colloid use in the critically ill. Consensus statement of the subcommittee of the American Throracic Society Critical Care Assembly. American Journal of Respiratory and Critical Care Medicine, 170, 1247–1259.

channels. Mobilizes water from body tissues and increases urinary output. Initial 500 mL may be given rapidly. Remainder of any desired daily dose should be evenly distributed over 8 to 24 hours (Gahart & Nazareno, 2008).

High molecular weight Dextran 70 approximates colloidal properties of human albumin. Dilutes total serum proteins and hematocrit values. Used as adjunct in treatment of impending shock or shock states related to burns, hemorrhage, surgery or trauma (McEvoy, 2007). The rate of administration is variable depending on indication, present blood volume, and patient response. Initial 500 mL may be given at 20 to 40 mL/min if hypovolemic. If additional high molecular weight dextran is required reduce the flow rate to lowest possible (Gahart & Nazareno, 2008).

It is important to monitor the patient's pulse, blood pressure, and urine output every 5 to 15 minutes for the first hour of administration of dextran and then every hour after that.

These products are used when blood or blood products are not available. Not a substitute for whole blood or plasma proteins. Hydration status is important.

ADVANTAGE

- Intravascular space is expanded in excess of the volume infused.

DISADVANTAGES

- Possibility of hypersensitivity reactions (i.e., anaphylaxis)
- Increased risk of bleeding
- Circulatory overload
- For I.V. use only

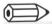 NURSING FAST FACT!

Dextran is contraindicated in patients with severe bleeding disorders, congestive heart failure, and renal failure. It is important to draw blood for typing and cross-matching before administering dextran.

Refer to Table 4-3 for dextran osmolarity, expansion and side effects.

Hydroxyethyl Starches: Hetastarch and Pentastarch

Hetastarch (hydroxyethyl glucose) is a synthetic colloid made from starch and is similar to human albumin. It is available under the name Hespan® as a 6% or 10% solution, diluted in isotonic sodium chloride in a 500-mL container. These starches are not derived from donor plasma and are therefore less toxic and less expensive. Hetastarch is equal in plasma volume expansion properties to 5% human albumin.

Pentastarch is another polydisperse formulation of hydroxyethyl starch with a lower molecular weight. Pentastarch has a greater colloid osmotic pressure than hetastarch. In 2007 the FDA approved Voluven®, a 6% hydroxyethyl starch injection, for the prevention and treatment of dangerously low blood volume (McEvoy, 2007).

> *EBNP In clinical trials of 10% pentastarch with 5% albumin, it was found that pentastarch over 5% albumin may provide greater plasma volume expansion for the volume infused, with faster onset and more rapid elimination than albumin or hetastarch (Brutocao, Bratton, Thomas, et al., 1996).*

ADVANTAGES

- Hetastarch and Pentastarch do not interfere with blood typing and crossmatching, as do other colloidal solutions.
- Provides hemodynamically significant plasma volume expansion in excess of the amount infused for about 24 hours (Gahart & Nazereno, 2008).
- Permits retention of intravascular fluid until hetastarch is replaced by blood proteins.

DISADVANTAGES

- Possibility of allergic reaction including anaphylaxis.
- Anemia and/or bleeding due to hemodilution and/or factor VIII deficiency, and other coagulopathies, including DIC.
- Increased intracranial bleeding.

 NURSING FAST FACT!

Use hetastarch cautiously in patients whose conditions predispose them to fluid retention.

Refer to Table 4-3 for hydroxyethyl starches, osmolarity expansion and side effects.

Mannitol

Mannitol is a hexahydroxy alcohol substance that is available in concentrations of 5%, 10%, 15%, 20%, and 25% and is classified as an osmotic diuretic. This solution is limited to the extracellular space, where it draws fluid from the cells due to its hypertonicity (275–1375 mOsm). Mannitol increases the osmotic pressure of the glomerular filtrate, thereby inhibiting reabsorption of water and electrolytes.

Administration of this solution causes excretion of water, sodium, potassium chloride, calcium phosphorus and magnesium, urea and uric acid. It is usually dosed by kilograms of body weight (Deglin & Vallerand, 2007; Gahart & Nazereno, 2008).

ADVANTAGES

- Used to promote diuresis in patients with oliguric acute renal failure
- Promote excretion of toxic substances in the body
- Reduce excess cerebrospinal fluid (CSF)

- Reduce intraocular pressure, and to treat intracranial pressure and cerebral edema.
- Administration of mannitol can reduce excess CSF within 15 minutes.

DISADVANTAGES

- Fluid and electrolyte imbalances are the most common and may be severe.
- Mannitol may induce dehydration with hyperkalemia, hyponatremia, hypokalemia, or hyponatremia.
- This solution is irritating to the vein intima and may cause phlebitis. Extravasation of mannitol may lead to skin irritation and tissue necrosis (Deglin & Vallerand, 2008).
- Mannitol may interfere with laboratory tests.

NOTE > This solution requires cautious use for patients with impaired cardiac or renal system. Use mannitol cautiously for patients with impaired cardiac or renal systems. It is contraindicated in the presence of anuria, severe pulmonary and cardiac congestion and intracranial bleeding.

 NURSING FAST FACT!

The nurse needs to monitor the administration of mannitol for crystal formation, it is recommended that an in-line filter be used during administration of 15%, 20%, and 25% solutions (Deglin & Vallerand, 2007).

Gelatins

Gelatin is the name given to the proteins formed when the connective tissue of animals are boiled. They have the property of dissolving in hot water and forming a jelly when cooled. Gelatin is thus a large molecular weight protein formed from hydrolysis of collagen. Several modified gelatin products are available; they have been collectively called the New-generations Gelatins. There are three types of gelatin solutions currently in use: succinylated or modified fluid gelatins (e.g., Gelofusine®, Plasmagel®, Plasmion®); urea-crosslinked gelatins (e.g., Polygeline®) and oxypolygelatins (e.g., Gelifundol®; McEvoy, 2007). They have no preservatives and all Gelatins have a recommended shelf-life of 3 years when stored at temperatures less than 30°C. It is rapidly excreted by the kidney following infusion. Gelatins (GEL) have the advantage of their unlimited daily dose recommendation and minimal effect on hemostasis (Grocott, Mythen, & Gan, 2005; Van de Linden, Hert, & Cromheecke, 2005).

ADVANTAGES

- Gelatins are used for replacement of intravascular volume due to acute blood loss.
- Priming heart-lung machines.
- Least effect on hemostasis (Grocott, Mythen, & Gan, 2005).

Disadvantages

- Gelatins are associated with anaphylactic reactions, and may also cause depression of serum fibronectin.
- Urea-linked gelatin has much higher calcium and potassium levels than succinylated gelatin (Kelley, 2005).
- Risks associated with bovine-derived gelatin because of the association between new-variant Creutzfeldt–Jakob disease and bovine spongiform encephalitis. There are no known cases of transmission involving pharmaceutical gelatin preparations, but awareness of this issue is important (Grocott, Mythen, & Tan, 2005).

Refer to Table 4-3 for gelatins osmolarity, expansion and side effects.

NURSING POINTS-OF-CARE
COLLOID ADMINISTRATION

Nursing Assessments
- Carefully assess for history of allergic responses.
- Assess vital signs.
- Assess urinary output for renal function.

Key Nursing Interventions
1. Monitor for signs and symptoms of localized allergic reaction.
2. Monitor laboratory values (serum protein levels, sodium, serum hemoglobin and hematocrit).
3. Monitor central venous pressure (CVP) or jugular venous distention when appropriate.
4. Monitor infusion rate frequently.
5. Monitor and record input & output (I & O).
6. Monitor for the need of additional fluid in the dehydrated patients.
7. Monitor for signs of fluid overload.
8. Monitor/assess bleeding postinfusion.
9. Auscultate breath sounds for development of crackles.

AGE-RELATED CONSIDERATIONS
The Pediatric Client
Factors Affecting Fluid Needs in Pediatric Clients
The most common cause of increased fluid and calorie needs in children is temperature elevation. An increase in temperature of 1 degree increases a child's calorie needs by 12%. Fluid requirements of a child who is hypothermic decrease by 12% (Hockenberry & Wilson, 2006). In children, loss of GI fluids, ongoing diarrhea, and small intestinal drainage can seriously affect fluid balance.

Continued

NURSING FAST FACT!

> *To ensure accuracy in determining fluid needs, most pediatric patients should be on strict intake and output monitoring, including diaper weighing. When weighing an infant's diaper, consider the weight of the diaper before it was wet. The weight difference between a dry and a wet piece of linen represents the amount of liquid that it has absorbed. The weight of the fluid measured in grams is the same as the volume measured in milliliters (Hockenberry & Wilson, 2006).*

There are three general methods for assessment of 24-hour maintenance of fluids for the pediatric client: meter square, caloric, and weight. (Note these are general formulas and each specific age group has different fluid/electrolyte/replacement needs.)

1. Meter Square Method

For calculation of maintenance of fluid requirements, use the following formula:

1500 mL/m² per 24 hours

Example: If a child's surface area is 0.5 m², then 1500 mL × 0.5 m² = 750 mL/24 hr

A nomogram used to determine the **body surface area** (BSA) of the patient is the meter square method. To use a nomogram in this method, draw a straight line between the point representing the patient's height on the left vertical scale to the point representing the patient's weight on the right vertical scale. The point at which the line intersects indicates the body surface area in square meters:

The following are advantages of the meter square method:

• Provides calculation of body surface area to help determine the amount of fluid and electrolytes to be infused and assists with computing rate of infusion.
• Helps to calculate adult and pediatric dosage of I.V. medications.
• Is simple to calculate

The following is a disadvantage of the meter square method:

• Difficulty in accessibility to visual nomogram

2. Weight Method

The **weight method** uses the child's weight in kilograms to estimate fluid needs. This method uses 100 to 150 mL/kg for estimating maintenance fluid requirements and is most useful in children weighing less than 10 kg (use of the meter square method is recommended for children weighing more than 10 kg)

The following is an advantage of the weight method:

• Simple to use

The following is a disadvantage of the weight method:

• Inaccurate in children who weigh more than 10 kg

3. Caloric Method

The formula for calculating fluid requirement is:

100–150 mL/100 calories metabolized

Example: If the weight of the child is 30 kg and the child expends 1700 cal/day, fluid requirement is 1700–2550 mL/24 hours.

The **caloric method** calculates the usual metabolic expenditure of fluid. It is based on the following metabolic expenditure:

Children weighing 0 to 10 kg expend approximately 100 cal/kg per day

Children weighing 10 to 20 kg expend approximately 1000 cal/kg per day plus 50 cal/kg for each kilogram over 10 kg.

Children weighing 20 kg or more expend approximately 1500 calories, plus 20 cal/kg for each kilogram over 20 kg.

The following is an advantage of the caloric method:

• Easy to calculate

The following is a disadvantage of the caloric method:

• Not totally accurate unless actual calorie requirements and energy intake are continuously assessed (Broyles, Reiss, & Evans, 2007; London, Ladewig, Ball, & Bindler, 2007).

The Older Adult

With the older adult, be aware of the increased dangers of administering sodium chloride solutions to elderly patients, patients with severe dehydration, and patients with chronic glomerulonephritis.

Geriatric clients have a higher risk of developing dehydration than younger clients do (Ferry, 2005). Dehydrated geriatric clients who are to undergo surgery should receive I.V. fluids preoperatively in an effort to prevent complications from dehydration (Phillips, 2004).

Dextrose administered without a pump to elderly patients can lead to cerebral edema more rapidly than in younger patients.

Home Care Issues

Many infusion medications or fluids can be administered in the home setting including antimicrobials, chemotherapy, total parenteral nutrition, opioid analgesics, blood products, and hydration fluids.

Intravenous fluids may be administered for patients who are dehydrated, resulting from:

• Hyperemesis gravidarum
• Intractable diarrhea
• Drug related side effects (e.g., chemotherapy [before and after])
• Short bowel syndrome
• Short-term therapy lasts from 1 to 7 days and is usually administered via a peripheral lock or long-term access device, if there is one also in place.
• Educate patients about the need for therapy, aseptic technique, setup and administration of specific solution, and possible complications.

Patient Education

- Instruct the patient on the reason for therapy (e.g., replacement fluid, vitamins, nutrition, volume replacement).
- Instruct the patient to report signs and symptoms of complications (e.g., burning at infusion site, redness, any discomfort).
- Explain the need for increased oral intake if appropriate.
- Teach the patient how to follow sodium and fluid restriction if appropriate.
- Teach the patient to weigh self daily.
- Review signs and symptoms of dehydration and overhydration with patient.
- Teach the patient to change positions slowly if any dizziness or lightheadedness occurs.
- Teach the patient to report to the nurse any pain, swelling, leaking, redness, or harness at the I.V. site.

▉ Nursing Process

The nursing process is a five- or six-step process for problem-solving to guide nursing action. Refer to Chapter 1 for details on the steps of the nursing process related to vascular access. The following table focuses on nursing diagnoses, nursing outcomes classification (NOC), and nursing intervention classification (NIC) for patients with parenteral fluid needs. Nursing diagnoses should be patient specific and outcomes and interventions individualized. The NOC and NIC presented here are suggested direction for development of outcomes and interventions.

Nursing Diagnoses Related to Parenteral Solution Administration	NOC: Nursing Outcomes Classification	NIC: Nursing Intervention Classification
Fluid volume deficit related to: Abnormal loss of body fluids	Fluid and electrolyte balance, hydration	Fluid management
Fluid volume excess related to: Volume expansion	Electrolyte and acid–base balance, fluid balance, hydration	Fluid monitoring, fluid management
Knowledge deficit related to: Inadequate information: new procedure and maintaining infusion therapy	Knowledge of disease process; infusion therapy treatment regimen	Teaching: Disease process, treatment
Tissue integrity, impaired related to: Damage tissue (irritating solutions on the intima of the vein)	Tissue integrity: Skin	Skin care, skin surveillance, wound care

Nursing Diagnoses Related to Parenteral Solution Administration	NOC: Nursing Outcomes Classification	NIC: Nursing Intervention Classification
Tissue perfusion ineffective, risk for: Cerebral–renal related to fluid volume imbalance	Fluid balance, hydration	Circulatory care: Renal perfusion, cerebral perfusion
Collaborative problem Allergic reaction related to hypersensitivity and release of mediators to specific substances (antigens) secondary to colloid administration	Allergic response: Systemic	Allergy management

Sources: Ackley & Ladwig (2008); Carpenito-Moyet (2008); Heitz & Horne (2005); McCloskey, Dochterman, & Bulechek (2004); Moorhead, Johnson, & Maas (2004); NANDA-I (2007).

Chapter Highlights

- Three main objectives of I.V. therapy are to:
  - Maintain daily requirements
  - Replace previous losses
  - Provide fluids and electrolytes to restore ongoing losses
- Solutions have an osmolarity of hypotonic, isotonic, or hypertonic:
  - Hypotonic is 250 mOsm/L or below.
  - Isotonic ranges from 250 to 375 mOsm/L.
  - Hypertonic is above 375 mOsm/L.
- Give hypertonic solutions slowly to prevent circulatory overload.
- As the acidity of the solution increases, irritation to the vein wall increases.
- Do not play "catch-up" with I.V. solutions that are behind schedule; recalculate the infusion.
- Always check compatibility before adding medication to dextrose solutions.
- Do not give potassium solutions to any patient unless kidney function has been established.
- Infusates are categorized as:
  - Crystalloids: Solutions that are considered true solutions and whose solutes, when placed in a solvent, mix, dissolve, and cannot be distinguished from the resultant solutions. Crystalloids are able to move through membranes. Examples are dextrose and sodium chloride solutions and lactated Ringer's solution.
  - Colloids: Substances whose particles, when submerged in a solvent, cannot form a true solution because their molecules cannot dissolve, but remain suspended and distributed in the fluid. Examples are dextran, albumin, mannitol, hetastarch, and gelatins.

■■ Thinking Critically: Case Study

Over a 16-hour period of one hour, a 6-year-old child was inadvertently given 800 mL of 3% sodium chloride solution instead of the prescribed 0.33% sodium chloride. She developed lethargy, convulsions, and coma before the error was discovered. Despite resuscitative efforts the child died.

1. Identify the mEq of each electrolyte in the I.V. solutions.
2. Identify the osmolality/tonicity of each of the electrolyte solutions.
3. Refer to Chapter 1 on legal aspects for factors involved in malpractice. Who was liable?
4. What types of safeguards should be in place for the pediatric patient receiving I.V. fluids?

Refer to Chapter 6 for pediatric peripheral infusions.

 Media Link: Answers to the case study and more critical thinking activities are provided on the CD-ROM.

Post-Test

1. The patient admitted to the emergency department with intractable vomiting and was started on 5% dextrose and 0.9% sodium chloride to support which of the following objectives of infusion therapy?

    a. Maintenance of daily requirements
    b. Replacement of current losses
    c. Restore ongoing losses

2. The functions of glucose in parenteral therapy include which of the following? (*Select all that apply.*)

    a. Provides calories for energy.
    b. Helps to prevent negative nitrogen balance.
    c. Reduces catabolism of protein.
    d. Serves as vehicle for blood transfusions.

3. Maintenance solutions are used for patients who are:

    a. Ingesting nothing by mouth for a short period of time
    b. Experiencing hemorrhage
    c. Dehydrated from GI losses
    d. Experiencing draining fistulas

4. What is the most commonly used balanced electrolyte solution?

    a. 5% dextrose in water
    b. 0.9% sodium chloride
    c. Lactated Ringer's solution
    d. 5% dextrose and sodium chloride

5. Which of the following is the *most* common complication of the colloid dextran?

   a. Fluid overload
   b. Hypersensitivity reactions
   c. Hyponatremia
   d. Hyperkalemia

6. What is the purpose of a colloid solution?

   a. To expand the interstitial compartment
   b. To replace electrolytes
   c. To expand the intravascular compartment
   d. To correct acidosis

7. Dextrose and hypotonic sodium chloride solutions are considered hydrating fluids because:

   a. They provide more water than is required for excretion of sodium.
   b. The water they provide equals that needed for excretion of sodium.
   c. They maximize retention of potassium in the cell.
   d. They maximize the retention of sodium.

8. The expected outcome of administering a hypertonic solution is to:

   a. Shift ECF from intracellular space to plasma
   b. Hydrate cells
   c. Supply free water to vascular space

9. Which of the following solutions are used to prime the administration set when blood is to be administered?

   a. 5% dextrose in water
   b. Lactated Ringer's
   c. 0.9% sodium chloride
   d. 5% dextrose and 0.45% sodium chloride

10. Before administering a prescribed intravenous solution that contains potassium chloride, the nurse should assess for:

    a. Poor skin turgor with "tenting"
    b. Behaviors indicating irritability and confusion
    c. A urinary output of 200 mL during the previous shift
    d. An oral intake of 300 mL of fluid during the previous shift.

Media Link: Answers to the Chapter 4 Post-Test and more test questions together with rationales are provided on the CD-ROM.

■ References

Ackley, B.J., & Ladwig, G.B. (2008). *Nursing diagnosis handbook: An evidence-based guide to planning care*. St. Louis, MO: Mosby Elsevier.

Broyles, B.E., Reiss, B.S., & Evans, M.E. (2007). *Pharmacological aspects of nursing care* (7th ed.). Clifton Park, NY: Thomson Delmar Learning.

Brutocao, D., Bratton, S.L., Thomas, J.R., et al. (1996). Comparison of hetastarch with albumin for postoperative volume expansion in children after cardiopulmonary bypass. *Journal of Cardiothoracic and Vascular Anesthesia, 10*(3), 348–351.

Carpenito-Moyet L.J. (2008). *Nursing diagnosis: Application to clinical practice* (12th ed.). Philadelphia: Lippincott, Williams & Wilkins.

Cook, L.S. (2003). IV fluid resuscitation. *Journal of Infusion Nursing, 26*(5), 2003.

Deglin, J.H., & Vallerand, A.H. (2007). *Davis's drug guide for nurses* (11th ed.). Philadelphia: F.A. Davis.

Ferry, M. (2005). Strategies for ensuring good hydration in the elderly. *Nutrition Reviews, 63*(6), S22.

Finfer, S., Bellomo, R., Boyce, N., et al. (2004). A comparison of albumin and saline for fluid resuscitation in the intensive care unit. *New England Journal of Medicine, 350*, 2247–2256.

Gahart, L., & Nazareno, A.R. (2008). *2008 Intravenous medications* (24th ed.). St. Louis, MO: Mosby Elsevier.

Grocott, M., Mythen, M.G., & Gan, T.J. (2005). Perioperative fluid management and clinical outcomes in adults. *International Anesthesia Research Society, 100*, 1093–1096.

Hankins, J. (2006). The role of albumin in fluid and electrolyte balance. *Journal of Infusion Nursing, 29*(5), 260–265.

Heitz, U., & Horne, M.M. (2005). *Pocket guide to fluid, electrolyte, and acid-base balance* (5th ed.). St. Louis, MO: C.V. Mosby.

Hill, J.W., & Petrucci, R.H. (2004). *General chemistry: An integrated approach* (3rd ed.). Upper Saddle River, NJ: Prentice-Hall.

Hockenberry, M.J., & Wilson D. (2006). *Wong's nursing care of infants and children* (8th ed). St. Louis, MO: Mosby/Elsevier.

Holliday, M.A., & Segar, W.E. (1957). The maintenance need for water in parenteral fluid therapy. *Pediatrics, 19*, 823–832.

Hospira (2006). 20%, 30%, 40%, 50%, and 70% dextrose injection, USP. Retrieved from www.hospira.com (Accessed January 8, 2008).

Jordan, K.S. (2000). Fluid resuscitation in acutely injured patients. *Journal of Intravenous Nursing, 23*(2), 81–87.

Kelley, D.M. (2005). Hypovolemic shock: An overview. *Critical Care Nurse, 28*(1), 2–19.

Kraft, P.A. (2000). The osmotic shift. *Journal of Intravenous Nursing, 23*(4), 220–224.

London, M.L., Ladewig, P.W., Ball, J., & Bindler, R.C. (2007). *Maternal and child nursing care* (2nd ed.). Upper Saddle River, NJ: Pearson Prentice Hall.

Martin, G.S., & Matthay, M.A. (2004). Evidence-based colloid use in the critically ill. Consensus Conference Statement subcommittee of the American Thoracic Society Critical Care Assembly. *American Journal of Respiratory and Critical Care Medicine, 170* (11), 1247–1259.

McCloskey-Dochterman, J.C., & Bulechek, G.M. (2004). *Nursing interventions classification* (NIC) (4th ed.). St. Louis, MO: C.V. Mosby.

McEvoy, G.K. (2007). *AHFS drug information 2007.* Bethesda, MD: American Society of Health System Pharmacists.

Metheny, N.M. (1997). Focusing on the dangers of D5W. *Nursing 97, 10,* 55–59.

Metheny, N.M. (2000). *Fluid and electrolyte balance: Nursing considerations* (4th ed.). Philadelphia: Lippincott Williams & Wilkins.

Moorhead, S., Johnson, M., & Maas, M. (2004). *Nursing outcomes classification* (NOC) (3rd ed.). St. Louis, MO: C.V. Mosby.

NANDA-I. (2007). *Nursing diagnoses: Definitions and classification,* 2007–2008. Philadelphia: Author.

O'Keeffe, S.T., & Lavan, J.N. (1996). Subcutaneous fluid in elderly hospital patient with cognitive impairment. *Gerontology, 42,* 36–39.

Phillips, N. (2004). *Berry & Kohn's operating room technique* (10th ed.). St. Louis, MO: C.V. Mosby.

Popcock, G., & Richards, C.D. (2000). *Human physiology: The basis of medicine.* Oxford: Oxford University Press.

Porth, C.M., & Martin, G. (2008). *Pathophysiology: Concept of altered health states* (8th ed.). Philadelphia: Lippincott Williams & Wilkins.

Revell, M., Porter, K., & Greaves, I. (2002). Fluid resuscitation in prehospital trauma care: A consensus view. *Emergency Medicine Journal, 19*(6), 494–499.

Roberts, J.S., & Bratton, S.L. (1998). Colloid volume expanders: Problems, pitfalls and possibilities. *Drugs, 55*(5), 621–630.

Scalea, T.M., & Boswell, S.A. (2002). Initial management of traumatic shock. In: K.A. McQuillen, K.T. Von Rueden, R.I. Hartsock, et al. (Eds.). *Trauma nursing: From resuscitation through rehabilitation* (3rd ed.). Philadelphia: W.B. Saunders.

Siegel, A.J. (2007). Hypertonic (3%) sodium chloride for emergent treatment of exercise-associated hypotonic encephalopathy. Conference paper. *Sports Medicine, 37*(94–95), 459–462.

Slesak, G., Schnurle, J.W., Kinzel, E., et al. (2003). Comparison of subcutaneous and intravenous rehydration in geriatric patients: A randomized trial. *Journal of the American Geriatric Society, 51,* 155–160.

Turner, T., & Cassano, A.M. (2004). Subcutaneous dextrose for rehydration of elderly patients – an evidence-based review. *BMC Geriatrics 4,* 2. Retrieved from www.pubmedcentral.nih.gov/article (Accessed January 10, 2008).

van der Linden, P.J., Hert, S.G., Cromheecke, S., et al. (2005). Hydroxyethyl starch 130/0.4 versus modified fluid gelatin for volume expansion in cardiac surgery patients: The effects on perioperative bleeding and transfusion needs. *International Anesthesia Research Society, 101,* 629–634.

van Wissen, K., & Breton, C. (2004). Perioperative influences on fluid distribution. *MEDSURG Nursing, 13*(5), 304–311.

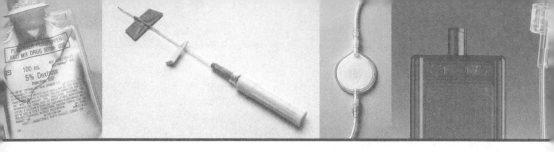

Chapter **5**

Infusion Equipment

*All our elaborate scientific equipment will not save us if the intellectual and
spiritual elements in our art are subordinated to the mechanical, and if the
means come to be regarded as more important than ends.*
—Isabel M. Stewart, 1929

Chapter Contents

▪ LEARNING OBJECTIVES   *On completion of this chapter, the reader will be able to:*

1. Define the terminology related to I.V. equipment.
2. Identify the types and characteristics of infusate containers.
3. Identify the use of vented and nonvented administration sets with the appropriate solution containers.
4. Identify the types and characteristics of peripheral and central infusion devices.
5. State the major advantages and disadvantages associated with over-the-needle catheters and scalp vein needles.
6. Identify the characteristics and uses of electronic infusion devices (EIDs)
7. Describe the use of filters in the infusion of solutions and blood products.
8. Describe the use of miscellaneous adjuncts to aid in the administration of safe infusions.
9. Identify the Infusion Nurses Society (INS) and the Centers for Disease Control and Prevention (CDC) recommendations for standards of practice related to equipment safety and use.

▷ GLOSSARY

Cannula   A flexible tube that may be inserted into a duct, cavity, or blood vessel to deliver medication or drain fluid. It may be guided by a sharp, pointed instrument (stylet).

Catheter (intravenous)   A cannula inserted into a vein to administer fluids or medications or to measure pressure

Check valve   A device that functions to prevent retrograde solution flow; also called a backcheck valve

Coring   Visible, as well as microscopic, particles of rubber bung displaced by the spike during piercing of the glass container or needle during access of implanted vascular access devices

Drip chamber   Area of the intravenous administration set usually found under the spike where the solution drips and collects before running through the I.V. tubing

Drop factor   The number of drops needed to deliver 1 mL of fluid

Elastomeric pump   A portable infusion device with a balloon made of soft rubberized material capable of being inflated to a predetermined volume

Electronic infusion device   An automated system of introducing a fluid into a vein. The device may have programmable settings that control the amount of fluid to be infused, rate, low-volume notification level and keep-vein-open rate

Filter   A special porous device used for eliminating certain elements as in particles of a certain size in a solution

Gauge   Size of cannula opening—a standard of measurement

Hub   Female connection point of an I.V. cannula where the tubing or other equipment attaches

Implanted port   A catheter surgically placed into a vessel or body cavity and attached to a reservoir

Infusate   Any liquid introduced into the body

Locking device   A capped resealable diaphragm that may have Luer-Lock or Luer-Slip connection. This diaphragm can be accessed multiple times, also called PRN device or saline lock

Lumen   The space within a tubular structure, such as an artery, vein, or catheter

Macrodrop   In I.V. therapy, an administration set that is used to deliver measured amounts of I.V. solutions at a specific flow rate based on the size of the drops of the solution

Microaggregate   Microscopic collection of particles, such as platelets, leukocytes, and fibrin that can exist in stored blood

Microdrop   In I.V. therapy, an administration set that delivers small amounts of I.V. solutions. Drop factor of 60 drops/mL

Midline   Peripherally inserted catheter with the tip terminating in the proximal portion of the extremity, usually 6 inches in length

Multichannel pump   Electronic infusion device that delivers multiple drug or solutions simultaneously or intermittently from bags, bottles, or syringes

Needleless system   A system for administering intravenous solutions that permits intravascular access without the necessity of handling a needle

Over-the-needle catheter   A flexible tube that enables passage of fluid from or into a blood vessel. Consists of needle with a catheter sheath

Patient-controlled analgesia (PCA)   A drug delivery system that dispenses a preset intravascular dose of a narcotic analgesic when the patient pushes a switch on a electric cord

Peripherally inserted central catheter (PICC)   Long (20–24 in.) I.V. access device made of a soft flexible material inserted into one of the superficial veins of the peripheral vascular system and advanced to the superior vena cava

Port   Point of entry

Primary administration set   Device used for delivery of large volume parenterals.

Psi   Pounds per square inch; a measurement of pressure: 1 psi equals 50 mm Hg or 68 cm H_2O

Radiopaque   Material used in I.V. catheter that can be identified by radiographic examination

Rubber bung   Stopper of glass container composed of numerous substances including rubber, chemical particles, and cellulose fibers

Secondary administration set   Administration set that has short tubing used for delivery of 50 to 150 mL of infusion attached to primary administration set for intermittent delivery of medication or solutions.

Stylet   Needle or guide that is found inside a catheter used for vein penetration

Syringe pump   Piston driven pumps that provide precise infusion by controlling the rate of drive speed and syringe size.

Tunneled catheter   A catheter designed to have a portion lie within a subcutaneous passage before exiting the body

▪ Infusion Therapy Equipment

The nurse's role in infusion therapy equipment use includes the decision-making process of equipment acquisition; knowledge of operation of equipment to ensure safe, effective delivery of infusion therapy; and financial accountability. There is a relationship between the industry that manufacturers the equipment, healthcare providers, and the patient that is collaborative and mutually dependent.

The public holds industry, medical institutions, and professionals accountable for the safe and effective delivery of health care. Medical products and equipment are the collaborative responsibility of industry and medical professionals.

▪ Infusion Delivery Systems

Two infusion systems are available for delivery of fluids: the glass system and the plastic system (Fig. 5-1). Sterile evacuated glass containers became available in 1929. The rigid glass containers are composed of a standard mix of materials, glass, metal, and rubber. The combination of materials is a disadvantage because of incompatibilities with fluids and additives and the breakdown of the materials during heat sterilization. In 1950, plastic containers became accessible for the storage and delivery of blood products. Today, the plastic system is used 90% to 95% of the time for administering solutions and blood products.

The Glass System

The glass system available in the United States is the closed glass system. Individual plastic systems are made of the same materials, rather than a combination of glass, plastic, rubber, and metal found in the glass system. The glass system has a partial vacuum and requires an air vent. In the closed-glass system, air is filtered into the container via vented administration tubing. The closed-glass system must use vented tubing to allow air into the container. Although plastic containers are used in most situations, the glass system remains the container of choice for infusates that cannot adapt to plastic bags because of incompatibilities with the chemical or properties of plastic.

The closed glass system has a stopper, also called the **rubber bung**. During insertion of the administration set, **coring** can occur, which results

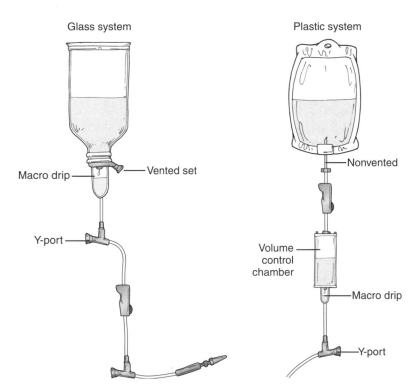

Figure 5-1 ■ Comparison of glass and plastic infusion delivery systems.

in the introduction of fragments of the rubber core into the solution. Twisting the spike through the rubber bung can displace visible and microscopic particles of the rubber bung. Because of the combination of materials in the glass system, some disadvantages have been experienced when using this system during heat sterilization procedures.

Checking the Glass System for Clarity

To ensure safety in the administration of solutions, the nurse must check the solution's clarity and expiration date before connecting it to the administration set. To check the glass system, hold the glass bottle up to the light and check for flashes of light, floating particles, or discoloration. The glass system should be crystal clear; if it is not, mark the container as contaminated and return it to the central supply station. Check the expiration date on the label.

Advantages

- Crystal clear; allows good visualization of contents
- Graduations on glass easy to read.
- Inert; has no plasticizers

Disadvantages

- Breakage and shattering of glass
- Storage problems
- Coring (because of the rubber bung)
- Cumbersome disposal
- Rigidity
- Container constructed of mixed materials

NOTE > Once the glass system is opened by a pharmacist during introduction of an admixture it is sealed with a tamper proof closure to prevent alteration of the infusate. The nurse must check the closure for integrity and if torn must not use and consult the pharmacy.

The Plastic System

Most commonly **infusate** solutions are packaged in plastic containers that are flexible or semirigid (Fig. 5-2). The flexible plastic container has several unique features. The entire structure that comes in contact with the fluid, including the closure, is made of the same material, the most common material for plastic system is polyvinylchloride (PVC), though some non-PVC materials are emerging. There is no combination of metal, rubber, or glass as in the rigid glass system. The plastic system is a truly closed system. The solution containers are provided in 1000-mL and 500-mL bags for primary infusions, and 50- to 150-mL bags for secondary infusions.

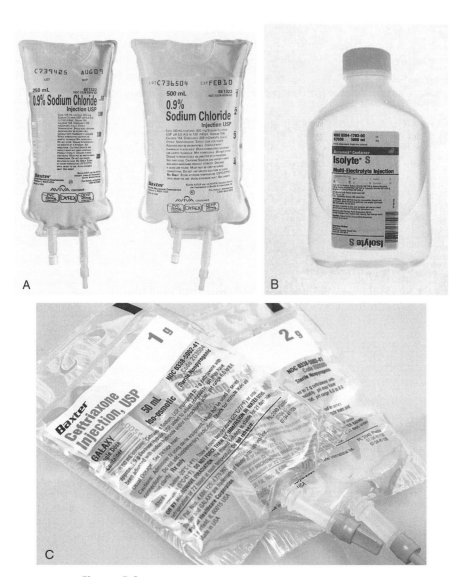

Figure 5-2 ■ Plastic infusion system. I.V. solutions are available in both *(A)* a flexible plastic container (Courtesy of Baxter Healthcare Corp., Round Lake, IL) and *(B)* a more rigid type of container (Courtesy of D. Anderson, Chico, CA). C, Secondary solution container of 50 mL. (Courtesy of Baxter Healthcare Corp., Round Lake, IL.)

NOTE > Use of PVC plastic solution containers has been accompanied by concerns of compatibility, specifically with the di(2-ethylhexyl) phthalate (DEHP). Many manufacturers are providing non-DEHP PVC fluid containers.

The plastic system does not contain a vacuum; therefore, the containers must be flexible and collapsible. The plastic system does not need air to replace fluid flowing from the container. Either a vented or a nonvented administration set is acceptable for delivery of the infusate. Depending on the manufacturer, there may be one or two extensions protruding from the bottom of the bag. If there are two, one is the administration set port, encased in protective easily removable plastic pigtail that maintains the port's sterility before spiking with the administration set. The second extension is an injection port for adding medication. A membrane seals both the medication and the administration ports of the container, and entry of air into this system is prevented. Because there is no rubber bung on the plastic system, spiking the system can be accomplished by means of a simple twisting motion. Because the plastic can be easily perforated during use, careful attention should be paid to the integrity of this container during preparation and infusion delivery.

NOTE > As with glass systems, tamper-proof additive caps are available for use with the plastic system. The cap fits over the medication port and indicates that a pharmacist has added medication to the infusate.

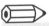 *NURSING FAST FACT!*

Never write directly on a flexible plastic bag with a ballpoint or indelible marker; the pen may puncture the bag and the marker ink may absorb into the plastic.

The outer wrap must remain on until use with PVC bags due to IV fluids lost through the bag. Non-PVC bags do not contain an outer wrap, but have a multilayer film.

The advantages of the semirigid, hard plastic unit are that it is made of polyolefin, contains no plasticizers, and the fluid level marks are easier to read, and impermeable to moisture. Semirigid containers crack easier and do not do well being exposed to temperature extremes. Semirigid containers must be vented to add air to the infusion system.

ADVANTAGES

- Closed system
- Flexible
- Lightweight
- Container composed of one substance
- Better storage

DISADVANTAGES

- Punctures easily
- Fluid level difficult to determine

- Composed of plasticizers
- Not completely inert (potential for leaching)
- Environmentally unsafe

Checking the Plastic System for Clarity

The plastic container should be held up to the light and checked for clarity. If the plastic system is not crystal clear, any discoloration or floating particles in the solution should be identified and labeled as contaminants. The plastic system must be squeezed to check for pinholes. Check the expiration date on the label to ensure patient safety and be sure the outer wrap of the plastic system is free of pooled solution.

 NURSING FAST FACT!

> *It is important that the nurse providing infusion therapy be able to read and identify information provided on the solution bag. Refer to Figure 5-3 for identification of solution bag information.*

Use-Activated Containers

Use-activated containers (Fig. 5-4) are compartmentalized with premeasured ingredients that form an admixture when mixed. The containers are useful for high-use infusions that have a short shelf life after admixture. These systems initially were useful in the emergency department because they enable ease of use in acute situations (such as in an ambulance), in field use, and during transport. However, they are now used commonly

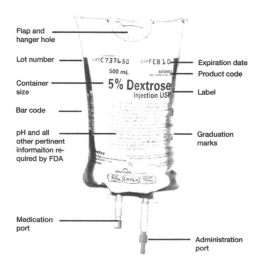

Figure 5-3 ■ Sample solution bag with information identified. (Courtesy of Baxter Healthcare Corp., Round Lake, IL.)

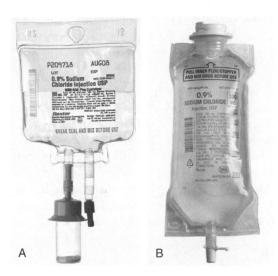

Figure 5-4 ◼ *A*, Medication additive system®. (Courtesy of Baxter Healthcare Corp., Round Lake, IL.) *B*, ADD-Vantage® system allows drugs to be reconstituted quickly and safely in an appropriate amount of diluent immediately before use. (Courtesy of Hospira, Inc., Lake Forest, IL.)

on all nursing departments. The ambulatory and home care settings also benefit from use-activated systems. These systems are more expensive.

To activate the container, the nurse deliberately ruptures the container's seal or diaphragm by compressing opposing parts or applying pressure to rupture the internal reservoir. The primary disadvantage of the system occurs when this step is not completed appropriately and that the med will not be added to the solution.

 NURSING FAST FACT!

A concern with use-activated containers is the belated rupture of the medication reservoir with a potentially harmful concentration of drug being administered .

◼ Administration Sets

The tubing choices or administration sets are manufactured with varying materials. The common types are PVC or non-PVC (usually polyolefin). Administration set choices include:

1. PVC with DEHP: Used for a majority of administration sets; however, not compatible with lipid and some drugs
2. PVC without DEHP: Used for administration of lipids and some drugs

3. Non-PVC lined (polyethylene-lined): Inner lumen is lined with non-PVC material, used for administration of nitroglycerin
4. Non-PVC: Is more rigid plastic than PVC; may not be compatible with some IV infusion pumps

The most frequently used administration sets (primary, secondary, Y-set) vary among manufacturers all have the basic components but vary in drop factor (Fig. 5-5).

◼ Single-line sets, which include primary (standard) sets, secondary sets (also called "piggyback" sets), and volume-controlled (also called metered-volume) sets
◼ Primary Y sets, which are used for rapid infusion or for administration of more than one solution and for administration of blood components with 0.9% sodium chloride.

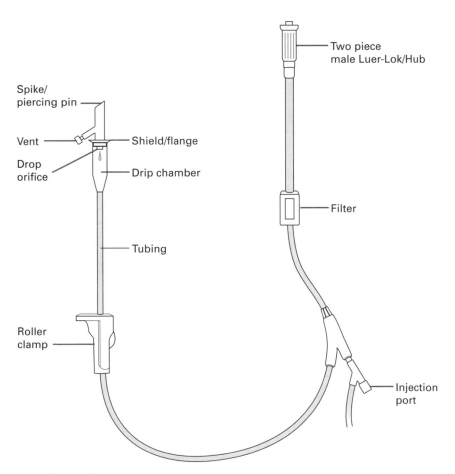

Figure 5-5 ◼ Basic administration system components.

Basic Components of Administration Sets

The basic components of administration sets include:

1. *Spike/piercing pin:* The spike/piercing pin is a sharply tipped plastic tube designed to be inserted into the infusate container. It is connected to the flange, drop orifice, and drip chamber.
2. *Flange:* The flange is a plastic guard that helps prevent touch contamination during insertion of the spike.
3. *Drop orifice:* The drop orifice is an opening that determines the size and shape of the fluid drop. The size of this drop orifice determines the **drop factor**.
4. *Drip chamber:* The drip chamber is a pliable, enlarged clear plastic tube that contains the drop orifice. It is connected to the tubing.
5. *Tubing:* The plastic tubing connects to the drip chamber. Depending on the manufacturer, the tubing may have a variety of clamps, ports, connectors, or filters built into the system. The average length of primary tubing is 66 to 100 inches. The length of secondary administration sets averages from 32 to 42 inches.
6. *Clamp:* The flow clamp control device operates on the principle of compression of the tubing wall. Each manufacturer supplies a clamp (roller, screw, or slide), and all operate on the principle of compression. The roller and screw clamps are equally reliable. The slide clamp is viewed as less reliable in controlling flow.
7. *Injection ports:* Injection ports serve as an access into the tubing and are located at various points along the administration set. Usually the ports are used for administration of medication. These are accessed with needleless and most are Luer activated mechanical valves.
8. *Backcheck valve:* The valve allows the primary solution to resume after the piggyback is completed.
9. *Hub:* The adaptor to connect the administration set to the I.V. catheter or a needleless system is also called the male Luer-Lok or Luer-slip.
10. *Final filter:* The final filter removes foreign particles from the infusate. It can be purchased as part of the administration set tubing, or filters can be added on.

Single-Line Administration Sets

Single-line sets have only one spike that extends proximally from the drip chamber. Only one main bag of infusate is used with this system. The tubing distal to the **drip chamber** terminates in one male-adapter end that connects to the **hub** of a vascular access device.

Primary Sets

Primary sets are referred to as standard or basic sets, and are available as vented or nonvented. Vented sets have an air filter attached to the spike pin that allows air to enter the container. Vented sets must be used on the closed-glass system. Nonvented sets have a straight spike pin without an air vent device. Refer to Figure 5-6. Nonvented sets can be used on any open-glass or plastic system. Primary sets are available in **macrodrip** form (10–20 drops/mL) or in **microdrip** form (60 drops/mL).

Primary sets can have one, two, or three access ports, and often have inline filters with backcheck valves (Schiff, 2001). The drop factor is clearly specified on the box of each administration set, as well as in the accompanying literature. The microdrip set, also called a minidrip or pediatric set, is used when small amounts of fluid are required (Fig. 5-7).

A **check valve** (also called backcheck valve) is a device that functions to prevent retrograde flow of the fluid. When the fluid is flowing in the proper direction, from the bag to the patient, the valve is open. If the fluid flows in the wrong direction, from the patient toward the solution container the valve closes. Check valves are most commonly used to administer secondary medications. The piggyback is attached to the injection port on the upper third of the primary administration set. The check valve

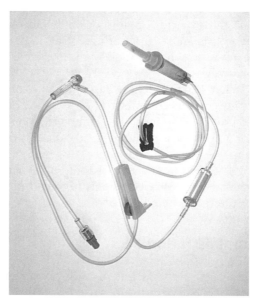

Figure 5-6 ■ Primary administration set. (Courtesy of Baxter Healthcare Corp., Round Lake, IL.)

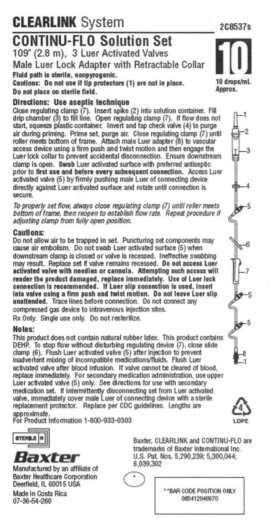

CLEARLINK System   2C8537s

CONTINU-FLO Solution Set

109" (2.8 m), 3 Luer Activated Valves
Male Luer Lock Adapter with Retractable Collar

Fluid path is sterile, nonpyrogenic.
Cautions: Do not use if tip protectors (1) are not in place.
Do not place on sterile field.

10 drops/mL
Approx.

Directions: Use aseptic technique

Close regulating clamp (7). Insert spike (2) into solution container. Fill drip chamber (3) to fill line. Open regulating clamp (7). If flow does not start, squeeze plastic container. Invert and tap check valve (4) to purge air during priming. Prime set, purge air. Close regulating clamp (7) until roller meets bottom of frame. Attach male Luer adapter (8) to vascular access device using a firm push and twist motion and then engage the Luer lock collar to prevent accidental disconnection. Ensure downstream clamp is open. **Swab Luer activated surface with preferred antiseptic prior to first use and before every subsequent connection.** Access Luer activated valve (5) by firmly pushing male Luer of connecting device directly against Luer activated surface and rotate until connection is secure.

To properly set flow, always close regulating clamp (7) until roller meets bottom of frame, then reopen to establish flow rate. Repeat procedure if adjusting clamp from fully open position.

Cautions:
Do not allow air to be trapped in set. Puncturing set components may cause air embolism. Do not swab Luer activated surface (5) when downstream clamp is closed or valve is recessed. Ineffective swabbing may result. Replace set if valve remains recessed. **Do not access Luer activated valve with needles or cannula. Attempting such access will render the product damaged, replace immediately. Use of Luer lock connection is recommended. If Luer slip connection is used, insert into valve using a firm push and twist motion. Do not leave Luer slip unattended.** Trace lines before connection. Do not connect any compressed gas device to intravenous injection sites.
Rx Only. Single use only. Do not resterilize.

Notes:
This product does not contain natural rubber latex. This product contains DEHP. To stop flow without disturbing regulating device (7), close slide clamp (6). Flush Luer activated valve (5) after injection to prevent inadvertent mixing of incompatible medications/fluids. Flush Luer activated valve after blood infusion. If valve cannot be cleared of blood, replace immediately. For secondary medication administration, use upper Luer activated valve (5) only. *See directions for use with secondary medication set.* If intermittently disconnecting set from Luer activated valve, immediately cover male Luer of connecting device with a sterile replacement protector. Replace per CDC guidelines. Lengths are approximate.
For Product Information 1-800-933-0303

STERILE R

Baxter
Manufactured by an affiliate of
Baxter Healthcare Corporation
Deerfield, IL 60015 USA
Made in Costa Rica
07-36-54-260

Baxter, CLEARLINK and CONTINU-FLO are trademarks of Baxter International Inc.
U.S. Pat. Nos. 5,290,239; 5,300,044; 6,039,302

**BAR CODE POSITION ONLY
085412048970

LDPE

Figure 5-7 ▪ Primary administration set package. (Courtesy of Baxter Healthcare Corp., Round Lake, IL.)

is between the site and the primary fluid container, this prevents the secondary medication from flowing into the primary infusion container. The primary container must hang lower than the secondary container. Check valves are inline components of many primary administration sets. Refer to Figure 5-8.

> *EBNP A study of the timing of intravenous administration set changes demonstrated that intravenous administration sets containing crystalloids can be changed in patients every 72 hours or more without increasing the risk of blood-stream infection (BSI; Gilles, O'Riordan, Wallen, et al., 2004).*

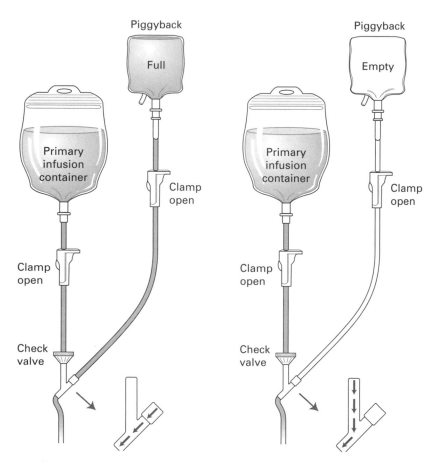

Figure 5-8 ■ Check valve (also called backcheck valve) acts to prevent retrograde solution flow.

INS Standard Primary and secondary *continuous* administration sets shall be changed every 72 hours and immediately on suspected contamination or when the integrity of the product or system has been compromised. All administration sets shall be of Luer-Lok™ design. If a primary *intermittent* administration set is used, it should be changed every 24 hours and immediately on suspected contamination or when the integrity of the product or system has been compromised. (INS, 2006, 48; O'Grady, Alexander, Dellinger, et al., 2002)

Secondary Administration Sets

Two types of secondary administration sets are available: the piggyback set and the volume-controlled set.

Piggyback Set/Secondary Set

The piggyback set has short tubing (30–36 inches) with a standard drop factor of 10 to 20 drops/mL. It is used to deliver 50 to 100 mL of infusate. These sets are widely used because of the administration of multiple drug therapies to patients. They are connected with a needleless adapter into an **injection port** immediately distal to the backcheck valve of the primary tubing. In setting up the piggyback set, the primary infusion container is positioned lower than the secondary container, using the extension hook provided in the secondary line box. Refer to Figure 5-9.

Volume-Controlled Set

The volume-controlled set, also called a metered-volume chamber set, is designed for intermittent administration of measured volumes of fluid with a calibrated chamber. These sets are calibrated in much smaller in- crements than other infusion devices, thus limiting the amount of solution available to the patient (usually for reasons of safety). Most chambers hold 100 to 150 mL of solution, but neonatal chambers may hold only 10 to 50 mL. The volume-controlled set is most frequently used for pedi- atric patients and critically ill patients when small, well-controlled deliv- ery of medication or solution is needed (Fig. 5-10).

> **INS Standard** Primary *intermittent* administration sets shall be changed every 24 hours and immediately upon suspected contamina- tion or when the integrity of the product or system has been compro- mised. (INS, 2006, 48)

Primary Y Administration Sets

The primary Y administration set is used for rapid infusion or for ad- ministration of more than one solution at a time. Each leg of the Y set is capable of being the primary set. The Y set has two separate spikes with a separate drip chamber and short length of tubing with individual

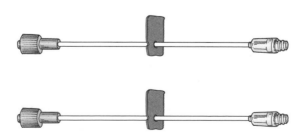

Figure 5-9 ■ Secondary administration set. (Courtesy of Baxter Healthcare Corp., Round Lake, IL.)

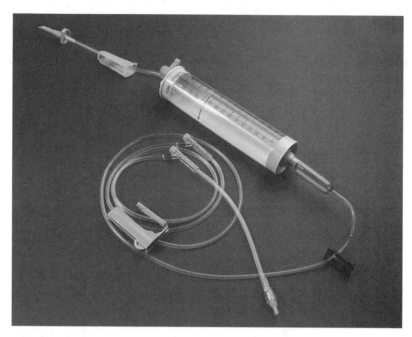

Figure 5-10 ■ Volume chamber control set for intermittent infusion. (Courtesy of Baxter Healthcare Corp., Round Lake, IL.)

clamps. Primary Y sets are made up of large-bore tubing because the purpose of this tubing is to infuse large amounts of fluid in acute situations. Blood components can be administered through primary Y sets. A Y set allows for priming of the administration set before the blood is administered. Most blood administration Y sets contain inline filters with a pore size of 170 to 260 microns and have a drop factor of 10 to allow for the safe infusion of blood cells (American Association of Blood Banks [AABB], 2008). Refer to Figure 5-11.

> **INS Standard** Administration sets and add-on filters that are used for blood and blood components shall be changed after administration of each unit or at the end of 4 hours, whichever comes first. (INS, 2006, 48)

Pump-Specific Administration Sets

Pump-specific administration sets are made specifically for use with electronic infusion devices (EIDs). These sets also come in a number of configurations, with each set specific for respective electronic delivery systems. For specifics on each pump administration set, see the literature that accompanies each EID.

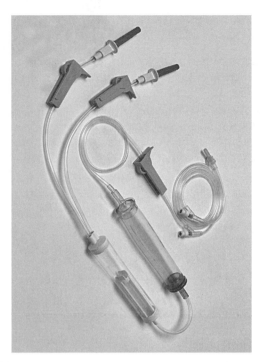

Figure 5-11 ■ Y administration set used for blood administration. (Courtesy Teleflex Medical, Research Triangle Park, NC.)

Lipid Administration Sets (Intravenous Fat Emulsion [IVFE])

Lipids or fat emulsions are supplied in glass containers and require special vented tubing that is supplied by the manufacturer. Lipid-containing infusates have been known to leach phthalates from bags and tubing made of PVC. Fat emulsions are supplied in glass containers with non-PVC infusion sets.

Special Medication Administration Sets

Some drugs (nitroglycerin and Taxol specifically) readily migrates into many plastics, including PVC plastics. Nitroglycerin absorption by PVC tubing is increased when the tubing is long, the flow rates are low, and the nitroglycerin concentration of the solution is high. Nitroglycerin should be used with non-PVC sets and glass containers. Taxol solutions should be stored in glass or polyolefin plastic container and administered through polyethylene-lined administration sets (Trissel, 2006). Special administration sets are used for propofol infusions, and the CDC (2002) recommend replacing sets every 6 to 12 hours, when the vial is changed, per the manufacturer's recommendation.

INS Standard When units of intravenous fat emulsion (IVFE) are administered consecutively, the administration set shall be changed every 24 hours; IVFE administration sets shall be changed immediately upon suspected contamination or when the integrity of the product or system has been compromised.

When a unit of IVFE is administered intermittently, a sterile administration set shall be attached to each new container. (INS, 2006, 48)

 NURSING FAST FACT!

> It is important that all administration sets be changed using aseptic technique, that they be of Luer-Lok™ design and be anti-free-flow.

Accessory Devices/Add-On Devices

Accessory, or add-on, devices for administration sets include:
- Securement devices
- Extension tubings
- Filters
- Injection and access caps
- Stopcocks

When an add-on device is used, it should be of a Luer-Lok configuration. Aseptic technique and infection control measures must be followed for all add-on device changes. Adding accessories to an existing administration set is referred to as breaching the infusion line. Whenever an infusion line is breached, the possibility of introduction of contaminates exists.

INS Standard When add-on devices are used, they should be changed with each catheter or administration set replacement, or whenever the integrity of either product is compromised. (INS, 2000, 35)

Securement Devices

Securement devices are those that secure tubing and/or a catheter to the patient. Historically, nonsterile tape has been used to secure peripheral IV catheters (Maki, 1991). The complications that result from this method of securement have been documented in hospital and home care settings. The complications include dislodgement, disconnection, infiltration, phlebitis, skin damage, unscheduled dressing changes, and unscheduled catheter restarts (Sheppard, LeDesma, Moris, & O'Connor, 1999).

Newer securement devices are available for better patient outcomes to reduce complications associated with catheter movement (e.g., infection, phlebitis and infiltration). Many new securement devices are on the market now: StatLock® (C.R. Bard), Grip-Lok™ (Zefon Medical), and Tegaderm™ securement dressing (3M). Many of the securement devices include custom-formulated acrylic adhesive and precision-molded engagement parts.

> *EBNP A prospective study of two intravenous catheter securement techniques found that the use of a securement device (StatLock®) reduced complications associated with managing vascular access devices (Sheppard, LeDesma, Moris, & O'Connor, 1999).*

Refer to Figure 5-12.

NOTE > Tape should not be used as a means of junction securement (INS, 2006, 29).

INS Standard Catheter stabilization shall be used to preserve the integrity of the access device and to prevent catheter migration and loss of access.

Products used to stabilize the catheter should include manufactured catheter stabilization devices, sterile tapes, and surgical strips. Whenever feasible, using a manufactured catheter stabilization device is preferred. (INS, 2006, 43)

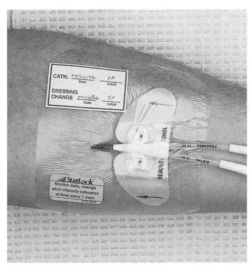

Figure 5-12 ■ Securement device, StatLock®. (Courtesy of Bard Access Systems, Covington, GA.)

Extension Tubing Sets

Extension tubing is an add-on administration set used to add length. The short tubing is usually connected to an intermittent locking device and then connected to the hub of the catheter. Refer to Figure 5-13. Extension tubing is also frequently used as primary tubing for syringe pumps and ambulatory pumps. Disadvantages are an added cost and an additional site for bacteria to enter the system.

Filters

Inline Infusion Solution Filters

Inline **filters** are used during the infusion of intravenous medications to prevent the administration of any particulate matter, air, or microorganisms that may be in the I.V. line. Particles of 5 to 20 microns and larger have the capability of obstructing blood flow through pulmonary capillaries. Foreign particles can also cause phlebitis at the injection site and filters may help to reduce the incidence of phlebitis. The use of inline filtration in intravenous infusions guards against inadvertent infusion of particulate matter; air and lipid emboli; endotoxins; and microorganisms such as bacteria, protozoa, and fungi. There are two groups of particulate

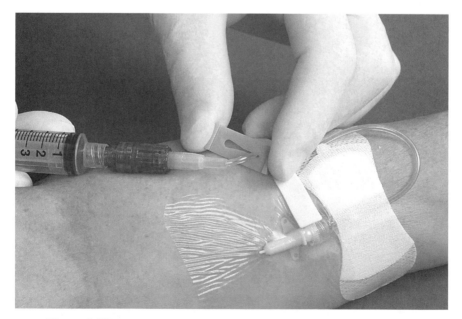

Figure 5-13 ■ Extension tubing connected to access device and hub of catheter, with slide clamp. (Courtesy of Baxter Healthcare Corp., Round Lake, IL.)

matter: (1) nonviable contaminants such as particles of metal, lint, asbestos, rubber, cotton, dust, and glass and (2) viable contaminants, consisting of bacteria and fungi. In addition, inline filters remove undissolved drug powders or crystals and precipitates from incompatible admixtures.

The Infusion Nurses Society standards (2006) favor the inline filters for removal of bacteria, fungi, particulate matter, air, and some endotoxins from I.V.-delivered fluids. The National Coordinating Committee on Large Volume Parenteral has established priorities for the use of filters and recommends the use of filters with tissue plasminogen activator (TPN) admixtures; for immunodeficient or immunocompromised patients; and for I.V. infusions containing additives, especially those that are heavily precipitated.

Inline filters are available in a variety of forms, sizes, and materials:

- Filters measuring 170 microns remove most debris from blood.
- Filters measuring 0.5 to 1.2 microns remove most particulate matter but do not remove fungi or bacteria.
- Filters measuring 0.45 micron remove fungi or bacteria.
- Filters measuring 0.2 micron remove all fungi and bacteria but can reduce flow rates.

Refer to Figure 5-14 for an example of a 0.22-micron filter.

The smallest human capillary is slightly larger than a red blood cell (approximately 6 microns). Well mixed infusate solutions may contain microprecipitates in the range of 1 to 50 microns. The use of inline filters ensures removal of particles that can pass rigorous visual inspection. Infusion-related phlebitis, a common complication occurring in patients receiving I.V. therapy, can be attributed to physical (microprecipitates and particulate matter) and chemical (irritating pharmaceuticals and additives) causes, as well as increased manipulation of I.V. sets and materials (Maki & Mermel, 2007).

Multiple organ failure (MOF) is one of the most serious disease complexes in contemporary intensive care medicine. Experimental studies indicate that from a pathophysiological point of view MOF is a problem of microcirculation. One of the components of MOF is adult respiratory distress syndrome (ARDS). In ARDS pathogenetic mechanisms lead to microthrombus formation. It is hypothesized that the contaminants in intravenous infusions, both of particulate and endotoxin nature may significantly contribute to the microcirculatory disturbances (Pall, 2008).

EBNP A study by Kirkpatrick (1992) concluded that data from in vivo and in vitro studies support the view that high-risk groups, such as intensive care patients, be protected from contaminants from intravenous infusions by effective filtration systems, for both particulate matter and endotoxins.

EBNP A study of 88 neonates (76 preterm, 12 term) randomized to receive IV fluids and medications through an endotoxin-retentive intravenous filter (Pall Posidyne ELD96™, 0.2 micron) or unfiltered showed a 50% reduction in sepsis with decreased cost in nursing time (van Lingen, Baerts, Marquering, & Ruijs, 1997).

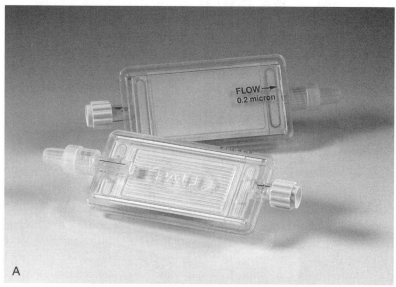

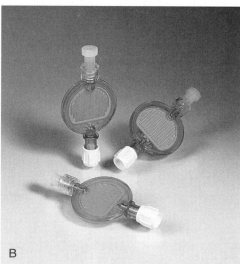

Figure 5-14 ◼ *A*, Posidyne® ELD 0.2 micron filter. *B*, The Supor® AE NT 0.2-micron filter set for removal of inadvertent particulate debris and bacterial contamination with minimal drug binding. (Courtesy of Pall Corp., Ann Arbor, MI.)

INS Standard A 0.22-micron filter is considered a bacterial/particulate retentive, air-eliminating filter and is recommended for use to decrease the potential of air emboli, reduce the risk of phlebitis, and prevent bacterial contamination. To achieve final filtration, the filter should be located as close to the **cannula** site as possible. The filter should be an integral part of the administration set. (INS, 2006, 32)

Membrane Filters

Membrane filters are screen filters with uniformly sized pores. Filters range in size from 170 microns (largest) to 0.22 micron (smallest). They allow liquids but not particles to pass through them. The finer the membrane, the more fully it will filter the liquid. A 5-micron screen will retain on the flat portion of the membrane all particles larger than 5 microns. Filters of 0.2 microns are for bacteria, fungus, and air retention. The 0.22-micron air-venting filters automatically vent air through a nonwettable (hydrophobic) membrane and permit uniform high-gravity flow through large wettable (hydrophilic) membrane.

To be effective, an infusion membrane filter must have the ability to:
- Maintain high flow rates
- Automatically vent air
- Retain bacteria, fungi, particulate matter, and endotoxins
- Tolerate pressures generated by infusion pumps
- Act in a nonbinding fashion to drugs

Membrane filters are used when:

1. An additive has been combined with the solution.
2. The injection port on the tubing is used.
3. The patient is susceptible to infusion phlebitis.
4. The infusion is given centrally.
5. The solution is a three-in-one TPN solution.

Prescribed therapies in which a 0.2-micron filter is contraindicated include administration of blood or blood components, lipid emulsions, and low-dose (less than 5 micron/mL) solutions. Other contraindications include the administration of low-volume medications (total amount less than 5 mg over 24 hours), I.V. push medications, medications in which pharmacologic properties are altered by the filter membrane, and medications that adhere to the filter membrane.

All filters have a certain pressure value at which they will allow the passage of air from one side of a wetted hydrophilic membrane to the other. This pressure valve is called the bubble point. Filters are also rated according to the pounds per square inch (**psi**) of pressure they can withstand. The filter should withstand the psi exerted by the infusion pump or rupture may occur. If the psi rating of the housing is less than that of the membrane, excess force will break the housing.

INS Standard When using a positive-pressure EID, consideration should be given to the psi rating of a filter. The psi exerted by the device should never exceed the psi capacity of the filter. (INS, 2006, 32)

Filters for Crystalloid Intravenous Therapy

An air-eliminating 0.22-micron filter set designed for 96-hour bacteria and endotoxin retention is indicated for use with I.V. administration sets for the removal of inadvertent particulate debris, microbial contaminants, and their associated endotoxin, and entrained air that may be found in solutions intended for I.V. administration (Pall, 2008). Ideally, a 0.2-micron filter provides low protein binding with minimal adsorption while containing no external wetting agents or surfactant to introduce unwanted extractables, and is free or natural rubber latex. The 0.2-micron filter can be used with continuous infusions or intermittent infusions or injections.

Lipid Filter Set

A filter set for total nutritional admixture administration has a 1.2-micron air-eliminating filter. This filter set is indicated for use with any nutritional I.V. administration containing lipids for the removal of inadvertent particulate debris, fungal contaminants, and entrained air (Pall, 2008; Fig. 5-15). These filters retain oversized lipid droplets.

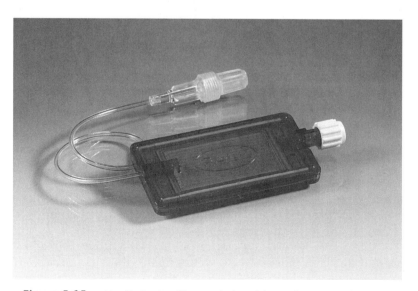

Figure 5-15 ■ Air-eliminating filter set designed for total nutrient admixture solutions. This filter has a 1.2-micron nylon membrane that provides an effective barrier for the patient from inadvertent particulate contamination, uncontrollable precipitate contamination, and entrained air. (Courtesy of Pall Corp., Ann Arbor, MI.)

Neonatal and Infant Filters

This filter is designed for the neonatal intensive care unit and offers protection against particles, microbes, endotoxins, and entrapped air (Pall, 2008). The device is small with a round housing, making the 0.2-micron filter easy to secure and comfortable for pediatric patients. Refer to Figure 5-16.

Blood Filters

The American Association of Blood Banks states that blood must be transfused through a sterile, pyrogen-free transfusion set that has a filter capable of retaining particles that are potentially harmful to the recipient (AABB, 2008). Commercially available filters include the standard clot filter, the microaggregate filter, and the leukocyte depletion filter. For further details on blood filters, see Chapter 11.

> **INS Standard** Blood and blood by product filters, appropriate to the therapy, shall be used to reduce particulate matter, microaggregates, or leukocytes in infusions of blood and blood products. (INS, 2006, 32)

Standard Clot Filter

Blood administration sets have a standard clot filter of 170 to 260 microns. They are intended to remove coagulated products, microclots, and debris resulting from collection and storage. These filters allow passage of

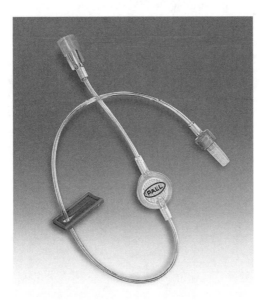

Figure 5-16 ■ Neonatal filter. (Courtesy of Pall Corp., Ann Arbor, MI.)

smaller particles called microaggregates, which are composed of nonviable leukocytes, primarily granulocytes, platelets, and fibrin strands. The microaggregates can cause pulmonary dysfunction (ARDS) when large quantities of stored bank blood are infused.

Microaggregate Filters

A supplementary filter (transfusion filter) can be added to an in-use administration set, permitting infusion of blood, easy replacement of the filter (if clogging occurs), and multiple infusions of blood units. The 20- to 40-micron **microaggregate** blood filters remove most debris from the transfusion product but can slow the administration of blood to an undesirable rate. The 40-micron filter allows blood to be transfused easily in the specified period of time; however, filtration is less refined. The 80-micron filter is the filter of choice in many institutions because of its safe level of filtration and high flow rate potential. A microaggregate filter is a free-flow, low priming volume device that provides a 40-micron rated screen filter medium for the removal of potentially harmful blood components, microaggregates, and nonblood component particulate matter (Fig. 5-17).

Leukocyte Depletion Filters

Leukocyte depletion filters are used to remove leukocytes (including leukocyte-mediated viruses) from red blood cells and platelets. Leukocyte-poor filters are classified according to efficiency level, not micron size. These filters can be used to remove 99.9% of leukocytes from red blood cells, platelets, and plasma (Pall, 2008). Additional information on leukocyte depletion filters is provided in Chapter 11. Refer to Figure 5-18.

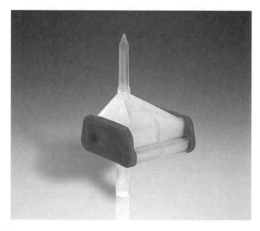

Figure 5-17 ■ Microaggregate blood transfusion filter. (Courtesy of Pall Corp., Ann Arbor, MI.)

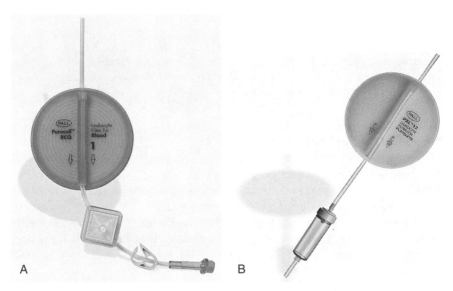

Figure 5-18 ■ Leukocyte depletion filters. *A*, Purecell® RCQ for blood and *B*, PXL 12 Leukocyte™ filter for platelets. (Courtesy of Pall Corp., Ann Arbor, MI.)

Websites

Pall Medical Filter information: www.pall.com/medical

Stopcocks

A stopcock is a device that controls the direction of flow of an infusate through manual manipulation of a direction-regulating valve. A stopcock is usually a three- or four-way device. A three-way stopcock connects two lines of fluid to a patient and provides a mechanism for either one to run to the patient (similar to a faucet). With a four-way stopcock, the valve can be manipulated so that one or both lines can run to the patient, alone, or in combination.

The general use of stopcocks used for medications, administration of I.V. infusions, and collection of blood samples represent a potential portal of entry for microorganisms and are strongly discouraged because of the issue of contamination (O'Grady, Alexander, Dellinger, et al., 2002). When the stopcock portals are uncapped they are vulnerable to touch contamination. The stopcock itself is small and requires handling in such a way that sterility can easily be compromised. Syringes are frequently attached to I.V. push administration, and the portal is poorly protected after use.

INS Standard A stopcock should be changed with each catheter change and should be covered with a sterile cap when not in use. (INS, 2006, 29)

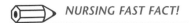 NURSING FAST FACT!

> Caution should be exercised when using a stopcock because of the risk of contamination of the I.V. system or accidental disconnection if a Luer-Lok™ connection is not used or if the stopcock is accidentally turned. Also, the infusion might be interrupted or administered incorrectly.

Needleless Systems

The Needlestick Safety and Prevention Act, which took effect in April of 2001, reinforces the need to use safe needles to reduce injuries. Numerous studies have documented the efficacy of needleless I.V.-access devices in reducing the risk of I.V.-related injuries. Needleless systems and needle safety systems are the state-of-the-art technology of needle systems and are used to connect I.V. devices, administer infusates and medications, and sample blood.

The use of protected needles or needleless equipment significantly decreases the risk of needlestick injuries (ECRI, 2003). An increasing number and variety of needle devices with safety features are now available. Examples of safety device designs include:

- Needleless valves and caps
- Protected needle connectors
- Needles that retract into a syringe or vacuum tube holder
- Hinged or sliding shields attached to phlebotomy needles, winged steel needles
- Protective encasements to receive an I.V. stylet
- Sliding needle shields attached to disposable syringes and vacuum tube holders
- Self-blunting phlebotomy and winged steel needles
- Retractable finger/heel-stick lancets

Figure 5-19 is an example of a needleless injection system (NIS) with a Luer mechanism.

Luer Access Valve/Injection Ports

A **locking device** is a capped resealable diaphragm that has a Luer-Lok™ connection, and is part of a NIS or needleless access port (NAP). Refer to Figure 5-20 for three examples of positive displacement valves. The use of NIS has reduced the risk of needlestick injuries to healthcare workers (O'Grady, Alexander, Dellinger, et al., 2002). This type of device can convert a continuous I.V. infusion to an intermittent device when the NIS valve or cap is inserted into the cannula hub. The resealable lock is used for flushing to maintain catheter patency or delivery of intermittent fluid or medications.

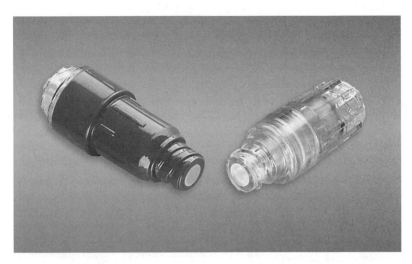

Figure 5-19 ▪ Needleless I.V. access devices. Luer mechanical valve. Clearlink® & Flolink®. (Courtesy of Baxter Healthcare Corp., Round Lake, IL.)

There are currently several types of NIS/NAP, differentiated by the type of fluid movement through them. Refer to Figure 5-21 for chart.
- Blunt cannula split–septum (negative displacement)
- Luer access mechanical valve (negative displacement)
- Luer access mechanical valve with positive displacement feature
- Neutral displacement needleless system

The blunt cannula split-septum is penetrated by a blunt cannula to become the fluid path. The Luer mechanical valve has an internal mechanism actuated with a standard male Luer (syringe tip or administration set) to open a fluid path. The Luer access mechanical valve with positive displacement feature has an additional fluid reservoir that creates positive displacement on disconnection. The positive displacement needleless injection system will reserve a small amount of fluid to push toward the catheter tip at disconnection of the syringe or tubing, thus preventing blood from remaining inside the lumen. The neutral displacement needleless system has slight refluxing but generally will not allow fluid to move in either direction when tubing or a syringe is disconnected (Hadaway, 2006). The New V-Link™ (Baxter, IL) device with VitaShield™ is the first needless I.V. connector containing an antimicrobial coating on the inner and outer surfaces with proprietary silver technology. The V-Link is a Luer-activated device (Baxter, 2008). Refer to Figure 5-22.

 NURSING FAST FACT!

Negative and positive displacement devices are dependent upon flushing technique. It is important that all nurses using NIS understand which type of device is being used.

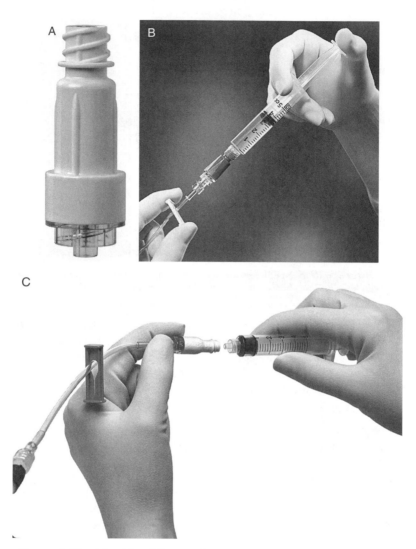

Figure 5-20 ■ Needleless I.V. access devices. Luer with positive displacement features. *A*, Ultrasite®. (Courtesy of B. Braun Medical, Inc., Bethlehem,PA.). *B*, Posiflow™. (Courtesy of Becton Dickinson, Sandy, UT.) *C*, Smart Site Plus Alaris. (Courtesy of Cardinal Health Co., San Diego, CA.)

Flushing Techniques

When a negative-displacement device is used one of the positive pressure flushing techniques is required. Refer to Chapter 6 for steps in flushing NIS. INS defines positive pressure as a constant, even force within a catheter lumen preventing reflux of blood by clamping during injection or by withdrawing from the catheter hub while injecting (INS, 2006).

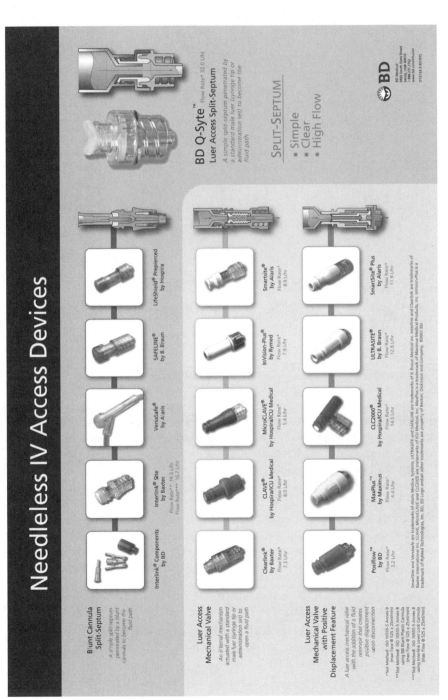

Figure 5-21 ■ Chart negative and positive displacement devices. (Courtesy of Becton Dickinson, Sandy, UT.)

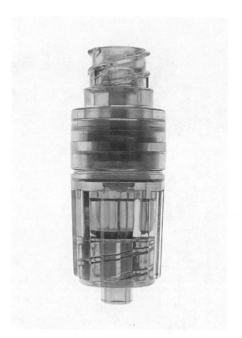

Figure 5-22 ■ V-Link™ Luer activated device with antimicrobial coating interior and exterior surfaces, flat swabable surface. (Courtesy of Baxter Healthcare Corp., Round Lake, IL.)

When a positive-displacement NIS is used, the nurse must disconnect the tubing or syringe, allow sufficient time for the positive fluid displacement, and then close the catheter clamp. Using a positive-pressure flushing technique on a positive displacement NIS will prevent proper function of the positive displacement NIS.

A disadvantage of a valve or cap is that it can separate at the hub or plug junction allowing bacteria to enter the system, or development of biofilm from gram-negative bacteria inside NIS from collection of whole blood cells within the silicone valve (Hadaway, 2006).

- The CDC recommends changing needleless devices in the same interval as the I.V. administration set (O'Grady, Alexander, Dillinger, et al., 2002).
- The Infusion Nurses Society allows for changing at least every 7 days (INS, 2006, 35).
- Some studies recommend changing valve/caps every 2 days rather than once per week to decrease BSI (Do, Ray, Banerjee, et al., 1999).

Refer to Evidence-Based Care Box 5-1 for a description of a study on disinfection of NAPs.

NOTE > Further research is needed to identify the factors associated with NIS and BSI.

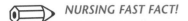 *NURSING FAST FACT!*

Emphasis on appropriate disinfection of injection port with each connection using a twisting motion with 70% alcohol or 3.1% chlorhexidine/70% alcohol for 15 seconds using friction (twisting motion) is strongly recommended (Kaler & Chinn, 2007).

EVIDENCE-BASED CARE BOX 5-1

Time and Friction Study—Disinfection of Needleless Access Ports (NAPs)

Kaler, W., & Chinn, R. (2007). Successful disinfection of needleless access ports: A matter of time and friction. JAMA, 12(3), 140–142.

The ports of four models of needleless access ports were inoculated with bacteria (*Staphylococcus epidermidis, Staphylococcus aureus, Pseudomonas aeruginosa and Candida albicans*). After inoculation, the membranous septa were allowed to air dry for 18 hours. The ports were then disinfected for 15 seconds with 70% alcohol alone or 3.15% chlorhexidine/70% alcohol. Saline flush solutions were collected and cultured.

Results: Disinfection with either 70% alcohol alone or with 3.15% chlorhexidine/ 70% alcohol for 15 seconds were effective. All models of needleless access ports were effectively disinfected using these two methods.

INS Standard Injection or access caps attached to a catheter shall be of Luer-Lok™ design.

To prevent entry of microorganisms into the vascular system, the injection or access port should be aseptically cleansed with an approved antiseptic solution immediately before use; antiseptic solution of single-use package should be used. Whenever an injection or access cap is removed from a catheter, it should be discarded and a new sterile injection or access cap should be attached. (INS, 2006, 35)

■ Peripheral Infusion Devices

Several types of peripheral infusion devices are commercially available: scalp vein needles, over-the-needle catheters (peripheral-short catheters), single- and dual-**lumen** catheters, and midline catheters. The catheter-type devices usually have **radiopaque** material or stripping added to ensure radiographic visibility. Radiopacity aids in the identification of a catheter embolus, a rare complication. The hub of a cannula is plastic and color coded to indicate the length and **gauge**. A short peripheral catheter is defined as one that is smaller than 3 inches in length.

Catheters are made of various biocompatible materials such as steel polytetrafluoroethylene (Teflon), polyurethane, silicone, and Vialon™ (Becton Dickinson). Teflon is less thrombogenic and less inflammatory than polyurethane or PVC, and Vialon is a newer material that is non-hemolytic and free of plasticizers. Teflon, a polyurethane material, has been shown to provide low cost, low rates of infiltration, and comparatively low rates of phlebitis. Vialon is slick when wetted and softens after insertion, minimizing venous trauma and clot induction. For a comparison of the types of peripheral infusion devices, see Table 5-1.

> *EBNP Teflon over-the-needle catheters tend to increase the risk of infusion-related phlebitis with small peripheral venous catheters over Vialon catheters (Maki & Ringer, 1991).*

> Table 5-1 **COMPARISON OF PERIPHERAL INFUSION DEVICES**

Cannula	Advantages	Disadvantages	Uses
Scalp-Vein Needle	Excellent for one-time I.V. medication, blood withdrawal, in patients allergic to nylon or Teflon Wings allow ease of insertions and secure taping. Attached extension permits easy tubing change.	Needle increases the risk of infiltration Not recommended for use in flexor areas Needle not flexible Repuncture by contaminated needle possible	Infants and children Elderly and other adults with small veins Adults receiving short-term therapy
Over-the-Needle	Easy to insert Stays patent longer Catheter tip tapered to prevent peel-back Radiopaque feature makes radiographic detection easy Infiltration rare Winged cannula easy to tape Stable; allows for greater patient mobility	Depending on the hub, sometimes difficult to secure with tape Long inflexible stylet increases the risk of accidental puncture; pressure marks from hub Some catheters drag through the skin on insertion. Increased risk of phlebitis	Long-term therapy Delivery of viscous liquids: Blood and total parenteral nutrition Arterial monitoring

> Table 5-1	COMPARISON OF PERIPHERAL INFUSION DEVICES—cont'd		
Cannula	Advantages	Disadvantages	Uses
Through-the-Needle	Permits insertion of catheter into the SVC Less likely to damage veins Stable	Needle remains secured outside the skin; risk of catheter embolus Plastic catheter may support infection or trigger phlebitis in central veins Central venous pressure monitoring	Long-term therapy Delivery of viscous liquid Delivery of drugs

Vialon, an elastomer of polyurethane, is a high-strength material that provides a smooth-surfaced catheter for easy insertion. After it is inside a vein, Vialon becomes soft and pliable, permitting the catheter to float in the vein rather than against the intima of the vein wall. Vialon is also designed to minimize local reactions under conditions of extended use.

INS Standard The catheter selected shall be of the smallest size and the shortest length possible to accommodate the prescribed therapy. All catheters shall be radiopaque. (INS, 2006, 38)

Scalp-Vein Steel Needles

The wing-tipped or butterfly needles are types of scalp-vein steel needles. Scalp-vein needles are made of stainless steel with odd-numbered gauges (i.e., 17-, 19-, 21-, 23-, 25-) and lengths of 0.5 to 1.0 inch. The wings attached to the shaft are made of rubber or plastic, and the flexible tubing extending behind the wings varies from 3 to 12 inches long (Fig. 5-23).

These needles are most frequently used for short-term therapy, usually in patients with expected indwelling catheter times of less than 24 hours, such as with single-dose therapy, I.V. push medications, or blood sample retrieval. Steel needles are biocompatible, and low rates of inflammation or phlebitis have been documented. Steel cannulas do not flex or yield with resistance; therefore, the steel tip can easily puncture the vasculature after placement, increasing the risk of infiltration.

INS Standard The use of steel-winged infusion sets should be limited to short-term or single-dose administration. (INS, 2006, 38)

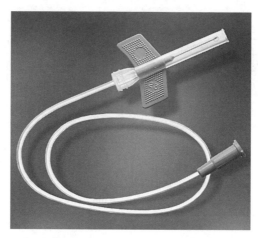

Figure 5-23 ■ Butterfly winged scalp vein needle. (Courtesy of Becton Dickinson, Sandy, UT.)

Over-the-Needle Catheters

The most widely used infusion device is the **over-the-needle catheter** (ONC), which consists of a two-part flexible catheter in tandem with a rigid needle or stylet that is used as a guide to puncture and insert the catheter into the vein. The stylet connects with a clear chamber that allows for visualization of blood return indicating successful venipuncture. The hub of the catheter is plastic and color coded to indicate length and gauge. Refer to Figure 5-24 for hubs and examples of over-the-needle catheters. The point of the stylet extends beyond the tip of the catheter. After venipuncture, the needle (**stylet**) is withdrawn and discarded, leaving a flexible catheter within the vein. The peripheral-short catheter consists of a catheter with a length of 0.5 to 3.0 inches and gauges of even numbers ranging from 12 to 24. Use the following as a guide regarding when to use the different gauge catheters:

- 14- to 16-gauge: Multiple trauma, heart surgery, transplantation procedures
- 18-gauge: Major trauma or surgery, blood administration
- 20-gauge: Minor trauma or surgery, blood administration
- 22- to 24-gauge: Pediatric use, person with small veins, administration of platelets or plasma in limited situations.

 NURSING FAST FACT!

With any catheter, use the shortest length and the smallest gauge to deliver the ordered therapy. Also, use a vein large enough to sustain sufficient blood flow because this will decrease irritation to the vein wall.

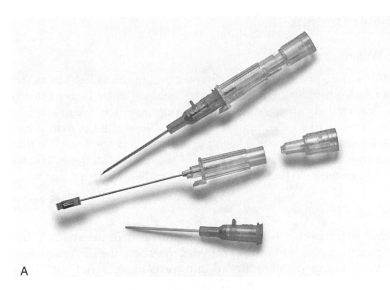

A

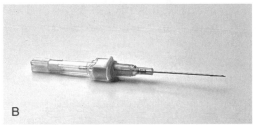

B

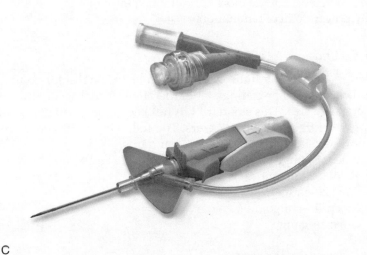

C

Figure 5-24 ■ Over-the-needle catheters. *A*, Introcan® safety I.V. catheter with passive safety. (Courtesy of B. Braun Medical Inc., Bethlehem, PA.) *B*, Addvantive® ONC®. (Courtesy of Smith Medical Critical Care, Carlsbad, CA.) C, Nexiva™ closed I.V. catheter system. (Courtesy of Becton Dickinson, Sandy, UT.)

Catheter Designs

Thin-Walled

The thin-walled over-the-needle catheter is constructed of plastic and its thinner wall provides higher flow rates because of its larger internal lumen. Thin-walled catheters are smoother on insertion because they have a more tapered fit to the inner stylet. The thin-walled construction also causes the catheter to become less able to hold its shape once it is inserted and warmed to body temperature. This soft, "flimsy" catheter is easier on the intima of the vein but collapses with negative pressure.

Flashback Chambers

The flashback chamber is a small space at the hub of the stylet. When the stylet punctures the vein during catheter insertion, the increased pressure in the vein is immediately relieved into the catheter stylet with a flow of blood in the flashback chamber. This allows the nurse to see that the blood return is continuing as the catheter is advanced and secured. The safest catheters use a flashback chamber that allows the rapid return of blood but prohibits any blood spillage.

Addition of Wings

Adding wings to the design of I.V. catheters and scalp-vein needles is intended to improve insertion technique and catheter stabilization. The wings are usually flexible plastic protrusions from the hub of the device. Winged catheters provide more control when the catheter is manipulated, thereby preventing contamination.

Color Coding

The peripheral catheter hubs incorporate international color-coding standards. Universal color-coding standards allow visual recognition of the catheter gauge size. This standard has not been applied to gauge sizes of midline or central infusion catheters. The following color codes are common; however, they are not industry standards.

- Blue: 24-gauge
- Yellow: 22-gauge
- Pink: 20-gauge
- Green: 18-gauge
- Gray: 16-gauge

 NURSING FAST FACT!

Looking at color-coding should never substitute for reading the package label.

Needle Protection: Active and Passive Sharps Safety

The Needlestick Safety and Prevention Act of April 2001 mandates that U.S. healthcare workers be engaged in new safer sharps. The OSHA blood-borne pathogens standards as of July 1, 2004 mandate protected needles. Two categories of safer needle devices incorporate prevention techniques for intravenous catheters: the active design and passive design.

The active design safety needles require healthcare workers to activate a safety mechanism after use to protect against accidental needlesticks. The user can bypass these safety mechanisms, leaving him or her at risk for injury. If a nurse forgets to activate the safety mechanism or if the safety mechanism fails to activate once the needle is removed from the patient, the nurse is at risk. The passive design deploys automatically during use. The FDA defined "passive devices" as those requiring no user activation, thus offering a sharps injury prevention feature that is an integral part of the device: one that cannot be deactivated and remains protective through disposal. Healthcare workers cannot bypass this mechanism; they remain protected from pre- through postusage (Shelton & Rosenthal, 2004). Refer to Figure 5-25.

> **EBNP** *A study in 2003 demonstrated that over a 6-month period, in 87,000 usages, no needlestick injuries occurred when a passive design was used (Mendelson, Chen, Solomon, et al., 2003).*

INS Standard Peripheral-short catheters and steel-winged infusion sets should be equipped with a safety device with engineered sharps injury protection. (INS, 2006, 38)

Dual-Lumen Peripheral Catheters

The dual-lumen peripheral catheter is available in a range of catheter gauges with corresponding lumen sizes. Two totally separate infusion channels exist, making it possible to infuse two solutions simultaneously. They are available as 16-gauge catheters with 18- and 20-gauge lumens or as 18-gauge catheters with 20- and 22-gauge lumens. Dual-lumen catheters are also available as midlines.

 NURSING FAST FACT!

> *Controversy still exists regarding simultaneous infusions of known incompatible solutions or medications through a dual-lumen peripheral catheter because of the limited hemodilution achievable in any peripheral vessel.*

Midline Catheters

Midline catheters were introduced in the 1950s by the Desert Medical Corporation and used for surgical patients who often needed 1 week of

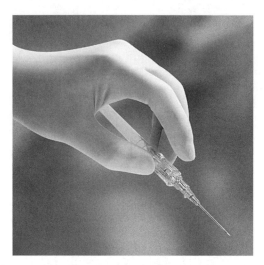

Figure 5-25 ■ Insyte® with Authoguard. (Courtesy of Becton Dickinson, Sandy, UT.)

infusate therapy. In the early 1980s improvements were made in the design to incorporate a split-away plastic introducer and evolved to its current design. Any catheter placed between the antecubital area and the head of the clavicle is called a midline catheter.

Midline catheters are designed for intermediate-term therapies of up to 4 weeks of isotonic or near isotonic therapy. Refer to Figure 5-26. The catheters are between 3 and 8 inches long and are made of polyurethane or silicone. It is placed midline in the antecubital region in the basilic, cephalic, or median antecubital site and is then advanced into the larger vessels of the upper arm for greater hemodilution. The catheter is placed using sterile technique and a traditional breakaway peripheral introducer or via a

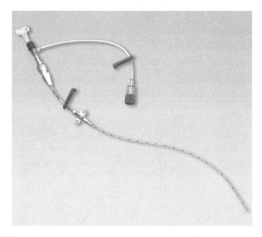

Figure 5-26 ■ Midline catheter. (Courtesy of Teleflex Medical, Research Triangle Park, NC.)

modified Seldinger technique (Anderson, 2004). Midine catheters can be placed with ultrasound guidance. The midline catheter should never be readvanced.

Radiologic confirmation of the tip location is recommended in the following clinical situations:

Advantages

The major advantages over the convention peripheral-short catheter have been

- Drug hemodilution
- Improved dwell times
- Dwell time 1 to 4 weeks

Disadvantages

- Potential for phlebitis
- Previous coatings have caused some reports of anaphylaxis (Mermel & Tow, 1995)

INS Standard The midline catheter is indicated for those peripheral infusion therapies prescribed for a duration of one to four weeks. For those therapies requiring catheter dwell times greater than four weeks, extension of catheter dwell should be based on the professional judgment of the nurse after consideration of the following factors including, but not limited to, length of therapy remaining, peripheral venous status, patient condition, condition of the vein in which the catheter is placed, and skin integrity. (INS, 2006, 49)

Vein Illumination Devices

The use of illumination devices has affected the practice of intravenous access and infusion therapy for patients who are in need of I.V.s but have veins that can neither be seen nor palpated. The transilluminator works by directing a high-intensity cool light down into the subcutaneous tissue and creating a uniform area of orange-like reflection from the fatty tissue. The light is flush with the skin; by moving it around the extremity, a dark line can be seen. The vein's deoxygenated blood absorbs the light, whereas the fatty tissue reflects the light. Refer to Figure 5-27.

Ultrasound

Ultrasound allows for real-time imaging of selected blood vessels and nearby anatomic structures before and during placement of midline catheters and peripherally inserted central catheter (PICCs). Use of ultrasound guided catheter insertion requires training. An understanding of the vascular system, and the veins accessed (basilic, brachial, and cephalic), is necessary (Hunter, 2007). Refer to Figure 5-28.

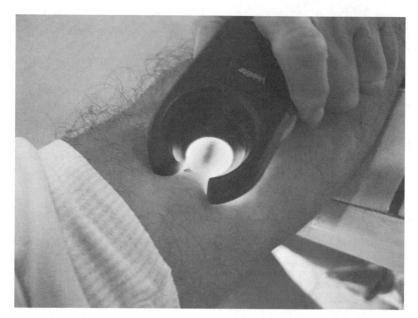

Figure 5-27 ■ Transillumination device Veinlite®. (Courtesy of Translite LLC, Sugar Land, TX.)

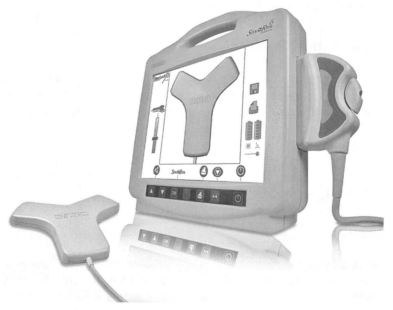

Figure 5-28 ■ Ultrasound bedside device for catheter placement: Siterite®. (Courtesy of Bard Access Systems, Salt Lake City, UT.)

Central Infusion Devices

Long-term infusion therapy may require venous access over weeks, months, or even years. Special central venous catheters have been designed specifically for long-term access, patient comfort, and decreased complications associated with multiple therapies. There are two categories of central venous catheters (CVCs): short term and long term. The short term include the nontunneled percutaneous catheters with a 7- to 10-day dwell time and the peripherally inserted central catheter (PICC) with dwell time up to 1 year. The long-term catheters include the tunneled-cuffed catheters and the implanted ports.

Central catheters are made of soft, medical grade silicone elastomers or thermoplastic polyurethane, and are commercially available in many designs. Polyurethane catheters are the most commonly used catheters because of the material's versatility, malleability (tensile strength and elongation characteristics), biocompatibility with the range in size from 24 gauge, 3 ½ inches to 14 gauge, 12 inches. Central catheters are radiopaque with single, or multiple lumens. New technologies such as the power injectable central catheters, catheter coatings, and addition of impregnated cuffs are addressed in Chapter 8.

NOTE > Refer to Chapter 8 for additional information on catheter materials and designs.

Short-Term Central Catheters

Nontunneled Percutaneous Catheters

In 1961, the first I.V. catheter for accessing the central circulation was introduced. The nontunneled percutaneously inserted catheter may consist of polyurethane, a stiffer material, which makes the catheter easy to advance, allowing catheter insertion outside the operating room. The percutaneous catheter is placed by an infraclavicular approach through the subclavian vein or the external, internal jugular or femoral vein and secured by suturing. The final tip location should be in the superior vena cava (SVC). The catheter may remain in place up to 10 days. This type of catheter provides access to larger venous circulation for the delivery of hypertonic solutions. These catheters can have single, double, triple, or quadruple lumen. Refer to Figure 5-29.

Peripherally Inserted Central Venous Catheters

A **peripherally inserted central catheter** (PICC) is a percutaneous IV composed of silicone elastomers or polyurethane. Silicone elastomer is soft, flexible, nonthrombogenic, and biocompatible (Fig. 5-30). It may be

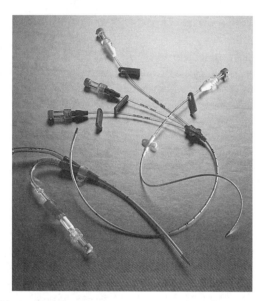

Figure 5-29 ■ Nontunneled percutaneous catheters. (Courtesy of Teleflex Medical, Research Triangle Park, NC.)

single or multiple lumens. PICCs ranges in sizes of 16 to 23 gauge and 50 to 60 cm in length. Insertion, using sterile technique, is performed by a trained competency-documented registered nurse using a traditional breakaway peripheral introducer or via a modified Seldinger technique with a peelaway needle or a modified Seldinger technique with tip location in the superior vena cava (SVC). This catheter usually ranges

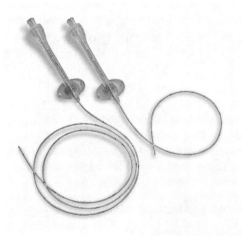

Figure 5-30 ■ Examples of peripherally inserted central catheter compared to a midline catheter. (Courtesy of Becton Dickinson, Sandy, UT.)

from 16 to 26 gauges and from 20 to 24 inches in length. The peripheral catheter is inserted into a peripheral site in the antecubital area and advanced into the SVC. To reach the SVC in the average adult, a catheter at least 20 inches long is required. External jugular peripherally inserted central catheters (EJ PICC) are catheters placed through the external jugular vein and advanced into the SVC. EJ PICCs are used for nonemergent access when other veins cannot be accessed (INS, 2008).

A PICC may be used to deliver all types of therapy. It is the appropriate choice for parenteral nutrition with dextrose content greater than 10%, continuous infusion of vesicant medications or medications with the ability to cause necrosis if they infiltrate, therapies with extreme variations in tonicity of pH, or anticipated extended infusion therapy. A new product is the PowerPicc™, which combines efficacy of PICC and maximum injection rates with a new bifurcation design, and easy to read labeling and is rated to 300 psi and 5 mL/second injection (Fig. 5-31).

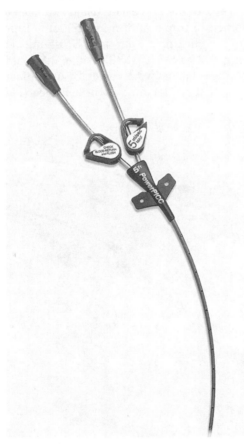

Figure 5-31 ■ Power PICC®. (Courtesy of Bard Access Systems, Salt Lake City, UT.)

INS Standard Site selection should be routinely initiated in the region of the antecubital fossa; veins that should be considered for peripherally inserted central cannulation are the basilic, median cubital, cephalic and brachial veins. (INS, 2006, 37)

Long-Term Central Catheters

Tunneled-Cuffed Central Catheters

Central venous **tunneled catheters** (CVTCs) are made of soft, medical grade silicone elastomers. CVTs have a Dacron cuff near the subcutaneous exit site of the catheter that anchors it in place, acts as a securing device, and serves as an antimicrobial barrier. CVTCs are surgically inserted through percutaneous cutdown under local or general anesthesia. The distal catheter tip is advanced into the vessel and is placed in the SVC. The proximal end is subcutaneously tunneled to an incisional exit site on the anterior or posterior trunk of the body. The usual exit sites for CVTCs are the mid- to lower thoracic or upper abdominal regions. Types of tunneled catheters include Broviac, Hickman, Raaf, and Groshong. These catheters are 20 to 30 inches long and have a 17- to 22-gauge internal lumen diameter. The thickness of the silicone wall varies by manufacturer. Silicone catheters can be single, dual, triple, or quadruple lumen (Fig. 5-32).

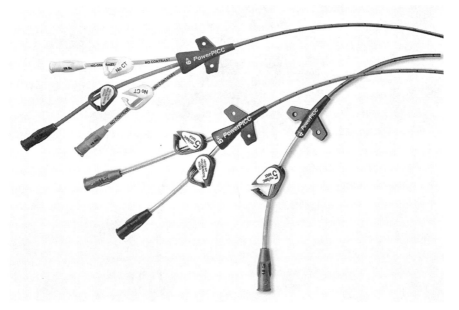

Figure 5-32 ■ Example of multilumen catheters: Single-, double-, and triple-lumen. (Courtesy of Bard Access Systems, Salt Lake City, UT.)

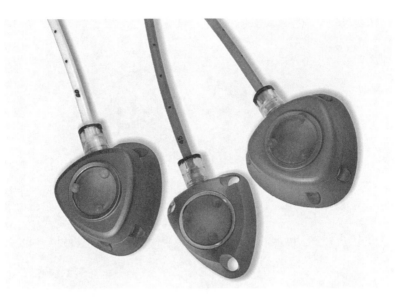

Figure 5-33 ■ Examples of ports. (Courtesy of Bard Access Systems, Salt Lake City, UT.)

Implantable Venous Access Ports

The implantable venous access port (IP) is a completely closed system consisting of an implanted device with a drug reservoir, or port, with a self-sealing system connected to an outlet catheter. The device is surgically implanted into a convenient body site in a subcutaneous pocket. The self-sealing septum can withstand up to 2000 needle punctures. This device provides venous access for blood withdrawal, intravenous infusions of hypertonic solutions, blood components, and chemotherapy. Refer to Figure 5-33. The **implanted port** must be accessed with a Huber needle (noncoring) for safe and proper penetration of the septum of the port. Because these are noncoring needles, they contribute to the long lifetime of the port. The needles are sized from 19 to 24 gauge and range from 1 to 2 inches in length. The needles are available in 90-degree or straight-needle designs (Fig. 5–34).

> **INS Standard** Introducers for percutaneous nontunneled and tunneled catheters, and implanted ports should be equipped with a safety device with engineered sharps injury protection. (INS, 2006, 38)

■ Infusion Regulation Devices

Introduction to Regulation Device Technology

Historically, infusion systems were regulated with a roller clamp, which the nurse adjusted manually with the roller or screw clamp on

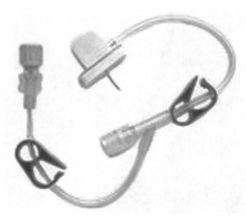

Figure 5-34 ■ Gripper® Huber needle. (Courtesy of Smith Medical, Carlsbad, CA.)

the administration set. Today numerous mechanical and electronic infusion devices (EIDs) are available to assist nurses in maintaining an accurate infusion rate. EIDs regulate infusions either as gtt/min or mL/hr. An infusion pump delivers fluids, medications, or nutrients into a patient's circulatory system. EIDs are generally used via the intravenous route; however, subcutaneous, arterial, and epidural infusions are occasionally used. There are two basic classes of pumps: large-volume pumps and small-volume pumps. Within these classes, some pumps are designed to be portable, others stationary.

Pump Programming

The user interface of pumps usually requests details on the type of infusion from the nurse that sets them up.

- *Rate:* Amount of time over which a specific volume of fluid is delivered. Infusion pumps deliver in increments of milliliters per hour. The most common rate parameters for regular infusion pumps are 1 to 999 mL/hr. Many newer pumps are capable of setting rates that offer parameters of 0.1 mL in increments of 0.1 to 99.9 mL, then in 1-mL increments up to 999 mL. Many newer pumps are capable of setting rates that satisfy both regular infusion and microinfusion needs. Better-quality pumps that offer combination rates do not allow the rate to be set above 99.9 without a deliberate act to enter the adult values.
- *Volume infused:* Measurement that tells how much of a given solution has been infused. This measurement is used to monitor the amount of fluid infused in a shift. It can also be used in home

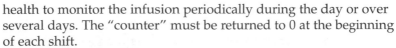

health to monitor the infusion periodically during the day or over several days. The "counter" must be returned to 0 at the beginning of each shift.

- *Volume to be infused:* Usually the amount of solution hanging in the solution container. A pump is designed to sound an alarm when the volume to be infused is reached.
- *Tapering or ramping:* These are terms that are used to describe the progressive increase or decrease of the infusion rate. Pumps that will increase or taper infusion rates are gaining popularity. The pump can use its own program to mathematically calculate the ramping rate once the duration of infusion and total volume to be infused is given.
- *Timed infusion:* This refers to an infusion governed by a 24-hour clock within the device. With timed infusion, the device must have a sufficient internal backup battery to maintain the clock accurately at all times. Timed infusions are used for ramping and tapering, automatic piggybacking, and intermittent dosing.

Alarm Terminology

- *Air-in-line:* Designed to detect only visible bubbles or microscopic bubbles. This alarm is necessary for all positive-pressure pumps and infusion controllers. Volumetric pumps are usually equipped with air-in-line detectors.
- *Occlusion:* Standard alarm for infusion devices. Controllers may be able to indicate only "no flow." With an occlusion alarm, controllers are able to indicate upstream (between pump and container) or downstream (between patient and pump) occlusion by absence of flow. Many newer pumps are able to differentiate between upstream (or proximal) and downstream (or distal) occlusions. This is often detected by changes in pressure.

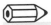 *NURSING FAST FACT!*

In a number of EIDs, the pressure is "user" selectable from 0.10 to 10 psi. Occlusion alarms at low psi settings are common because the pumps are sensitive to even slight changes in pressure and very small I.V. catheter or patient movement. Many of the current EIDs infuse fluids using very low infusion pressures, often lower than the pressure of a gravity delivery. These devices are not, however, designed to detect infiltrations. When an infiltration occurs, the inline pressure may actually drop; therefore, the EID will not detect the infiltration. Visual monitoring of the I.V. site by a professional nurse is mandatory for patients with EIDs.

- *Infusion complete:* Alarm triggered by a preset volume limit ("infusion complete"). These alarms are helpful in preventing the fluid container from running dry because they can be set to sound before the entire solution container is infused.

- *Low battery or low power:* Gives the user ample warning of the pump's impending inability to function. A low-battery alarm means that the batteries need to be replaced or external power source needs to be connected. As a protective measure, when low-battery and low-power alarms are continued over a preset number of minutes, the pumps usually convert to a keep-vein-open (KVO) rate. The preset KVO rate is usually between 0.1 and 5 mL.

- *Nonfunctional or malfunctional:* Alarm that means the pump is operating outside parameters and the problem cannot be resolved. When this alarm sounds, the pump should be disconnected from the patient and returned to biomedical engineering or to the manufacturer for evaluation. The alert signifying a nonfunctional alarm may be worded in many ways, depending on the manufacturer.

- *Not infusing:* Indicates that all of the pump infusion parameters are not set. This feature prevents tampering or setting changes from happening accidentally. The pump must be programmed or changed and then told to "start."

- *Parameters or timed-out:* Reminds the programmer that all settings have not been completed.

- *Tubing:* Used generally with controllers. Ensures that the correct tubing has been loaded into the pump. If tubing is incorrectly loaded, this alarm will also sound.

- *Door:* Indicates that the door that secures the tubing is not closed. Cassette pumps may give a "cassette" alarm if the cassette is unable to infuse within device operating parameters.

- *Free flow:* Detects the rapid infusion of fluid, which can occur when the set is removed from the pump. Disengaging the tubing from the pump requires a deliberate act. Most newer devices have free-flow protection, meaning that when the door is opened accidentally, there should be no fluid flow to the patient without nurse intervention.

Many other functions have been added to newer pumps. These include:

- Preprogrammed drug compatibility
- Retrievable patient history data
- Central venous pressure monitor
- Positive pressure fill stroke
- Modular self-diagnosing capability
- Printer read-out
- Nurse call system
- Remote site programming
- Syringe use for secondary infusion

- Adjustable occlusion pressures
- Secondary rate settings
- Lock level for security
- Barcoding

Smart Pump Electronic Infusion Device Enhancements

Thirty-five percent of all medication errors that result in significant harm are the result of infusion pump errors, with the most common error being incorrect programming of the infusion parameters into the pump (Tourville, 2003). Manual programming errors cause two out of three infusion pump-related deaths in hospitals each year. New sophisticated infusion systems (smart pumps) introduced in 2001 provide advanced technologies for safety. The computerized large-volume pumps incorporate software that can be customized for each hospitals best practices for infusion therapy.

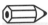 *NURSING FAST FACT!*

In October of 2002, Health Devices, published by ECRI evaluated all currently marketed general-purpose infusion pumps and concluded that only pumps that had "dose error reduction software" should be considered for purchase (ECRI, 2003).

The ECRI has established Smart Pumps criteria. Refer to Table 5-2.

On-Board Drug Library

The new smart pumps contain advanced drug libraries that allow a facility to list medications in department-specific categories, establish standardized concentrations for these medications and set minimum and maximum dosing parameters for each medication (Jacobs, 2006).

Drug Specific-Dosing Limits

The pump is programmed with dosing parameters. Alerts will prompt the nurse to confirm and authorize the dosage if the rate entered is outside the parameters. This double check significantly improves I.V. medication safety (Jacobs, 2006).

Refer to Figures 5-35 and 5-36 for examples of smart pump technology.

INS Standard The flow control device selected shall be based on patient age, condition, prescribed infusion therapy, type of vascular access device and care setting.

Dose-error reduction systems shall be considered in the selection and use of electronic infusion devices. Anti-free-flow administration sets shall be considered in the selection and use of administration delivery systems. (INS, 2006, 33)

> Table 5-2	ECRI SMART PUMP CRITERIA

Minimum of 8 profiles or "areas of use"
Comprehensive drug library including:
    Drug names/concentrations
    Dosing units
    Hard and soft dose limits
    Maximum weight, maximum rate, maximum volume per profile
Forced function to select new patient and area of use
Continuous display of drug name/dose on infusion pump
Continuous indicator of doses infused outside of limit (soft)
Comprehensive log to record Smart alerts
Support structure to assist in Smart pump implementation

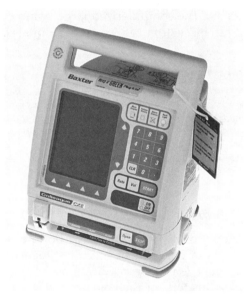

Figure 5-35 ■ Volumetric infusion pump. Colleague CX™ has guardian feature. Provide simple infusions to medication therapies requiring complex dose calculations. Dose calculator accommodates nine different delivery modes. Label library includes 64 drug and therapy labels. Guardian feature helps reduce medication errors by alerting staff when programmed doses are not met within institutional limits. (Courtesy of Baxter Healthcare Corp., Round Lake, IL.)

Mechanical Gravity Devices

Flow-regulating mechanisms that attach to the primary infusion administration sets are called mechanical gravity control devices (or mechanical controllers). They are manually set to deliver specified volumes of fluid per hour. They are available as dials, with clocklike faces, or a barrel-shaped device with cylindrical controls. Flow markings on the dials help

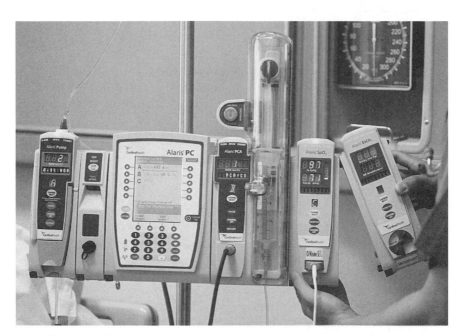

Figure 5-36 ■ Alaris® medication safety system: Modular point-of-care computer. Medley medication safety system. (Courtesy of Cardinal Health Co., San Diego, CA.)

to approximate the drops per minute, based on the set drop factor, but should be verified by counting the drops (Fig. 5-37).

Electronic Infusion Devices

The use of electronic infusion devices (EIDs) or flow-control devices should be guided by the patient's age and condition, setting, and prescribed therapy. These devices provide an accurate flow rate, are easy to use, and have alarms that signal problems with the infusion. However, hourly assessment, responsibility, and accountability for safe infusion still lie with the professional nurse. To use these devices effectively, the nurse should know (1) indications for their use, (2) their mechanical operation, (3) how to troubleshoot, (4) their psi rating, and (5) safe usage guidelines.

Infusion control devices have come a long way since their introduction in 1958. The very early models had serious accuracy and safety problems: air embolisms, fluid containers that ran dry, and clogged catheters were common. The pumps were large, hard to troubleshoot, and limited in their reliability and usability.

IVAC Corporation introduced the concept of the rate controller in 1972; today there are many models and types on the market, including:
■ Positive-pressure infusion pumps
■ Volumetric pumps

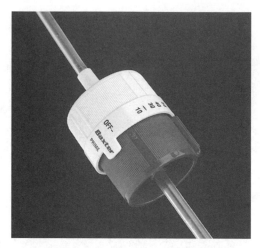

Figure 5-37 ■ Mechanical controller: Rate flow regulator. (Courtesy of Baxter Healthcare Corp., Round Lake, IL.)

- Peristaltic pumps
- Syringe pumps
- Patient-controlled analgesia (PCA) systems
- Multichannel and dual channel pumps
- Ambulatory pumps
- Disposable pumps (elastomeric balloon pumps)

 NURSING FAST FACT!

Because of the many pumps on the market, refer to the manufacturer's recommendations for troubleshooting guidelines for setup and of each EID.

Controllers

Controllers operate strictly on gravity flow and do not exert positive pressure greater than the head height of the infusion bag, which is usually 2 psi. Some controllers can reach a psi of 5, but this pressure is uncommon. The maximum flow rate is affected by how high the I.V. container is hung above the I.V. site. Controllers cannot detect infiltrations. After the I.V. catheter leaves the vein and infiltrates into the tissues, the pressure drops. Because the infusion device is "looking" for pressure to signal an infiltration, it may be a long time with significant fluid accumulation before the infuser actually detects infiltration. It is always best to recommend that the nurse monitor the infusion visually and not rely on the infusion device to detect infiltrations.

 NURSING FAST FACT!

One psi and 50 mm Hg exert the same amount of pressure.

A drop sensor and electric feedback mechanism regulate the gravity flow of the fluid. Controllers reduce the potential for rapid infusion of large amounts of solution (runaways) and empty bottles. Controllers assist the nurse in detecting infiltrations and maintaining accurate flow rates.

The I.V. bag is usually hung 36 inches above a patient's head for adequate gravity pressure. When there is resistance to the flow, the controller's alarm will sound, signaling that it cannot maintain the preset rate. Resistance can occur when the patient is restless and frequently changing positions, if the catheter tip is at a flexion point, or if the patient lies on the tubing. Many of the newer controllers can deliver blood components safely.

Positive-Pressure Infusion Pumps

Positive-pressure infusion pumps average 10 psi, with up to 15 psi considered to be safe, although newer technology has the psi set as low as 0.1 psi. Older pumps still in use may pump at dangerous pressures of 16 to 22 psi. Pressures greater than 15 to 20 psi should be used with extreme caution.

Positive-pressure infusion pumps are used for delivering high volumes and complex therapies in high-acuity situations. The pumps are more precise than controllers; accurately deliver the fluid as programmed; and have many features, such as the ability to keep track of fluid amounts and to sound alarms for various malfunctions. These pumps totally control the flow rate.

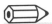 *NURSING FAST FACT!*

> All positive-pressure pumps should have an "anti–free-flow" alarm to prevent inadvertent free-flowing solution.

Volumetric Pumps

Volumetric pumps calculate the volume delivered by measuring the volume displaced in a reservoir that is part of the disposable administration set. The pump calculates every fill and empty cycle of the reservoir. The reservoir is manipulated internally by a specific action of the pump. The industry standard for the accuracy of electronic volumetric infusion pumps is plus or minus 5%.

Pressure terminology includes the terms "fixed" and "variable." With fixed infusion pressure, the pump is set internally to infuse up to a certain psi but not more (occlusion limit). Variable-pressure pumps allow individual judgment about the psi needed to safely deliver therapy. Nurses can adjust a variable-pressure pump through programming. Variable-pressure devices have a conservative upper limit (usually 10 psi) and a lower limit of 2 psi similar to that of a controller. A psi setting of 4 to 8 is common.

Volumetric pumps have proved invaluable in neonatal, pediatric, and adult intensive care units, where critical infusions of small volumes of fluid or doses of high-potency drugs are indicated. A cartridge pumps the solution to be delivered; therefore, blood and red blood cells can be administered without damage to the blood cells.

Many pumps use microprocessor technology for a more compact unit and for easier troubleshooting. All volumetric pumps require special tubing.

 NURSING FAST FACT!

> *To ensure safe, efficient operation, review the literature that accompanies the pump to become familiar with the operation of the pump. Observe all precautions.*

Peristaltic Pumps

Peristaltic refers to the controlling mechanisms: a peristaltic device moves fluid by intermittently squeezing the I.V. tubing. The device may be rotary or linear. In a rotary peristaltic pump, a rotating disk or series of rollers compresses the tubing along a curved or semicircular chamber, propelling the fluid when pressure is released. In a linear device, one or more projections intermittently press the I.V. tubing. Peristaltic pumps are used primarily for the infusion of enteral feedings.

Syringe Pumps

Syringe pumps are piston-driven infusion pumps that provide precise infusion by controlling the rate by drive speed and syringe size, thus eliminating the variables of the drop rate. Syringe pumps are valuable for critical infusions of small doses of high-potency drugs. A lead, screw motor-driven system pushes the plunger to deliver fluid or medication at a rate of 0.01 to 99.9 mL/hr. It is a precisely accurate delivery system that can be used to administer very small volumes. Some models have program modes capable of administration in mg/kg per minute, mcg/min, and mL/hr. The syringe is usually filled in the pharmacy and stored until used.

These pumps are used most frequently for delivery of antibiotics and small-volume parenteral therapy. Syringe pump technology was applied to PCA infusion devices. Syringe pumps are used frequently in the areas of anesthesia, oncology, and obstetrics.

The volume of the syringe pump is limited to the size of the syringe; a 60-mL syringe is usually used. However, the syringe can be as small as 5 mL. The tubing usually is a single, uninterrupted length of kink-resistant tubing with a notable lack of Y injection ports. Syringe pumps can use primary or secondary sets, depending on the intended use) (Fig. 5-38).

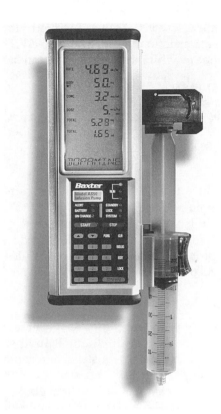

Figure 5-38 ■ Syringe pumps. Autosyringe® AS50 infusion pump.
(Courtesy of Baxter Healthcare Corp., Round Lake, IL.)

Patient-Controlled Analgesia Pumps

PCA pumps have been developed to assist patients in controlling their pain at home or in the hospital. PCA pumps can be used to deliver medication through I.V., epidural, or subcutaneous routes. These pumps are different from other infusion devices in that they have a remote bolus control in which the patient or nurse can deliver a bolus of medication at set intervals. PCA pumps are available in ambulatory or pole-mounted models.

There are three types of PCA pumps: basal, continuous, and demand. All three afford some type of pain control with varying degrees of patient interaction.

■ The basal mode is designed to achieve pain relief with minimal medication with intermittent dosing, thus allowing the patient to remain alert and active without sedation.

■ The continuous mode of therapy is designed for patients who need maximum pain relief; it usually does not fluctuate from hour to hour and should completely relieve pain or achieve a constant effect.

- The demand mode dose is delivered by intermittent infusion when a button attached to the pump is pushed. The demand dose can be used alone or with the basal type of infusion.

 NURSING FAST FACT!

Patient-controlled analgesia pumps must be programmed with parameters to prevent overmedication. These pumps are designed with a special key or locking device for security of the medications.

INS Standard Patient education, consent, assessment and monitoring should be ongoing during PCA.

The RN should have knowledge of analgesic pharmacokinetics, and equianalgesic dosing, contraindications, side effects and their management, appropriate administration modalities, and anticipated outcomes. (INS, 2006, 67)

Multichannel Pumps

Multiple-drug delivery systems are computer generated, and many use computer-generated technology. **Multichannel pumps** can deliver several medications and fluids simultaneously or intermittently from bags, bottles, or syringes. Multichannel pumps (usually with two to four channels) require manifold-type sets to set up all channels, whether or not they are in use; each channel must be programmed independently. Programming a multichannel pump can be challenging (Fig. 5-39).

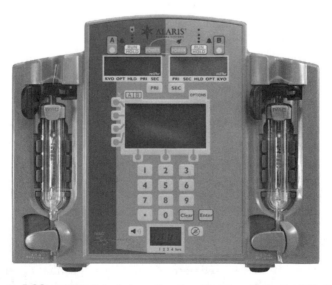

Figure 5-39 ■ Alaris® dual-channel pump. (Courtesy of Cardinal Health Co., San Diego, CA.)

Dual-channel pumps offer a two-pump mechanism assembly, with a common control and programming panel. This type of pump uses one administration set for each channel.

Ambulatory Pumps

Ambulatory pumps are lightweight, compact infusion pumps. These have made a significant breakthrough in long-term care. This device allows the patient freedom to resume a normal life. Ambulatory pumps range in size and weight; most weigh less than 6 lb and are capable of delivering most infusion therapies. Features include medication delivery, delivery of several different dose sizes at different intervals, memory of programs, and safety alarms. The main disadvantage of ambulatory pumps is limited power supply; they function on a battery system that requires frequent recharging (Fig. 5-40).

Nonelectric Disposable Pumps

Nonelectric disposable infusion pumps have been in clinical use for more than 20 years. Disposable infusion pumps are extensively used in home care settings. A wide range of disposable pumps is available. Application of disposable pumps include:

1. Continuous analgesia for postoperative pain management
2. Patient-controlled analgesia
3. Delivery of chemotherapy drugs and opioids for cancer treatment
4. Delivery of antimicrobials in the home
5. Pediatric applications (Skryabina & Dunn, 2006)

All nonelectric disposable pumps exploit the same physical principles: mechanical restriction within the flow path determines the speed of pressurized fluid. The pressure on the fluid is generated by a variety of mechanisms using nonelectric power, including a stretched elastomer or compressed spring (Bayne, 1997), pressure generated during a chemical reaction, and pressure supplied from a cartridge of pressurized gas (Nowak, 2004). The restriction of flow in all disposable pumps is caused by narrow-bore tubing. Tubing diameter has a determining influence on the device's flow rate.

Elastomeric Infusion Pumps

The elastomeric balloon pump system is a portable device with an elastomeric reservoir, or balloon, that works on flow restrictions. The balloon, which is made of a soft rubberized material capable of being inflated to a predetermined volume, is safely encapsulated inside a rigid, transparent container. When the reservoir is filled, the balloon exerts positive pressure to administer the medication with an integrated flow restrictor that controls

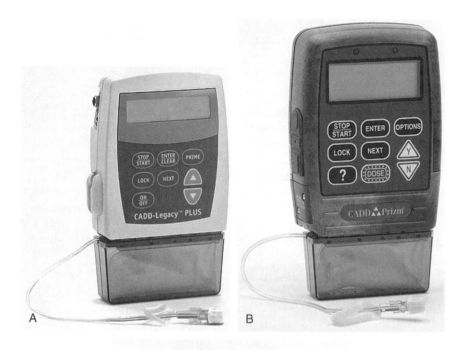

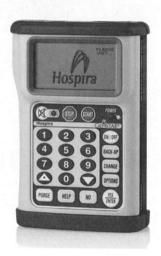

Figure 5-40 ■ Ambulatory pumps. *A*, CADD™ Legacy-Plus system. *B*, CADD™ Prizm. (Courtesy of Smith Medical, Carlsbad, CA.) *C*, Hospira ambulatory pump. (Courtesy of Hospira, Inc., Lake Forest, IL.)

the flow rate. This system requires no batteries or electronic programming and is not reusable (Fig. 5-41).

Elastomeric balloon devices are used primarily for the delivery of antibiotics. The typical volume for these devices is 50 to 100 mL, but these balloons are available in sizes up to 250 mL. Elastomeric pumps operate

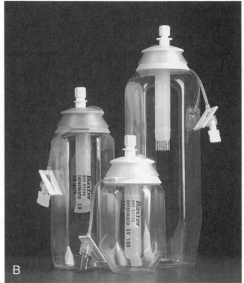

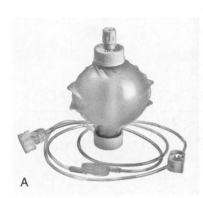

A

B

Figure 5-41 ■ Disposable pumps. *A*, Eclipse™ elastomeric pump. (Courtesy of B. Braun Medical Inc., Bethlehem, PA.) *B*, Intermate® in a variety of different sizes (50–500 mL). (Courtesy of Baxter Healthcare Corp., Round Lake, IL.)

with a drive pressure of 260 to 520 mm Hg and infuse at rates of 0.5 to 500 mL/hr (Skryabina & Dunn, 2006).

ADVANTAGES

- Portability
- Simplicity
- Disposability

DISADVANTAGES

- Temperature effect on performance due to drug viscosity changing with temperature.
- Viscosity of fluid will have an inverse effect on flow rate.
- Atmospheric pressure can affect flow accuracy.
- Changing the pump's position relative to the infusion site might affect accuracy.
- Partial filling of a disposable pump can affect the internal pressure of an elastomeric balloon.
- Storing pumps at a lower than recommended temperature result in lower flow rates (Skryabina & Dunn, 2006).

Additional nonelectric disposable pumps include spring-powered infusion pumps, negative-pressure infusion pumps, and disposable PCA pumps.

NURSING FAST FACT!

Allow nonelectric infusion pumps to warm after storage and before infusion for accurate flow rate.

NURSING POINTS-OF-CARE
MANAGEMENT OF INFUSION EQUIPMENT

Focus Assessment
■ Knowledge of therapies and equipment used to deliver therapy
■ Suitable vascular access device for length and type of therapy
■ Adequate level of consciousness and compliance

Key Nursing Interventions
1. Monitor the patient for:
   a. Breaks in the integrity of the infusion equipment
   b. Patient's knowledge of equipment
2. Help the patient and/or family identify potential areas of conflict; cultural mores, or cost.
3. Follow the manufacturer's guidelines on the setup and maintenance of specific EIDs.
4. Select and prepare infusion pumps as indicated.
5. Set alarm limits on equipment as appropriate.
6. Respond to equipment alarms appropriately.
7. Consult with other healthcare team members and recommend equipment and devices for patient use.
8. Compare machine-derived data with nurse's perception of the patient's condition.
9. Follow INS Standards of Practice in rotation of I.V. sites, fluid container, administration set, and dressing changes.
10. Maintain the integrity of the infusion site and equipment at all times.
11. Use filters when appropriate.
12. Use appropriate administration set (vented or nonvented) with the appropriate fluid container.
13. Inspect fluid containers, administration sets, and cannulas for integrity before use.

Developing and Participating in Product Evaluation

Product Problem Reporting

In 1990, the Medical Device Act was amended to clearly place responsibility for ensuring that medical devices in domestic commercial distribution are safe and effective for their intended purposes. A medical device is defined as any instrument, apparatus, or other article that is used to prevent, diagnose, mitigate, or treat a disease or to affect the structure or function of the body, with the exception of drugs. Clinical investigations of medical devices must comply with the U.S. Food and Drug Administration (FDA) informed consent and Institutional Review Board (IRB) regulations (FDA, 1998). The infusion nurse specialist plays an important role in the product selection and evaluation processes. Ongoing evaluation of products in use is important in the delivery of high-quality patient care. The infusion nurse specialist's participation with his or her colleagues from other departments enhances commitment to the specialty and to the facility. The FDA regulates products in the United States, including over-the-counter and prescription drugs and pharmaceuticals, food, cosmetics, veterinary products, biologic devices, and medical devices. Nurses use many medical devices and are usually the primary reporters of device problems.

The following are examples of medical device problems related to infusion therapy practice:

- Loose or leaking catheter hubs
- Occluded cannula
- Defective infusion pumps
- Contaminated infusates
- Misleading labeling
- Inadequate packaging
- Cracked or leaking I.V. solution bag

When to Report

Participation in product evaluation is an ongoing responsibility of professional practitioners. Inappropriate use of medical devices may contribute to pain and suffering. The FDA evaluates approximately 2000 medical devices each month. Devices are inspected on three levels:

1. Good manufacturing controls
2. Application for a device existing before 1976 and in common use
3. Implantable or hazardous devices

The simple act of "gerryrigging" or otherwise manipulating a device to overcome a small problem results in the liability for problems arising from use of that piece of equipment residing with the institution. The law states that the responsibility shifts to the institution when a practitioner interferes with the design of a piece of equipment. Nurses have a critical role in reporting the failure of a device. When a device failure is noted, it is important to follow the following steps:

1. Identify previously recorded lot numbers and expiration dates of products.
2. Complete a designated internal report.
3. Inform the supervisor.
4. Notify the Risk Management Department.

It is the responsibility of the Risk Management Department to notify the manufacturer and the FDA and file the appropriate FDA MedWatch Form #3500A. Completion of these steps satisfies the legal requirement of identifying and reporting products that may have caused a patient harm (Deacon, 2004).

What to Report

Report any problems with medical devices if the event observed involves, or has the potential to cause, a death, serious injury, or life-threatening malfunction. In 1992, a congressional hearing focused on needle safety, a needleless system, and safe medical devices. Since this hearing, the Occupational Safety and Health Administration (OSHA) and the Centers for Disease Control and Prevention (CDC), along with the FDA, have been collaboratively reviewing the issue of safe medical devices. OSHA expects hospitals to have an ongoing system in place to evaluate safer medical devices.

Report a complete description of the problem. Information regarding the device needs to be submitted, including:

■ Product name
■ Manufacturer's name and address
■ Identification numbers of the device (lot number, model number, serial number, expiration date)
■ Problem noted
■ Name, title, and practice specialty of the device's user

How to Report

The ECRI discontinued the Computerized Problem Reporting System (CPRS) in 2007. In 2008 the MedWatch forms became available from the FDA. Instructions for completing a voluntary or mandatory report can be downloaded from the FDA Web site.

 Website

www.fda.gov/medwatch
www.ecri.org/PatientSafety

Mandatory reporting forms (MDR forms) can be sent to FDA:
MDR Reporting
Center for Devices and Radiological Health
Food and Drug Administration
P.O. Box 3002
Rockville, MD 20847-3002
Voluntary reporting forms (FDA voluntary reporting form 3500) can be mailed to:
MedWatch
FDA Safety Information and Adverse Event Reporting Program
Food and Drug Administration
5600 Fishers Lane
Rockville, MD 20852-9787

INS Standard The nurse shall be involved in the evaluation of infusion-related technologies. The evaluations shall include, but are not limited to, product reliability, clinical application, performance, infection control, safety, efficacy, efficiency, and cost. (INS, 2006, 15)

Home Care Issues

Home care infusion devices are designed to allow the patient maximum portability and freedom of movement. The aim is small, quiet, lightweight infusion pumps with pouches that enclose both the pump and the infusion container. Equipment and supplies used at home must offer safety features, as the patient or a caregiver are expected to participate in their care.
Equipment and supplies used in home care management may include:
• Medical teaching dolls: Facilitate visual, hands-on approach to educate patients of all ages and families about vascular access site, equipment, and procedures.
• Vascular access devices: Required for home infusion therapy; the most common VAD used in home care is the peripherally inserted central catheter (PICC).
• Infusion administration supplies: I.V. tubing, injection caps/valves, alcohol wipes, site care kits including disinfectant, sterile gloves, mask, dressings, and tape.
• Infusion delivery systems: Syringe pumps, elastomeric infusers, ambulatory pumps.
• Premixed medications: Saline/heparin syringes for flushing (usually prefilled)
• Transport storage pouch

NOTE > Reimbursement is an important issue to be addressed while planning for home care. The home care agency and the home infusion pharmacy are resources for reimbursement questions and will assess and verify reimbursement sources, and potential patient co-payments, before providing home care.

Patient Education

Patient education in the hospital and home care settings is necessary for patient safety and to decrease anxiety related to high technical equipment. The following is important in equipment education.

- Instruct the patient by demonstrating the preparation and administration of therapy.
- Teach the patient and family how to operate equipment, as appropriate.
- Advise the patient regarding pump alarms and advise him or her to contact the nurse if the alarm is triggered in the hospital setting.
- Instruct the patient and family on the use of PCA pumps for pain control.
- Teach the patient and family the expected patient outcomes and side effects associated with using the equipment.
- Document the patient's and family's understanding of the education provided to them.

◼ Nursing Process

The nursing process is a five- or six-step process for problem-solving to guide nursing action. Refer to Chapter 1 for details on the steps of the nursing process. The following table focuses on nursing diagnoses, nursing outcomes classification (NOC), and nursing intervention classification (NIC) for patients using infusion equipment. Nursing diagnoses should be patient specific and outcomes and interventions individualized. The NOC and NIC presented here are suggested direction for development of outcomes and interventions.

Nursing Diagnoses Related to Management of Infusion Equipment	NOC: Nursing Outcomes Classification	NIC: Nursing Intervention Classification
Anxiety (mild, moderate, or severe) related to: New equipment technology.	Coping	Anxiety reduction techniques
Knowledge deficit related to: Equipment: Unfamiliarity with information resources, cognitive limitation, and information misinterpretation.	Knowledge treatment procedure (equipment use), health resources	Teaching: Use written educational materials, demonstrate equipment with return demonstration, observe ability and readiness to learn.

Nursing Diagnoses Related to Management of Infusion Equipment	NOC: Nursing Outcomes Classification	NIC: Nursing Intervention Classification
Risk for injury (external) related to: Physical environmental conditions: Equipment	Patient safety behavior Safe home environment	Accuracy of patient identification Effectiveness of communication Medication safety Education on equipment

Source: Ackley & Ladwig (2008). Heitz & Horne (2005); McCloskey, Dochterman, & Bulecheck 2004; Moorhead, Johnson, & Maas (2004); NANDA. I (2007).

Chapter Highlights

- Types of infusion delivery systems include glass and plastic (rigid and flexible).
- Check all solutions for clarity and expiration date. Squeeze to check for leaks, floating particles, and clarity.
- Concerns over PVC and DEHP: The plasticizer phthalate (DEHP) is added to some infusion products for flexibility. EPA warns that PVC leaches into I.V. solutions and toxic absorption can occur. Many new products are on the market that do not contain DEHP.
- Administration sets
  - Single-line sets: Most frequently used; follow INS standards for frequency of set changes. Available in vented and nonvented sets.
  - Primary (standard) set, volume-controlled sets
  - Primary Y sets: Most often used with blood components
  - Pump-specific sets: Used with EIDs
  - Lipid administration sets: Used with fat emulsion, which are supplied in glass containers with special vented tubing
  - Nitroglycerin administration sets
- Filters
  - Inline I.V. solution filters
  - Depth: Filters in which pore size is not uniform
  - Membrane (screen): Air-venting, bacteria-retentive, 0.22-micron filter
  - Blood filters
  - Standard clot: 170 to 220 microns; used on blood administration sets to remove coagulated products, microclots, and debris
  - Microaggregate: 20, 40, and 80 microns; can be added to an in-use blood administration set, permitting infusion of blood and easy replacement of the filter for delivery of multiple units
  - Leukocyte depletion: Used to remove 95% to 99.9% of leukocytes from red blood cells
- Stopcocks
  - Control the direction of flow of an infusate through manual manipulation of a direction regulation valve. Can be sources of infection. Should have sterile cap at all times.

- (PRN device)
  - Attach to the hub of the catheter and convert the cannula into an intermittent device
- Needleless systems
  - State-of-the-art technology to replace needles to connect I.V. devices and administer infusates
- Infusion devices (catheters)
  - Scalp vein needles: For short-term therapy; odd-numbered gauges
  - Over-the-needle catheters: For peripheral therapy, made from Teflon, Vialon; even-numbered gauges
  - Midline catheters: 6 inches long; indwelling time, 28 days
- Central infusion devices: Short and long term
  - Nontunneled catheters
  - Peripherally inserted central catheters (PICCs): Inserted peripherally and threaded to the SVC; can be placed by physicians or nurses
  - Central venous tunneled catheters (CVTCs)
  - Implantable ports: Closed system composed of implanted device with reservoir, port, and self-sealing system; require the use of a noncoring needle to access port
- EIDs
  - Pumps
    - Volumetric: Calibrated in milliliters per hour; require special cassette or cartridge to be used with the machine, very accurate, and used in delivery of high-potency drugs.
    - Peristaltic: Calibrated in milliliters per hour; used primarily for delivery of enteral feedings; have a rotary disk or rollers to compress tubing
    - Syringe: Piston-driven pump that controls rate of infusion by drive speed and syringe size
    - Patient-controlled analgesia (PCA): Can be used at home or in hospital to deliver pain medication
    - Ambulatory infusion: Lightweight, compact infusion pumps
    - Elastomeric balloons: Portable device designed with an elastomeric reservoir for delivery of medication
  - Product evaluation: When a device failure is noted, it is important to follow the following steps.
    - Identify previously recorded lot numbers and expiration dates of products.
    - Complete a designated internal report.
    - Inform the supervisor.
    - Notify the Risk Management Department.

Report a complete description of the problem. Information regarding the device needs to be submitted, including
  - Product name
  - Manufacturer's name and address

- Identification numbers of the device (lot number, model number, serial number, expiration date)
- Problem noted
- Name, title, and practice specialty of the device's user

■■ Thinking Critically: Case Study

A 45-year-old woman postoperative hysterectomy patient has an order to convert her continuous I.V.™ to an intermittent locking device. The Luer-activated device the hospital uses is a Posiflow (BD) mechanical valve.

1. What type of device is this NIS?
   a. Luer access mechanical valve (negative displacement),
   b. Luer access mechanical valve with positive displacement feature, or
   c. Neutral displacement needleless system (refer to chart on NIS).

2. What are the steps in flushing this device?

3. What BSI prevention technique should be used prior to access the NIS each time?

 Media Link: Answers to the case study and more critical thinking activities are provided on the CD-ROM.

Post-Test

1. Match the term in Column I with the definition in Column II.

   Column I

   A. Cannula

   B. Drip chamber

   C. Lumen

   D. Hub

   E. Port

   Column II

   a. A female connection point of an I.V. cannula where the tubing or other equipment attaches

   b. Point of entry

   c. Area of the I.V. tubing usually found under the spike where the solution drips and collects

   d. Space within an artery, vein, or catheter

   e. A tube or sheath used for infusing fluids

2. When using a flexible plastic system, what type of administration set could you choose?

   a. Vented
   b. Nonvented
   c. Vented or nonvented; both work with this system

3. Which of the following situations would be appropriate for a 0.22-micron filter? (*Select all that apply.*)

   a. An additive has been combined with the solution
   b. The patient is immunocompromised and receiving irritation medication

   c. Infusion of 10% dextrose and amino acids via central line.
   d. Total parenteral nutrition with lipids.

4. The standard blood administration set has a clot filter of how many microns?

   a. 170
   b. 40
   c. 20
   d. 10

5. Microaggregate filters are used for:

   a. Administration of protein solutions
   b. Administration of whole blood and packed cells stored more than 5 days
   c. Removal of bacteria for infusion
   d. Filtering air from the set

6. A disadvantage of the glass system is that it:

   a. Is breakable and difficult to store
   b. Reacts with some solutions and medications
   c. May be difficult to read fluid levels
   d. May develop leaks

7. The nurse flushing technique for a negative displacement device would be. (*Select all that apply.*)

   a. No special flushing technique is needed.
   b. Disconnect the tubing or syringe, allow sufficient time for the positive fluid displacement, then close the catheter clamp.
   c. As the last 0.5 to 1 mL of fluid is flushed inward, withdraw the syringe.
   d. Flush all fluid into the catheter lumen. Maintain force on the syringe plunger as a clamp on the catheter or extension is closed, then disconnect.

8. Which of the following technologies assist in the reduction of needle-stick injuries?

   a. Elastomeric pumps
   b. Luer locks
   c. Needleless systems
   d. Three-way stopcocks

9. The limit to operating pressure at which an alarm is triggered on an electronic infusion device is known as the:

   a. Air-in-line alarm
   b. Parameters or timed-out
   c. Occlusion alarm
   d. Not infusing alarm

10. The nurse identifies errors in programming an infusion pump. What should the nurse do? (*Select all that apply.*)

    a. Report the device malfunction to the supervisor.

    b. Fill out appropriate hospital form.

    c. Notify ECRI on appropriate form.

    d. Notify the Risk Manager.

 Media Link: Answers to the Chapter 5 Post-Test and more test questions together with rationales are provided on the CD-ROM.

▪ REFERENCES

Ackley, B.J., & Ladwig, G.B. (2008). *Nursing diagnosis handbook: An evidence-based guide to planning care.* St. Louis, MO: Mosby Elsevier.

American Association of Blood Banks (AABB). (2008). *Technical manual* (14th ed.). Bethesda, MD: Author.

Anderson, N.R. (2004). Midline catheters: The middle ground of intravenous therapy administration. *Journal of Infusion Nursing, 27*(5), 313–321.

Baxter Healthcare Corporation. (2008). Baxter receives 510(K) clearance from FDA for V-Link with VitaShield, new antimicrobial intravascular technology. Retrieved from http://www.baxter.com (Accessed September 10, 2008).

Bayne, C.G. (1997). Removing the confusion about infusion. *Nursing Management, 28,* 15–23.

Bennion, D., & Martin, K. (1991). In-line filtration. *Pediatric Nursing,* June, 20–21.

Deacon, V.L. (2004). The safe medical device act and its impact on clinical practice. *Journal of Infusion Nursing, 27*(1), 31–36.

Do, A., Ray, B., Banerjee, S., et al (1999). Bloodstream infection associated with needleless device use and the importance of infection-control practices in the home healthcare setting. *Journal of Infectious Diseases, 179*(2), 442–448.

ECRI. (2003). *Sharps safety & needlestick prevention* (2nd ed.). World Health Organization. Retrieved from www.ecri.org (Accessed August 18, 2008).

Gilles, D., O'Riordan, L., Wallen M., et al. (2004). Timing of intravenous administration set changes: A systematic review. *Infection Control & Hospital Epidemiology, 25*(3), 240–250.

Hadaway, L. (2006). Technology of flushing vascular access devices. *Journal of Infusion Nursing, 29*(3), 137–145.

Heitz., U., & Horne, M.M. (2005). *Pocket guide to fluid, electrolyte, and acid-base balance* (5th ed.). St. Louis, MO: C.V. Mosby.

Hunter, M. (2007). Peripherally inserted central catheter placement at the speed of sound. *Nutrition in Clinical Practice, 22,* 406–411.

Infusion Nurses Society (INS). (2006). Infusion Nursing Standards of Practice. *Journal of Infusion Nursing, 29*(1S), 32–36.

Infusion Nurses Society (INS). (2008). The role of the registered nurse in the insertion of external jugular peripherally inserted central catheters (EJ PICC) and external jugular peripheral intravenous catheters (EJ PIV). Position Paper. Norwood MA: Author.

Jacobs, B. (2005). Pump away high-risk infusion errors. *Nursing Management.* December, 40–44.

Kaler, W., & Chinn, R. (2007). Successful disinfection of needleless access ports: A matter of time and friction. *JAMA, 12*(3), 140–142.

Kirkpatrick, C.J. (1992). Microcirculatory problems in multiple organ failure: the role of endotoxins and particulate contamination. Proceedings of the symposium Managing the complications of intravenous therapy. Retrieved from www.pall.com (Accessed August 16, 2008).

Maki, D. (1991). Infection caused by intravascular devices: Pathogenesis, strategies for prevention. In: D.G. Maki (Ed.), *Improving catheter site care* (pp. 3–27). New York: Royal Society of Medicine Services.

Maki, D.G., & Mermel, L.A. (2007). Infection due to infusion therapy. In: W.R. Jarvis (Ed.). *Bennett and Brachman's hospital infections* (5th ed.). Philadelphia: Lippincott Williams & Wilkins.

Maki, D., & Ringer, M. (1991). Risk factor for infusion-related phlebitis with small peripheral venous catheters. *Annals of Internal Medicine, 114,* 845–854.

McCloskey-Dochterman, J.C., & Bulecheck, G.M. (2004). *Nursing interventions classification* (NIC) (4th ed.). St. Louis, MO: C.V. Mosby.

Mendelson, M., Chen, L., Solomon, R., et al. (2003). Study of Introcan Safety I.V. Catheter for the prevention of percutaneous injuries in healthcare workers. Society for Healthcare Epidemiology of America Annual Meeting. March 2003. Wake Forest University, Winston-Salem, NC.

Mermel, L.A., & Tow, S.M. (1995). The risk of midline catheterization in hospitalized patients: A prospective study. *Annals of Internal Medicine, 123*(1), 841–844.

Moorhead, S., Johnson, M., & Maas, M. (2004). *Nursing outcomes classification* (NOC) (3rd ed.). St. Louis, MO: C.V. Mosby.

Nowak, R. (2004). Scuba valve inspires cheap drug delivery. *New Science, 25,* 2474.

O'Grady, N.P., Alexander, M., Dellinger, E.P., et al. (2002). Guidelines for the prevention of intravascular catheter-related infections. *Morbidity and Mortality Weekly Report MMWR 51* (RR-10).

Pall Biomedical Corporation (2008). New York: Pall Biomedical Products Corporation.

Schiff, L. (2001). IV administration sets. *RN, 11*(64), 61.

Shelton, P., & Rosenthal, K. (2004). A safer needle. *Nursing Management, 6,* 27–30.

Sheppard, K., LeDesma, M., Moris, N., & O'Connor, K. (1999). A prospective study of two intravenous catheter securement techniques in a skilled nursing facility. *Journal of Infusion Nursing, 22*(3), 151–156.

Skryabina, E.A., & Dunn, T.S. (2006). Disposable infusion pumps. *American Journal of Health-System Pharmacy, 63*(7), 1260–1268.

Tourville, J. (2003). Automation and error reduction: How technology is helping Children's Medical Center of Dallas reach zero-error tolerance. *US Pharmacist, 28*(6), 80–86.

Trissel, L.A. (2006). *Handbook on injectable drugs* (14th ed.). Bethesda, MD: American Society of Health-System Pharmacists.

U.S. Food and Drug Administration (FDA). (1995). Supplement guidance on the content of premarket notification submissions for medical devices with sharps injury prevention features. Rockville, MD: Author.

U.S. Food and Drug Administration (FDA) (1998). Medical devices. Information sheets. Retrieved from www.fda.gov (Accessed August 16, 2008).

van Lingen, R.A., Baerts, W., Marquering, A.C., & Ruijs, G.J. (1997). The use of in-line intravenous filters in sick newborn infants result in significantly fewer infectious complications at lower cost. *Journal of Clinical Microbiology and Infection, 3,* 122.

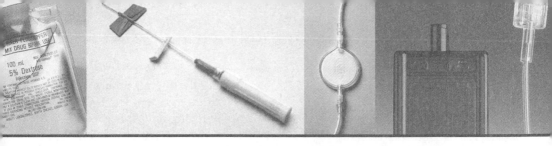

Chapter **6**

Techniques for Initiation and Maintenance of Peripheral Infusion Therapy

The proficient nurse learns from experience what typical events to expect in a given situation and how plans need to be modified in response to these events.
—*Patricia Benner*

■ **LEARNING OBJECTIVES**

On completion of this chapter, the reader will be able to:

1. Define the terminology related to peripheral venous access.
2. Recall the anatomy and physiology related to the venous system.
3. Identify the five tissue structures that the infusion nurse must penetrate for a successful venipuncture.
4. Identify the peripheral veins appropriate for venipuncture.
5. List the factors affecting site selection.
6. Demonstrate Phillips' 15-step approach for initiating peripheral-short infusion therapy.
7. List the three sites appropriate for labeling.
8. Identify the key components of the documentation process for peripheral infusion therapy.
9. Be familiar with the Infusion Nurses Society (INS) Standards of Practice for peripheral infusions and Centers for Disease Control and Prevention (CDC) guidelines for prevention of catheter-related bloodstream infections.
10. Recall the steps in performing a saline lock flush.
11. Describe the advantages and disadvantages of resealable locking devices.
12. Identify the risks and benefits of lidocaine and topical creams for initiating infusion therapy.
13. Describe techniques to assist with venipuncture visualization and dilation in patients with sclerotic veins, alterations in skin integrity, obesity, and edema.
14. Identify physiologic characteristics that differentiate infusion therapy for neonates, infants, children, and older adults.
15. Locate the most appropriate sites for venipuncture in pediatric and older adult patients.
16. Identify the types of needles and catheters available for pediatric patients.
17. Describe special considerations for successful venipuncture of neonates, infants, and older adults.

⧉ GLOSSARY

Antimicrobial   An agent that destroys or prevents the growth of microorganisms

Bevel   Slanted edge on opening of a needle or cannula device

Dermis   The corium layer of the skin composed of connective tissue, blood vessels, nerves, muscles, lymphatics, hair follicles, and sebaceous and sudoriferous glands

Distal   Farther from the heart; farthest from the point of attachment (below the previous site of cannulation)

Drop factor   The number of drops needed to deliver 1 mL of fluid

Endothelial lining   A thin layer of cells lining the blood vessels and heart

Epidermis   The outermost layer of skin covering the body, which is composed of epithelial cells and is devoid of blood vessels

Gauge   Size of a cannula (catheter) opening; gradual measurements of the outside diameter of a catheter

Macrodrop   I.V. tubing with a drop factor of 10 to 20 drops per milliliter (mL)

Microabrasion   Superficial break in skin integrity that may predispose the patient to infection

Microdrop   I.V. tubing with a drop factor of 60 drops/mL

Midline Catheter   A flexible catheter measuring 3.1 to 8 inches in length with the distal tip dwelling in the basilic, cephalic, or brachial veins, level with the axilla and distal to the shoulder.

Palpation   Examination by touch

Peripheral infusion (PIV)   Catheter inserted into the peripheral veins in outer extremities (usually arms and hands) for delivery of short-term infusion therapies.

Prime   To flush the air from the administration set with a solution before use

Proximal   Nearest to the heart; closest point to attachment (above the previous site of cannulation)

Spike   A sharp object (piercing pin) used to puncture an object (e.g., a bag of intravenous fluid) permitting fluids within the object (bag) to flow out.

Transillumination   Passage of light through a solid or liquid substance for diagnostic examination

■ Anatomy and Physiology Related to I.V. Practice

In order to perform **peripheral infusion (PIV)** therapy with the goal of providing positive vascular access outcomes, the nurse must understand the anatomy and physiology of the skin and venous system and be familiar with the physiologic responses of veins to heat, cold, and stress. It is also important to become familiar with the skin thickness and consistency at various sites to perform venous access proficiently.

Skin

The skin consists of two main layers, the **epidermis** and the **dermis**, which overlie the superficial fascia. The epidermis, composed of squamous cells that are less sensitive than underlying structures, is the first line of defense against infections. Two types of cells are common to the epidermis: Merkel and Langerhans cells. Merkel cells are receptors that transmit stimuli to axons through a chemical synapse. Langerhans' cells are believed to play a significant role in cutaneous immune system reactions. The epidermis is thickest on the palms of the hands and soles of the feet and is thinnest on the inner surfaces of the extremities. Thickness varies with age and exposure to the elements, such as wind and sun.

The dermis, a much thicker layer, is located directly below the epidermis. The dermis consists of blood vessels, hair follicles, sweat glands, sebaceous glands, small muscles, and nerves. As with the epidermis, the thickness of the dermis varies with age and physical condition. The skin is a special-sense touch organ, and the dermis reacts quickly to painful stimuli, temperature changes, and pressure sensation. This is the most painful layer during venipuncture because of the large amount of blood vessels and the many nerves contained in this sheath (Smeltzer, Bare, Hinkle, & Cheever, 2008).

The hypodermis, or fascia, lies below the epidermis and dermis and provides a covering for the blood vessels. This connective tissue layer varies in thickness and is found over the entire body surface. Because any infection in the fascia, called superficial cellulitis, spreads easily throughout the body, it is essential to use strict aseptic technique when inserting infusion devices. This superficial tissue layer connects with deeper fascia (Fig. 6-1).

Sensory Receptors

There are five types of sensory receptors, four of which affect the initiation of infusion therapy. The sensory receptors transmit along afferent fibers. Many types of stimulation, such as heat, light, cold, pain, pressure, and sound, are processed along the sensory receptors. Sensory receptors related to peripheral intravenous therapy include:

1. Mechanoreceptors, which process skin tactile sensations and deep tissue sensation (**palpation** of veins)
2. Thermoreceptors, which process cold, warmth, and pain (application of heat or cold)

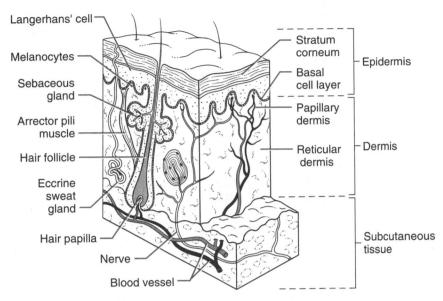

Figure 6-1 ■ Anatomy of skin.

3. Nociceptors, which process pain (puncture of vein for insertion of the cannula)
4. Chemoreceptors, which process osmotic changes in blood and decreased arterial pressure (decreased circulating blood volume) (Smeltzer, Bare, Hinkle, & Cheever, 2008).

> **NURSING FAST FACT!**
>
> To decrease the patient's pain during venipuncture, keep the skin taut by applying traction to it and move quickly through the skin layers and past the pain receptors.

Venous System

The blood transport system, circulatory system, has two main subdivisions—the cardiopulmonary and the systemic systems. The systemic circulation, particularly the peripheral veins, is used in infusion therapy. Veins function similarly to arteries but are thinner and less muscular (Table 6-1).

The wall of a vein is only 10% of the total diameter of the vessel, compared with 25% in the artery. Because the vein is thin and less muscular, it can distend easily, allowing for storage of large volumes of blood under low pressure. Approximately 75% of the total blood volume is contained in the veins.

> Table 6-1 | **COMPARISON OF ARTERY AND VEIN**
Artery*	Vein*
Thick-walled	Thin-walled
25% of arterial wall	10% of vein wall
Lacks valves	Greater distensibility
Pulsates	Valves present approximately every 3 in.

*Has three tissue layers.

Some veins have valves, particularly those that transport blood against gravity, as in the lower extremities. Valves, made up of endothelial leaflets, help prevent the **distal** reflux of blood. Valves occur at points of branching, producing a noticeable bulge in the vessel (Smeltzer, Bare, Hinkle, & Cheever, 2008). Arteries and veins have three layers of tissue that form the wall: the tunica intima, tunica adventitia, and tunica media (Fig. 6-2).

Venous blood flows slower in the periphery and increases in turbulence in the larger veins of the thorax. This increased flow rate is an important aspect in administering hypertonic fluids in larger vasculatures. The following is the amount of blood flow in milliliters per minute through each of the major veins used to deliver intravenous solutions:

- Cephalic and basilic veins: 45 to 95 mL/min
- Subclavian vein: 150 to 300 mL/min
- Superior vena cava: 2000 mL/min

Tunica Adventitia

The outermost layer, called the tunica adventitia, consists of connective tissue that surrounds and supports a vessel. The blood supply of this layer, called the vasa vasorum, nourishes both the adventitia and media

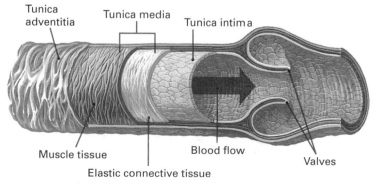

Figure 6-2 ■ Anatomy of a vein. (Courtesy of Medical Economics Publishing, Montvale, NJ, with permission.)

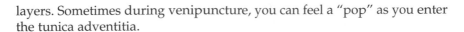

layers. Sometimes during venipuncture, you can feel a "pop" as you enter the tunica adventitia.

Tunica Media

The middle layer, called the tunica media, is composed of muscular and elastic tissue with nerve fibers for vasoconstriction and vasodilation. The tunica media in a vein is not as strong and rigid as it is in an artery, so it tends to collapse or distend as pressure decreases or increases. Stimulation by change in temperature or mechanical or chemical irritation can produce a response in this layer. For instance, cold blood or infusates can produce spasms that impede blood flow and cause pain. Application of heat promotes dilatation, which can relieve a spasm or improve blood flow.

 NURSING FAST FACT!

> *During venipuncture, if the tip of the catheter has nicked the tunica adventitia or is placed in the tunica media layer, a small amount of blood will appear in the catheter; however, the catheter will not thread because it is trapped between layers. If you cannot get a steady backflow of blood, the needle might be in this layer, so advance the stylet of the cannula slightly before advancing the catheter.*

Tunica Intima

The innermost layer, called the tunica intima, has one thin layer of cells, referred to as the **endothelial lining**. The surface is smooth, allowing blood to flow through vessels easily. Any roughening of this bed of cells during venipuncture while the catheter is in place, or on discontinuing the system, fosters the process of thrombosis formation and discomfort. (Refer to Chapter 9 for complications.)

Veins of the Hands and Arms

The venous system of the hands and arms is abundant with acceptable veins for cannulation (Figs. 6-3 and 6-4). When selecting the best site, many factors must be considered, such as ease of insertion and access, type of needle or catheter that is to be used, and comfort and safety for the patient. Table 6-2 provides information on identifying and selecting the most effective I.V. site for the clinical situations.

◼ Approaches to Venipuncture: Phillips 15-Step Peripheral-Venipuncture Method

Performing a successful venipuncture requires mastery and knowledge of infusion therapy as well as psychomotor clinical skill. Many aseptic approaches to venipuncture techniques provide safe parenteral therapy.

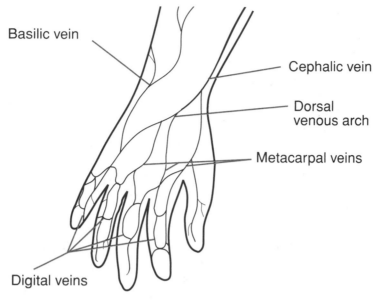

Basilic vein

Cephalic vein

Dorsal
venous arch

Metacarpal veins

Digital veins

Figure 6-3 ■ Superficial veins of the dorsum of the hand. (Courtesy of Becton Dickinson, Sandy, UT.)

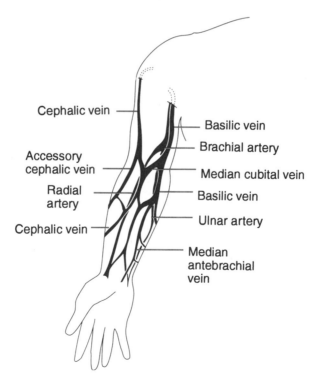

Cephalic vein

Accessory
cephalic vein

Radial
artery

Cephalic vein

Basilic vein

Brachial artery

Median cubital vein

Basilic vein

Ulnar artery

Median
antebrachial
vein

Figure 6-4 ■ Superficial veins of the forearm. (Courtesy of Becton Dickinson, Sandy, UT.)

> Table 6-2	SELECTING AN INSERTION SITE FOR THE SUPERFICIAL VEINS OF THE DORSUM OF THE HAND AND THE ARM	
Vein and Location	**Insertion Device**	**Considerations**
Digital Lateral and dorsal portions of the fingers	Small-gauge cannula 20- to 22-gauge catheter 21- to 25-gauge steel needle	Use a padded tongue blade to splint the cannula. Use only solutions that are isotonic without additives because of the risk of infiltration.
Metacarpal Dorsum of the hand formed by union of digital veins between the knuckles	20- to 22-gauge to ¾–1 inch in length over the needle catheter 21- to 25-gauge steel needle (short-term)	Good site to begin therapy Usually easily visualized Avoid if infusing antibiotics, potassium chloride, or chemotherapeutic agents.
Cephalic Radial portion of the lower arm along the radial bone of the forearm	18- to 22-gauge cannulas, usually over-the-needle catheter	Large vein, easy to access First use most distal section and work upward for long-term therapy Useful for infusing blood and chemically irritating medications
Basilic Ulnar aspect of the lower arm and runs up the ulnar bone	18- to 22-gauge, usually over-the-needle catheter	Difficult area to access Large vein, easily palpated, but moves easily; stabilize with traction during venipuncture. Often available after other sites have been exhausted.
Accessory Cephalic Branches off the cephalic vein along the radial bone	18- to 22-gauge, usually over-the-needle catheter	Medium to large size and easy to stabilize May be difficult to palpate in persons with large amounts of adipose tissue Valves at cephalic junction may prohibit cannula advancement Short length may prohibit cannula use
Upper Cephalic Radial aspect of upper arm above the elbow	16- to 20-gauge, usually over-the-needle catheter	Difficult to visualize Excellent site for confused patients.
Median Antebrachial Extends up the front of the forearm from the median antecubital veins	18- to 22 gauge, usually over-the-needle catheter	Area has many nerve endings and should be avoided Infiltration occurs easily.

> Table 6-2   **SELECTING AN INSERTION SITE FOR THE SUPERFICIAL VEINS OF THE DORSUM OF THE HAND AND THE ARM—cont'd**

Vein and Location	Insertion Device	Considerations
Median Basilic Ulnar portion of the forearm	18- to 22-gauge, usually over-the-needle catheter	Medium to large size vein, good for phlebotomy or emergency access
Median Cubital Radial side of forearm; crosses in front of the brachial artery at the antecubital space	16- to 22-gauge, usually over-the-needle catheter	Medium to large size vein, good for phlebotomy or emergency access
Antecubital In the bend of the elbow	All sizes especially 16- to 18-gauge; used for midline catheters and peripherally inserted central catheters and blood collection	Should be reserved for blood draws for laboratory analysis only, unless in an emergency Uncomfortable placement site, owing to the arm extending in an unnatural position Area difficult to splint with armboard

The Phillips 15-step venipuncture method, outlined in Table 6-3 and explained in detail in this chapter, is an easy-to-remember step approach for beginning practitioners.

> Table 6-3   **PHILLIPS 15-STEP PERIPHERAL-VENIPUNCTURE METHOD**

Precannulation

1. Checking physician's or authorized provider's orders
2. Hand hygiene following standard precautions
3. Equipment inspection and preparation
4. Patient assessment, psychological preparation, and patient identification.
5. Site selection and vein dilation

Cannulation

6. Catheter selection
7. Gloving
8. Site preparation – 30 seconds and let dry
9. Vein entry, direct versus indirect
10. Catheter stabilization and dressing management

Postcannulation

11. Labeling
12. Equipment disposal
13. Patient education
14. Rate calculations
15. Documentation

Guidelines supporting quality client care have been published by the Occupational Safety and Health Administration (OSHA) and the Centers for Disease Control and Prevention (CDC). The Infusion Nurses Society (INS) Standards of Practice (2006a) were developed to address patients' infusion needs based on research and evidence-based practice. As a nurse initiating infusion therapy, be aware of these standards, as well as those of your own institution.

NOTE > Current INS standards have been integrated throughout the 15 steps.

Precannulation

Before initiating cannulation, you must follow steps 1 through 5: checking the physician's or authorized prescriber's order, handwashing, preparing the equipment, assessing and preparing the patient, and selecting the vein and the site of insertion.

Step 1: Authorized Prescriber's Order

An authorized prescriber order is necessary to initiate infusion therapy. The order should be clear, concise, legible, and complete.

NOTE > The use of electronic order entry has assisted with the prevention of transcription errors.

All parenteral solutions should be checked against the authorized prescriber's order. The order should include:
- Date and time of the day
- Infusate name
- Route of administration
- Dosage of administration
- Volume to be infused
- Rate of infusion
- Duration of infusion
- Signature of authorized prescriber

INS Standard Verbal orders written by a nurse in the medical record in a hospital setting should be signed by the prescriber within an appropriate time frame in accordance with state and federal regulations and organizational polices and procedures. (INS, 2006a, 9)

The Joint Commission (TJC) in their 2003 National Safety Goals to improve communication by verifying the complete order or test result by having the person receiving the order or test "read-back" the complete order or test result (TJC, 2003).

Step 2: Hand Hygiene

Hand hygiene has been shown to significantly decrease the risk of contamination and cross-contamination. Touch contamination is a common cause of transfer of pathogens. Soap and water are adequate for handwashing before the insertion of a catheter; however, an antiseptic solution such as chlorhexidine may be used. Wash hands for 15 to 20 seconds before equipment preparation and before insertion of a catheter. Do not apply hand lotion after handwashing (Siegel, Rhinehart, Jackson, & Chiarello, 2007).

The CDC recommends the following for hand hygiene:

- Decontaminate hands after removing gloves.
- Before eating and after using a restroom, wash hands with a non-antimicrobial soap and water or with antimicrobial soap and water.
- Antimicrobial-impregnated wipes may be considered as an alternative to washing hands with non-antimicrobial soap and water.
- When using an alcohol-based hand gel, apply product to palm of one hand and rub hands together, covering all surfaces of hands and fingers until hands are dry (Siegel, Rhinehart, Jackson, & Chiarello, 2007).

INS Standard   Handwashing shall be performed before and immediately after all clinical procedures and before and after removal of gloves. (INS, 2006a, 20)

- Do not wear artificial fingernails or extenders when having direct contact with patients at high risk (those in intensive care units or operating rooms). Keep natural tips ¹/₄ inch long (Siegel, Rinehart, Jackson, & Chiarello, 2007).

> *EBNP Numerous studies have been published in the last decade that focus on fingernails and infection control. Studies by Moolenaar, Crutcher, San Joaquin, et al. (2000) and by Parry, Grant, Yukna, et al. (2001) indicated Pseudomonas aeruginosa and Candida outbreaks had correlations to use of artificial nails. The evidence-based practice demonstrated that workers who wear artificial nails are more likely to harbor pathogens than those who do not.*

Several studies have demonstrated that skin underneath rings is more heavily colonized than comparable areas of skin on fingers without rings.

Consideration should be given to limiting jewelry when delivering health care to patients who are immunocompromised or at high risk for infection (CDC, 2002).

> EBNP A study by Trick, Vernon, Hayes, et al. (2003) demonstrated the impact of ring wearing on hand contamination and comparison of hand hygiene agents in a hospital. It was found that the presence of rings on nurses' hands resulted in an increased frequency of hand carriage of S. aureus, gram-negative bacilli, or Candida species and that for any transient organism, there was a larger increase when several rings were worn.

Step 3: Equipment Collection and Preparation

Step 3 follows hand hygiene so that the equipment preparation following aseptic technique. If the order is for delivery of a primary or secondary solution:
- Gather infusate ordered and appropriate administration set, catheters, stabilization device (sterile tape or securement device), dressing, and prep solution. There are many prepackaged I.V. start packs on the market.
- Inspect the infusate container at the nurses' station, in the clean utility, or in the medication room. In today's practice, two systems are available: glass system and plastic system (rigid or soft).

To check the glass system:
- Hold the container up to the light to inspect for cracks as evidenced by flashes of light. Glass systems are crystal clear.
- Rotate the container and look for particulate contamination and cloudiness.
- Inspect the seal and check the expiration date.

To check a plastic system:
- The outer wrap of the plastic system should be dry.
- Gently squeeze the soft plastic infusate container to check for breaks in the integrity of the plastic; squeeze the system to detect pinholes.
- Inspect the solution for any particulate contamination. The plastic systems are not crystal clear, but slightly opaque.
- Check the expiration date.

If the order is for an intermittent infusion device:
- Gather catheters, prep solution, stabilization device (tape or securement/dressing device) and/or dressing, along with 3 mL of sodium chloride for flush. Must be a single-use syringe for the flush.

Select either a vented or nonvented primary tubing set or a secondary set, depending on the rationale for infusion. It is wise to "**spike**" the solution container and "**prime**" the administration set in the clean utility area or nurse's station to detect defective equipment before taking into the patient care area. Choose the correct administration set to match the solution delivery system. For the closed glass, use vented only; for the plastic, use either vented or nonvented. (See Chapter 5 for more detailed information on I.V. equipment.) Refer to Figure 6-5 for spiking and priming.

Step 4: Patient Assessment, Psychological Preparation, and Identification

Before assessment of the patient, the nurse must use at least two patient identifiers (neither to be the patient's room number) whenever providing treatments or procedures (TJC, 2003).

Selection of the vascular access device and insertion site requires integration of data obtained from the patient care issues, patient assessment, and the specific infusion therapy prescribed. Selection of the vascular access device requires collaboration efforts with input from physician, nurse, client, and caregiver. It is important to use step 4 to gather the necessary information needed to perform a successful venipuncture and infusion therapy.

First, provide privacy for the patient. Explain the procedure to minimize his or her anxiety. Instruct the patient regarding the purpose of the intravenous therapy, the procedure, what the physician has ordered in the infusate and why, the mobility limitations, and signs and symptoms of potential complications.

Evaluate the patient's psychological preparedness for the peripheral intravenous procedure by talking with him or her before assessing the vein. The nurse should consider aspects such as autonomy, handedness, and

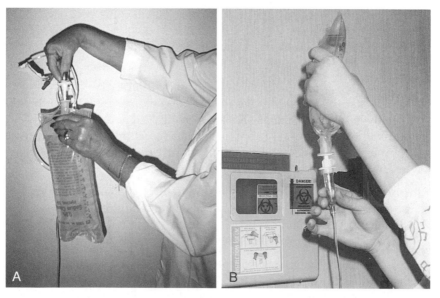

Figure 6-5 ■ *A*, Spiking and *B*, priming plastic system.

independence, along with invasion of personal space when I.V. placement is necessary. Often the patient has a fear of pain associated with venipuncture, or the memory of a previously negative encounter related to necessity of the therapy.

Step 5: Site Selection and Vein Dilatation

SITE SELECTION

Assessment is the first step in the nursing process, and is the first step for successful infusion therapy. The site selection is based on a thorough assessment of patient's condition, age, diagnosis, vascular condition, history of previous access devices, and type and duration of therapy.

According to the INS Standards of Practice (2006a) the following should be taken into consideration during site selection.

1. Consideration needs to be given to manufacturer's labeled use(s) and directions for catheter device insertion.
2. Veins for assessment for peripheral cannulation are those found on the dorsal and ventral surfaces of the upper extremities.
3. For pediatric infusion additional site selection can include the veins of the head, neck, and lower extremities. Refer to the section in this chapter on pediatric peripheral intravenous techniques.
4. Veins of the lower extremities should not be used routinely in the adult population due to risk of embolism and thrombophlebitis.
5. Assess previous venipunctures and subsequent injury to the vein.
6. Routinely initiate venipuncture in the **distal** areas of the upper extremities; subsequent cannulation should be made **proximal** to the previously cannulated site.
7. Choice of alternative site due to inadvertent infiltration or extravasation of infusate(s) should require assessment as to type of infusate, pH and osmolality, estimated volume of the infusate, and vein condition.
8. Site selection should avoid areas of flexion.
9. Blood pressure cuffs or tourniquets should not be used during periods of infusion on an extremity with an indwelling peripheral short catheter.
10. A physician should be consulted and an order obtained before cannulation of an arm of a patient who has undergone breast surgery requiring axillary node dissection.
11. Therapies not appropriate for peripheral-short catheters include continuous vesicant therapy, parenteral nutrition, infusates with pH less than 5 or greater than 9, and infusates with an osmolality greater than 600 mOsm/L.
12. Peripheral-short catheters should not be used routinely for blood drawing. The exception is short-term use, that is, anticipated need less than 48 hours, in which case the peripheral-short

catheter should be used only for blood withdrawal, not for infusion of fluids or medications.

13. Consideration should be given to use of visualization technologies that aid in vein identification and selection. (INS, 2006a, 37)

Additional information must be considered before initiation of infusion therapy and is part of step 4 in completing a thorough assessment. Patient assessment should be ongoing and requires the nurse to evaluate and use critical thinking skills to achieve positive patient outcomes (Phillips, 2008).

The following factors help nurses make competent choices for site selection and should be part of the data gathering nursing process step.

1. *Type of solution*: Fluids that are hypertonic (i.e., more than 375 mOsm), such as antibiotics and potassium chloride, are irritating to vein walls. Select a large vein in the forearm to initiate this therapy.

2. *Condition of the vein*: A soft, straight vein is the ideal choice for venipuncture. Palpate the vein by moving the tips of the fingers down the vein to observe how it refills. The dorsal metacarpal veins in elderly patients are a poor choice because blood extravasation (i.e., hematoma) occurs more readily in small, thin veins. When a patient is hypovolemic, peripheral veins collapse more quickly than larger veins.
   Avoid:
   ■ Bruised veins
   ■ Red, swollen veins
   ■ Veins near previous site of phlebitis and infiltration
   ■ Sites near a previously discontinued site

3. *Duration of therapy*: Choose a vein that supports I.V. therapy for at least 72 hours. Start at the best, lowest vein. Use the hand only if a nonirritating solution is being infused. Long courses of infusion therapy make preservation of veins essential. Perform venipuncture distally with each subsequent puncture **proximal** to previous puncture and alternate arms.
   Avoid:
   ■ A joint flexion
   ■ A vein too small for cannula size

4. *Cannula size*: Hemodilution is important. The **gauge** of the cannula should be as small as possible.

5. *Patient age*: Infants do not have the accessible sites that older children and adults have owing to infants' increased body fat. Veins in the hands, feet, and antecubital region may be the only accessible sites. Veins in elderly persons are usually fragile; approach venipuncture gently and evaluate the need for a tourniquet.

6. *Patient preference:* Consider the patient's personal feelings when determining the catheter placement site. Evaluate the extremities, taking into account the dominant hand.
7. *Patient activity:* Ambulatory patients using crutches or a walker will need cannula placement above the wrist so the hand can still be used.
8. *Presence of disease or previous surgery:* Patients with vascular disease or dehydration may have limited venous access. Avoid phlebitis-infiltrated sites or a site of infection. If a patient has a condition with poor vascular venous return, the affected side **must be avoided**. Examples are cerebrovascular accident, mastectomy, amputation, orthopedic surgery of the hand or arm, and plastic surgery of the hand or arm.
9. *Presence of shunt or graft:* Do not use a patient's arm or hand that has a patent graft or shunt for dialysis.
10. *Patients receiving anticoagulation therapy:* Patients receiving anticoagulant therapy have a propensity to bleed. Local ecchymoses and major hemorrhagic complications can be avoided if the nurse is aware that the patient is taking anticoagulant therapy. Precautions can be taken when initiating infusion therapy. Venous distention can be accomplished with minimal tourniquet pressure. Use the smallest catheter that will accommodate the vein and deliver the ordered infusate. The dressing must be removed gently using alcohol or adhesive remover. On discontinuation of infusion therapy for patients on anticoagulation, direct pressure must be applied over the site for 10 minutes.

 NURSING FAST FACT!

> If the veins are fragile or if the patient is taking anticoagulants, avoid using a tourniquet; constricted blood flow may overdistend fragile veins, causing vein damage, vessel hemorrhages, or subcutaneous bleeding.

11. *Patient with allergies:* Determine whether a patient has allergies. Allergies to iodine need to be identified because iodine is contained in products used to prep the skin before venipuncture. Question the patient regarding allergies to shellfish. If there is a doubt, use chlorhexidine gluconate or 70% isopropyl alcohol to prep the skin and cleanse the ports. Other allergies of concern to delivery of safe patient care include allergies to lidocaine, other medications, foods, animals, latex, and environmental substances.

Refer to Table 6-4 for tips in selecting veins for peripheral infusions.

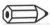

> Table 6-4   **TIPS FOR SELECTING VEINS**

- A suitable vein should feel relatively smooth, pliable with valves well spaced.
- Veins will be difficult to stabilize in a patient who has recently lost weight.
- Debilitated patients and those taking corticosteroids have fragile veins that bruise easily.
- Sclerotic veins are common among narcotics addicts.
- Sclerotic veins are common among the elderly population.
- Dialysis patients usually know which veins are good for venipuncture.
- Start with distal veins and work proximally.
- Veins that feel bumpy, like running your finger over a cat's tail, are usually thrombosed or extremely valvular.

NURSING FAST FACT!

Always question the patient regarding allergies before administering medications, especially those given by intravenous route. Question patients on latex allergy.

CULTURAL AND ETHNIC CONSIDERATIONS: PERFORMING INFUSION THERAPY

Transcultural nursing is becoming a specialty field; however, every nurse must use transcultural knowledge to facilitate culturally appropriate care. Practitioners performing I.V. therapy must make every effort to deliver culturally sensitive care that is free of inherent biases based on gender, race, and religion.

Culturally diverse nursing care must take into account six cultural phenomena that vary with application and use, yet are evident in all cultural groups: (1) communication, (2) space, (3) social organization, (4) time, (5) environmental control, and (6) biologic variations.

In preparing to perform I.V. therapy–related procedures on patients from different cultures, it is important to remember some key guidelines:
- Plan care based on the communicated needs and cultural background.
- Learn as much as possible about the patient's cultural customs and beliefs.
- Encourage the patient to share cultural interpretations of health, illness, and health care.
- Be sensitive to the uniqueness of the patient.
- Identify sources of discrepancy between the patient's and your own concepts of health and illness.
- Communicate at the patient's personal level of functioning.
- Modify communication approaches to meet cultural educational needs.
- Understand that respect for the patient and his or her communication needs is central to the therapeutic relationship.
- Communicate in a nonthreatening manner.
- Follow acceptable social and cultural amenities.

Continued

- Adopt special approaches when the patient speaks a different language (e.g., translators or AT&T).
- Use a caring tone of voice and facial expression.
- Speak slowly and distinctly but not loudly.
- Use gestures, pictures, and play acting to help the patient understand.
- Repeat the message in a different way.
- Be alert to words the patient seems to understand and use them frequently.
- Keep messages simple and repeat them.
- Avoid using technical medical terms and abbreviations.
- If available, use an appropriate language dictionary.
- Use interpreters to improve communication (Giger & Davidhizar, 2004; Munoz & Luckmann, 2005).

Vein Dilatation

There are many ways to increase the flow of blood in the upper extremities. Factors affecting the capacity for dilatation are blood pressure, presence of valves, sclerotic veins, and multiple previous I.V. sites. Refer to Table 6-4 for tips for dilating veins.

The following list provides ways to dilate veins.

1. *Gravity*: Position the extremity lower than the heart for several minutes.
2. *Clenching/pumping fist*: Instruct the patient to open and close his or her fist. Squeezing a rubber ball or rolled washcloth works well.
3. *Stroking the vein*: Lightly stroke the vein downward or use light tapping with index finger to cause dilation of vein.
4. *Warm compresses*: Apply warm towels to the extremity for 10 minutes. A new technology available is a passive warming mitt, which is not heated and can be used for 15 minutes before venipuncture and during the venipuncture procedure.

> EBNP In a study by Walling and Lenhardt (2003) it was documented that the success rate for cannula insertion was 94% with active warming.

NOTE > Do not use a microwave oven to heat towels; the temperature can become too hot and cause a burn.

5. *Blood pressure cuff*: This is an excellent choice for vein dilatation. Pump the cuff up slightly (e.g., about 30 mm Hg). This method prevents constriction of the arterial system.

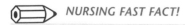 *NURSING FAST FACT!*

Care must be exercised when using a blood pressure cuff not to start the I.V. too close to the cuff, which causes excessive back pressure.

6. *Tourniquet*: Apply the tourniquet 6 to 8 inches above the venipuncture site if the blood pressure is within the normal range. If the patient is hypertensive, the tourniquet should be placed high on the extremity; occasionally, the tourniquet is not needed in the case of severely hypertensive patients because the veins are readily visible and palpable. With hypotensive patients, move the tourniquet as close as possible to the venipuncture site without contamination of the prepped area.

 NURSING FAST FACT!

Tourniquets shall be single-patient use and material should be considered with regard to potential latex allergy (INS, 2006a, 36).

7. *Multiple tourniquet technique*: Applying additional tourniquets to increase the oncotic pressure and bring deep veins into view. This technique is useful for clients with extra adipose tissue. Refer to Table 6-5 for the steps. Refer to Figure 6-6 for a picture of a multiple tourniquet.
8. *Transillumination*: **Transillumination** has been used for imaging of subsurface veins and some structures. The classic method of transillumination involves shining a light through a part of the body and observing the veins; this side-transillumination method shines light into the skin from outside the field of view

> Table 6-5   **MULTIPLE TOURNIQUET TECHNIQUE**

- Assess patient's arms for appropriate vascular access. Explain reasons for use of multiple tourniquet technique and that there may be some pressure discomfort for a short period of time. Verify the patient's understanding of the explanation.
- Place one tourniquet high on the arm for 2 minutes and leave in place. The arm should be stroked downward toward the hand.
- After 2 minutes, place a second tourniquet at midarm just below the antecubital fossa for 2 minutes. By increasing the **oncotic** pressure inside the tissue, blood is forced into the small vessels of the periphery
- The practitioner should assess for collateral circulation. If soft collateral veins do not appear in the forearm, a third tourniquet may be placed near the wrist.
- Tourniquets must not be left on longer than 6 minutes.
- *Use Multiple Tourniquet Technique*: If the peripheral vessels are hard and sclerosed because of a disease process, personal misuse, or frequent drug therapy, venous access is difficult.

Note: The multiple tourniquet technique helps novices learn the differences between collateral veins and sclerosed vessels. Usually, veins appear in the basilic vein of the forearm and the hands when this approach is used.

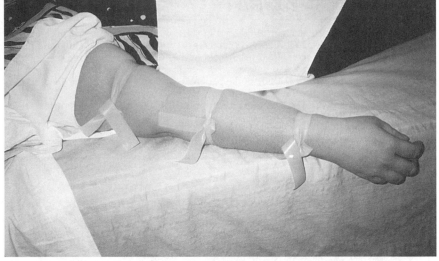

Figure 6-6 ■ Multiple tourniquet technique.

so that it is pointed toward the center at a depth of approximately 2 cm. The depth of visualization of veins is between 3 and 6 mm depending on the color of the light used. Transillumination light frequencies are greatly absorbed by deoxygenated hemoglobin in venous blood and show up as dark areas in the skin (Translite, 2008). Added use transillumination with a penlight or to illuminate veins in patients with dark skin. Veinlite® by TransLite (Sugar Land, TX) and Venoscope II Transilluminator (The Vein Finder) are two transilluminator devices. Refer to Table 6-6 for information on how to use a transilluminator or penlight. Refer to Figure 6-7 for techniques for transillumination.

 NURSING FAST FACT!

> To enhance vein location, use adequate lighting. Bright, direct overhead examination lights may have a "washout" effect on veins. Instead, use side lighting, which can add contour and "shadowing" to highlight the skin color and texture and allow visualization of the vein shadow below the skin.

●● CULTURAL AND ETHNIC CONSIDERATIONS: SKIN COLOR

Skin color is the most significant biological variation in terms of nursing care. When caring for patients with highly pigmented skin, establish the baseline color by daylight. Give dark-skinned individuals a window to provide access to sunlight (Giger & Davidhizar, 2004).

> Table 6-6 | **TRANSILLUMINATION**

- Take precautions in patients with alterations in skin surfaces caused by lesions, burns, or a disease process. Patients with altered skin integrity are often photosensitive and need additional protection of their already damaged tissue. This indirect lighting does not flatten veins or cause damage to the skin.
- Use a light directed toward the side of the patient's extremity to illuminate the blue veins and provide a guide for venipuncture.

For Veinlite and Venoscope II see manufacturer's guidelines for use of the product penlight:

- Turn down the light in the room.
- Use penlight on the side of the forearm to illuminate any veins.

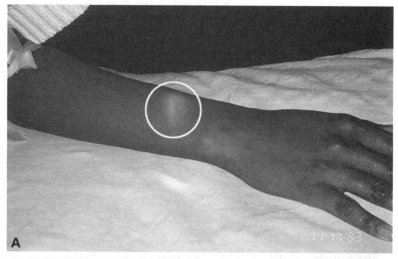

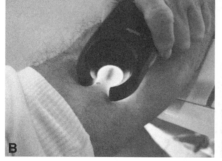
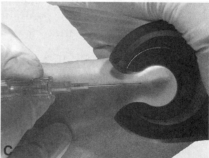

Figure 6-7 ▪ Transillumination techniques. *A*, Tangential lighting using flashlight to illuminate veins of dark skin individual. *B*, Veinlite® LED assisted vein finder. *C*, Veinlite® LED assisted vein finder. (Courtesy of Translite LLC, Sugar Land, TX.)

9. Ultrasonography can be used to place peripheral intravenous catheters for short-term therapy when traditional landmark methods for placement fail. However, special training in use of ultrasound for placement of PIV is recommended (LaRue, 2000).

Table 6-7 presents a summary of tips for the difficult venous access.

Cannulation

Cannulation involves steps 6 through 10: selecting the appropriate catheter, gloving, preparing the site, direct or indirect entry into the vein, and stabilizing the catheter and managing the dressing.

Nursing goals for choosing an appropriate site include the following:
- The site must tolerate the rate of flow.
- The site must be capable of delivering the medications or solutions ordered.
- The site must tolerate the gauge of cannula needed.
- The patient must be comfortable with the site chosen.
- The site must be one that least limits the patient's activities of daily living.

Step 6: Catheter Selection

Nursing criteria for choosing an appropriate type of catheter include the following:
- The patient's vascular access needs based on the prescribed therapy
- Length of treatment (over 3–7 days) for a short-peripheral catheter three inches in length or less.
- Resources available to care for device (acute care facility, home care, or long-term care).
- A **midline catheter** is considered when the length of therapy is beyond 6 days but does not extend past 4 to 6 weeks. The length of midline is 3.1 to 8 inches with the distal tip dwelling in the basilic, cephalic, or brachial vein level with the axilla and distal to the shoulder.

> Table 6-7 | **TECHNIQUES TO ASSIST WITH DIFFICULT VENOUS ACCESS**

- Alterations in skin surfaces: Use tangential lighting.
- Hard sclerosed vessels: Use multiple tourniquet technique.
- Obesity: Use 2-inch catheter, lateral veins, and multiple tourniquet technique.
- Edema: Displace edema with digital pressure.
- Fragile veins: Maintain traction using one-handed technique. Be gentle.
Use blood pressure cuff, or digital pressure with assistance from another nurse.

INS Standard All catheters must be radiopaque, and the cannula selected shall be the smallest **gauge** and shortest length to accommodate the prescribed therapy.

The nurse shall select a catheter with the fewest number of lumens for the infusion management of the patient. (INS, 2006a, 38)

Peripheral intravenous therapy is most often delivered with safety over-the-needle catheters. (See Chapter 5 for catheter choice and sizes.) The choice of catheter depends on the purpose of the infusion and the condition and availability of the veins.

Most hospitals, clinics, and home care agencies have policies and procedures for the selection of catheters. Table 6-8 presents the recommended gauges and color codes for catheters.

The tip of the catheter should be inspected for integrity before venipuncture to note the presence of burrs on the needle, peeling of catheter material, or other abnormalities.

Step 7: Gloving

The CDC (2007) recommends following standard precautions whenever exposure to blood or body fluids is likely. Wear gloves with fit and durability appropriate to the task.

Remove gloves after contact with a patient and/or the surrounding environment (including medical equipment) using proper technique to prevent hand contamination.

NOTE > Do not wear the same pair of gloves for the care of more than one patient, and do not wash gloves for the purpose of reuse because this practice has been associated with transmission of pathogens. Change gloves during patient care if the hands will move from a contaminated body-site to a clean body-site (Siegel, Rhinehart, Jackson, & Chiarello, 2007).

> Table 6-8 **RECOMMENDED GAUGES AND COLOR CODES OF CATHETERS**

Gauges	Color Code
16-gauge for trauma	16-gauge: gray
18- to 20-gauge for infusion of hypertonic or isotonic solutions with additives	18-gauge: green
	20-gauge: pink
18- to 20-gauge for blood administration	18-gauge: green
	20 gauge: pink
22- to 24-gauge for pediatric patients	22-gauge: yellow
	24-gauge: blue
22-gauge for fragile veins in elderly persons if unable to place a 20-gauge catheter	24-gauge: yellow
24- to 26-gauge for neonate	24-gauge: blue

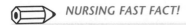 *NURSING FAST FACT!*

Latex and the powder used in the gloves are associated with potentially severe allergic reactions in susceptible persons. Avoid using this material if you have experienced any reactions to their use. (For more information on latex allergy, see Chapter 2 under occupational risks.)

INS Standard Gloves will be worn during all infusion procedures that will potentially expose the nurse to blood and body fluids. (INS, 2006a, 19)

Local Anesthetic Agents

If the policy and procedures of the agency and assessment of the patient support use of local anesthesia, consideration should be given to offering the patient this option before prepping the site for venipuncture. Local anesthetic agents include lidocaine, iontophoresis, low-frequency ultrasonography, pressure-accelerated lidocaine, or topical transdermal agents.

INS Standard Use of topical anesthetics prior to painful dermal procedures in children should be encouraged, in addition to use of adjunctive and less invasive anesthetics and anxiolytic therapies. (INS, 2006a, 40)

NOTE > The duration required for activation will depend on which agent is used.

Lidocaine

Lidocaine has been used in clinical practice since 1948 and is one of the safest anesthetics. Lidocaine is an amide that works by stopping impulses at the neural membrane. The anesthetized site is numb to pain, but the patient perceives touch and pressure and has control of his or her muscles. The anesthetic becomes effective within 15 to 30 seconds and lasts 30 to 45 minutes. The nurse must have knowledge of the actions and side effects associated with lidocaine. A history of previous allergies precludes the administration of lidocaine.

The process of using 1% lidocaine (without epinephrine) before venipuncture is as follows:

1. Review the authorized prescriber's order or the standardized procedure in the facility for use of lidocaine prior to venipuncture.
2. Check for patient allergy and lidocaine sensitivity.

3. Verify patient's identity using two independent identifiers.
4. Select the appropriate arm for infusion therapy, apply the tourniquet, and select a suitable vein.
5. Draw up 0.3 mL of 1% lidocaine (without epinephrine) in a 1 mL TB syringe.
6. Don gloves.
7. Prep the site with alcohol for 30 seconds and allow it to dry.
8. Reapply the tourniquet. The vein should be fully dilated, pulled taut by stretching, and stabilized while the local anesthetic is administered.
9. Insert the needle bevel up at a 15- to 25-degree angle. Aspirate to confirm no blood return.
10. Inject the lidocaine intradermally into the side of the vein next to the desired insertion site. Do not nick the vein.
11. Withdraw the needle. Allow 5 to 10 seconds for the anesthetic to take effect.
12. Continue with the Phillips' step 8 in starting the I.V. Refer to Figure 6-8.

Transdermal Analgesia

ELA-Max (Ferndale Laboratories) by prescription and EMLA (Astra), which is over the counter, creams are examples of transdermal analgesic

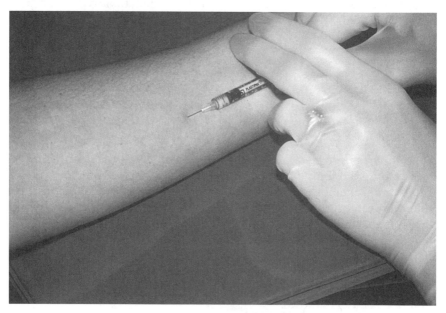

Figure 6-8 ■ Intradermal lidocaine administered before venipuncture using 0.1–0.2 mL of 1% lidocaine and a tuberculin syringe entering the skin at a 15- to 25-degree angle.

topical creams. ELA-Max contains 4% lidocaine. ELA-Max® contains microscopic, phospholipid spheres called Accusomes™. Accusomes™ act as microscopic vessels that help deliver the drug through the skin. It is not necessary to cover the area after application, but it is recommended when using on young children to prevent accidental ingestion or removal of the cream. This transdermal analgesic takes effect in 30 minutes.

Follow these steps when applying ELA-Max® cream:

1. Check for allergies to lidocaine.
2. Don gloves and use clean technique.
3. Prepare the affected area by washing with mild soap and water. Do not use alcohol or acetone.
4. Apply a small amount of cream and gently massage it into the skin. Next, squeeze enough cream to cover the affected area completely so that no skin is visible beneath the cream
5. The cream should remain undisturbed for 30 to 60 minutes.
6. Remove the occlusive dressing, if one is used; remove the cream by wiping with a clean gauze or tissue. Additional skin preparation or cleaning may now be performed.

Figure 6-9 shows application of a transdermal analgesic agent. With ELA-Max® cream an occlusive dressing does not have to be used.

Iontophoresis

Iontophoresis is a drug delivery method that uses a small external electric current to deliver water-soluble, charged drugs into the skin. Iontocaine (Numby Stuff®, IOMED, Salt Lake City, UT) is lidocaine 2% HCl and epinephrine 1:100,000, which are both positively charged with a pH of 4.5 and both drugs are delivered simultaneously by the Phoresor System from the positive electrode to provide dermal anesthesia. Iontocaine is actively pushed into the skin by a low-level direct current. The area of skin under the electrode is anesthetized within 7 to 10 minutes and has a penetration

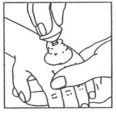

A   **B**

Figure 6-9 ■ *A*, Application of EMLA cream to the intended venipuncture site. *B*, Placement of an occlusive dressing over the cream. (Courtesy of Astra Pharmaceutical Products, Inc., Westborough, MA.)

depth of 10 mm. Iontophoresis of iontocaine causes a transient, local blanching. Iontocaine is indicated for production of local dermal analgesia. Iontocaine is contraindicated in patients with a known history of hypersensitivity to local anesthetics of the amide type (Numby Stuff, IOMED, 2008).

The following are key points with regard to iontophoresis:

- Iontophoretic drug delivery systems and Numby Stuff electrodes are designed to operate safely when used together.
- Electrodes are disposable; discard after use.
- Iontophoresis can cause skin irritation or burns.
- Iontophoresis can cause transient erythema under either electrode.
- Do not apply electrodes over or across the right and left temporal regions.
- Ask the patient or caregiver about drug allergies. (IOMED, 2008)

Step 8: Site Preparation

Hair should be removed only with scissors or clippers. Shaving is not recommended because of the potential for **microabrasions**, which increase the risk of infection. The use of depilatories is not recommended because of the potential for allergic reactions. Electric hair removal devices are not used unless they are effective and meet the criteria for preservation of skin integrity (INS, 2006a, 41).

Cleansing the insertion site reduces the potential for infection. The following **antimicrobial** solutions may be used to prepare the cannula site:

- 2% Chlorhexidine gluconate with alcohol (ChloraPrep®, Cardinal Health)
- Iodophor (povidone-iodine)
- 70% Isopropyl alcohol

NOTE > These must be single-unit use configuration.

The CDC (2002) recommends preference be given to the use of chlorhexidine-based preparation to disinfect clean skin before catheter insertion and during dressing changes. Povidone-iodine and 70% alcohol can be used. Allow the antiseptic to remain on the insertion site and air-dry before catheter insertion. Povidone-iodine must remain on skin for 2 minutes, or longer if it is not yet dry before insertion (O'Grady, Alexander, Dellinger, et al., 2002).

In reviewing time-kill kinetic evaluation of chlorhexidine/alcohol-based preparations, microorganisms were reduced ≥99.99% from baseline at 15 seconds (Kaler & Chinn, 2007; Maki, Ringer, & Alvarado, 1991).

NOTE > In preparing the site, the process for applying the chosen antiseptic agent is dependent on and should be consistent with the manufacturer's labeled use and directions.

 NURSING FAST FACT!

Prep the insertion site for peripheral infusions for a minimum of 30 seconds, allowing the site to dry completely before insertion of the catheter. Use a back and forth friction scrub of the site.

EBNP A recent analysis of four pivotal and two comparative clinical trials concluded that ChloraPrep® [a combination of 2% chlorhexidine (CHG) gluconate and 70% isopropyl alcohol (IPA)] and another combination of CHG and isopropyl alcohol demonstrated significant persistent (residual) and/or cumulative antimicrobial activity over IPA alone, 2% aqueous CHG alone, 4% CHG (Hibiclens) alone, or povidone-iodine alone (Hibbard, 2005).

Refer to Evidence-Based Care Box 6-1 and Figure 6-10.

INS Standard Alcohol should not be applied after the application of povidone-iodine preparation. (INS, 2006a, 41)

Alcohol negates the effects of povidone-iodine.

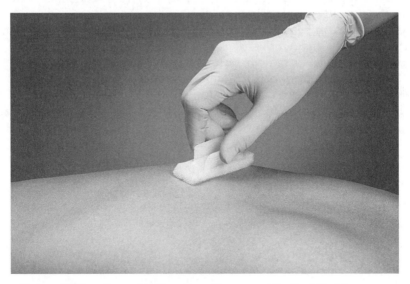

Figure 6-10 ■ Prep with ChoraPrep. (Courtesy of Cardinal Health, San Diego, CA.)

NOTE > The use of chlorhexidine gluconate in infants weighing less than 1000 grams has been associated with contact dermatitis and should be used with caution in this patient population (Garland, Alex, Mueller, et al., 2001).

EVIDENCE-BASED CARE BOX 6-1

Use of Chlorhexidine Compared with Povidone-Iodine in Prevention of Catheter-Related BSIs

Chiyakunapruk, N., Veenstra, D., Lipsky, B., & Saint, S. (2002). Chlorhexidine compared with povidone-iodine solution for vascular catheter-site care: A meta analysis. Annals of Internal Medicine, 136, 792–801.

This study evaluated the efficacy of skin disinfection with chlorhexidine gluconate compared with povidone-iodine solution in preventing catheter-related bloodstream infection.

Results: The results suggested that incidence of bloodstream infections is significantly reduced in patients with catheters who receive chlorhexidine gluconate versus povidone-iodine for insertion-site skin disinfection.

Step 9: Vein Entry

Gloves should be in place before venipuncture and kept on until after the cannula is stabilized. Gloves should be removed only after the risk of exposure to body fluids has been eliminated. Venipuncture can be performed using a direct (one-step) or indirect (two-step) method. The direct method is appropriate for small-gauge needles and fragile hand veins or rolling veins and carries an increased risk of causing a hematoma. The indirect method can be used for all venipunctures. Procedures Display 6-1 at the end of the chapter describes the steps to initiate a peripheral-short infusion by a direct or indirect technique.

Traction is important to maintain stability of the vein in either direct or indirect approach. Refer to Figure 6-11. Refer to Figures 6-12 and 6-13 for diagrams of insertion of a catheter into a vein and threading the cannula (catheter) into the vein and removing the stylet.

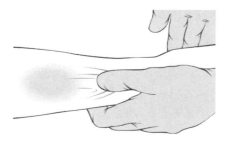

Figure 6-11 ■ Application of traction to the skin.

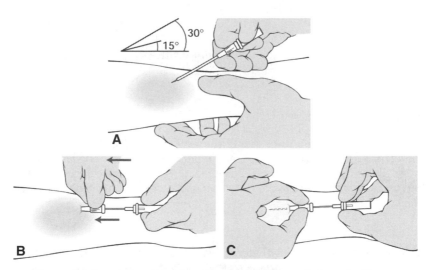

Figure 6-12 ■ *A,* Insertion of needle at a 30-degree angle through skin. *B,* Threading catheter into vein. *C,* Removing stylet from catheter.

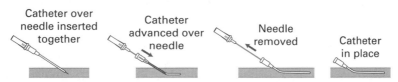

Figure 6-13 ■ Steps in insertion of an over-the-needle catheter once through the skin into the vein.

TROUBLESHOOTING TIPS

Common reasons for failure of venipuncture include:

- Failure to release the tourniquet promptly when the vein is sufficiently cannulated.
- Use of a "stop and start" technique by beginners who may lack confidence; this tentative approach can injure the vein, causing bruising.
- Inadequate vein stabilization. Not using traction to hold the vein causes the stylet to push the vein aside.
- Failure to recognize that the catheter has gone through the opposite vein wall.
- Stopping too soon after insertion so only the stylet, not the catheter, enters the lumen (intima) of the vein. Blood return disappears when the stylet is removed because the catheter is not in the lumen.
- Inserting the cannula too deeply, below the vein. This is evident when the catheter won't move freely because it is

imbedded in fascia or muscle. The patient also complains of severe discomfort.

■ Failure to penetrate the vein wall because of improper insertion angle (too steep or not steep enough), causing the catheter to ride on top of or below the vein.

 NURSING FAST FACT!

Only two attempts at venipuncture are recommended because multiple unsuccessful attempts cause unnecessary trauma to the patient and limit vascular access. When aseptic technique is compromised (i.e., in an emergency situation), the cannula is also considered compromised and a new catheter should be placed within 48 hours.

Safety features on all catheters must be activated once the stylet is removed from the catheter. Refer to Figure 6-14 for passive button activation to retract the stylet.

Step 10: Catheter Stabilization and Dressing Management

CATHETER STABILIZATION

The purpose of catheter stabilization is to preserve the integrity of the access device and to prevent the catheter migration. The catheter should be stabilized in a manner that does not interfere with visualization and evaluation of the site. Stabilization reduces the risk of complications related to

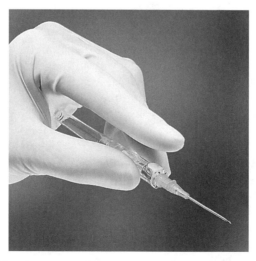

Figure 6-14 ■ Insyte Autoguard. Passive needle safety system button. Push to activate once stylet is removed from the catheter. (Courtesy of Becton Dickinson, Sandy, UT.)

peripheral intravenous therapy such as phlebitis, infiltration, sepsis, and cannula migration (Moureau & Lannucci, 2003; Smith, 2007).

There are several methods appropriate for stabilization of the catheter hub including the use of a dressing and securement device. In addition, another method of catheter securement became available in the 1990s as an alternative to the traditional tape and/or suture securement. This new method is an adhesive pad with an integrated posted retainer designed to hold the catheter in place more securely than allowed by tape. The StatLock® (C.R. Bard) is one manufacturer of this sort of adhesive anchor/built-in retainer.

Refer to Figure 6-15 and Evidence-Based Care Box 6-2 for evidence-based support for use of securement device.

> *EBNP A summary of product trials of a pool of 10,164 patients in 24 university teaching hospitals and 59 community hospitals using the StatLock® catheter securement found a 67% reduction in total patient complications in the stabilizing device group, as compared with the tape group. It was also found that unscheduled PIV restarts were reduced by 76% with the stabilizing device (Schears, 2006).*

INS Standard Whenever possible use a manufactured catheter stabilization device. Whenever sterile tapes or surgical strips are used, they should be applied only to the catheter adapter and should not be placed directly on the catheter-skin junction site. (INS, 2006a, 43)

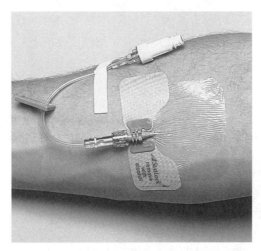

Figure 6-15 ■ Stabilization device: Statlock®. (Courtesy of Bard Access Systems, Covington, GA.)

EVIDENCE-BASED CARE BOX 6-2

Use of Catheter Securement Methods

Smith, B. (2006). Peripheral intravenous catheter dwell times: A comparison of 3 securement methods for implementation of a 96-hour scheduled change protocol. Journal of Infusion Nursing, 29(1), 14–17.

A prospective, sequential clinical trial was done to determine whether any of three methods of peripheral IV catheter (PIV) securement could extend the average survival time of catheters. Nonsterile tape, StatLock and HubGuard were evaluated. This study was not a randomized, controlled trial.

Results: The use of nonsterile tape securement resulted in an 8% PIV survival rate, HubGuard produced a 9% PIV survival rate, and StatLock produced a 52% PIV survival rate.

A dressing securement device such as the IV House UltraDressing with flexible fabric to wrap around a patient's hand after the I.V. is started can be used. Refer to Figure 6-16.

JUNCTION SECUREMENT

Policies and procedures regarding add-on devices and junction securement should be in place to implement practice guidelines in each organization. Add-on devices such as stopcocks, extension sets, manifold sets, extension loops, solid cannula caps, injection or access caps, needleless systems, and filters should have Luer-Lok™ junction securement. The use of junction securement minimizes the risk of complications related to infusion therapy.

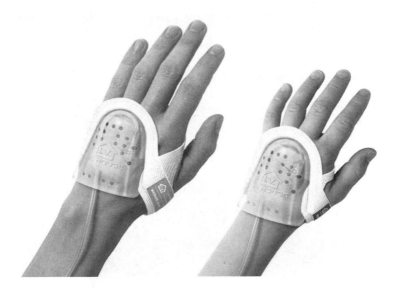

Figure 6-16 ■ I.V. House UltraDressing® that consists of flexible fabric with thumb holes and a polyethylene dome that wraps around a patient's hand after an I.V. is started. This prevents accidental snagging of the loop or catheter hub. (Courtesy of I.V. House, Inc., Chesterfield, MO.)

INS Standard   Tape should not be used as a means of junction securement. (INS, 2006a, 29)

ARM BOARDS

Every attempt should be made not to use arm boards. An arm board can be used to facilitate infusion delivery when the catheter is placed in or adjacent to an area of flexion. If arm boards are used they should be considered single-patient use.

NOTE ＞   If an arm board is used for the purpose of stabilization at an area of flexion, it is not considered a restraint.

DRESSING MANAGEMENT

There are two methods for dressing management: (1) a gauze dressing secured with tape and (2) a transparent semipermeable membrane dressing (TSM). A sterile gauze dressing can be applied aseptically with edges secured with tape. The dressing and catheter should be replaced together, unless the integrity of the dressing is impaired; then removal of the dressing with replacement of a new sterile TSM is required. Do not use ointment of any kind under a TSM dressing. The TSM dressing should be applied only to the cannula hub and wings.

To apply a TSM:

1. Cleanse the area of excess moisture after venipuncture.
2. Center the transparent dressing over cannula site and partially over the hub.
3. Press down on the dressing, sealing the catheter site.
4. A piece of tape can be added to loop the administration set tubing to secure it to the skin below TSM. Refer to Figure 6-17.

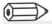   *NURSING FAST FACT!*

   Do not put tape over the TSM dressing, because it is difficult to remove the dressing if the dressing needs to be changed due to break in the integrity of dressing.

Advantages of TSM dressings include that they allow continuous inspection of the site, are more comfortable than gauze and tape, and permit patients to bathe and shower without saturating the dressing.

EBNP Many studies have been done comparing gauze and tape versus TSM dressing (conventional and those with high moisture vapor transmission rate). The rate at which dressing changes occurred was significant build up of skin flora. Gauze and tape should be changed every 2 days and polyurethane dressings every 5 days (Makl, Stolz, Wheeler, et al., 1994).

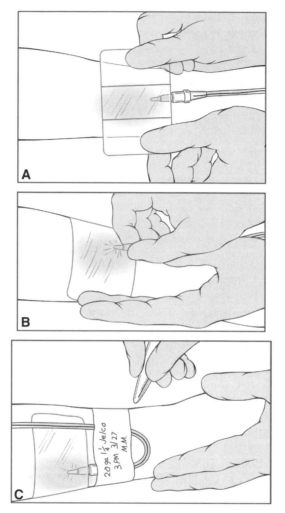

Figure 6-17 ▪ *A* and *B*, Steps in applying transparent semipermeable dressing directly over the I.V. catheter hub and insertion site. *C*, Label site below TSM.

INS Standard Gauze dressings that prevent visualization of the insertion site should be changed routinely every 48 hours on peripheral and central catheter sites and immediately if the integrity of the dressing is compromised.

A TSM dressing on the peripheral vascular access device should be changed at the time of catheter site rotation and immediately if the integrity of the dressing is compromised. (INS, 2006a, 44)

Refer to Figure 6-18 for an example of a peripheral I.V. site dressed with TSM dressing.

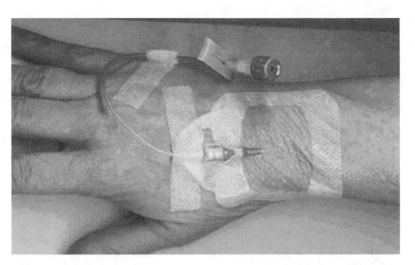

Figure 6-18 ■ Application of Tegaderm dressing. (Courtesy of 3M Health Care Division, St. Paul, MN.)

Postcannulation Insertion

Step 11: Labeling

For peripheral infusions, labels need to be applied to three areas: the insertion site, the tubing, and the solution container, which can be time stripped.

1. The venipuncture site should be labeled on the side of the transparent dressing or across the hub. Do not place the label over the site because this obstructs visualization of the site. Include on the insertion site label:
   - Date and time
   - The type, size, and length of the catheter (e.g., 20-gauge, 1-inch)
   - The nurse's initials
     (INS, 2006a, 44)
2. Label the administration set according to agency policy and procedure so that practitioners on subsequent shifts will be aware of when the tubing must be changed.
3. Labeling the solution container with a strip of tape or a preprinted strip is still practiced in some areas of the country. Place a time strip on all parenteral solutions with the name of the solution and additives, initials of the nurse, and the time the solution was started if included in the policy and procedure of the institution.

 NURSING FAST FACT!

> *Time strips are helpful as a quick method to visually assess whether the solution is on schedule. They are not used in all institutions.*

Step 12: Equipment Disposal

Equipment disposal need to follow CDC guidelines for biohazards. Recapping needles increases the risk of needlestick injuries to the practitioner. In accordance with the Occupational Safety and Health Administration (OSHA), needles and stylets should not be recapped, broken, or bent (NIOSHA, 2004). Needles and stylets should be disposed of in nonpermeable, puncture-resistant, tamper-proof container. All devices should have engineered sharps injury protection mechanisms; these mechanisms should be activated before disposal (ECRI, 2003). After venipuncture is complete, dispose of non-sharp items exposed to blood in a biohazard container. Refer to Figure 6-19 for examples of tamper-proof biohzard containers.

> **INS Standard** All blood contaminated and sharp items including needles or stylets, surgical blades, and syringes, shall be discarded in a nonpermeable puncture-resistant, tamper-proof biohazard container. (INS, 2006a, 25)

Step 13: Patient Education

The nurse has a responsibility to educate the patient, caregiver, or legally authorized representative relative to the prescribed infusion therapy. The plan of care as part of the nursing process includes: developing a plan for teaching and implementing the plan under interventions. Documentation of teaching is a mode of communication among the members of the health team (Phillips, 2008). The nurse must document, as part of intervention the education of the client, or caregivers.

> **INS Standard** The nurse shall educate the patient, caregiver, or legally authorized representative relative to the prescribed infusion therapy and plan of care including, but not limited to potential complications associated with treatment or therapy, and risks and benefits. (INS, 2006a, 11)

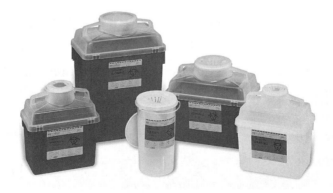

Figure 6-19 ◼ Tamper proof biohazard containers. (Courtesy of Becton Dickinson, Sandy, UT.)

NURSING FAST FACT!

> *Attention should be given to age, developmental (psychosocial as well as psychomotor) and cognitive levels, and cultural and linguistic sensitivity.*

Patient education begins before initiation of infusion therapy with discussion of potential complications with risks and benefits of therapy. Once the catheter is stabilized and dressing applied, the following information should be included in education and documented:

- Inform the patient of any limitations on movement or mobility.
- Explain all alarms if an electronic control device is used.
- Instruct the patient to call for assistance if the venipuncture site becomes tender or sore or if redness or swelling develops.
- Advise the patient that the venipuncture site will be checked by the nurse routinely.

 NURSING FAST FACT!

> *It is important to validate the patient's understanding and ability to perform infusion-related self-care procedures. Written and verbal instructions should be documented.*

Step 14: Rate Calculations

Many clinical environments require delivery of primary, secondary infusions or infusions with delivery of medications. over a period of time. Calculating the proper infusion rate for medication and solution delivery can be time intensive. All infusions should be monitored frequently for accurate flow rates and complications associated with infusion therapy.

NOTE > Practice problems are included in the chapter along with extra practice problems on DavisPlus.

Refer to Worksheet 6-2.

The following presents the basic formulas for calcuation of drip rates of intravenous solutions.

PRIMARY AND SECONDARY INFUSIONS

The ability to calculate infusion rates is essential in many clinical environments. The nurse must determine the manner in which the infusion is to be administered. Infusions may be delivered by gravity or by electronic infusion device (EID). The rate of infusion can be calculated as drops per minute or milliliters per hour. Factors to include in learning accurate rate calculations include:

1. **Drop factor** of tubing
2. An authorized prescriber's hourly rate.
3. Whether an EID will be used to deliver the infusion

DROP FACTOR OF TUBING

For macrodrop sets:

To calculate the drip rate correctly, note the drop factor of the administration set. This is usually located on the side, front, or back of the administration package. Drop factors provided by the administration set for **macrodrop** tubing are as follows:

Primary (macrodrop) sets:

- 10 drops = 1 mL
- 15 drops = 1 mL
- 20 drops = 1 mL

Use macrodrop sets whenever (1) a large amount of fluid is ordered to be infused over a short period of time or (2) the microdrips per minute are too many, making counting too difficult.

FORMULA FOR I.V. FLOW RATES USING DROPS PER MINUTE

After the drop factor of the tubing and the amount of solution to be infused are known, the following formula can be used to calculate the drop rate per minute:

mL per hour × drops per mL (drop factor [DF]) ÷ 60 (minutes in an hour) = drops per minute

$$\text{Formula: } \frac{\text{mL/hr} \times \text{DF}}{\text{minutes}} = \text{drop (gtt)/min}$$

Macrodrop Infusion. Example: Physician orders are for 125 mL/hr and the primary tubing selected has a drop factor of 15. Two steps are needed.

$$\text{Formula: } \frac{\text{mL/hr} \times \text{DF}}{\text{minutes}} = \text{gtt/min}$$

$$\text{Step 1: } \frac{125 \times 15}{60} = \text{gtt/min}$$

$$\text{Step 2: } = 31 \text{ gtt/min}$$

Microdrop Sets. Special administration sets such as pediatric (**microdrop**) sets and transfusion administration sets are also available. All manufacturers of microdrip sets are consistent in having 60 drops equal 1 mL.

Pediatric (microdrop) sets:

- 60 drops = 1 mL

Use microdrop sets whenever (1) the I.V. is to be administered over a long period of time, (2) a small amount of fluid is to be administered, or (3) the macrodrops per minute are too few.

FORMULA FOR I.V. FLOW RATES USING AN ELECTRONIC RATE CONTROL DEVICE

Calculations are particularly important when an electronic rate control device is not being used or when an electronic controller is used that does not have a mechanism to dial in milliliters per hour.

Microdrop Infusion. When using a microdrip (pediatric tubing) that is 60 drops/mL, the drops per minute equal the milliliters per hour, so only one step is needed.

Example: The physician orders 35 mL of 0.45% sodium chloride solution per hour for a 2-year-old girl. You would set up your rate calculation as follows, using only one step.

$$\text{Formula: } \frac{\text{mL/hr} \times \text{DF}}{\text{minutes}} = \text{gtt/min}$$

$$\text{Step 1: } \frac{35 \times 60}{60} = \text{gtt/min} = 35 \text{ gtt/min}$$

NOTE > Refer to Table 6-9 for conversion chart and rate calculation.

INTERMITTENT MEDICATION OR SOLUTION CALCULATIONS

Secondary infusions to be infused in less than 1 hour are usually medications that have been added to small amounts of I.V. fluid (usually 50–150 mL). The rate of I.V. administration must be adjusted during the administration to the time indicated by the pharmacist or pharmaceutical

> Table 6-9	**CONVERSION CHART: RATE CALCULATION**		

	Drop Factors		
Order: mL/hr	10 Drops/mL	15 Drops/mL	20 Drops/mL	60 Drops/mL
---	---	---	---	---
10	2	3	3	10
15	3	4	5	15
20	3	5	7	20
30	5	8	10	30
50	8	13	17	50
75	13	19	25	N/A
80	13	20	27	N/A
100	17	25	33	N/A
120	20	30	40	N/A
125	21	31	42	N/A
150	25	38	50	N/A
166	27	42	55	N/A
175	29	44	58	N/A
200	33	50	67	N/A
250	42	63	83	N/A
300	50	75	100	N/A

Microdrip tubing is not appropriate for rates greater than 50 mL/hr.

manufacturer. The rate of infusion of most I.V. medications is determined to prevent the possible deleterious effects of too rapid a medication delivery.

Example: Kefzol 0.5 g in 100 mL of dextrose in water to run intravenous piggyback (IVPB) over 30 minutes. Administration set is 20 drop factor.

$$\text{Formula: } \frac{\text{mL/hr} \times \text{drops per mL (drop factor)}}{\text{Hourly volume (varies)}} = \text{drop per minute}$$

$$\frac{100 \text{ mL} \times 20}{30 \text{ minutes}} = 2000$$

$$= 67 \text{ gtt/min}$$

Step 15: Documentation

After implementation of infusion therapy, the procedure should be documented in the medical records. Patient education is lacking in most audits of charts; therefore, documentation of patient response to the procedure needs to be included in the charting format. This needs to be addressed in narrative charting, by check-off format or by the more common electronic documentation medical records, which includes the status of the patient, the reason for restart, the procedure used, and comments.

Documentation of peripheral intravenous therapy procedure generally includes:

- Date and time of insertion
- Manufacturer's brand name and style of device (in some settings lot number)
- The gauge and length of the device
- Specific name and location of the accessed vein
- The infused solution and rate of flow
- Infusing by gravity or pump
- The number attempts for a successful I.V. start
- Condition of extremity before access
- The patient's specific comments related to the procedure
- Patient response, excessive anxiety, patient movement, or an untoward response
- Signature of the nurse

Documentation should be legible, accessible to healthcare professionals, and readily retrievable.

INS Standard Nursing documentation in the patient's medical record shall contain complete information regarding infusion therapy and vascular access in the patient's permanent medical record. Documentation shall include factors related to assessment, intervention, and the patient's response to that intervention. (INS, 2006a, 14)

Table 6-10 provides a summary of steps in initiating peripheral infusion.

> Table 6-10	**SUMMARY OF STEPS IN INITIATING PERIPHERAL I.V. THERAPY**

Precannula Insertion

1. Check physician or authorized prescribers orders; confirm all parts of the order for accuracy.
2. Hand hygiene for 15–20 seconds using CDC 2007 guidelines.
3. Equipment collection and preparation: Prepare equipment: Check for breaks in integrity and check expiration date; spike and prime the infusion system.
4. Patient assessment, psychological preparation and patient identification: Provide privacy.
   Explain the procedure to the patient.
   Evaluate the patient's psychological preparation for PIV therapy by talking with patient prior to touching to assess veins. Consider autonomy, handedness, independence. Evaluate fear of pain associated with venipuncture
5. Site selection and vein dilation:
   Assess both arms keeping the factors for vein selection in mind.
   Make a choice whether to use blood pressure cuff or tourniquet for dilatation.
   Use other methods for venous distension, such as warm packs, gravity, or tapping, multiple tourniquet or tangential lighting if necessary.

Cannula Insertion

6. Choose the appropriate catheter for duration of infusion and type of infusate based on facility policy and procedure. Rewash hands.
7. Use gloves, following standard precautions for exposure to blood or body fluids. Use full barrier protection if needed.
   Note: If using lidocaine prep site with alcohol and instill 0.3 mL of 1% lidocaine intradermally. Allow 30 seconds for effect of anesthetic to begin.
8. Prepare site by using recommended chlorhexidine gluconate with alcohol to cleanse the site. Let the chlorhexidine air dry. Do not remove. Do not retouch. Put on gloves before venipuncture.
9. Insert the over-the-needle catheter with the direct or indirect method. Thread the catheter while removing the stylet needle. Connect the catheter hub to administration set or a locking device – needleless valve.
10. Stabilize the catheter hub with stabilization device. There are two methods of dressing management: (1) 2-inch × 2-inch gauze with all edges taped; change every 48 hours or (2) TSM applied with aseptic technique and changed at 72 hours when catheter site is rotated, or if the integrity of the dressing is compromised.

Postcannula Insertion

11. Label the insertion site with cannula size, date, time, and initials; label the tubing with the date and time; strip the solution.
12. Dispose of equipment using OSHA standards for disposal of the stylet in sharps container and the rest of equipment in biohazard container.
13. Explain to the patient the limitations, provide information on the equipment being used, and give instructions for observation of the site.
14. Calculate drip rate: Remember when doing rate calculations that if a roller clamp or electronic controller is used, the drops per minute should be calculated based on the drop factor.
15. Document the procedure: Monitor the patient for response to prescribed therapies. Document the procedure performed, how the patient tolerated the venipuncture, and what instructions were given to the patient.

NOTE > Refer to Procedures Display 6-1 at end of chapter for detailed instructions on inserting an over-the-needle catheter by the direct and indirect method.

■ Intermittent Infusion Therapy

Intermittent infusion devices or resealable caps/valves are used when converting a continuous infusion to intermittent access. This method of intermittent access, also called saline locks or heparin locks, is also used for emergency access. The access cap is changed when the catheter is changed, or when injection port is contaminated. TH access cap are made of Luer-Lok™ design. Flushing is performed to ensure and maintain patency of the catheter and prevent mixing of medications and solutions that are incompatible. Review flushing procedures in this chapter. Routine flushing shall be performed with the following:

- Administration of blood and blood components
- Blood sampling
- Administration of incompatible medications or solutions
- Administration of medication
- Intermittent therapy
- When converting from continuous to intermittent therapies.

Intermittent infusion devices have both advantages and disadvantages. Refer to Figure 6-20 for an example of an intermittent infusion device.

ADVANTAGES

- Provide access to the vascular system, allowing for more flexibility than hanging I.V. fluids
- Allow for reduced volume of fluid administered, which can be important for cardiac patients

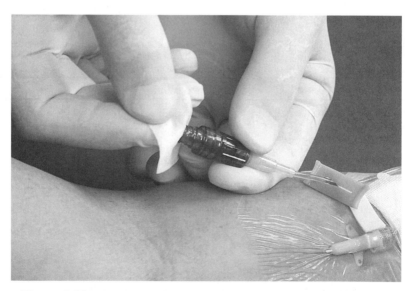

Figure 6-20 ■ Intermittent infusion device. (Courtesy of Baxter Healthcare Corp., Round Lake, IL.)

- On initiation of PIV to collect blood sample
- In phlebotomy setting to collect blood glucose tolerance test (interval blood collections)
- Provide access for delivery of emergency medications

Disadvantages

- Occlusion or blood clotting within the lock
- Possibility of speed shock due to the medication being rapidly introduced into the circulation. (Note: speed shock is covered in Chapter 9.)

NOTE > Refer to Procedures Display 6-2 for converting continuous infusion to intermittent access device at the end of this chapter.

Midline Catheters

A midline catheter (MLC) is a peripheral catheter that is placed between the antecubital fossa and the head of the clavicle. It is defined as one that is between 3 inches and 8 inches in length. Unlike the peripherally inserted central catheter (PICC) or the peripheral-short catheter, the midline is the bridge between the two (Anderson, 2004). It is advanced into a large vessel below the axilla where there is good hemodilution using an introducer. The length of the catheter allows for appropriate placement without alteration of tip integrity; caution should be used and manufacturer's labeled use(s) and directions should be strictly adhered to when tip alteration is required.

It is intended for intermediate-term from 6 days to 4 weeks for the delivery of most infusion products except vesicant therapy, parenteral nutrition, infusates with pH lower than 5 or greater than 9, and infusates with osmolarity greater than 600 mOsm/L.

NOTE > The midline catheter is often used for patients requiring 4 weeks of therapy in home care settings (Gorski, 2005).

Site Selection

The three prominent antecubital veins are ideal insertion sites for the midline catheter (basilic, cephalic, and median cubital). The basilic vein is the preferred vessel because it is larger and follows a straighter path. Insertion site is one fingerbreadth below or three fingerbreadths above the bend of the arm. Refer to Figure 6-21.

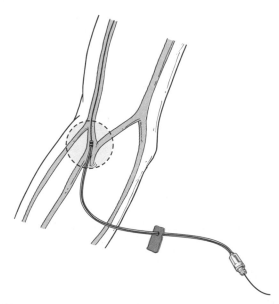

Figure 6-21 ▪ Insertion site for midline catheter. (Courtesy of Baxter Health-care Corp., Round Lake, IL.)

Patient Assessment

Before placing a midline catheter it is necessary to assess the anatomy of the patient's skin, subcutaneous tissues, and veins. Follow the criteria in step 4 of the Phillips 15-step method for initiating a short-peripheral catheter to guide assessment. Owing to variations in patient size and vessel anatomy, it is recommended that the arm be premeasured.

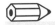 *NURSING FAST FACT!*

Optimal catheter tip location is level with the axilla, just distal to the shoulder and deltoid muscle. Using a measuring tape, measure from the intended insertion site to the axilla and write down the distance.

INS Standard   Midline catheters should be removed if the tip location is no longer appropriate for the prescribed therapy. (INS, 2006a, 49)

INS Standard   Midline catheters should not be used routinely for blood drawing. (INS, 2006a, 37)

The goal of infusion therapy using midline catheters is to complete a patient's infusate delivery 80% of the time without a complication and a second venipuncture. A study done by Anderson (2004) demonstrated a goal of 86% of midlines completed infusion therapy without complications.

NOTE > The key to successful delivery of peripheral infusion therapy is early vascular access assessment.

■ Peripheral Infusion Site Care and Maintenance (Peripheral-Short and Midline Catheters)

The Nursing Process for Patients Receiving Peripheral Infusion

The nursing process is central to nursing actions in any setting because it is an efficient method of organizing thought processes for clinical decision-making and problem solving. Use of the nursing process framework (assessment, diagnosis, planning, interventions, and evaluation) is beneficial for both the patient and the nurse because it helps ensure that care is planned, individualized, and reviewed over the period of time that the nurse and patient have formed a professional relationship (Phillips, 2008).

Monitoring of the patient should include cannula, exit site, and surrounding area; flow rate; clinical data; patient response; and compliance to the prescribed therapy. The site assessment should be done and documented every 4 hours. The frequency of monitoring provides for patient protection and is an integral part of quality and risk management. Information that is obtained by monitoring should be communicated to other healthcare professionals responsible for the patient's care by documentation. Observation of the patient and the delivery of infusion therapy provide data for nursing interventions. Assessment and key nursing interventions are presented under Nursing Points-of-Care: Adult Peripheral Infusions.

Peripheral intravenous monitoring and site care includes observations of the site and the infusion, administration set change, catheter removal criteria, flushing standards, and catheter site care.

Administration Set Change

Administration set change best practices are the same for short-peripheral catheters and midline catheters.

CONTINUOUS INFUSIONS

The primary and secondary *continuous* administration sets and add-on devices, according to CDC (2009) should be replaced no more frequently than at 96-hour intervals, and up to 7 days, unless catheter-related infection is suspected (Gillies, O'Riordan, Wallen, et al., 2005; O'Grady, Alexander, Dellinger, et al., 2002).

INS Standard Primary and secondary continuous administration sets shall be changed no more frequently than every 72 hours and immediately upon suspected contamination or when the integrity of the product or system has been compromised. All administration sets shall be of Luer-Lok™ design. (INS, 2006a, 48)

Secondary Intermittent Infusions

When intermittent infusions of antibiotics, and with other cyclic medications, the integrity of the administration sets can be compromised over the 24 hours due to interruptions to the closed system. The intermittent sets need to be changed every 24 hours. The administration sets and needleless device should be aseptically maintained between medication dosages.

INS Standard Intermittent administration sets shall be changed every 24 hours and immediately upon suspected contamination. (INS, 2006a, 48)

NOTE > Administration sets used to administer blood components or lipid emulsions are covered in Chapters 11 and 12.

Catheter Removal Criteria

Inappropriate catheter care is an independent risk factor for catheter-related infections, and phlebitis formation. Clear policies and procedures for peripheral-short catheter changes should be established and documented in the patient's medical records. Studies have supported the removal of short peripheral catheters before 4 days to decrease the risk of phlebitis and the risk of phlebitis and catheter-related infections.

EBNP A study of 1054 peripheral I.V. catheters using the Kaplan–Meier risk for phlebitis found that risk for phlebitis exceeded 50% by the fourth day after PIV catheterization (Maki & Ringer, 1991).

INS Standard A peripheral-short catheter in an adult patient shall be removed every 72 hours and immediately on suspected contamination, complication, or therapy discontinuation. (INS, 2006a, 49)

INS Standard Removal of a midline catheter should be determined by patient condition and diagnosis, type and duration of therapy administered, presence of infectious or inflammatory process, and catheter malposition. (INS, 2006a, 49)

INS Standard A peripheral-short catheter placed in an emergency situation where aseptic technique has been compromised shall be replaced as soon as possible and no later than 48 hours. (INS, 2006a, 49)

NOTE > Refer to Procedures Display 6-4 at the end of the chapter for discontinuation of a peripheral I.V. catheter.

Peripheral Flushing Standards for Intermittent Infusion Devices

Nurses must be knowledgeable about medication and solution incompatibilities and the process to flush a peripheral catheter to maintain patency and prevent incompatibilities between medications.

Peripheral vascular access devices need to be flushed with 0.9% preservative-free sodium chloride (USP) at established intervals. The minimum volume of flush solution should be equal to at least twice the volume capacity of the catheter and add-on devices.

- Flush peripheral catheters with a minimum of 2 mL of 0.9% preservative-free sodium chloride (USP) before and after administration of medication and at least every 12 hours if the catheter is not in use (INS, 2008).

INS Standard Flushing with 0.9% preservative-free sodium chloride (USP) injection solution to ensure and maintain patency of an intermittently used peripheral vascular catheter should be performed at established intervals. (INS, 2006a, 50)

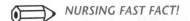 *NURSING FAST FACT!*

Push–pause method of flushing: *When flushing a peripheral catheter a rapid succession of push–pause–push–pause movements should be exerted on the plunger of the syringe barrel. This recreates a turbulence within the catheter lumen that causes a swirling effect to move any debris (residues of fibrin, or medication) attached to the catheter lumen.*

NOTE > Refer to Procedures Display 6-3 at the end of the chapter for flushing technique and protocols.

Accessing Needle-Free Injection Systems (NIS)/ Needle-Free Access Port (NAP)

Recent documentation of sepsis from injection ports has caused concern about the buildup of biofilm from gram-negative bacteria inside NIS/NAP. The CDC (2002) guidelines recommend changing needleless devices at least as frequently as the administration set. All components of a NIS must be compatible to minimize leaks and breaks in the system. Before any attempt to access an injection port (valve), strict technique in cleansing the site must be followed, using an appropriate antiseptic (chlorhexidine preferred) (O'Grady, Alexander, Dellinger, et al., 2002). Follow these steps every time the injection port is accessed.

1. Use proper hand hygiene
2. Disinfection of injection port with each connection using a twisting motion with 70% alcohol or 3.1% chlorhexidine/70% alcohol for 15 seconds using friction (twisting motion) is strongly recommended. The technique is similar to juicing an orange (Kaler & Chinn, 2007).
3. Let the alcohol/chlorhexidine dry (drying kills bacteria).
4. Then follow flushing guidelines (Rosenthal, 2007).

NOTE > Refer to Procedures Display 6-3 at the end of the chapter for a peripheral-short flush procedure.

EBNP A study by Kaler and Chinn (2007) provided evidence that when access ports are subjected to a disinfection time of 15 seconds with friction, alcohol alone or chlorhexidine/alcohol is effective in sterilizing NIS/NAP ports inoculated with a 10^5 colony-forming units (CFU) suspension of microorganisms, regardless of whether the NIS/NAP were constructed using positive, negative, or neutral displacement technologies.

Midline Catheter Flush

Midline catheter requires a minimum of 3 mL of preservative-free 0.9% sodium chloride for each flush procedure. Use the same technique as with peripheral-short catheters except with midline catheters it is recommended that final locking is with heparin solution. The procedure for flushing a midline catheter is as follows.

Follow procedure from the short-peripheral technique with the following.

■ Use 3 mL of 10 units/mL heparin to lock the device

NOTE > This would be the *SASH method* for locking intermittent infusion device. Saline–(clear catheter and check patency). Administer medication –Saline (clear medication)–Heparin (administer 3 mL/10 units heparin/mL).

Discontinuation of the Peripheral Infusion Devices

Documentation of infusion discontinuation of therapy is an important legal responsibility of the nurse. Documentation of a peripheral infusion device removal should include the site condition; integrity and length of the catheter; any complications incurred; date, time, and reason for discontinuation of therapy; and initials of the person removing the device and patient response (INS, 2006a, 52). Infusion therapy should be discontinued if the integrity of the cannula is compromised or the authorized prescriber orders the discontinuation of therapy. Sterile occlusive dressing should be applied to the access site. Refer to Procedures Display 6-4 at the end of the chapter for steps in discontinuation of a peripheral catheter.

Notify the physician if resistance is encountered when a midline catheter is being removed. The condition, length, and site of the catheter should be ascertained on removal; nursing interventions should be implemented as necessary; and observations and actions should be documented in the patient's permanent medical record.

INS Standard After midline catheter removal, the dressing should be changed and access site assessed every 24 hours until the site is epithelialized. (INS, 2006a, 49)

NURSING PLANS-OF-CARE
ADULT PERIPHERAL INFUSION

Nursing Assessments
- Interview the patient regarding previous experiences with venipunctures
- Review the purpose of the infusion and patient diagnosis
- Assess venipuncture sites taking into consideration physical condition of sites, any disease processes, cultural issues.
- Review trends in vital signs.

Key Nursing Interventions
Verify the authorized prescriber's written or electronic orders for infusion therapy.
1. Educate the client about the procedure before initiation of therapy.
2. Maintain Standard Precautions.

Continued

3. Adhere to hand hygiene practices.
4. Use strict aseptic technique during insertion and maintenance of the cannula.
5. Inspect the solution for type, amount, expiration date, character of solution, and integrity of container.
6. Determine compatibility of all infusion fluids and additives, consulting the appropriate literature.
7. Select and prepare EID as indicated.
8. Choose an appropriate size catheter for delivery of infusion.
9. Apply the catheter stabilization device.
10. Monitor the I.V. site for local complications during therapy and for postinfusion phlebitis.
11. Maintain the integrity of I.V. equipment.
12. Document the procedure and observations of the site.

AGE-RELATED CONSIDERATIONS

Pediatric Peripheral Infusion Therapy

Physiologic Characteristics

A **neonate** is a child in the period of extrauterine life up to the first 28 days after birth. Low-birth-weight and premature infants have decreased energy stores and increased metabolic needs compared with those of full-term, average-weight newborns.

A premature infant's body is made up of approximately 90% water; the full-term infant's is 70% to 80%, and the adult's is about 60%. **Infants** have proportionately more water in the extracellular compartment than do adults. Therefore, any depletion in these water stores may lead to dehydration. As an infant becomes older, the ratio of extracellular to intracellular fluid volume decreases.

Although infants have relatively greater total body water content, this does not protect them from excessive fluid loss. Infants are more vulnerable to fluid volume deficit because they ingest and excrete a relatively greater daily volume of water than adults do (Metheny, 2000). Any condition that interferes with normal water and electrolyte intake or that produces excessive water and electrolyte losses will produce a more rapid depletion of water and electrolyte stores in an infant than it will in an adult.

Illness, increased muscular activity, thermal stress, congenital abnormalities, and respiratory distress syndrome influence metabolic demands as well. The metabolic demand of an infant is two times higher per unit of weight than that of adults (Hockenberry & Wilson, 2006).

In most cases, 100 to 120 cal/kg per day maintains a normal infant and provides sufficient calories for growth. For high-risk infants who require increased handling for procedures, the calorie requirement is up to 100% higher than that of a normal newborn. Heat production increases calorie expenditure by 7% per degree of temperature elevation. Infants and young children cannot store protein as well as adults; therefore, preventive nutritional support is needed (Metheny, 2000).

Young children have immature homeostatic regulating mechanisms that need to be considered when water and electrolyte replacement is needed. Renal functioning, acid–base balance, body surface area differences, and electrolyte concentrations all must be taken into consideration when planning fluid needs.

Newborns' renal functions are not yet completely developed. Infants' kidneys appear to become mature by the end of the neonatal period. An infant's kidneys have a limited concentrating ability and require more water to excrete a given amount of solutes. Infants are less likely to be able to regulate fluid intake and output.

The buffering capacity to regulate acid–base balance is lower in newborns than in older children. Neonates, with an average pH of 7.0 to 7.38, are slightly more acidotic than adults. The base bicarbonate deficit is thought to be related to high metabolic acid production and to renal immaturity.

The integumentary system in neonates is an important route of fluid loss, especially in illness. This must be considered when determining fluid balance in infants and young children because their body surface area is greater than those of older children and adults. Any condition that produces a decrease in intake or output of water and electrolytes affects the body fluid stores of the infant. Because the gastrointestinal (GI) membranes are an extension of the body surface area, relatively greater losses occur from the GI tract in sick infants (Hockenberry & Wilson, 2006).

Plasma electrolyte concentrations do not vary strikingly among infants, small children, and adults. The plasma sodium concentration changes little from birth to adulthood. The potassium and chloride concentrations are higher in the first few months of life than at any other time. Magnesium and calcium levels are both low in the first 24 hours after birth. The serum phosphate level is elevated in the early months of infancy, which contributes to a low calcium level. Newborn infants are vulnerable to disrupted calcium homeostasis when stressed by illness or by an excess phosphate load and are at risk for hypocalcemia (Metheny, 2000).

CULTURAL AND ETHNIC CONSIDERATIONS: DECISION-MAKING

In many cultures, women can express an opinion regarding the care of a child; however, many others consider women to be subservient to men; and the men (e.g., the husband or the eldest son) make all decisions. Be sure to be sensitive to lines of communication (Giger & Davidhizar, 2004; Munoz & Luckmann, 2005).

Continued

Physical Assessment

A physical assessment should be performed on pediatric patients before I.V. therapy is initiated. Table 6-11 presents the components of a pediatric assessment. Risk factors that must be considered during the assessment phase include prematurity, catabolic disease state, hypothermia, hyperthermia, metabolic or respiratory alkalosis or acidosis, and other metabolic derangements.

Site Selection

When selecting the venipuncture site, keep in mind that the main goal of infusion therapy is to provide the treatment with safety and efficiency while meeting the child's emotional and developmental needs.

Consider the following factors before selecting a site for venipuncture:

- Age of the child
- Size of the child
- Condition of veins
- Objective of the infusion therapy (hydration, administration of medication, etc.)
- General patient condition
- Mobility and level of activity of child
- Gross and fine motor skills (e.g., sucks fingers, plays with hands, holds bottle, draws)
- Sense of body image
- Cognitive ability of the child (i.e., can understand and follow directions)

Peripheral Routes

Peripheral routes for pediatric I.V. therapy include scalp veins and the veins in the dorsum of the hand, forearm, and foot. Refer to Table 6-12 for comparison of selected insertion sites.

SCALP VEINS

The major superficial veins of the scalp can be used. Scalp veins can be used in children up to age 18 months; after that age, the hair follicles mature and

> Table 6-11	COMPONENTS OF THE PEDIATRIC PHYSICAL ASSESSMENT

Measurement of head circumference (up to 1 year)
Height or length
Weight
Vital signs
Skin turgor
Presence of tears
Moistness and color of mucous membranes
Urinary output
Characteristics of fontanelles
Level of child's activity related to growth and development

> Table 6-12	PEDIATRIC INFUSION SITES		
Veins and Site	Age Appropriate	Advantages	Disadvantages
Scalp			
Superficial temporal Frontal Occipital Posterior auricular Supraorbital	Infant	Easily accessed and monitored Readily dilates Keeps feet and hands free No valves	Hair must be trimmed or clipped. Infiltrates easily Difficult to achieve device securement Increase familial anxiety May have cultural issues.
Foot			
Saphenous Median marginal Dorsal arch	Infant	Readily dilates Hands kept free Easily restrained/ splinted	Decreased mobility Catheter gauge restricted Located near arterial structures Risk of phlebitis is increased.
Hand			
Metacarpal Cephalic and basilic accessory	All ages	Easily accessible/ visible May accommodate a larger gauge Distal location May not require splinting	Uncomfortable Difficult to anchor/ stabilize May impede child's activities (thumbsucking/ schoolwork)
Forearm			
Cephalic Basilic Median antebrachial	All ages	Same as for hand Keeps hands free	Difficult to observe/ palpate in chubby toddlers

the epidermis toughens. There are four scalp veins used most commonly for I.V. access: frontal (best access), preauricular, supraorbital, and occipital. Refer to Figure 6-22.

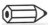 *NURSING FAST FACT!*

> *The choice of a scalp vein for placement of I.V. therapy is often traumatic for the parents because removal of hair may have cultural and religious significance. In addition, maintaining patency of this site can be difficult at times.*

The I.V. catheter must be placed in the direction of blood flow to ensure that the I.V. fluid will flow in the same direction as that of the blood returning to the heart. In the scalp, venous blood generally flows from the top of the head down.

NOTE > Shaving is not recommended; if necessary, clip the hair on infants.

Continued

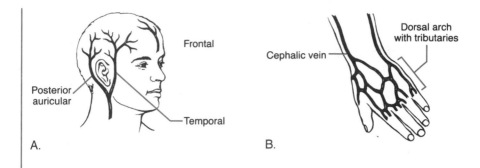

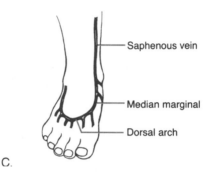

Figure 6-22 ■ *A*, Superficial veins of scalp; *B*, dorsum of hand and *C*, foot.

CULTURAL AND ETHNIC CONSIDERATIONS: USING SCALP VEINS

People in the Hmong culture believe the spirit (soul) of the child can be released from the head. Be sure to check with an elder family member before choosing a site for venipuncture (Giger & Davidhizar, 2004; Munoz & Luckmann, 2005).

DORSUM OF THE HAND AND FOREARM

Because the veins over the metacarpal area are mobile and not well supported by surrounding tissue, the limb must be immobilized with a splint and taped before cannulation. This site can be used in children of all ages.

The antecubital fossa should not be routinely used because of the use of the antecubital area for blood drawing and the mobility problems resulting from use of this site. However, the antecubital area can be used for placement of peripherally inserted central catheters (PICCs).

DORSUM OF THE FOOT

The foot is used as a venipuncture site for infants and toddlers but should be avoided in children who are walking. The curve of the foot, especially around the ankle, makes entry and cannula advancement difficult. The veins used are the saphenous, median, and marginal dorsal arch. Because neonates have very little subcutaneous adipose tissue, the veins are easily identified and cannulated just beneath the skin.

 NURSING FAST FACT!

> *The foot should be secured on a padded board with a normal joint position.*

Selecting the Equipment

A nurse must be aware of the special needs of pediatric patients when selecting appropriate equipment for administering fluids and medication. When choosing administration equipment, the safety of the child requires that the activity level, age, and size of the patient be considered. For safe delivery of I.V. therapy in pediatric patients, the following equipment is recommended:

- An electronic infusion device for administration of therapy
- A solution container with a volume based on the age, height, and weight of the patient containing no more than 500 mL of fluid (preferably 250 mL)
- Special pediatric equipment, such as volume control chamber for the delivery of therapy.
- Plastic fluid containers (preferable to glass because of possible breakage)
- Microdrip tubing (60 gtt/min)
- Visible cannula site
- A 0.2-micron air-eliminating filter set (Fig. 6-23) is available for neonates and infants to provide 96-hour bacterial and associated endotoxin retention for patient protection.

It is necessary to monitor at least every 2 hours or more frequently, depending on the patient's age and size or type of therapy.

Needle Selection

The choice of needle depends on the site selected. In children, peripheral over-the-needle type catheters are preferred with gauges of 26 to 21. A 27- to 19-gauge scalp vein (butterfly) needle is easy to insert and can be used, but has the risk of infiltrating easily. For neonates, 26- to 24-gauge needles are used; for children, 24- to 22-gauge are most common. Over-the-needle cannulas usually last longer than scalp vein metal needles. These catheters are also easier to stabilize. Use a small-size, short-length catheter, appropriate for the prescribed therapy (INS, 2008).

Equipment

- A child's I.V. container should contain no more than 500 mL of I.V. fluid. A 250-mL solution container should be used for children younger than 12 months of age.
- Obtain a volume control chamber (metered volume containers should be used for hourly rates of less than 50 mL/hr).

Continued

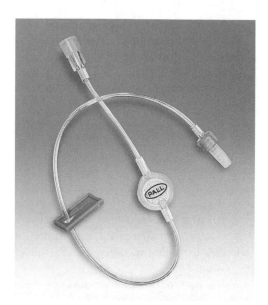

Figure 6-23 ■ 0.2 Micron air-eliminating filter set. (Courtesy of Pall Corp., Ann Arbor, MI.)

NOTE > Fill the cylinder with enough fluid to prime the tubing plus fluid for a *maximum* of 2 hours.

- A 0.2 micron air-eliminating and particulate-retentive filter should be used for neonates and infants. Refer to Figure 6-23.
- All infusion administrative equipment should be of Luer-Lok design.
- All EIDs must be accurate, have anti-free-flow protection alarms, and lock-out protection to prevent tampering. Dose error reduction systems should be considered for EIDs (INS, 2008).

Venipuncture Techniques

The methods for venipuncture are the same for children as for adults; a direct or indirect method can be used. Keep in mind the following safety guidelines when setting up an I.V. for a child.

Tips

The following tips on technique are unique to pediatric patients:

1. Venipuncture should be performed in a room separate from the child's room. The child's room is his or her "safe space."
2. For the scalp vein position, the head is in a dependent position.
3. Use a pacifier for neonates and infants.
4. A smaller tourniquet is preferred for neonates and pediatric clients.

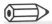 *NURSING FAST FACT!*

A tourniquet is not used in premature infants (INS, 2008).

5. Use mummy and clove-hitch immobilizers as needed. Infants should be covered with a blanket to minimize cold stress. If the dorsum of the hand is used, place the extremity on an armboard before venipuncture.
6. A flashlight or transilluminator device placed beneath the extremity helps to illuminate tissue surrounding the vein; the veins are then outlined for better visualization
7. Warm hands by washing them in hot water before gloving.
8. Use a saline-filled syringe with a scalp vein infusion device.
9. Minimizing pain during venipuncture is a goal of nursing care. Two commonly used methods are the use of a topical cream (EMLA or Numby Stuff) or ethyl chloride spray (an assistant is needed to spray). Apply 1 to 4 hours before IV access (Otto, 2005).
10. Flush the needle immediately with saline if a backflow of blood occurs.
11. Use surgical lubricating jelly to help secure the tape around a scalp I.V. by applying a small amount under the tape.
12. Stabilize the catheter with manufactured stabilization devices, sterile tapes, or surgical strips.
13. Use only hypoallergenic or paper tape. When you are ready to remove the tape, apply warm water; the tape will then lift off easily.

NOTE > Use colored stickers or drawings on the I.V. site as a reward. **Always have extra help**.

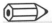 *NURSING FAST FACT!*

■ *When securing a child's extremity to an armboard, use clear tape for visualization of the I.V. site and digits or skin immediately adjacent to the site.*
■ *Use of a paper cup to cover the infusion site on the **scalp is not** recommended.*

Stabilizing and maintaining the patency of I.V. cannula sites can be a challenge. Poorly secured IV access sites may result in dislodgements or infiltrations requiring I.V. restarts. Refer to Figure 6-24. Products are available to help stabilize pediatric I.V.s, while maintaining visualization. The IV House® (Progressive IVs, Inc.) is a clear, one-piece unit that protects any I.V. site (Fig. 6-25).

For children, illness and hospitalization constitute major life crises. Children are vulnerable to the crises of illness and hospitalization because stress represents a change from the usual state of health and environmental routine and because children have a limited number of coping mechanisms to resolve the stressful events.

Continued

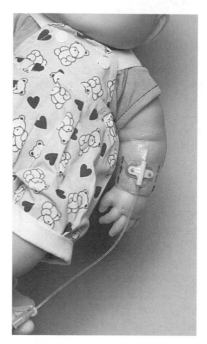

Figure 6-24 ■ StatLock® pediatric securement device. (Courtesy of Bard Access Systems, Inc., Covington, GA.)

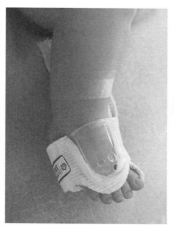
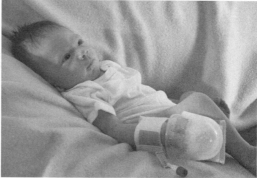

Figure 6-25 ■ IV House Ultradressing® Pediatric. (Courtesy of IV House, Inc., Chesterfield, MO.)

Children's understanding of, reaction to, and methods of coping with illness or hospitalization are influenced by the significance of individual stressors during each developmental phase. The major stressors are separation, loss of control, and bodily injury.

Site Care and Maintenance

Inspect and monitor the vascular access device, connections, infusate prescribed, and pump functions including flow rate. In a small child, site checks every hour should be done with minimum frequency. Assess the range of motion of the cannulated extremity, taking into consideration the child's developmental age. Monitor the patient's overall response to therapy. Peripheral-short catheters should be rotated every 72 to 96 hours and as necessary.

Flushing Protocols

Flushing protocols have recently been developed by the Infusion Nurses Society for adult as well as pediatric patients. Refer to Table 6-13 for flush standards for peripheral-short and midline catheters in children.

Medication Administration

Delivering medication to children requires that the nurse have expert knowledge of the techniques for the delivery of medication and for the calculation of formulas. Most infusion complications in pediatric patients are attributed to dosing, fluid administration, or both. A nurse administering infusion therapy to pediatric patients must possess the knowledge necessary to verify, calculate, administer, and accurately control the rate of the prescribed therapy.

Strategies for safe delivery of medications to children include:

- Purchase and use only scales that measure weight in kilograms.
- Develop a method (flow sheets) of documenting weight changes. Include weight changes in shift reports.
- Perform staff competency checks annually in weighing children, using scales on the unit.

> Table 6-13   **FLUSHING GUIDELINES FOR PEDIATRIC PATIENTS**

Peripheral I.V. catheters with approximate priming volume (APV) of 0.05–0.07 mL have the following guidelines for flushing:

Locking Device

NICU patient: 1 mL of preservative-free saline every 6 hours
Pediatric patient: 1–3 mL preservative free saline every 8 hours
■ Medication pre- and postadministration: 2 times administration tubing and add-on set.

Midline Flushing Standards (Fr = French)

3 Fr: 0.16 APV
4 Fr: 0.19 APV
5 Fr: 0.22 APV

■ 2 Fr: 1 mL preservative free saline + 10 units/mL heparin every 6 hours
■ 2.6 Fr and larger: 2–3 mL preservative free saline + 10 units/mL of heparin every 12 hours.
■ Medication pre- and postadministration: 2 times administration tubing and add-on set volume

Source: INS Flushing Protocols (2008), with permission.

Continued

- Collaborate with biomedical engineers regarding the frequency of quality assurance and calibration checks of scales.
- Require nurses to verify accuracy in dose recommendations and calculations on the original drug and I.V. fluid prescription forms.
- Acquire current medication manuals that provide necessary information for safe administration of I.V. medications.
- Develop charts of frequently used drugs that provide practical information of medication concentrations, drug dosing, and administration requirements.

NOTE > Pediatric medication calculations and formulas are covered in Chapter 7, with worksheets. Calculating drug dosages by body weight, body surface area, and intermittent infusion by volume control chamber (VCC) is covered in Chapter 7, along with formulas.

Four methods are used to deliver intravenous medications and solutions to the pediatric client: I.V. push or bolus, by volume control chamber (VCC), retrograde method, and by syringe pump.

NOTE > The child's developmental stage is an important factor to consider when planning to administer medications.

I.V. Push or Bolus
Direct I.V. push delivers small amounts of medication over a short period of time, usually 5 minutes or less. The advantage of this method is its speed, the nurse is present during the complete administration of the medication, and the immediate response to the drug can be assessed. This is the method of choice for administering I.V. pain medications.

Volume Control Chamber
Volume control chambers (VCCs) are used frequently with children for safety in delivery of medication and solutions. This administration set is best practice, along with a 250- to 500-mL solution container to ensure decreased risk of fluid overload. This method allows up to 100 mL of solution to be admitted into the VCC at any one time. Frequent monitoring and refilling of the VCC by the nurse is required (Broyles, Reiss, & Evans, 2007).

Retrograde Infusions
Retrograde infusion is an alternative to drug administration by syringe pumps, used in the general pediatric area and neonatal intensive care units. A specific retrograde administration set is required for this purpose. The tubing volume varies but generally holds less than 1 mL. A three-way

stopcock or access port is at each end of the tubing. To use retrograde infusion, follow these steps:

1. Attach the retrograde tubing and prime along with the primary administration set. The tubing functions as an extension set when it is not used to administer medication.
2. To administer the medication, attach a medication-filled syringe to the port proximal to the patient and connect an empty syringe to the port most distal from the patient.
3. Make sure the clamp between the port and the child is closed and then inject the medication distally up the tubing (this prevents your patient from getting medication as a bolus dose). The fluid in the retrograde tubing is displaced upward into the tubing and the empty syringe.
4. Remove both syringes and open the lower clamp. The medication is then infused into the patient at the prescribed rate by the electronic infusion device.

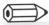 *NURSING FAST FACT!*

Do not use this method with volumes of medication greater than 1 mL. Injecting larger volumes by retrograde can put excess pressure on the I.V. tubing (Hadaway, 2005).

Syringe Pump
The fourth method of infusing drugs is called the syringe pump, which is the method of choice for administering most medications greater than 2 mL in volume and for those that cannot be administered by the I.V. push method. Many new pumps on the market contain safety features. Refer to Chapter 5 for a discussion of infusion equipment.

NOTE > Parenteral nutrition and transfusion therapy are also frequently administered to the pediatric client. Special considerations for the delivery of blood products and parenteral nutrition are discussed in Chapters 11 and 12.

Alternative Administration Routes
Alternative routes for administration of infusion therapy in pediatric patients are intraosseous and umbilical veins and arteries. These routes are addressed in Chapter 10.

NURSING POINTS-OF-CARE
PEDIATRIC PERIPHERAL INFUSION

Nursing Assessments
- Interview the patient's parents/caregiver for the patient's current health status.
- Measure height and weight for calculation of body surface area and drug dosages.
- Note the developmental level.
- Identify the purpose of the infusion.

Key Nursing Interventions
1. Maintain Standard Precautions.
2. Monitor for
   a. Intake and output
   b. I.V. site every hour minimally and document
   c. Fluid overload
   d. Alterations in vital signs
3. Explain the procedure and equipment and rationales for treatment to the parents and child if appropriate.
4. Provide opportunities for non-nutritive sucking in infants.
5. Encourage parents to provide daily care of the child.
6. Maintain the daily routine during hospitalization.
7. Provide a quiet, uninterrupted environment during nap time and nighttime as appropriate.
8. Immobilize when appropriate for venipuncture.
9. Use appropriate equipment for delivery of safe infusions (volume control chamber, EID, syringe pump for small volumes).
10. Calculate drug dosage correctly and double check the dosage calculation with another licensed nurse before administration.
11. Follow best practices for use of safety equipment in delivery of medications and solutions to pediatric patients.

Peripheral Infusion Therapy in The Older Adult
The impact of the baby-boom generation reaching the older adult stage will impact delivery of infusion therapy. Competency in the care of the elderly patient, particularly the frail elder, is important due to the significant impact on nursing, especially in light of the nursing shortage (Zwicker, 2003). The infusion nurse is in a pivotal position to proactively improve outcomes related to infusion therapy practices for the elder population.

Aging is dependent on nutritional, environment, education, socioeconomic, genetic, physiologic, and spiritual factors (Walther, 2008). The older adult is classified in three major groups to help in the assessment process of the older adult:

- Young old: 65 to 74 years
- Middle old: 74 to 84
- Frail elderly: 85 years and older

Physiologic Changes
Aging occurs on all levels of bodily function: cellular, organic, and systemic. "Loss of cells and loss of physiologic reserve make up the dominant processes of aging" (Smeltzer, Bare, Hinkle, & Cheever, 2008). The major system changes the nurse must be aware of related to infusion therapy are homeostatic changes, immune system and cardiovascular changes, and skin and connective tissue changes.

Homeostasis is the body's ability to maintain a stable internal environment. As a person ages, his or her homeostatic mechanism become less efficient, and reserve power is lost. For example, when external stressors such as trauma or infection occur, there is minimal reserve capacity. This creates a situation in which the person is more vulnerable to disease.

Two immune processes change with aging:

1. The immune system becomes hyporesponsive to foreign antigens (e.g., decreased numbers of circulating lymphocytes and cells have fewer receptors to decrease ability to generate energy).
2. The immune system becomes hyperresponsive to itself.

Cardiovascular changes related to arteriosclerosis become clinically recognizable. With aging, three functions of the heart are affected: (1) the ability to oxygenate the cardiac muscle decreases, (2) diastolic filling decreases, and (3) left ventricular wall thickness increases. Arteries show progressive chemical and anatomic changes, with an increase in cholesterol, other lipids, and calcium. The intima increases, which increases resistance and decreases compliance of veins and arteries. The elastic fibers progressively straighten, fray, split, and fragment. There is an increase in density and amount of collagen fibers in the vessel walls, along with decreasing elasticity of these walls.

The skin is one of the first systems to show signs of the aging process. The epidermis and dermis are visible markers of aging and greatly affect the placement of peripheral catheters. As a person ages, a loss of subcutaneous supporting tissue and resultant thinning of the skin occur. The turnover rate for the production of new cells slows: at the age of 20 years, turnover of new cells takes 3 weeks; at age 30 years, 6 weeks; and after age 30 years, 2 months. Folds, lines, wrinkles, and slackness appear as the skin ages. **Purpura** and ecchymoses may appear owing to the greater fragility of the dermal and subcutaneous vessels and the loss of support for the skin capillaries. Minor trauma can easily cause bruising.

Continued

A common symptom in older people is pruritus or "itchiness." This is usually caused by dry skin and by medications and should be considered when preparing the patient for parenteral therapy.

 NURSING FAST FACT!

> *Alcohol if used as a preparatory aid will add to the drying effect on the skin.*

The dermis becomes relatively dehydrated and loses strength and elasticity. This layer has underlying papillae that hold the epidermis and dermis together; this means that as one ages, the older skin loosens. Older skin has decreased flexibility in the collagen fibers, increased fragility of the capillaries, and fewer capillaries. Older skin feels dryer because of loss of subcutaneous fat and decreased production of sebum and sweat (Smeltzer, Bare, Hinkle, & Cheever, 2008). Refer to Figure 6-26.

 Website

American Geriatrics Society: www.americangeriatrics.org

Venipuncture Techniques

Special venipuncture techniques are required to successfully place and maintain infusion therapy in older patients. The potential complications associated with trauma, surgery, and illness in elderly people, along with the

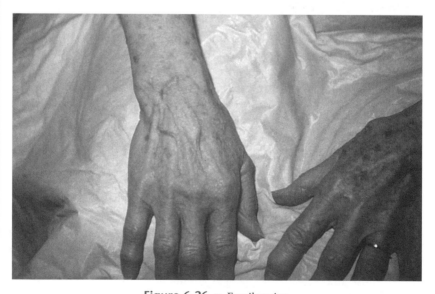

Figure 6-26 ■ Fragile veins.

physiologic changes mentioned previously, require that nurses be knowledgeable in the special skills associated with delivery of care.

The older adult client may be at greater risk for potential complications related to infusion therapy and may require more frequent monitoring.

Vascular Access Device Selection

Consider the skin and vein changes of older adults before initiating PIV. Also, consider catheter design and gauge size. Softer, more flexible materials and those that soften after insertion into the vein may allow increased indwelling time and prevent or reduce complications. The bevel-tip design of the peripheral catheter's needle may help to decrease trauma to vein.

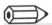 *NURSING FAST FACT!*

> *To reduce insertion-related trauma use a 22- to 24-gauge catheter.*

Selecting Administration Equipment

Because of the risk of over-administration or under-administration of infusion therapy, the type of infusion equipment selected should provide safe, consistent delivery of medication and fluids. Advanced technology provides uses of stationary and ambulatory electronic monitoring devices. Monitoring devices must have safety features to protect high-risk patients from fluid volume overload.

 NURSING FAST FACT!

> *To prevent fluid overload, use a microdrip administration set when appropriate. Because of the fragile nature of the veins of elderly patients, be aware of the potential complications associated with pressures generated from mechanical infusion devices (see Chapter 5 for a discussion of safety features associated with programmable pumps).*

Selecting a Vein

Selecting a vein that can support I.V. therapy for at least 72 to 96 hours can be a challenge for nurses caring for the older adult. Initial venipuncture should be in the most distal portion of the extremity, allowing for subsequent venipunctures to move progressively upward. However, in older adults, the veins of the hands may not be the best choice for the initial site because of the loss of subcutaneous fat and thinning of the skin. Physiologic changes in the skin and veins must be considered when a site is selected. Areas for PIV access should have adequate tissue and skeletal support. Avoid flexion areas and areas with bruising because the oncotic pressure is increased in these areas and causes vessels to collapse.

Use a tourniquet to help distend and locate appropriate veins, but avoid applying it too tightly because it can cause vein damage when the vein is punctured. During venous distention, palpate the vein to determine its condition. Veins that feel ribbed or rippled may distend readily when a tourniquet

Continued

is applied, but these sites are often impossible to access, causing pain for the patient. Refer to the summary of tips for fragile veins in Table 6-14.

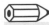 *NURSING FAST FACT!*

- *Place a tourniquet over a gown or sleeve to decrease the sheering force on fragile skin*
- *To thread a catheter through an inflexible valve, reduce the catheter size by several gauges.*

Valves become stiff and less effective with age. Bumps along the vein path (i.e., valves) may cause problems during attempts at vein access. Venous circulation may be sluggish, resulting in slow venous return, distention, venous stasis, and dependent edema. A catheter may not thread into a vein with stiff valves.

Small surface veins appear as thin tortuous veins with many bifurcations (Fig. 6–11). Appropriate catheter gauge and length selection is critical to successful I.V. access placement in these veins.

Cannulation Techniques

In elderly patients, stabilization of the vein is critical. The vessels may lack stability as a result of the loss of tissue mass and may tend to roll. Techniques to perform a venipuncture in elderly patients include:

1. Use of traction by placing the thumb directly along the vein axis about 2 to 3 inches below the intended venipuncture site. The palm and fingers of the traction hand serve to hold and stabilize the extremity. Using the index finger of the hand, provide traction to further stretch the skin above the intended venipuncture site. Maintain traction throughout venipuncture.

2. Insert the catheter, using either the direct or indirect technique. When the direct technique is used, insert the catheter at a 20- to 30-degree angle in a single motion, penetrating the skin and vein simultaneously. Do not stab or thrust the catheter into the skin; this could cause the catheter to advance too deeply and accidentally damage the vein. Use the indirect method (two-step) for patients with small, delicate veins. An alternative method is to have another nurse apply digital pressure with the hand above the site of venipuncture and release it after the vein has been entered.

> Table 6-14   **TIPS FOR THE OLDER ADULT WITH FRAGILE VEINS**

The following are tips for clients with fragile veins (age or disease process related)
- To prevent hematoma, avoid overdistention of the vein with tourniquet or BP cuff.
- Avoid multiple tapping of the vein.
- Use the smallest gauge catheter for the therapy prescribed.
- Lower the angle of approach into the vein.
- Pull the skin taut and stabilize the vein throughout venipuncture.
- Use the one-handed technique: advance the catheter off the stylet into the vein.
- Use warm compress to dilate vein if needed – be aware the older adult is more sensitive to heat.

NURSING POINTS-OF-CARE
OLDER ADULT PERIPHERAL INFUSION

Nursing Assessments
- Interview the patient regarding previous experiences with venipunctures.
- Review the purpose of the infusion and patient diagnosis, history, or comorbidities.
- Assess venipuncture sites taking into consideration the physical condition of skin, any disease processes, and cultural issues.
- Review trends in vital signs.

Key Nursing Interventions
1. Maintain standard precautions.
2. Use techniques to dilate veins that maintain the integrity of the skin (consider blood pressure cuff).
3. Explain procedures, keeping in mind sensory or auditory deficits.

Home Care Issues

Peripheral catheters are generally indicated for short-term infusion therapy (7–10 days) or intermittent infusions (e.g., monthly infusion) of nonirritating drugs and fluids. Home care issues related to the initiation and maintenance of peripheral I.V. administration include technical procedures, such as infusion administration and site rotation, as well as monitoring for expected effects and potential adverse reactions.

The technical procedures that the patient is expected to learn and perform depend on his or her cognitive ability, willingness to learn, and the specific technique being taught. Reimbursement often poses limitations. For example, with managed care payers, there may be a limited number of authorized home visits, as the expectation is that the patient or a caregiver will learn most aspects of infusion administration (Gorski, 2005).

- In alternative care settings, such as the home, the nurse may have to adapt to poor lighting, homes that are not clean, disorganized environments, and pets. It is important that the nurse work with the patient to establish a safe place for storage of supplies and a safe and efficient space for infusion administration. Many times the kitchen table is a good place with a cleanable surface and better lighting.
- Concern for latex-related allergic reactions. Many common household items contain latex. Synthetic rubber, polyethylene, silicone, or vinyl can be used effectively in the home care setting.
- Territoriality (i.e., the need for space) serves four functions: security, privacy, autonomy, and self-identification. People tend to generally feel safer in their own territory because it is arranged and equipped in a familiar manner.

Continued

Home Care Issues—cont'd

Most people believe there is a degree of predictability associated with being in one's own personal space and that this degree of predictability is hard to achieve elsewhere (Giger & Davidhizar, 2004).

- For patients with peripheral I.V. catheters, patients or their caregivers are usually instructed in and expected to:
  - Administer solutions or medications with some exceptions. For example, chemotherapy drugs are generally administered by the home care nurse.
  - Change administration sets.
  - Set up or monitor pump equipment.
  - Call the home health agency if there is pain, swelling, or redness at the peripheral I.V. site.
- The patient and his or her family must be taught standard precautions and aseptic technique in the home care setting.

Pediatric Patients in the Home

The home care environment must be assessed to be sure that infusion therapy can be carried out safely. In the home, children are more mobile and active. The parents must be educated about the use and care of therapy and accept involvement in and responsibility for the treatment regimen.

- Focus on the psychosocial and developmental needs of the child and family in planning home infusion therapy.
- The best infusion device is one that is portable and easy for the child and family to operate. A syringe pump and positive-pressure devices such as an elastomeric infusion device are examples of easy-to-use equipment.
- Keep in mind that parents need support from a home care agency.
- Identify alternate caregivers.

Older Adult Patients in the Home

Educating older adults in the administration of home infusion therapy can present challenges. The patient may be less ready to adapt to environmental changes, especially relating to independence.

The teaching of complex drug admixtures, tubing connections, PIV maintenance, and pump programming requires patience and step-by-step approaches. All equipment should be user friendly. Written teaching materials, video programs, and demonstrations, including return demonstrations, can be helpful.

- Evaluation of language or cultural differences can dramatically affect understanding of necessary healthcare concepts.
- Sensory changes occur with aging (e.g., in vision, hearing, and manual dexterity). Observe the patient while working with various devices (the needleless system may eliminate the risk of needlestick injuries) to ensure proficiency. Consider ways to simplify the procedure if the patient has functional limitations. For example, elastomeric infusion devices are more expensive and some organizations may try to use a more cost-effective method such as a simple gravity drip infusion. However, changing to the elastomeric device, which is very easy to use, may result in patient independence, reducing the need for frequent nursing visits.

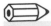

NURSING FAST FACT!

■ *The home care nursing staff is responsible for the routine restarts of PIV or blood draws. (In some areas, home laboratory services are also available for routine phlebotomy for needed laboratory studies.)*
■ *The principle diagnosis is critical for medical reimbursement, and the record must reflect total patient care, including the assessment, care plan, evaluations, implementation of care, and outcomes.*

Patient Education

Adult Clients
■ Instruct on the purpose of I.V. therapy.
■ Educate regarding limitations of movement.
■ Instruct to notify the nurse if pump alarms.
■ Instruct to report discomfort at the infusion site

Pediatric Clients
Education of the family including the child when appropriate should cover the following:
■ Child's participation in sports with the catheter in place
■ Purpose of I.V. therapy
■ Instruction on equipment
■ Verbal and written instructions on who, when, where, and how to call for assistance in an emergency or with significant concerns about infusion therapy
■ Instruction materials tailored to age and comprehension level (Otto, 2005)
■ Documentation should include the responses of the patient's family and caregiver to teaching. All infusion therapy modalities should be explained to all those involved in patient care.

INS Standard When a patient requires continued care in his or her home, the nurse shall provide comprehensive education to the patient and caregiver that includes the behavioral domains of cognitive, affective, and psychomotor, along with a written set of instructions on all pertinent aspects of treatment. (INS, 2006a, 11)

■ Nursing Process

The nursing process is a five- or six-step process for problem-solving to guide nursing action. Refer to Chapter 1 for details on the steps of the nursing process related to vascular access. The following two tables focuses on nursing diagnoses, nursing outcomes classification (NOC), and nursing intervention classification (NIC) for peripheral infusion therapy in adults and pediatric patients. Nursing diagnoses should be patient specific and outcomes and interventions individualized. The NOC and NIC presented here are suggested directions for development of specific outcomes and interventions.

Nursing Diagnoses Related to Peripheral Infusion Therapy in Adults	NOC: Nursing Outcomes Classification	NIC: Nursing Intervention Classification
Infection, risk for, related to: Inadequate acquired immunity; inadequate primary defenses (broken skin, traumatized tissue); inadequate secondary defenses; increased environmental exposure to pathogens	Immune status: Infection control, risk control, risk detection	Infection control and infection protection
Knowledge deficit related to: Cognitive limitation; information misinterpretation; lack of exposure; lack of interest in learning; lack of recall; unfamiliar with information resources regarding peripheral infusion therapy	Knowledge regarding health behavior, health resources, infection control, medication, personal safety and treatments	Teaching: Disease process, reasons for infusion therapy, treatment
Mobility, physical, impaired related to: Activity intolerance; altered cellular metabolism; prescribed movement restrictions secondary to I.V. therapy	Mobility, self-care: Activities of daily living (ADLs)	Joint mobility, positioning
Risk for injury related to: Disturbed sensory perception—the older adult		
Skin integrity impaired risk for: Physical immobilization; medications/solutions; fluid status	Immobility consequences: Physiological	Positioning: Pressure prevention, skin surveillance

Sources: Ackley & Ladwig (2008); McCloskey-Dochterman & Bulechek (2004); Moorhead, Johnson, & Maas (2004); NANDA-I (2007).

Nursing Diagnoses Related to Peripheral Infusion Therapy in Pediatric Patients	NOC: Nursing Outcomes Classification	NIC: Nursing Intervention Classification
Anxiety, related to: Role status; situational crises; unmet developmental needs	Anxiety level, coping	Anxiety reduction strategies for parents and child
Diversional activity deficit related to: Environmental lack of diversional activity—age appropriate	Play participation, social involvement	Recreational play therapy— age appropriate
Family process interrupted related to: Shift in health status of family member; situation transition secondary to hospitalization	Family coping, family social climate, family functioning	Family integrity promotion, family process maintenance, family therapy, support system enhancement
Fear related to: Loss of control, autonomy, independence, competence and self esteem; language barrier; separation from support system; unfamiliar with environmental experiences	Fear self-control	Anxiety reduction, coping enhancement and security enhancement strategies
Fluid volume deficit related to: Deviations affecting access fluids and intake of fluids; excessive losses through normal routes (diarrhea, vomiting); extremes of weight; medications	Fluid balance, hydration, nutritional status	Fluid management
Infection, risk for, related to: Inadequate acquired immunity; inadequate primary defenses (broken skin, traumatized tissue); inadequate secondary defenses; increased environmental exposure to pathogens	Immune status: Infection control, risk control, risk detection	Infection control and infection protection
Mobility, physical, impaired related to: Cultural beliefs regarding age-appropriate activity; prescribed movement restrictions secondary to I.V. therapy	Mobility, developmental self-care, activities of daily living	Joint mobility, positioning
Parenting, impaired related to: Illness; separation from parents	Family functioning, parent–infant attachment; role, safe home environment, social support	Family support, infant– parenting promotion, spiritual support, environmental management (safety)
Skin integrity, impaired related to: Physical immobilization; medications/solutions; fluid status	Tissue integrity: Skin	Skin surveillance, venipuncture site care

Sources: Ackley & Ladwig (2008); McCloskey-Dochterman & Bulechek (2004); Moorhead, Johnson, & Maas (2004); NANDA-I (2007).

Chapter Highlights

- The first step is an understanding of the anatomy and physiology of the venous system. The five layers in the approach to successful venipuncture are the epidermis, dermis, tunica adventitia, tunica media, and tunica intima.
- A working knowledge of the veins in the hand and forearm is vital so the practitioner can successfully locate an acceptable vein for venipuncture and cannula placement. Keep in mind the type of solution, condition of vein, duration of therapy, patient age, patient preference, patient activity, presence of disease, previous surgery, presence of shunts or grafts, allergies, and medication history.
- The steps in performing the placement of a catheter that can support PIV therapy for 72 hours are as follows:

Precannulation

- Step 1: Check the physician's order.
- Step 2: Wash hands.
- Step 3: Prepare equipment.
- Step 4: Assess the patient and his or her psychological preparedness, and verify patient identity.
- Step 5: Select the site and dilate the vein.

Cannula Placement

- Step 6: Needle selection
- Step 7: Gloving
- Step 8: Site preparation – 30 seconds and let dry
- Step 9: Vein entry
- Step 10: Catheter stabilization and dressing management

Postcannulation

- Step 11: Labeling
- Step 12: Equipment disposal
- Step 13: Patient instructions
- Step 14: Rate calculation
- Step 15: Documentation
- The choice of using heparin or saline to maintain intermittent injection ports is determined by the agency's policies and procedures and the physician's order. Check these before using the steps in heparin or saline lock flush.
- Locks must be flushed every 12 hours if not being used for medication administration.

- Use Xylocaine hydrochloride before venipuncture. Use 0.1 to 0.2 mL of 1% Xylocaine injected intradermal. Wait 5 to 10 seconds before continuing the steps of the venipuncture.
- Use topical transdermal analgesia cream, such as a combination of lidocaine 2.5% and prilocaine 2.5%. Apply in thick layer and cover with occlusive dressing for 1 hour.
- Rate calculations: To calculate drop rates of gravity infusions, I.V. nurses must know (1) the drop factor of the administration set and (2) the amount of solution ordered.

Macrodrip Sets

- 10 gtt = 1 mL
- 15 gtt = 1 mL
- 20 gtt = 1 mL

NOTE > Transfusion administration sets: usually 10 gtt = 1 mL

Microdrip Sets

- 60 gtt = 1 mL

Pediatric Infusion Therapy

- Children are not small adults. Physiologic differences must be kept in mind with particular focus on total body weight (85%–90% water) and heat production (increases caloric expenditure by 7% for each degree of temperature), and immature renal and integumentary systems important in regulation of fluid and electrolyte needs.
- Physical assessment of a pediatric patient includes measuring the head circumference (for patients up to 1 year of age) and checking height or length, vital signs, skin turgor, presence of tears, moistness and color of membranes, urinary output, characteristics of fontanels, and level of child's activity.
- Peripheral routes include the four scalp veins, dorsum of the hand and forearm, and dorsum of the foot.
- Selection of PIV equipment must keep in mind safety, activity, age, and size.
- Needle selection depends on the age of child: 26- to 24-gauge for neonates; 24- to 22-gauge for children.
- Use small volumes of solutions (250 or 500 mL). Use a volume control chamber (VCC) and, when indicated, infusion pumps.

- Always have extra help when starting an I.V. in a child.
- Perform venipuncture in a separate room, use a pacifier for neonates and infants, warm hands before applying gloves, and use stickers or drawing as rewards.
- Delivery of medications to children can be by intermittent infusion, retrograde infusion, or syringe pump.

The Older Adult

- Physiologic changes include homeostatic mechanisms becoming less efficient; immune system becoming hyporesponsive to foreign antigens; cardiovascular changes, including a change in elasticity of the vein walls; skin losses; subcutaneous support; and thinning of skin.
- Assessment guidelines include skin turgor, temperature, rate and filling of veins in hand or foot, daily weight, intake and output, center of tongue should be moist, postural blood pressure, swallowing ability, and functional assessment of patient's ability to obtain fluids if not NPO.
- Venipuncture techniques should take into consideration the skin and vein changes of elderly persons; use small-gauge catheters, use blood pressure cuff, or place loose tourniquet over clothing. Use warm compresses to visualize veins. Consider microdrip administration sets.

▪▪ Thinking Critically: Case Study

A 20-year-old obese, African American man is readmitted to the hospital with a diagnosis of osteomyelitis secondary from a gunshot wound in the right femur, obtained and treated a month earlier. The patient is to be medically managed with I.V. antibiotics for 4 to 6 weeks, and to receive a diet high in protein and hydration.

Decide which of the following access devices should be used to initiate therapy and give the rationale: a peripheral-short catheter, a midline catheter, or a peripherally inserted central catheter.

What should be taken into consideration during assessment of venous access sites?

What equipment might help you with a successful venipuncture?

Media Link:　Answers to the case study and more critical thinking activites are provided on the CD-ROM.

WORKSHEET 6-1
SUPERFICIAL VEINS OF THE UPPER EXTREMITIES

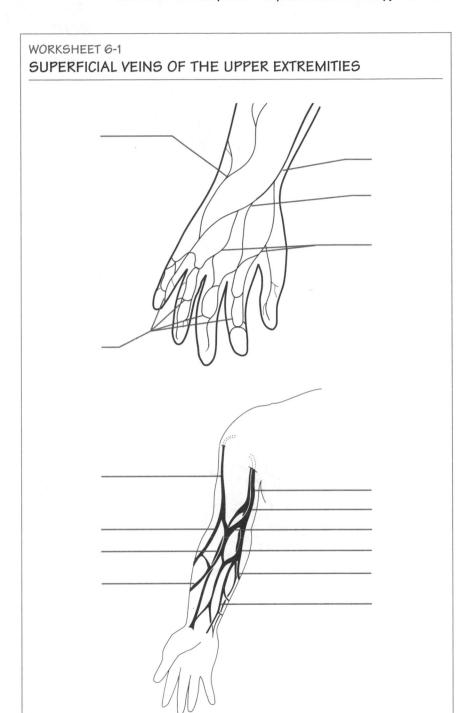

WORKSHEET 6-1 ANSWERS

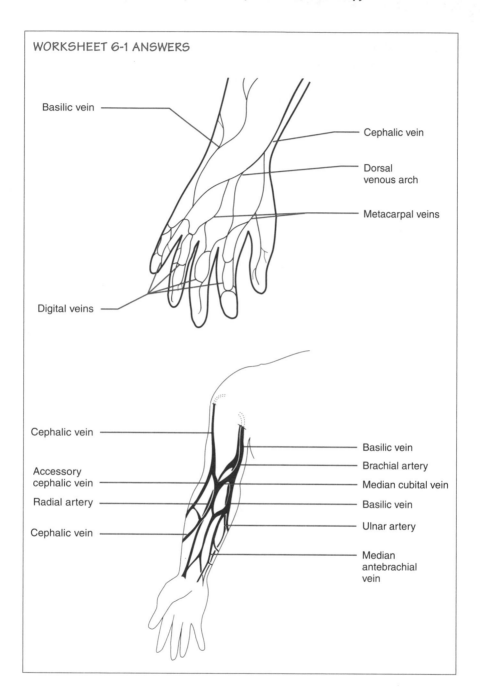

WORKSHEET 6-2

BASIC CALCULATION OF PRIMARY INFUSIONS

1. The order reads 1000 mL of 5% dextrose in water at 125 mL/h. You have available 20 drop factor tubing. Calculate the drops per minute.

2. The order is for 1000 mL of 5% dextrose and 0.45% sodium chloride at 150 mL/hr. You have available 15 drop factor tubing. Calculate the drops per minute.

3. The order is for 250 mL (1 U) of packed cells over 2 hours. Remember, blood tubing is always 10 drop factor. Calculate the drops per minute.

4. The order is for 45 mL/hr of 5% dextrose and 0.45% sodium chloride solution on an 8-month-old baby. Calculate the drops per minute if you have to use a controller that is drops per minute? (Remember, use microdrop tubing.) What else must be considered when administering this solution to an infant?

5. The order reads 3000 mL of a multiple electrolyte fluid over 24 hours. You have available 20 drop factor tubing. Calculate the drops per minute.

Intermittent I.V. Drug Administration

6. The physician orders a fluid challenge of 250 mL of 0.9% sodium chloride over 45 minutes. You have 20 drop factor tubing available. Calculate the drops per minute in order to accurately deliver the 250 mL over 45 minutes.

7. Administer 50 mg of vinblastine sulfate diluted in 50 mL of 0.9% sodium chloride over 15 minutes. You have available a 15 macrodrop infusion set.

8. Administer 500 mg of acyclovir in 100 mL of 5% dextrose in water over 1 hour. You have available macrodrop 20 gtt infusion set.

9. Administer trimethoprim–sulfamethoxazole 400 mg in 125 mL of dextrose in water over 90 minutes. You have available a microdrop set and macrodrip 15 gtt.

10. At 12 noon you discover that an infusion set to deliver 100 mL per hour from 7 A.M. to 5 P.M. has 400 mL left in the infusion bag. Recalculate the infusion using a 10 drop macrodrop infusion set.

Continued

ANSWERS TO WORKSHEET 6-2
USING FORMULA OR RATIO/PROPORTION

1. Formula: $\dfrac{\text{mL/hr} \times \text{DF}}{\text{minutes}} = \text{gtt/min}$

Step 1: $\dfrac{125 \times 20}{60} = \text{gtt/min}$

Step 2: $\dfrac{125}{3} = \textbf{42 gtt/min}$

2. Formula: $\dfrac{\text{mL/hr} \times \text{DF}}{\text{minutes}} = \text{gtt/min}$

Step 1: $\dfrac{150 \times 15}{60} = \text{gtt/min}$

Step 2: $\dfrac{150}{4} = \textbf{38 gtt/min}$

3. Formula: $\dfrac{\text{mL}}{\text{hours}} = \text{mL/h}$

Step 1: $250 \div 2 = 125 \text{ mL/hr}$

Formula: $\dfrac{\text{mL/hr} \times \text{DF}}{\text{minutes}} = \text{gtt/min}$

Step 2: $\dfrac{125 \times 10}{60} = \text{gtt/min}$

Step 3: $\dfrac{125}{6} = \textbf{21 gtt/min}$

4. Formula: $\dfrac{\text{mL/hr} \times \text{DF}}{\text{minutes}} = \text{gtt/min}$

Step 1: $\dfrac{45 \times 60}{60} = \textbf{45 gtt/min}$

Only one step is needed for microdrop infusions.
When using 60 gtt tubing the gtt/min = the amount of the hourly infusion volume.
In *addition:* All pediatric solutions and medications should be checked by another RN. Use volume control chamber and limit primary bottle to 500 mL container.

5. Formula: $\dfrac{\text{mL}}{\text{hours}} = \text{mL/hr}$

Step 1: $\dfrac{3000}{24} = 125 \text{ mL/hr}$

Formula: $\dfrac{\text{mL/hr} \times \text{DF}}{\text{minutes}} = \text{gtt/min}$

Step 2: $\dfrac{125 \times 20}{60} = \text{gtt/min}$

Step 3: $\dfrac{125}{6} = \textbf{42 gtt/min}$

6. Formula: $\dfrac{\text{mL/hr} \times \text{DF}}{\text{minutes}} = \text{gtt/min}$

Step 1: $\dfrac{250 \times 20}{45} = \text{gtt/min}$

Step 2: $\dfrac{250 \times 4}{9} = \dfrac{1000}{9} = \textbf{111 gtt/min}$

7. Formula: $\dfrac{\text{mL/hr} \times \text{DF}}{\text{minutes}} = \text{gtt/min}$

Step 1: $\dfrac{50 \times 15}{15} = \textbf{50 gtt/min}$

8. Formula: $\dfrac{\text{mL/hr} \times \text{DF}}{\text{minutes}} = \text{gtt/min}$

Step 1: $\dfrac{100 \times 20}{60} = \text{gtt/min}$

Step 2: $\dfrac{100}{3} = \textbf{33 gtt/min}$

9. Formula: $\dfrac{\text{mL/hr} \times \text{DF}}{\text{minutes}} = \text{gtt/min}$

Step 1: $\dfrac{125 \times 15}{90} = \text{gtt/min}$

Step 2: $\dfrac{125}{6} = \textbf{21 gtt/min}$

10. Formula: $\dfrac{\text{mL}}{\text{hours}} = \text{mL/hr}$

Step 1: $\dfrac{400}{5} = 80 \text{ mL/hr}$

Formula: $\dfrac{\text{mL/hr} \times \text{DF}}{\text{minutes}} = \text{gtt/min}$

Step 2: $\dfrac{80 \times 10}{60} = \text{gtt/min}$

Step 3: $\dfrac{80}{6} = \textbf{13 gtt/min}$

Post-Test

1. List the four steps in maintaining patency of a saline locking device when administering a medication by PIV.

   1.
   2.
   3.
   4.

2. Before equipment setup and venipuncture, how many seconds of hand hygiene procedure with an antimicrobial soap are recommended?

   a. 10 to 30
   b. 15 to 20
   c. 30 to 60
   d. 45 to 60

3. PIV therapy labels should be applied to:

   a. Catheter site, tubing, and solution container
   b. Tubing, solution container, and chart
   c. Solution container, catheter site, and patient's armband

4. What is the recommended frequency in which a patient receiving infusion therapy should be monitored?

   a. Systematic, ongoing, and documented
   b. Every 4 hours and documented
   c. Every shift or every 8 to 12 hours and documented
   d. Every 24 hours and documented

5. The preferred choice for peripheral infusion site in the young infant younger than age 9 months is the:

   a. Frontal vein in the scalp
   b. Dorsum of the foot
   c. Dorsum of the hand
   d. Occipital vein on the head

6. In a dark-skinned person, the best method for locating an accessible vein is:

   a. Multiple tourniquets
   b. Tangential lighting
   c. Direct overhead lighting
   d. Light application of a tourniquet

7. Which of the following is the most appropriate cannula size for use on a 2-month-old infant?

   a. 18-gauge over-the-needle catheter
   b. 23- to 25-gauge scalp vein needle

    c. 16-gauge scalp vein needle

    d. 22- to 24-gauge over-the-needle catheter

8. The most appropriate equipment for an infant receiving I.V. fluids includes:

    a. Microdrip tubing connected to a 50-mL infusate container

    b. Microdrip volume control cylinder attached to a 250-mL infusate container

    c. Macrodrip tubing connected to a volume control cylinder

    d. Any tubing or container as long as it is regulated with an electronic infusion device

9. Which of the following are techniques to dilate a vein for venipuncture in the older adult with fragile veins? (*Select all that apply.*)

    a. Apply the tourniquet loosely over the patient's sleeve.

    b. Apply multiple tourniquets.

    c. Use digital pressure to enhance vein filling.

    d. Use warm compresses before venipuncture.

10. The tunica intima of the vein is the layer: (*Select all that apply.*)

    a. With endothelial lining

    b. With nerve fibers for vasoconstriction or dilation

    c. Where thrombus formation can occur

    d. That is the outermost layer consisting of connective tissue

 Media Link: Answers to the Chapter 6 Post-Test and more test questions together with rationales are provided on the CD-ROM.

■ References

Ackley, B.J., & Ladwig, G.B. (2008). *Nursing diagnosis handbook: An evidence-based guide to planning care* (8th ed.). St. Louis, MO: Mosby Elsevier.

Anderson, N.R. (2004). Midline catheters: The middle ground of intravenous therapy administration. *Journal of Infusion Therapy, 27*(5), 313–321.

Broyles, B.E., Reiss, B.S., & Evans, M.E. (2007). *Pharmacological aspects of nursing care* (7th ed.). Clifton Park, NY: Thomson Delmar Learning.

Chiyakunapruk, N., Veenstra, D., Lipsky, B., & Saint, S. (2002). Chlorhexidine compared with povidone-iodine solution for vascular catheter-site care: A meta analysis. *Annals of Internal Medicine, 136,* 792–801.

Garland, J.S., Alex, C.P., Mueller, C.D., et al. (2001). A randomized trial comparing povidone-iodine to a chlorhexidine gluconate impregnated dressing for prevention of central venous catheter infections in neonates. *Pediatrics, 107*(6), 1431–1436.

Giger, J.N., & Davidhizar, R.E. (2004). *Transcultural nursing: Assessment and intervention* (4th ed.). St. Louis, MO: C.V. Mosby.

Gillies, D., O'Riordan, L., Wallen, M., et al. (2005). Optimal timing for intravenous administration set replacement. *Cochrane Database System Reviews* 4: CD 003588.

Gorski, L. (2005). *Pocket guide to home infusion therapy.* Sudbury, MA: Jones and Bartlett.

Hadaway, L. (2005). Giving medication by retrograde infusion. *Nursing 2005, 35*(11), 28.

Hibbard, J.S. (2005). Analyses comparing the antimicrobial activity and safety of current antiseptic agents: A review. *Journal of Infusion Nursing, 28*(3), 194–207.

Hockenberry, M.J., & Wilson, D. (2006). *Wong's nursing care of infants and children* (8th ed.). St. Louis, MO: C.V. Mosby

Infusion Nurses Society (INS). (2006a). Infusion nursing standards of practice. *Journal of Intravenous Nursing, 29* (1S).

Infusion Nurses Society (INS). (2006b). *Policies and procedures for infusion nursing* (3rd ed.). Norwood, MA: Author.

Infusion Nurses Society (INS). (2008). *Flushing protocols.* Norwood, MA: Author.

IOMED Clinical Systems. (2008). Iontocaine (product literature). Salt Lake City: Author.

IOMED, Inc. (2008). Retrieved from www.iomed.com/prod-numby.html (Accessed June 26, 2008).

Kaler, W., & Chinn, R. (2007). Successful disinfection of needleless access ports: A matter of time and friction. *JAVA, 12*(3), 140–142.

LaRue, G.D. (2000). Efficacy of ultrasonography in peripheral venous cannulation. *Journal of Intravenous Nursing, 23*(1), 29–34.

Maki, D.G., & Mermel, L.A. (2007). Infection due to infusion therapy. In: W. Jarvis (Ed.), *Bennett & Brachman's hospital infections* (5th ed., pp. 689–716). Philadelphia: Lippincott Williams & Wilkins.

Maki, D.G., & Ringer, M. (1991). Risk factors for infusion-related phlebitis with small peripheral venous catheters. *Annals of Internal Medicine, 114,* 845–854.

Maki, D.G., Ringer, M., & Alvarado, C.J. (1991). Prospective randomised trial of povidone-iodine, alcohol, and chlorhexidine for prevention of infection associated with central venous and arterial catheters. *Lancet, 228*(8763), 339–343.

Maki, D.G., Stolz, S.S., & Wheeler, S., et al. (1994). A prospective, randomized trial of gauze and two polyurethane dressings for site care of pulmonary artery catheters: Implications for catheter management. *Critical Care Medicine, 32,* 1729–1737.

McCloskey-Dochterman, J.C., & Bulechek, G.M. (2004). *Nursing interventions classification (NIC)* (4th ed.). St. Louis, MO: C.V. Mosby.

Metheny, N.M. (2000). *Fluid and electrolyte balance: Nursing considerations* (4th ed.). Philadelphia: J.B. Lippincott.

Moorhead, S., Johnson, M., & Maas, M. (2004). *Nursing outcomes classification (NOC)* (3rd ed.). St. Louis, MO: C.V. Mosby.

Moolenaar, R.L., Crutcher, J.M., San Joaquin, V.H., et al. (2000). A prolonged outbreak of *Pseudomonas aeruginosa* in a neonatal intensive care unit: Did staff fingernails play a role in disease transmission? *Infection Control and Hospital Epidemiology, 21*(2), 80–85.

Moureau, N., & Lannucci, A.L. (2003). Catheter securement: Trends in performance and complications associated with the use of either traditional methods or an adhesive device. *Journal of Vascular Access Devices, 8*(1), 29–33.

Munoz, C., & Luckmann, J. (2005). *Transcultural communication in nursing* (2nd ed.). Clifton Park, NY: Thomson Delmar Learning.

NANDA-I (2007). *Nursing diagnoses: Definitions and classification, 2007–2008.* Philadelphia: Author.

National Institute Occupational Safety and Health Administration (2004). Disposal of contaminated needles and blood tube holders used for phlebotomy. Washington, DC: US Department of Labor, OSHA. Available at www.osha.gov/dts/shib/shib101503.html. (Accessed June 12, 2008).

Parry, M.F., Grant, B.,Yukna, M., et al. (2001). Candida osteomyelitis and diskitis after spinal surgery: An outbreak that implicates artificial nail use. *Clinical Infectious Diseases, 32*(3), 352–357.

O'Grady, N.P., Alexander, M., Delllinger, E.P., et al. (2002). Guidelines for prevention of intravascular catheter-related infections. *Morbidity and Mortality Weekly Reports MMWR, 51* (RR-10).

Otto, S. (2005). *Infusion therapy: Pocket guide series* (5th ed.). St. Louis, MO: Mosby Elsevier.

Phillips, L.D. (2008). Reinforcing basic IV skills using nursing process. *Infusion Nurses Society Newsline, 30*(3), 8–14.

Rosenthal, K. (2007). *Infection prevention and needle-free devices.* Bethlehem, PA: B. Braun.

Schears, G.J. (2006). Summary of product trials for 10,164 patients: Comparing an intravenous stabilizing device to tape. *Journal of Infusion Nursing, 29*(4), 225–229.

Siegel, J.D., Rhinehart, E., Jackson, M., & Chiarello, L. (2007). Guideline for isolation precautions: Preventing transmission of infectious agents in healthcare settings 2007. Retrieved from www.cdc.gov/ncidod/dhqp/hai.html (Accessed June 19, 2008).

Smeltzer, S.C., Bare, B.G., Hinkle, J.L., & Cheever, K.H. (2008). *Brunner and Suddarth's textbook of medical-surgical nursing* (11th ed.). Philadelphia: Lippincott Williams & Wilkins.

Smith, B. (2006). Peripheral intravenous catheter dwell times: A comparison of 3 securement methods for implementation of a 96 hour scheduled change protocol. *Journal of Infusion Nursing, 29*(1), 14–17.

Smith, B. (2007). New standards for improving peripheral I.V. catheter securement. *Nursing 2007, 37*(3), 72–74.

The Joint Commission (TJC). (2003). National patient safety goals. Retrieved from http://www.jointcommission.org/PatientSafety (Accessed August 28, 2008).

Translite. (2008). Veinlite by Translite product information. Retrieved from www.veinlite.com/image.html (Accessed June 26, 2008).

Trick, W.E., Vernon, M.O., Hayes R.A., et al. (2003). Impact of ring wearing on hand contamination and comparison of hand hygiene agents in a hospital. *Clinical Infectious Diseases, 36*(11), 1383–1390.

Walling, A.D., & Lenhardt, R. (2003). Local warming and insertion of peripheral venous cannulas: Single blinded prospective randomized controlled trial and single blinded randomized crossover trial. *American Family Physician, 67*(2), 401.

Walther, K. (2008). Clinical concepts of infusion therapy: Infusion therapy and assessment of the older adult. *INS Newsline, 30*(3), 6.

Zwicker, C.D. (2003). The elderly patient at risk. *Journal of Infusion Nursing, 26*(3), 137–143.

PROCEDURES DISPLAY 6-1

Steps of Inserting a Peripheral-Short Over-the-Needle Catheter by Direct and Indirect Methods

Equipment Needed
Clean gloves
IV catheter (22-gauge, 20-gauge, 18-gauge) most common
Prep solution (chlorhexidine gluconate recommended)
Securement device
Needleless injection system
Primary administration set
Infusate
Non-latex tourniquet
Delegation:
This procedure can be delegated to LVN/LPN depending on their state nurse practice act for initiation of infusion therapy and agency policy.

Procedure	Rationale
1. Verify the authorized prescriber's order.	1. A written order is a legal requirement for infusion therapy.
2. Hand hygiene: Follow standards throughout the procedure.	2. Good hand hygiene is the single most important means of preventing the spread of infection.
3. Gather all equipment and check for integrity.	3. Having all equipment at hand will save time and lessen patient anxiety.
4. Introduce yourself to the patient.	4. Establishes nurse–patient relationship
5. Check patient ID using two forms (check ID bracelet and ask patient to state name).	5. The Joint Commission (2003) safety goal recommendation. Prepares patient for procedure. Safety
6. Assess patient (verify allergy status) and evaluate for psychological preparedness. Intruct patient on purpose of infusion or locking device. Apply tourniquet and evaluate both arms for best access site. Release tourniquet ■ Wash hands again before beginning procedure and don gloves.	6. Allows for dilation of veins and assessment of both extremities. Standard Precautions

PROCEDURES DISPLAY 6-1

Steps of Inserting a Peripheral-Short Over-the-Needle Catheter by Direct and Indirect Methods—cont'd

Procedure	Rationale
7. Help patient get into a comfortable position. Place linen saver under arm or hand.	7. Promotes cooperation with the procedure and facilitates your ability to perform the procedure. Protects bed linens.
8. Select the site and dilate the vein.	8. Choose the most distal veins of the upper extremity on the hand and/or arm so that you can perform subsequent venipunctures proximal to the previous site. Ensures preservation of veins.
9. Select the appropropriate catheter for therapy.	9. Chose the best needle gauge for the therapy and patient age.
10. Don clean gloves. Gloves must be left on throughout the entire procedure.	10. Standard precautions
11. Prepare the site using a circular technique, working from back and forth with friction for 30 seconds and let dry.	11. Prevents infection
12. Reapply the tourniquet.	12. Distend veins.
13. Insert the catheter by a direct or indirect method with a steady motion using traction to maintain an anchor on the vein.	13. Anchoring the vein properly is the key to successful catheter insertion.

For the Direct (One-Step) Method:
- A. Insert the catheter directly over the vein at a 20–30 degree angle
- B. Penetrate all layers of the vein with one motion.

Holding the catheter at a 20–30 degree angle allows you to pierce the skin without inadvertently piercing the back of the vein. Quickly gets through layers of epidermis and dermis, decreasing pain, and allows for adjustment to technqiue based on skin thickness.

Continued

PROCEDURES DISPLAY 6-1

Steps of Inserting a Peripheral-Short Over-the-Needle Catheter by Direct and Indirect Methods—cont'd

Procedure	Rationale
For the Indirect (Two-Step) Method:	Allows for repositioning of the catheter.
A. Insert the catheter at a 30-degree angle to the skin alongside the vien; gently insert the catheter distal to the point at which the needle will enter the vein.	The flashback of blood indicates that the vein has been cannulated.
B. Maintain parallel alignment and advance through the subcutaneous tissue.	Releasing the tourniquet restores full circulation to the patient's extremity.
C. Relocate the vein and decrease the angle as the catheter enters the vein.	

Note: Jabbing, stabbing, or quick thrusting should be avoided because such actions may cause rupture of delicate veins. For performing a venipuncture on difficult veins, follow these guidelines:

■ For paper-thin transparent skin or delecate veins: Use the smallest catheter possible (preferably 22-gauge); use direct entry; consider not using a tourniquet (blood pressure cuff); decrease the angle of entry to 15 degrees; apply minimal tourniquet pressure.

Catheter over needle inserted together   Catheter advanced over needle   Needle removed   Catheter in place

PROCEDURES DISPLAY 6-1

Steps of Inserting a Peripheral-Short Over-the-Needle Catheter by Direct and Indirect Methods—cont'd

Procedure   **Rationale**

- For an obese patient or if you are unable to palpate or see veins, create a visual image of venous anatomy and select a longer catheter (2 inch); use a multiple tourniquet technique.
- For veins that roll when venipuncture is attempted: Apply traction to the vein with the thumb during venipuncture, keeping skin taut; leave tourniquet on to promote venous distention; use a blood pressure cuff for better filling of vein; use 18-gauge catheter.

After the bevel enters the vein and blood flashback occurs, lower the angle of the catheter and stylet (needle) as one unit and advance into the vein. After the catheter tip and bevel are in the vein, advance the catheter forward off the stylet and into the vein.

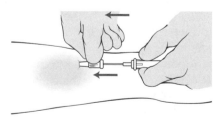

Continued

PROCEDURES DISPLAY 6-1

Steps of Inserting a Peripheral-Short Over-the-Needle Catheter by Direct and Indirect Methods—cont'd

Procedure

After the vein is entered, cautiously advance the catheter into the vein lumen. Hold the catheter hub with your thumb and middle finger and use your index finger to advance the catheter, maintaining skin traction. A one-handed technique is recommended to advance the catheter off the stylet so that the opposite hand can maintian proper traction on the skin and maintain vein alignment. (A two-handed technique can be used, but this increases the risk of vessel rupture during thread-ing of a rigid catheter in a nonstabilized vein.)

While the stylet is still partially inside the catheter, relase the tourniquet.

Remove the stylet and activate the passive or active safety feature of the catheter.

14. Connect the administration set or locking device with a twisting motion.
15. Stabilize the catheter with a stabilization device or apply transparent semipermeable membrane (TSM) dressing directly over the catheter and hub.

Rationale

14. Secures the Luer-Lok™ and prevents leakage and contam-ination.
15. Prevents movement of the catheter in the vein. Prevents microorganisms from entering the catheter–skin junction.

PROCEDURES DISPLAY 6-1

Steps of Inserting a Peripheral-Short Over-the-Needle Catheter by Direct and Indirect Methods—cont'd

Procedure	Rationale
16. Label the site with date, time; type and length of catheter; nurse's initials.	16. Legal protection of the patient and nurse.
17. Dispose of all equipment in appropriate receptacle.	17. To prevent contamination follow Standard Precautons.
18. Instruct the patient on use of an electronic infusion device (EID), what to report regarding site, and how often to expect the nurses will check the infusion site.	18. Knowledge of infusion therapy treatment assists in providing a positive outcome.
19. Calculate the infusion rate or dial in appropriate rate into EID.	19. To ensure correct delivery of prescribed solution or medications.
20. Document in the medical records: The date and time of insertion; type of device; gauge and length of the catheter; solution infusing and rate of flow; any additional equipment (EID); number of attempts; condition of extremity before access; patient's response; signature.	20. To maintain a legal record and communication with the healthcare team.

PROCEDURES DISPLAY 6-2

Converting a Primary Line to Intermittent Device

Equipment Needed

Luer-Lok™ needleless access port (NAP) (cap/valve)

Two syringes containing sodium chloride

Transparent semipermeable membrane (TSM) dressing

Stabilization device

Clean gloves

Alcohol

Delegation:

This procedure can be delegated to a LVN/LPN who is specially trained in I.V. therapy depending on their state nurse practice act for initiation of infusion therapy and agency policy. This cannot be delegated to nursing assistant personnel.

Procedure	Rationale
1. Confirm the authorized prescriber's order to discontinue continuous infusion.	1. A written order is a legal requirement for infusion therapy.
2. Introduce yourself to the patient.	2. Establishes the nurse–patient relationship.
3. Wash hands using friction for 15–20 seconds using an alcohol-based hand sanitizer.	3. Good hand hygiene is the single most important means of preventing the spread of infection.
4. Verify the patient's identity using two forms of ID (check ID bracelet and ask the patient to state name).	4. The Joint Commission (2003) safety goal recommendation.
5. Help the patient get into a comfortable position that provides access to the I.V. site.	5. Promotes cooperation and facilitates the nurse's ability to perform the procedure.
6. Apply clean gloves. Remove NAP from the package, and if appropriate flush the lock with the first syringe of sodium chloride. Place back in adapter sterile package.	6. Removes air from the lock.
7. Carefully remove the I.V. dressing and the tape that is securing the tubing.	7. Provides access to the I.V. catheter.

PROCEDURES DISPLAY 6-2

Converting a Primary Line to Intermittent Device—cont'd

Procedure	Rationale
8. Close the roller clamp on the administraiton set and if appropriate turn off the electronic infusion device (EID).	8. Prevents loss of I.V. fluid during the procedure.
9. With your nondominant hand, apply pressure over the catheter just above the insertion site.	9. Applying pressure over the vein stops blood from flowing from the catheter as you change the administration tubing to a lock.
10. Gently disengage the old tubing from the I.V. catheter. If it does not disengage easily, it may help to grip the catheter hub with a hemostat.	10. Prevents the catheter from becoming dislodged.
11. Quickly insert the lock adapter into the I.V. catheter.	11. Insert the adapter quickly to prevent blood from flowing from the I.V. catheter.
12. Cleanse the injection port of the adapter with an alcohol pad for 15 seconds.	12. Cleansing the port with alcohol helps prevent contamination by microorganisms when the adapter and I.V. catheter are flushed.
13. Flush the locking device with 2 mL of sodium chloride. Follow flush protocols.	13. Maintains patency of the lock.
14. Apply a fresh dressing.	14. Maintains occlusive dressing.
15. Discard the administration set in the appropriate biohazard container. Empty the I.V. solution in the nearest sink and discard it in a biohazard container.	15. Standard precautions
16. Remove gloves and wash hands.	16. Standard precautions

Continued

PROCEDURES DISPLAY 6-2

Converting a Primary Line to Intermittent Device—cont'd

Procedure	Rationale
17. Document the procedure with the date and time of conversion of primary solution infusion to locking device, amount of fluid infused, and how the patient tolerated the procedure.	17. Maintains a legal record and communication with the healthcare team.

PROCEDURES DISPLAY 6-3

Flushing a Peripheral-Short I.V. Catheter

Equipment Needed
3-mL syringe
Preservative-free 0.9% sodium chloride: 1 10 mL vial (single use)
Gloves
Sharps container
Antiseptic solution: 70% alcohol
Sterile injection or access cap

Delegation:
This procedure can be delegated to an LPN/LVN who is specially trained in I.V. therapy depending on the state nurse practice act for initiation of infusion therapy and agency policy and procedure. This cannot be delegated to nursing assistive personnel.

Procedure	Rationale
1. Confirm authorized prescriber's order for flushing or follow standardized procedure for the agency.	1. A written order is a legal requirement for infusion therapy.
2. Introduce yourself to the patient.	2. Establishes the nurse–patient relationship.
3. Wash hands using friction for 15–20 seconds using an alcohol-based hand sanitizer.	3. Good hand hygiene is the single most important means of preventing the spread of infection.

PROCEDURES DISPLAY 6-3

Flushing a Peripheral-Short I.V. Catheter—cont'd

Procedure	Rationale
4. Verify the patient's identity using two forms of ID (check ID bracelet and ask patient to state name).	4. The Joint Commission (2003) safety goal recommendation.
5. Identify whether the needleless injection cap/valve is a negative-displacement device, a postive-displacement device or a neutral-displacement device.	5. Negative and positve displacement devices are dependent on the flushing technique. A positive pressure technique is required with a negative-displacement device. With a positive-displacement device positive pressure flushing cannot be used. With neutral-displacement function of device is not dependent on the flushing technique.
6. Don gloves.	6. Prevents bacteria entry into the infusion system. Standard precautions.
7. Cleanse the catheter injection cap/valve with 70% isopropyl alcohol with a twisting motion for 15 seconds (10 twists). Allow to air-dry.	7. Prevents introduction of microorganisms into the system.
8. Attach a 3-mL syringe containing 2 mL of 0.9% preservative-free sodium chloride to the injection port via a needleless system.	8. To administer the irrigant and maintain patency of catheter.
9. Slowly aspirate until brisk postive blood return	9. To confirm catheter patency.
10. Irrigate the line with 0.9% sodium chloride using the push–pause method.	10. Maintains patency of catheter and prevents occlusion.

Continued

PROCEDURES DISPLAY 6-3

Flushing a Peripheral-Short I.V. Catheter—cont'd

Procedure	Rationale
Note: There are different types of NIS devices, be sure you know which devices are used in your facility. Negative and positive displacement devices are dependent on flushing technique.	
10a. For negative-displacement devices (positive-pressure flushing required) As the last 0.5–1 mL of solution is flushed inward, withdraw the syringe, allowing the last amount of flush solutions to fill the dead space. Flush all solution into the catheter lumen; maintain force on the syringe plunger as a clamp on the catheter or extension set is closed; then disconnect the syringe.	**10a.** Manufacturer requires positive pressure flushing technique to prevent reflux of blood.
10b. For positive-displacement device (positive pressure flushing technique cannot be used because it will overcome the positive displacement mechanism) Flush the catheter gently with solution, disconnect the syringe, and allow suffficent time for the positive fluid displacment; then close the catheter clamp.	**10b.** Manufacturer requires the catheter to be clamped before disconnection of syringe. A positive pressure technique on this system will prevent proper function of a positive-displacement system.
10c. For neutral-displacement device (not dependent on flush technique)	
11. Document the procedure on the patient record.	**11.** Maintains a legal record and communication with the healthcare team.

Sources: Hadaway (2006). Technology of flushing vascular access devices., JIN, 29(3), 137-145; INS (2006). Policies and procedures for infusion nursing; INS (2006). Standards of Practice.

PROCEDURES DISPLAY 6-4

Discontinuation of Peripheral-Short I.V. Catheter

Equipment Needed
Dressing materials: 2 × 2 gauze and tape
sharps container
Delegation:
This procedure can be delegated to an LPN/LVN who is specially trained in I.V. therapy depending on the state nurse practice act for initiation of infusion therapy and agency policy and procedure. This cannot be delegated to nursing assistive personnel.

Procedure	Rationale
1. Confirm the authorized prescriber's order for discontinuation of infusion therapy.	1. A written order is a legal requirement for infusion therapy.
2. Introduce yourself to the patient.	2. Establishes the nurse–patient relationship.
3. Wash hands using friction for 15–20 seconds.	3. Good hand hygiene is the single most important means of preventing the spread of infection.
4. Verify the patient's identity using two forms of ID (check ID bracelet and ask patient to state name).	4. The Joint Commission (2003) safety goal recommendation.
5. Assist the patient into a comfortable position.	5. Promotes cooperation and facilitates the nurse's ability to perform the procedure.
6. Place a linen-saver pad under the extremity that contains the I.V. catheter.	6. Protects bed linens.
7. Apply procedure gloves and close the roller clamp on the administration set if there is a continuous infusion running.	7. Standard precautions, and stops infusion of fluids.
8. Carefully remove the I.V. dressing, stabilization device, and the tape that is securing the tubing.	8. Allows access for catheter removal.

Continued

PROCEDURES DISPLAY 6-4

Discontinuation of Peripheral-Short I.V. Catheter—cont'd

Procedure	Rationale
9. Inspect the catheter–skin junction site.	9. Assess for signs of infection or phlebitis.
10. Apply a sterile 2 × 2 gauze pad above the I.V. insertion site and gently using even pressure remove catheter, directing it straight along the vein.	10. Could cause catheter to become detached from hub and embolize.
Note: Do not press down on the gauze pad while removing the catheter.	
11. Immediately apply firm pressure with the gauze pad over the insertion site once the catheter is removed. Hold for 2–3 minutes, longer if bleeding persists.	11. Prevents bleeding and hematoma formation.
12. Assess the integrity of the removed catheter. Compare length of catheter to original insertion length to ensure the entire catheter is removed.	12. Note the condition of site, including the presence of any site complications. To ensure full catheter length has been removed from the patient.
13. Dress the exit site. Secure fresh 2 × 2 gauze to the site with tape. Change dressing every 24 hours until the exit site is healed.	13. Keeps the venipuncture site clean.
14. Discard used supplies, and the I.V. catheter in sharps container, I.V. tubing, linen-saver pad, solution container, and gloves in appropriate trash receptacle according to institutional policy.	14. Follow OSHA standards of practice for biohazards.

PROCEDURES DISPLAY 6-4

Discontinuation of Peripheral-Short I.V. Catheter—cont'd

Procedure	Rationale
15. Remove gloves and then wash hands.	**15.** Standard precautions.
16. Document date and time that I.V. therapy was discontinued. Document any complications noted and interventions. If catheter defect is noted, report to the manufacturer and regulatory agencies.	**16.** Maintains a legal record and communication with the healthcare team.

Source: INS (2006). Policies and procedures for infusion nursing; INS (2006) Standards of Practice.

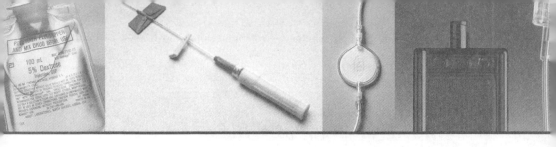

Chapter 7
Phlebotomy Techniques

*Medicine is not only a science, but also the art of letting our own individuality
interact with the individuality of the patient.*
—Albert Schweitzer

Chapter Contents

7-1 Collection of Blood in
    Evacuated Tube System
7-2 Collection of Blood Using
    a Winged or Butterfly
    Collection Set

7-3 Collection of Blood Using
    the Syringe Method

LEARNING
OBJECTIVES

On completion of this chapter, the reader will be able to:

1. List the various types of anticoagulants used in blood collection.
2. Identify the tube color codes for vacuum collection.
3. Describe phlebotomy safety supplies and equipment.
4. Identify the various supplies that should be carried on a specimen collection tray.
5. Identify the types of equipment needed to collect blood by venipuncture.
6. Describe the patient identification process.
7. List essential information for test requisitions.
8. Identify the most common sites for venipuncture for blood collection.
9. Describe the venipuncture procedure and steps for the evacuated tube method, winged infusion system, and syringe method.
10. State the order of draw for collection tubes.

GLOSSARY

Acid–citrate–dextrose (ACD) An additive commonly used in specimen collection for blood donations to prevent clotting. Ensures that the red blood cells maintain their oxygen-carrying capacity

Anticoagulant Substance introduced into the blood or a blood specimen to keep it from clotting

Assay Determination of the purity of a substance or the amount of any particular constituent of a mixture

Citrate–phosphate–dextrose (CPD) Anticoagulant typically used for blood donations.

Ethylenediaminetetraacetic acid (EDTA) Anticoagulant additive used to prevent the blood clotting sequence by removing calcium and forming calcium slats. EDTA prevents platelet aggregation and is useful for platelet counts and platelet function tests.

Hemoconcentration　Increased localized blood concentration of large molecules such as proteins, cells, and coagulation factors

Hemolysis　Rupture or lysis of the blood cells

Multiple-sample needle　Used with the evacuated tube method of blood collection; these needles are attached to a holder/adapter and allow for multiple specimen tube fills and changes without blood leakage.

National Committee for Clinical Laboratory Standards (NCCLS)　Nonprofit organization that recommends quality standard and guidelines for clinical laboratory procedures

National Phlebotomy Association (NPA)　Professional organization for phlebotomists that offers continuing education activities and certification examination for phlebotomists

Oxalates　Anticoagulants that prevent blood-clotting sequence by removing calcium and forming calcium salts

Phlebotomist　Individual who practices phlebotomy

Phlebotomy　Incision of a vein for blood collection

Single-sample needle　Used for collecting a blood sample from a syringe

Syringe method　Method of venipuncture whereby a syringe is used to collect blood that is then transferred to collection tubes

Vacuum (evacuated) tube system　Color-coded specimen collection tube that contains a vacuum so as to aspirate blood when a needle enters a patient's vein. The tubes are part of a blood collection method that also requires a double-pointed needle and special plastic holder (adapter).

▪ Introduction to Phlebotomy

Purpose of Phlebotomy

Blood and other specimen collections are important to the entire health assessment of the client. Laboratory analysis of a variety of specimens is used for three important purposes:

1. Obtain blood for diagnostic purposes and monitoring of prescribed treatment
2. Remove blood for transfusion at a donor center
3. Remove blood for therapeutic purposes such as treatment for polycythemia.

Professional Competencies

The term *phlebotomist* is applied to a person who has been trained in various techniques to perform phlebotomy procedures. The role of the nurse may include **phlebotomy**, along with the responsibility of preserving veins for infusion therapy (McCall & Tankersley, 2008). The nurse has the unique position of using a single venipuncture to permit both the withdrawal for blood and the initiation of an infusion, thereby preserving veins. Refer to Table 7-1 for duties and responsibilities of the nurse or phlebotomist.

Usually a **phlebotomist** or blood collector must complete a phlebotomy program.

Advances in laboratory technology are making point-of-care testing (POCT) more common. As many health professionals are being cross-trained to perform phlebotomy, the term "phlebotomist" is being applied to anyone who has been trained to collect blood specimens. The nurse performing phlebotomy procedures or the phlebotomist must have the knowledge base listed below to perform blood withdrawal procedures safely. Certification is evidence that an individual has mastered fundamental competencies of a technical area. Examples of national agencies that certify phlebotomists along with the title and corresponding initials awarded are listed as follows:

American Medical Technologists: Registered Phlebotomy
Technician RPT (AMT)
American Certification Agency: Certified Phlebotomy Technician
CPT (ACA)
American Society for Clinical Pathology: Phlebotomy Technician
PBT (ASCP)
National Center for Competency Testing: National Certified
Phlebotomy Technician NCPT (NCCT)
National Credentialing Agency: Clinical Laboratory Phlebotomist
CLPLB (NCA)
National Health Career Association: Certified Phlebotomy
Technician CPT (NHA)

> Table 7-1   **DUTIES OF THE NURSE OR PHLEBOTOMIST**

1. Prepare patients for blood collection procedures.
2. Collect routine skin puncture and venous specimens for testing.
3. Prepare specimens for transport.
4. Maintain Standard Precautions.
5. Maintain confidentiality.
6. Perform quality control checks while performing clerical, clinical, and technical duties.
7. Transport specimens to the laboratory.
8. Comply with all procedures instituted in the procedure manual.
9. Perform laboratory computer operations.
10. Collect and perform point-of-care testing.
11. Perform quality control checks on instruments.
12. Process specimens and perform basic laboratory tests.

Demonstrates knowledge of:
- Basic anatomy and physiology
- Medical terminology
- Potential sources of error
- Safety measures and infection control practices
- Standard operating procedures
- Fundamental biology

Selects appropriate:
- Courses of action
- Quality control procedures
- Equipment/methods and reagents
- Site for blood collection

Prepares patient and equipment
Evaluates:
- Specimen and patient situations
- Possible sources of error and inconsistencies

INS Standard The nurse shall have validation of competency in the knowledge and protocols for phlebotomy. (INS, 2006a, 66)

 NURSING FAST FACT!

In 1992 the Clinical Laboratory Improvement Amendments of 1988 became effective. This public law mandates that all laboratories must be regulated using the same standards regardless of location, type, or size (NCCLS, 1992).

Healthcare Worker Preparation

All healthcare workers must be familiar with current recommendations and hospital policies for handling blood and body fluids. All specimens should be treated as if they are hazardous and infectious.

NOTE > Review Chapter 2: Infection for Standard Precautions.

Before performing any type of specimen collection, the nurse or phlebotomist should have gathered the necessary protective equipment, phlebotomy supplies, test requisitions, writing pens, and appropriate patient information. Refer to Table 7-1 for a list of supplies that should be included in a blood collection tray.

Equipment for Blood Collection

Supplies for Venipuncture

Supplies for venipuncture differ according to the method used (i.e., syringe method, evacuated tube system). All methods of venipuncture involve the use of disposable gloves, a tourniquet, alcohol pads or disinfectants, cotton balls, bandages or gauze pads, glass microscope slides, needles, syringes, or evacuated tube holders. Refer to Table 7-2.

Vacuum (Evacuated) Tube Systems

Venipuncture with an **evacuated tube system (ETS)** is the most direct and efficient method for obtaining a blood specimen. It is a closed system in which the patient's blood flows through a needle inserted into a vein, directly into a collection tube without being exposed to the air or outside contaminants. The system allows for multiple tubes to be collected with a single venipuncture. Evacuated tube systems are available from several manufacturers. Refer to Figure 7-1 for traditional components of an evacuated tube system.

The evacuated tube system requires three components:
- The evacuated sample tube
- The double-pointed needle
- Plastic holder

> Table 7-2   **BLOOD COLLECTION TRAY CONTENTS**

Equipment carriers: Hand-held carriers, or phlebotomy carts
Gloves: Nonsterile, disposable latex, nitrile, neoprene, polyethylene, and vinyl exam gloves are acceptable. **NOTE:** A good fit is essential.
Marking pen or pencil
Watch
Antiseptics: Routine blood collection is 70% isopropyl alcohol; chlorhexidine gluconate or povidone-iodine is used for higher degree of antisepsis—for blood culture collection and blood gas collection.
Hand sanitizers: Alcohol-based hand sanitizers
Gauze pads/cotton balls (2 × 2 gauze pads)
Bandages (latex free): Adhesive bandages to cover site after bleeding stopped.
Paper, cloth, or knitted tape for use over cotton ball
Needles and sharps disposal containers
Vacuum tubes containing the anticoagulants
Safety holders for vacuum tubes (single-use disposable)
Needles for vacuum tubes and syringes
Tourniquets (latex and nonlatex)
Safety lancets
Microcollection blood serum separator tubes

Source: McCall & Tankersley (2008).

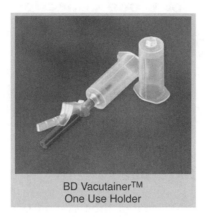

BD Vacutainer™
One Use Holder

Figure 7-1 ■ Traditional components of evacuated tube system. (Courtesy of Becton Dickinson, Franklin Lakes, NJ.)

The Tube Holder

The tube holder is a clear plastic, disposable cylinder with a small threaded opening at one end, where the needle is screwed into it, and a large opening at the other end where the collection tube is placed.

NOTE > OSHA regulations require that the tube holder with needle attached be disposed of as a unit after use and never removed from the needle and reused.

Double-Pointed Needle

One end of the double-pointed needle enters the vein; the other end pierces the top of the tube, and the vacuum aspirates the blood.

Evacuated Tubes

Vacuum tubes may contain silicone to decrease the possibility of **hemolysis**. Tubes have premeasured amounts of vacuum to collect a precise amount of blood. It is imperative that the expiration date be checked before using any blood collection tube. The tubes are available in different sizes and can be purchased in glass or unbreakable plastic. The Vacutainer system tubes are color coded according to the additive contained within the tube. The tubes are specifically designed to be used directly with chemistry, hematology, or microbiology instrumentation. The tube of blood is identified by its barcode and is pierced by the instrument probe, and some sample is aspirated into the instrument for analyses.

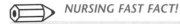 *NURSING FAST FACT!*

Use of closed systems minimizes laboratory personnel's risk of exposure to blood. The expiration dates of tubes must be monitored carefully.

Evacuated tubes can also be used for transferring blood from a syringe into the tubes. The syringe needle is simply pushed through the top of the tube, and blood is automatically pulled into the tube because of the vacuum. Place the vacuum tube in a rack before pushing the needle into the tube top. A safety syringe shielded transfer device needs to be used to avoid possible exposure to the patient's blood. See Figure 7-2 for an example of a safety feature.

The following are manufacturers of blood collection equipment:

- BD Vacutainer Systems™ (Becton Dickinson) have a protective shield so that blood collector can slide the protective shield over the needle and lock it in place after the needle is withdrawn from the puncture site.
- Eclipse™ (Becton Dickinson) is a single-use blood collection needle that allows the user to shield the needle after use.
- SIMS™ Venipuncture Needle-Pro (SIMS Portex Inc., Keene, NH) provides immediate containment of a used needle.
- VanishPoint™ (Retractable Technologies, TX) is a safety blood collection tube holder that provides for the needle to automatically retract into it after blood collection.
- Proguard II™ (KCK Medical) is a single-use vacuum tube/needle holder.
- Sarstedt, Inc. has the S Monovette™ (Sarstedt, Inc., Newton, NC) Blood Collection System, which is a safety device for vacuum collection or a syringe collection.

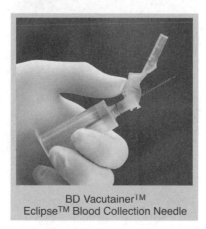

BD Vacutainer™
Eclipse™ Blood Collection Needle

Figure 7-2 ▪ BD Vacutainer Eclipse™ blood collection safety needle. (Courtesy of Becton Dickinson, Franklin Lakes, NJ.)

Summary of Tube Types and Their Uses

Anticoagulants

Most clinical laboratories use serum, plasma, or whole blood to perform various **assays**. Many coagulation factors are involved in blood clotting, and coagulation can be prevented by the addition of different types of anticoagulants. These anticoagulants often contain preservatives that can extend the metabolism and life span of the red blood cell. Refer to Figure 7-3 for examples of Vacutainer tubes.

Coagulation of blood can be prevented by the addition of one of the following four: oxalates, citrates, **ethylenediaminetetraacetic acid (EDTA),** or **heparin. Oxalates, citrates,** and **EDTA** prevent coagulation of blood by removing calcium and forming insoluble calcium salts. These four anticoagulants are the most common anticoagulants. These cannot be used in calcium determinations; however, citrates are frequently used in coagulation blood studies. EDTA prevents platelet aggregation and is used for platelet counts and platelet function tests. Heparin prevents blood clotting by inactivating the blood-clotting chemicals thrombin and thromboplastin.

NOTE > CLSI recommends spray-dried EDTA for most hematology tests because liquid EDTA dilutes the specimen and results in lower hemoglobin values (McCall & Tankersley, 2008).

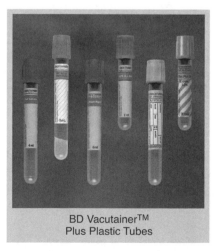

BD Vacutainer™
Plus Plastic Tubes

Figure 7-3 ▪ BD Vacutainer™ plastic tubes. (Courtesy of Becton Dickinson, Franklin Lakes, NJ.)

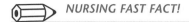 *NURSING FAST FACT!*

It is important to choose the correct anticoagulant tube for a specific laboratory assay, along with using the correct amount or dilution of anticoagulant in the blood specimen.

Special-Use Anticoagulants

Acid–citrate dextrose (ACD) is available in two formulations for immunohematology tests such as DNA testing and human leukocyte antigen (HLA) phenotyping used in paternity evaluation.

Citrate phosphate dextrose (CPD) is used in collection units of blood for transfusion.

Sodium polyanethol sulfonate (SPS) prevents coagulation by binding calcium. It is used for blood culture collection because in addition to being an anticoagulant, it reduces the action of a protein called complement that destroys bacteria, slows down phagocytosis, and reduces the activity of certain antibiotics. SPS tubes have yellow stoppers and require eight inversions to prevent clotting (McCall & Tankersley, 2008).

Color Coding

Tube stoppers are color-coded. Evacuated tubes are referred to as red tops, green tops and so forth. For most tubes, the stopper color identifies a type of additive placed in the tube by the manufacturer.

Red-Topped Tubes

Red-topped tubes that are glass indicate a tube without an anticoagulant; therefore blood collected in this tube will clot. The plastic red top tubes have a clot activator (silica). The red/light gray plastic do not have an additive and are used as discard tubes only. The red/black (tiger) tubes have clot activator and gel separator for chemistry.

Royal Blue-Topped Tubes

The royal blue-topped tubes are used to collect samples for nutritional studies, therapeutic drug monitoring, and toxicology. The royal blue-topped tube is the trace element tube. The royal blue-top tube with a lavender label has EDTA added; the green label has sodium heparin added.

Yellow-Topped Tubes

Yellow-topped tubes are used for blood cultures. The blood must be collected in a sterile container (vacuum tube, vial, or syringe) under aseptic conditions. The plastic tubes contain SPS for the microbiology tubes and acid-citrate dextrose (ACD) used specifically for yellow-topped tubes for blood band and immunohematology.

 NURSING FAST FACT!

Clotted specimens should not be shaken.

Green-Topped Tubes

The anticoagulants sodium heparin and lithium heparin are found in green-topped vacuum tubes. The green/gray (light green) also have a gel separator.

Gray-Topped Tubes

Gray-topped vacuum tubes usually contain either potassium oxalate and sodium fluoride or sodium fluoride and EDTA. This type of collection tube is used primarily for glycolytic inhibition tests. Gray-topped tubes are not used for hematology studies.

Light Blue-Topped Tubes

Tubes with light blue tops contain sodium citrate and are used for coagulation procedures. The sodium citrate comes in a concentration of 3.2% or 3.8%. It is preferable to use the 3.2% concentration to reduce false-negative or false-positive results.

Mottled-Topped, Speckled-Topped, and Gold-Topped Tubes

These tubes contain a polymer barrier that is present at the bottom of the tube. The specific gravity of this material lies between the blood clot and the serum. During **centrifugation**, the polymer barrier moves upward to the serum–clot interface, where it forms a stable barrier, separating the serum from fibrin and cells.

Pink or Lavender-Topped Tubes

The lavender or pink topped tubes contain EDTA. They are also used for hematology and blood bank.

Orange or Gray/Yellow-Topped Tubes

The organe or gray/yellow-topped tubes contain thrombin for chemistry.

Tan Glass- or Tan Plastic-Topped Tubes

The glass tan-topped tube contains sodium heparin and the plastic tan-topped tube contains EDTA.

Refer to Figure 7-4 for an illustration of a tube guide.

BD Vacutainer® Venous Blood Collection Tube Guide

Tubes with BD Hemogard™ Closure	Tubes with Conventional Stopper	Additive	Inversions at Blood Collection*	Laboratory Use
Gold	Red/Black	• Clot activator and gel for serum separation	5	For serum determinations in chemistry. May be used for routine blood donor screening and diagnostic testing of serum for infectious disease.** Tube inversions ensure mixing of clot activator with blood. Blood clotting time: 30 minutes.
Light Green	Green/Gray	• Lithium heparin and gel for plasma separation	8	BD Vacutainer® PST™ Tube for plasma determinations in chemistry. Tube inversions prevent clotting.
Red		• None (glass) • Clot activator (plastic)	0 5	For serum determinations in chemistry. May be used for routine blood donor screening and diagnostic testing of serum for infectious disease.** Tube inversions ensure mixing of clot activator with blood. Blood clotting time: 60 minutes.
Orange	Gray/Yellow	• Thrombin	8	For stat serum determinations in chemistry. Tube inversions ensure complete clotting, which usually occurs in less than 5 minutes.
Royal Blue		• Clot activator (plastic serum) • K_2EDTA (plastic)	8 8 0 5 8	For trace-element, toxicology, and nutritional chemistry determinations. Special stopper formulation provides low levels of trace elements (see package insert).
Green		• Sodium heparin • Lithium heparin	8 8	For plasma determinations in chemistry. Tube inversions prevent clotting.
Gray		• Potassium oxalate/ sodium fluoride • Sodium fluoride/ Na_2EDTA • Sodium fluoride (serum tube)	8 8 8	For glucose determinations. Oxalate and EDTA anticoagulants will give plasma samples. Sodium fluoride is the antiglycolytic agent. Tube inversions ensure proper mixing of additive and blood.
Tan		• K_2EDTA (plastic)	8 8	For lead determinations. This tube is certified to contain less than .01 µg/mL (ppm) lead. Tube inversions prevent clotting.
	Yellow	• Sodium polyanethol sulfonate (SPS) • Acid citrate dextrose additives (ACD): Solution A - 22.0 g/L trisodium citrate, 8.0 g/L citric acid, 24.5 g/L dextrose Solution B - 13.2 g/L trisodium citrate, 4.8 g/L citric acid, 14.7 g/L dextrose	8 8 8	SPS for blood culture specimen collections in microbiology. Tube inversions prevent clotting. ACD for use in blood bank studies, HLA phenotyping, and DNA and paternity testing.

BD Tube Guide. Courtesy and © 2008 Becton, Dickinson and Company.

Figure 7-4 ■ Blood collection tube top guide. (Courtesy of Becton Dickinson, Franklin Lakes, NJ.)

Continued

Tubes with BD Hemogard™ Closure	Tubes with Conventional Stopper	Additive	Inversions at Blood Collection*	Laboratory Use
Lavender		• Liquid K₃EDTA (glass) • Spray-coated K₂EDTA (plastic)	8 8	K₂EDTA and K₃EDTA for whole blood hematology determinations. K₂EDTA may be used for routine immunohematology testing and blood donor screening.*** Tube inversions prevent clotting.
White		• K₂EDTA with gel	8	For use in molecular diagnostic test methods (such as but not limited to polymerase chain reaction [PCR] and/or branched DNA [bDNA] amplification techniques).
Pink		• Spray-coated K₂EDTA	8	For whole blood hematology determinations. May be used for routine immunohematology testing and blood donor screening.*** Designed with special cross-match label for patient information required by the AABB. Tube inversions prevent clotting.
Light Blue Clear		• Buffered sodium citrate 0.105 M (≈3.2%) glass 0.109 M (≈3.2%) plastic • Citrate, theophylline, adenosine, dipyridamole (CTAD)	3-4 3-4	For coagulation determinations. CTAD for platelet function assays and routine coagulation determination. Tube inversions prevent clotting.
Clear	Red/Gray	• None (plastic)	0	For use as a discard tube or secondary specimen collection tube.

Partial-draw Tubes (2 ml and 3 mL: 13 x 75 mm)	Additive	Inversions at Blood Collection*	Laboratory Use
Red	• None	0	For serum determinations in chemistry. May be used for routine blood donor screening, immunohematology testing,*** and diagnostic testing of serum for infectious disease.** Tube inversions ensure mixing of clot activator with blood. Blood clotting time: 60 minutes.
Green	• Sodium heparin • Lithium heparin	8 8	For plasma determinations in chemistry. Tube inversions prevent clotting.
Lavender	• Spray-coated K₂EDTA (plastic)	8 8	For whole blood hematology determinations. May be used for routine immunohematology testing and blood donor screening.*** Tube inversions prevent clotting.

Small-volume Pediatric Tubes (2 mL: 10.25 x 47 mm, 3 mL: 10.25 x 64 mm)	Additive	Inversions at Blood Collection*	Laboratory Use
Light Blue	• 0.105 M sodium citrate (≈3.2%)	3-4	For coagulation determinations. Tube inversions prevent clotting.

* Invert gently, do not shake

** The performance characteristics of these tubes have not been established for infectious disease testing in general; therefore, users must validate the use of these tubes for their specific assay-instrument/reagent system combinations and specimen storage conditions.

*** The performance characteristics of these tubes have not been established for immunohematology testing in general; therefore, users must validate the use of these tubes for their specific assay-instrument/reagent system combinations and specimen storage conditions.

BD Tube Guide. Courtesy and © 2008 Becton, Dickinson and Company.

Figure 7-4—cont'd

Expiration Dates

Manufacturers guarantee reliability of additive and tube vacuum until an expiration date printed on the label, providing the tubes are handled properly and stored between 4° and 25°C.

With the use of plastic tubes, very few tubes are additive free. Even serum tubes need an additive to promote clotting if they are plastic. A few nonadditive red top tubes are still in existence, but most are in the process of being discontinued for safety reasons (McCall & Tankersley, 2008).

Syringe Systems

The evacuated tube system is the preferred method of blood collection, a syringe system is sometimes used for patients with small or difficult veins. This system consists of a sterile syringe needle called a hypodermic needle and sterile plastic syringe with a Luer-Lok™ tip. A newer syringe system component is an OSHA required syringe transfer device. This device is used to transfer blood from the syringe into ETS tubes.

The barrel of the syringe is in graduated measurements, usually milliliters. Sizes range from 0.2 to 50.0 mL; however, for specimen collection purposes, 5- to 20-mL syringes are most often used.

Needles

The gauge and length of a needle used on a syringe or a vacuum tube are selected according to specific tasks. Most multisample needles come in 1-inch or 1.5 inch lengths. Syringe needles come in many lengths; however, 1-inch and 1.5 inch are most commonly used for venipuncture. Butterfly needles are typically ½ to ¾ of an inch long. Some of the new safety needles come in slightly longer lengths to accommodate resheathing features. The needle gauges include 18-gauge needles, which are used for collecting donor units of blood and therapeutic phlebotomy; smaller 21- or 22-gauge needles are used for collecting specimens for laboratory assays. The 21-gauge 1-inch in length needle is considered the standard venipuncture needle for routine venipuncture. The 22-gauge multisample needle is used on older children and adult patients with small veins or syringe draws on difficult veins. The 23-gauge butterfly is used on infants and children and for difficult hand veins of adults. Needles are sterile and packaged by vendors in sealed shields that maintain sterility.

Different types of needles are used with vacuum collection tubes and the holder to allow for multiple tube changes without blood leakage within the plastic holder. The multisample needle has a rubber cover over the tube-top puncturing portion of the needle; this cover creates a leakage barrier. The single-sample needle is usually used for collecting blood with a syringe.

Winged Infusion Set

The winged infusion set or butterfly needle is the most commonly used blood collection set for small or difficult veins. The system consists of ½ to ¾ inch stainless steel needle permanently connected to a 5- to 12-inch length of tubing with either a Luer attachment for syringe use or a multisample Luer adapter for use with the evacuated tube system. Refer to Figure 7-5 for an example of a blood collection butterfly collection set.

 NURSING FAST FACT!

> *The first tube collected with a butterfly will underfill because of the air in the tubing.*

Microcollection Equipment

Lancets

Skin puncture blood-collecting techniques are used on infants. Skin puncture collection is indicated for adults and older children when they are severely burned, or have veins that are difficult to access because of their small size or location. The volume of plasma or serum that generally can be collected from a premature infant is approximately 100 to 150 µL, and about two times that amount can be taken from a full term newborn. Refer to Figure 7-6 for an example of a microcollection lancet.

Lancets for these sticks are available for two different incision depths, depending on the needs of the infant; the teal-colored BD Quikheel™. Quikheel has a depth of 1.0 mm and width of 2.5 mm, and the purple-colored Quikheel Preemie lancet has a preset incision depth of

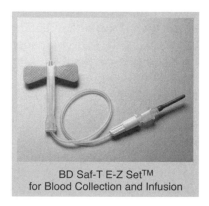

BD Saf-T E-Z Set™
for Blood Collection and Infusion

Figure 7-5 ■ BD Safe-T E-Z Set™ for blood collection. (Courtesy of Becton Dickinson, Franklin Lakes, NJ.)

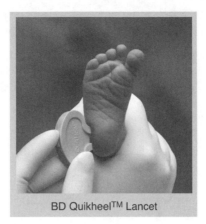

BD Quikheel™ Lancet

Figure 7-6 ▪ BD Quikheel™ Lancet. (Courtesy of Becton Dickinson, Franklin Lakes, NJ.)

0.85 mm and width of 1.5 mm. Most lancet blades retract permanently after activation to ensure safety for the healthcare worker.

 NURSING FAST FACT!

> *The recommended penetration depth of the lancet is no more than 2.0 mm on the heel.*
> *The National Committee for Clinical Laboratory Standards (NCCLS) recommends penetration depth of no more than 2.0 mm on heelsticks to avoid penetrating the bone (NCCLS, 2003a). Refer to Age-Related Considerations for more NCCLS guidelines on pediatric blood collection.*

▪ Blood Collection Procedure

Blood collection includes obtaining serum, plasma, or whole blood from the patient. Serum consists of plasma minus fibrinogen and is obtained by drawing blood in a dry tube and allowing it to coagulate. A majority of the diagnostic tests require serum. Plasma consists of stable components of blood minus cells. Anticoagulant tubes are used to prevent blood from clotting. Whole blood is required in many tests such as complete blood count and bleeding times.

In preparing for blood collection, the healthcare worker carries out essential steps to ensure a successful blood specimen collection. **The National Committee for Clinical Laboratory Standards** (2003a) has recommendations for safe blood collection. These steps may vary in individual facilities based on the characteristics of their patient populations. Some steps may be carried out simultaneously. The recommended steps include:

1. Review the test requisition.
2. Assess the patient and identify the patient using two identifiers (The Joint Commission [TJC], 2003).
3. Approach the patient.
4. Select a puncture site.
5. Select and prepare equipment and supplies.
6. Prepare the puncture site.
7. Choose a venipuncture method.
8. Collect the samples in the appropriate tubes and in the correct order.
9. Label the samples.
10. Assess the patient after withdrawal of the blood specimen.
11. Consider any special circumstances that occurred during the phlebotomy procedure.
12. Assess criteria for sample recollection or rejection.
13. Dispose of equipment in sharps or biohazard containers.
14. Transport the specimen to the laboratory.

Test Requisition

Laboratory tests must be ordered by a qualified healthcare practitioner. Test requisitions can be manual, three-part paper-based, or computer requisitions, which are more common in today's medical settings. The computer requisitions contain the actual labels that are placed on the specimen tubes immediately after collection. With computer generated requisitions, the phlebotomist is typically required to write the time of collection and his or her initials on the label after collection. Both the manual and computer requisitions may contain a bar code.

Bar code requisition contains a series of black stripes and white spaces of varying widths that correspond to letters and numbers. The stripes and spaces are grouped together to represent patient names, identification number, or laboratory tests. The requisition should contain the following information (McCall & Tankersley, 2008).

- Patient's first and last name and middle initial
- Physician or authorized prescriber's name
- Patient's identification or medical record number
- Patient's date of birth
- Room number and bed (if inpatient)
- Types of test to be performed
- Date of test

- Billing information and ICD-9 codes (if outpatient)
- Test status (timed, priority, fasting, etc.)
- Special precautions (potential bleeder, faints easily, latex sensitivity, etc.)

Drawing Station

A blood-drawing station is a dedicated area of a medical laboratory or clinic equipped for performing phlebotomy. In addition, blood is often collected from the patient in the acute care hospital at the bedside. A phlebotomy chair should be used at drawing stations where the patient sits during the blood collection procedure. Most have adjustable armrests that lock in place to prevent the patient from falling should fainting occur. Refer to Figure 7-7.

Assessment and Identification

The nurse or phlebotomist must be aware of the physical or emotional disposition of the patient, which can have an impact on the blood collection

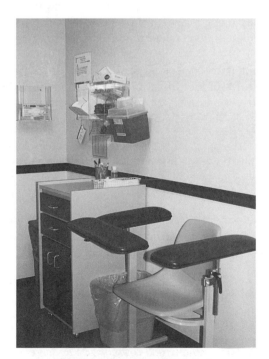

Figure 7-7 ■ Blood draw chair.

process. Cues that can help in the phlebotomy process include the following (Garza & Becan-McBride, 2002):

- *Diet:* It is important to note whether the patient has been fasting or not.
- *Stress:* A patient who is excessively anxious or emotional may need extra time.
- *Age:* The elderly may have more difficult or frail veins from which to choose for the venipuncture site. Pediatric patients often need additional support for venipuncture.
- *Weight:* Obese patient may require special equipment, such as a large blood pressure cuff for the tourniquet or a longer needle to penetrate the vein.

Patient Identification Process

The Joint Commission (TJC, 2003) National Patient Safety goals requires at least two patient identifiers (neither to be the patient's room number) whenever taking blood samples or administering medications or blood products. This reliably identifies the individual as the person for whom the service or treatment is intended; second, it matches the service or treatment to that individual.

Before any specimen collection procedure, the patient must be correctly identified by using a two-step process:

- The patient should be asked to state his or her first and last names.
- Confirm a match between patient's response, the test requisition, and some form of identification, such as hospital identification bracelet, driver's license, or another identification card.

NOTE > A hospitalized patient should always wear an identification bracelet indicating his or her first and last names and a designated hospital number.

Patients in outpatient clinics usually have the same procedures as inpatient clients, with use of identification bracelet or predistributed identification cards before any specimens are collected.

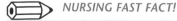 *NURSING FAST FACT!*

Technology has advanced such that many hospitals have one-and two-dimensional bar code technologies to enable more information to be encoded. Bar codes tend to be very accurate and cost-effective for larger organizations. The specimen labels are now bar coded. Refer to Figure 7-8.

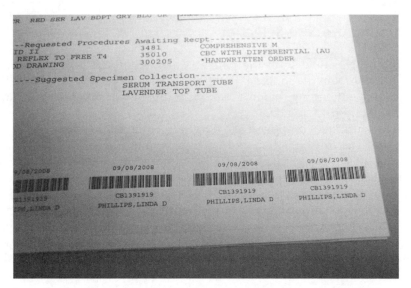

```
R   RED  SER  LAV  BDPT  GRY  BLU  OK

--Requested Procedures Awaiting Recpt----------------
ID II                      3481        COMPREHENSIVE M
REFLEX TO FREE T4          35010       CBC WITH DIFFERENTIAL (AU
D DRAWING                  300205      *HANDWRITTEN ORDER

----Suggested Specimen Collection------------------
                 SERUM TRANSPORT TUBE
                 LAVENDER TOP TUBE
```

Figure 7-8 ■ Sample bar code.

Blood specimen collection for blood banking, such as typing and crossmatching, may require additional patient identification procedures and armband application.

Care must be taken in identification of emergency room patients. Often when patients come to the emergency room, they are unconscious and/or unidentified. Each hospital has policies and procedures for dealing with these cases, which usually includes assigning the patient an identification tag with a hospital or medical record number.

INS Standard The nurse shall identify the patient by using at least two identifiers including, but not limited to, date of birth or photographs, prior initiation of therapy or procedure; neither identifier may be the patient's room number. (INS, 2006a, 66)

NOTE > Never attempt to collect a blood specimen from a sleeping patient. Such an attempt may startle the patient and cause injury to the patient or the phlebotomist.

Hand Hygiene/Gloving

Follow Standard Precautions by use of alcohol-based hand sanitizer before donning gloves for the procedure. When using hand sanitizers, it is important to use a generous amount and allow the alcohol to evaporate to achieve proper antisepsis. Don non-sterile gloves.

Venipuncture Site Selection

Position the patient with the patient's arm extended downward in a straight line from the shoulder to the wrist and not bent at the elbow. For the outpatient setting, blood is drawn with the patient sitting up in a special blood-drawing chair.

The tourniquet is applied 3 to 4 inches above the intended venipuncture site. The tourniquet should be tight enough to slow venous flow without affecting arterial flow. If a patient has prominent visible veins, tourniquet application can wait until after the site is cleaned and before insertion of the needle.

The most common site for venipuncture is in the antecubital area of the arm, where the median cubital veins lie close to the surface of the skin. Refer to Figure 7-9. The median cubital vein is most commonly used; the cephalic vein lies on the outer edge of the arm, and the basilic vein lies on the inside edge. The healthcare practitioner should palpate the veins to get an idea of the size, angle, and depth of the vein. The patient can assist in the process by closing his or her fist tightly (McCall & Tankersley, 2008).

The dorsal side of the hand or wrist should be used only if arm veins are unsuitable. Hand veins or the veins on the dorsal surface of the wrist are preferred over foot or ankle veins because coagulation and vascular complications may occur in the lower extremities, especially for diabetic patients. Position patients with hand well supported on the bed, rolled towel, or armrest.

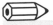 *NURSING FAST FACT!*

> ■ *Never draw above an infusing I.V.; this can alter the test results.*
> ■ *Use caution during venipuncture; although nerve damage during venipuncture is rare, it has been known to occur as a result of excessive needle probing and sudden movement of the patient.*
> ■ *Never place towels or washcloths in a microwave oven.*

INS Standard Blood samples should be obtained from the non-cannulated extremity. When this is not possible, the peripheral infusion should be stopped and the venipuncture should be made distal to the catheter location. (INS, 2006a, 66)

The venipuncture site may be warmed to facilitate vein prominence. A surgical towel or washcloth warmed to about 42°C and then wrapped around the site for 3 to 5 minutes can increase skin temperature. Encasing the towel or washcloth in a plastic bag or wrap helps to retain heat.

NOTE > According to NCCLS Standard H3-A5 (2003a) an attempt must have been made to locate the median cubital on both arms before considering an alternate vein, and due to possibility of nerve injury and damage to the brachial artery the basilic vein should not be chosen unless other vein is prominent.

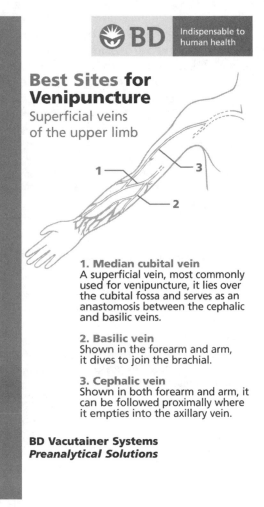

⊛**BD** | Indispensable to human health

Best Sites for Venipuncture
Superficial veins of the upper limb

1
2
3

1. Median cubital vein
A superficial vein, most commonly used for venipuncture, it lies over the cubital fossa and serves as an anastomosis between the cephalic and basilic veins.

2. Basilic vein
Shown in the forearm and arm, it dives to join the brachial.

3. Cephalic vein
Shown in both forearm and arm, it can be followed proximally where it empties into the axillary vein.

BD Vacutainer Systems
Preanalytical Solutions

Figure 7-9 ■ Best sites for venipuncture. (Courtesy of Becton Dickinson, Franklin Lakes, NJ.)

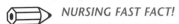 *NURSING FAST FACT!*

If the patient has sensitive skin or dermatitis, apply the tourniquet over a dry washcloth or gauze wrapped around the arm or a hospital gown sleeve.

Preparation of the Venipuncture Site

Once the site is selected, the site should be prepped with 70% isopropyl alcohol or chlorhexidine (ChloraPrep®) and allowed to dry. Alcohol is not recommended for use when obtaining a specimen for blood alcohol level determination. Chlorhexidine is recommended; however, check the institutional policy.

Povidone-iodine (Betadine) or chlorhexidine is usually used for drawing blood for blood gas analysis and blood cultures. Remove excess povidone-iodine from the skin with sterile gauze after prepping because iodine can interfere with some laboratory tests. Clean the site with a circular motion, starting at the point where you expect to insert the needle, and moving outward in ever-widening concentric circles until a 2- to 3-inch area is prepped (McCall & Tankersley, 2008).

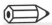 *NURSING FAST FACT!*

Do not touch the prepared venipuncture site after prepping. The alcohol should be allowed to dry (30–60 seconds). Do not fan the site with your hand or blow on it to hasten drying time.

Equipment Preparation and Venipuncture Technique

Place all collection equipment and supplies within easy reach, typically on the same side of the patient's arm as your free hand during venipuncture.

 NURSING FAST FACT!

Do not place the phlebotomy tray on patient's bed or any other place that could be considered contaminated.

Once the venipuncture site is prepped, and the tourniquet reapplied, the healthcare worker may hold the patient's arm below the site, pulling the skin tightly with the thumb (traction) to anchor the vein.

 NURSING FAST FACT!

For safety do not use a two-finger technique (also called "C") in which the entry point of the vein is straddled by the index finger above and the thumb below. If the patient pulls the arm back when the needle is inserted, there is a possibility that the needle may recoil as it comes out of the arm and spring back into the phlebotomist's index finger.

A safety syringe, butterfly, or Vacutainer system can be used for venipuncture. The needle should be lined up with the vein and inserted smoothly and quickly at approximately a 15- to 30-degree angle with the skin. The needle should be inserted with the bevel side upward and directly above a prominent vein or slightly below the palpable vein. Sometimes a slight "pop" can be felt when the needle enters the vein. Refer to Figure 7-10 for an illustration of how needle positioning can result in failure to draw blood.

The tourniquet can be released immediately after blood begins to flow so as not to collect blood that is **hemoconcentrated**. When a tourniquet is placed on the patient, the tourniquet pressure forces low molecular compounds and fluid to move into the tissues from the intravascular

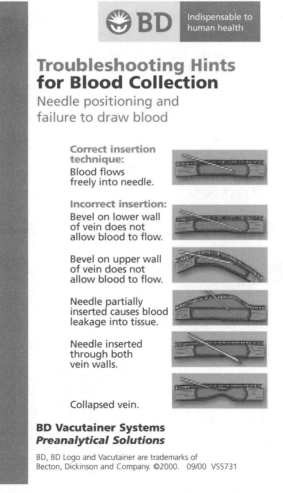

Figure 7-10 ■ Troubleshooting hints for blood collection. (Courtesy of Becton Dickinson, Franklin Lakes, NJ.)

space. Large molecules such as cholesterol and proteins cannot move through the capillary wall, and their blood levels increase as the tourniquet remains on the arm. In addition, the longer the tourniquet remains on the arm, the greater amount of potassium leakage occurs from tissue cells into the blood, increasing the chances of a false blood potassium level reading (Garza & Becan-McBride, 2002).

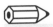 *NURSING FAST FACT!*

> ▪ *It is recommended that the tourniquet be released as the last tube is filling, but always before withdrawing the needle from the arm.*
> ▪ *If the patient continues to bleed, the healthcare practitioner should apply pressure until the bleeding stops.*

ETS Equipment Preparation and Venipuncture Technique

Select the appropriate ETS tubes based on requisition. Check the expiration date on each one of the tubes. Tap additive tubes lightly to dislodge any additive that may be adhering to the tube stopper. Inspect the seal of the needle, if broken discard. Twist the needle cover apart to expose the short or back end of the needle that is covered by a retractable sleeve. Screw this end of the needle into the threaded hub of an ETS tube holder. Place first tube in the holder and use a slight clockwise twist to push it onto the needle just far enough to secure it from falling out, but not far enough to release the tube vacuum. Refer to Figure 7-11.

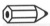 *NURSING FAST FACT!*

> ▪ *For beginners it is easier not to try to balance the tube in the holder before venipuncture. Access the vein and then pick up the tube and push it onto the inner needle.*
> ▪ *Vigorous handling of the blood tubes and sluggish propulsion of blood into the tube can cause hemolysis and separation of cells from liquid, which can affect the test results*
> ▪ *Some healthcare workers use the dominant hand to change tubes while the other hand keeps the needle apparatus steady.*

Refer to Procedures Display 7-1 at the end of this chapter for steps in performing the evacuated tube blood collection method.

When multiple sample tubes are to be collected, each tube should be gently removed from the Vacutainer holder and replaced with the next tube. Experienced healthcare workers are able to mix a full tube in one hand while holding the needle apparatus with the other hand. Multiple tubes can be filled in less than 1 minute if the needle remains stable in the vein and the vein does not collapse. The holder must be securely held while changing tubes so the needle is not pushed further into or removed from the vein.

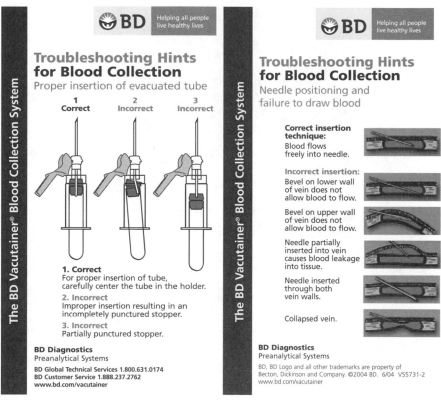

Figure 7-11 ■ Proper insertion of needle into Vacutainer holder. (Courtesy of Becton Dickinson, Franklin Lakes, NJ.)

After collection of the blood and removal of the last tube, the entire needle assembly should be withdrawn quickly. Safety devices should be activated immediately, depending on the manufacturer's specifications.

Winged Infusion Set Equipment Preparation and Venipuncture Technique

The 23-gauge winged set is most commonly used. Select the type of butterfly needle set either one with hub to attach a syringe or hub with a multisample Luer adapter that can be threaded onto an ETS tube holder. Refer to Figure 7-12. Verify the sterility of the packaging of needle before aseptically opening it. Attach the butterfly to the evacuated tube holder or syringe. Select small-volume tubes, larger tubes may collapse the vein or hemolyze the specimen. When using a butterfly needle on a hand vein, insert it into the vein at a shallow angle between 10 and 15 degrees. Use a 15- to 30-degree angle for antecubital vein.

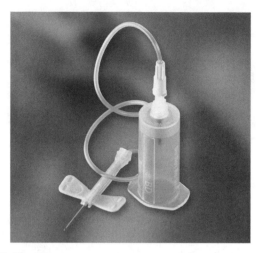

Figure 7-12 ■ Insertion of winged needle into ETS holder. (Courtesy of Becton Dickinson, Franklin Lakes, NJ.)

A winged infusion system can be used for particularly difficult venipunctures. This method is now used with safety equipment so as to decrease the risk of needlestick injuries to the healthcare worker. This method is sometimes useful for patients with:

- Small veins, such as the hand
- Pediatric or geriatric patients
- Restrictive positions, that is, traction, severe arthritis
- Patients with numerous needlesticks
- Patients with fragile skin and veins
- Short-term infusion therapy
- Patients who are severely burned

The needles range from ½ to ¾ inch in length and from 21- to 25-gauge in diameter. Attached to the needle is a thin tubing with a Luer adapter at the end so that it can be used on a syringe or an evacuated tube system from the same manufacturer.

 NURSING FAST FACT!

Because the tubing contains air, it will underfill the first evacuated tube by 0.5 mL. This affects the additive-to-blood ratio. A red-topped nonadditive tube should be filled before any tube with additives is filled.

Healthcare workers should be extra cautious as the needle is removed from the patient to activate the safety device that is built into the system. Use of the winged infusion or butterfly system requires training and practice. Failure to activate the safety devices correctly as described by the manufacturer may result in a higher incidence of needlestick injuries. Refer to Figure 7-13 for steps of push-button winged needle blood

BD Vacutainer® Push Button Blood Collection Set
In-Vein Needle Activation at the Push of a Button

General Use and Disposal (See package insert for detailed directions for use.)

   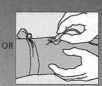

1a. Peel back packaging at arrow so that the back end of the wing set is exposed.

1b. With thumb and middle finger grasp the rear barrel of the wingset and remove from package. Be careful to avoid activating the button.

2. CAUTION - Never use a blood collection set without a holder or syringe attached.

Assemble to BD Vacutainer® One Use Holder or BD Syringe. (Disregard this step if pre-attached holder is used.)

3a. With thumb and index finger, grasp the wings together and access vein using standard needle insertion technique.

3b. If preferred by your institution, the body of the device can be held, instead of the wings, during insertion.

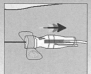 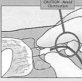

4. Proper access to the vein will be indicated by the presence of "flash" directly behind and below the button.

5a. The device is designed to be activated while the needle is still in the patient's vein. Place your gauze pad or cotton ball on the venipuncture site. Allow gauze pad or cotton ball to cover nose of front barrel. Following the collection procedure, and while the needle is still in the vein, grasp the body with the thumb and middle finger. Activate the button with the tip of the index finger.

5b. To ensure complete and immediate retraction of device, make sure to keep fingers and hands away from the end of the blood collection set during retraction. Do not impede retraction.

6. Apply pressure to the venipuncture site in accordance with your facility's protocol.

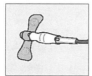

7. Confirm that the needle is in the shielded position prior to disposal.

8. Discard the entire shielded blood collection set and holder into an approved sharps disposal container.

Ordering Information

Facility Reference Number	BD Reference Number	Needle Gauge	Wing Color	Tubing Length	Configuration	Packaging
			BD Vacutainer® Push Button Blood Collection Sets with Pre-Attached Holder			
	367752	21		12"	with holder	20/Box 100/Case
	368656	23		12"	with holder	20/Box 100/Case
			BD Vacutainer® Push Button Blood Collection Sets			
	367338	21		7"	with luer	50/Box 200/Case
	367344	21		12"	with luer	50/Box 200/Case
	367326	21		12"	without luer	50/Box 200/Case
	367336	23		7"	with luer	50/Box 200/Case
	367342	23		12"	with luer	50/Box 200/Case
	367334	23		12"	without luer	50/Box 200/Case
	367341	25		12"	with luer	50/Box 200/Case
	367323	25		12"	without luer	50/Box 200/Case
			BD Vacutainer® One Use Holder			
Facility Reference Number	BD Reference Number	Description				Packaging
	364815	One Use Holder				250/Bag 1,000/Case

BD Global Technical Services: 1.800.631.0174
vacutainer_techservices@bd.com
BD Customer Service: 1.888.237.2762
www.bd.com/vacutainer

CAUTION:
Handle all biologic samples and blood collection "sharps" (lancets, needles, luer adapters, and blood collection sets) in accordance with the policies and procedures of your facility. Obtain appropriate medical attention in the event of any exposure to biologic samples (e.g., through a puncture injury) since samples may transmit viral hepatitis, HIV (AIDS), or other infectious diseases. Utilize any safety-engineered feature if the blood collection device provides one. Discard all blood collection "sharps" in biohazard containers approved for their disposal.

BD, BD Logo and all other trademarks are property of Becton, Dickinson and Company. © 2006 BD
05/06 VS7104-3

BD

Helping all people
live healthy lives

BD Diagnostics
Preanalytical Systems
1 Becton Drive
Franklin Lakes, NJ 07417
www.bd.com/vacutainer

Figure 7-13 ■ Vacutainer push button winged needle blood collection set steps. (Courtesy of Becton Dickinson, Franklin Lakes, NJ.)

collection. Refer to Procedures Display 7-2 at the end of this chapter for steps in using winged needle system for blood collection.

Syringe Equipment Preparation and Venipuncture Technique

Select a syringe and needle size compatible with the size and condition of the patient's vein and the amount of blood to be collected. Open the needle package aseptically then attach to the syringe. A blood specimen collected in a syringe will have to be transferred to ETS tubes.

When using a **syringe method** the same approach to needle insertion should be followed as is used for the evacuated tube method. Once the needle is in the vein, the syringe plunger can be drawn back gently to avoid hemolysis of the specimen until the required volume of blood has been withdrawn. The healthcare worker must be careful not to withdraw the needle from the vein while pulling back on the plunger.

 NURSING FAST FACT!

Turn the syringe so that the graduated markings are visible.
Refer to Procedures Display 7-3 at the end of this chapter for steps in the syringe method of blood collection.

Order of Tube Collection

The National Committee for Clinical Laboratory Standards (NCCLS, 2003b) recommends the following specific order when collecting multiple tubes of blood via the evacuated method or the syringe transfer method:

1. Blood culture tubes (yellow top), or blood culture vials or bottles
2. Coagulation tube (light blue top)
3. Red-topped glass nonadditive or plastic clot activator tubes (red topped)
4. Heparin tubes (green) or plasma separator tubes (PSTs) (green and gray, light-green plastic)
5. EDTA tubes (lavender or pink)
6. Oxalate/fluoride (glucose) tubes (gray)

Refer to Table 7-3 for order of draw for multiple tube collections.

Yellow–Light Blue–Red–Green–Lavender/Pink–Gray Tips

- Be meticulous about time, type of test, and the volume of blood required
- Blood cultures are always drawn first to decrease the possibility of bacterial contamination.
- When drawing just coagulation studies for diagnostic purposes, it is preferable that at least one other tube of blood be drawn before the coagulation test specimen. This diminishes contamination

> Table 7-3	ORDER OF DRAW FOR MULTIPLE TUBE COLLECTIONS	
Collection Tube	Mix by Inverting	Color
Blood cultures—SPS	8–10 times	Yellow
Coagulation Citrate tubes	3–4 times	Light blue
Serum tube (glass)	None glass	Red
Plastic clot activator tubes	5 times plastic	Red or red/gray rubber gold plastic
Plasma separator tubes (PSTs) with gel separator/ heparin	8–10 times	Green/gray Light-green plastic
Heparin tube	8–10 times	Green
EDTA tube	8–10 times	Lavender Pink
Oxalate/fluoride tubes	8–10 times	Gray

NOTE: Always follow your facility's protocol for order of draw.

Adapted courtesy of Becton Dickinson, Franklin Lakes, NJ.

with tissue fluids, which may initiate the clotting sequence Usually a nonadditive red top is used.

■ Coagulation tubes should be mixed as soon after collection as possible.

■ Minimize the transfer of anticoagulants from tube to tube by holding the tube horizontally or slightly downward during blood collection.

■ When a large volume (more than 20 mL) of blood has been drawn using a syringe, there is a possibility that some of the blood may be clotted.

■ If two syringes of blood have been withdrawn, NCCLS recommends taking blood from the second syringe for coagulation studies (NCCLS, 2003b).

■ Watch the "fill" rate and volume in each tube; evacuated tubes with anticoagulants must be filled to the designated level for the proper mix of blood with the anticoagulant.

NOTE > Partial fill tubes are available when it is suspected that the blood specimen will not be adequate.

Fill and Mix of Tubes

If the tube contains an additive, mix it by gently inverting it 3 to 8 times depending upon the type of additive and manufacturer's recommendations as soon as removed from the tube holder. Nonadditive tubes do not require mixing.

NOTE > Do not shake or vigorously mix blood specimens, as this can cause hemolysis.

Remove the last specimen tube from the holder before removing the needle from the vein. Gently but quickly remove the needle. After collection of the blood the entire blood collection assembly should be withdrawn quickly. Safety devices should be activated immediately, depending on the manufacturer's specifications.

A dry sterile gauze or cotton ball should be applied with pressure to the puncture site for several minutes or until bleeding has stopped. Keep the patient's arm straight, or elevate above the heart, if possible. A pressure bandage should be applied and the patient should be instructed to leave it on for at least 15 minutes.

Disposal of Equipment

All contaminated equipment should be discarded into appropriate containers. Paper and plastic wrappers can be thrown into a wastebasket. Needles and lancets should be placed into a sturdy puncture-proof disposable container following OSHA guidelines.

Any items, such as cotton or gauze, that have been contaminated with blood should be disposed of in biohazardous disposal containers following standard precautions.

Specimen Identification and Labeling

Specimens should be labeled immediately at the patient's bedside or ambulatory setting. Some laboratories require labels to be placed so that the label does not obscure the entire specimen. If using preprinted computer or bar code label, write the date, time, and your initials on label immediately after withdrawal from tube. Any handwritten labeling must be done with permanent ink pen with the following information:
- Patient's full name
- Patient's identification numbers
- Date and time of collection
- Healthcare worker's initials
- Patient's room number, bed assignment, or outpatient status are optional information.

Post-Procedure Patient Care

Once the last tube has been removed from the holder, fold a clean gauze square into fourths or use a cotton ball and lightly apply for venipuncture site. Do not press down until the needle is removed. Activate the safety feature of the needle according to the manufacturer's recommendations. Apply pressure to the site for 3 to 5 minutes or until the bleeding stops. Do not ask the patient to bend his or her arm.

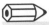 *NURSING FAST FACT!*

> *Folding the arm back at the elbow to hold pressure or keep the gauze in place after a blood draw actually increases the chance of bruising by keeping the wound open, or disrupting the platelet plug when the arm is lowered (McCall & Tankersley, 2008).*

Apply adhesive bandage (or tape and folded gauze or cotton ball) over the site. If the patient is allergic to adhesive bandage use paper tape and gauze. Instruct the patient to leave the bandage on for a minimum of 15 minutes, after which it should be removed to avoid irritation. Instruct an outpatient not to carry a purse or other heavy object for 1 hour.

 NURSING FAST FACT!

> *Failure to apply pressure or applying inadequate pressure can result in leakage of blood and hematoma formation.*
> *It is acceptable to have the patient hold pressure while you proceed to label tubes providing the patient is fully cooperative.*

Transport of the Specimen to the Laboratory

All specimens should be transported to the laboratory or designated pickup site in a timely fashion. The phlebotomist is typically responsible for verifying and documenting collection by computer entry or manual entry in a logbook (McCall & Tankersley, 2008).

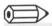 *NURSING FAST FACT!*

> *If the specimen cannot be transported to the laboratory within a reasonable time or if analysis is delayed, arrange for proper storage to prevent deterioration or contamination that can cause inaccurate results (Van Leeuwen, Kranpitz, & Smith, 2006).*

NURSING POINTS-OF-CARE
COLLECTION OF BLOOD SPECIMENS

Focus Assessment
- Assess the patient's understanding of the blood test.
- Assess the patient's degree of anxiety about the procedure.
- Assess the infant's or child's need for restraint and reassurance.

- Ensure that food, fluid, and medication restrictions have been followed.
- Verify the patient's identity using two identifiers.
- Assess both median antecubital sites for the appropriate venipuncture site.

Key Nursing/Phlebotomist Interventions

1. Select appropriate evacuated tubes, winged set or syringe.
2. Ensure the collected sample is valid by applying the tourniquet appropriately; avoid possible invalid testing caused by prolonged use of tourniquet, excessive suction on the syringe, or vigorous shaking of specimen in a tube.
3. Use aseptic technique.
4. Apply adhesive bandage after bleeding has stopped.
5. Provide support to the client if the puncture is not successful and another must be performed to obtain the blood sample.
6. Check the venipuncture site after 5 minutes for hematoma formation.
7. If the client is immunosuppressed, check the puncture site every 8 hours for signs and symptoms of infection.
8. Document in the patient medical record; include the amount of blood used for sampling and patient's response to the procedure (INS, 2006b).
9. Instruct the patient to leave the bandage over the site for a minimum of 15 minutes.

■ Complications

Hematoma

Hematoma formation is the most common complication of venipuncture. It is caused by blood leaking into the tissues during or after venipuncture and is identified by rapid swelling at or near the venipuncture site. Presence of a hematoma makes the site unacceptable for subsequent venipunctures.

If a hematoma forms during blood collection the draw should be discontinued, and pressure must be held over the site for 2 minutes. Cold compresses can be used for large hematomas to reduce swelling. Refer to Figure 7-14 for an example of hematoma formation after venipuncture.

NOTE > Ice can be applied for first 24 hours to help manage discomfort. After 24 hours heat or warm moist compresses can help reabsorb accumulated blood (McCall & Tankersley, 2008).

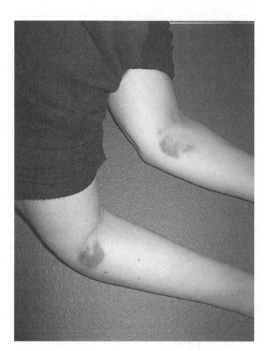

Figure 7-14 ■ Hematoma from multiple attempts at blood draw.

Iatrogenic Anemia

Blood loss as a result of blood removed for testing is called iatrogenic blood loss. Removing blood on a regular basis or in large quantities can lead to iatrogenic anemia in some patients, especially infants.

Infection

Although rare, infection at the site of venipuncture can occur. The risk of infection can be minimized by use of proper aseptic technique, hand hygiene and gloves.

Nerve Injury

Improper vein selection can lead to nerve injury during insertion of the needle too deeply or quickly. Movement by the patient as the needle is inserted can also cause nerve injury. Blind probing while attempting venipuncture can lead to injury of a main nerve.

 NURSING FAST FACT!

Extreme burning or pain, electric shock sensation, numbness of the arm, and pain that radiates up or down the arm are all signs of nerve involvement. Remove needle immediately. Applying an ice pack to the site can help reduce inflammation associated with nerve involvement (McCall & Tankersley, 2008).

Vein Damage

Numerous venipuncture in the same area over an extended period of time can cause a buildup of scar tissue and increase the difficulty of performing subsequent venipunctures. Blind probing and improper technique when redirecting the needle can also damage veins and impair patency (McCall & Tankersley, 2008).

AGE-RELATED CONSIDERATIONS
The Pediatric Client

Collection of blood by venipuncture from infants and children may be necessary for tests that require large amounts of blood (i.e., cross-matching and blood cultures).

- Venipuncture in children younger than the age of 2 should be limited to superficial veins. The accessible veins of infants and toddlers are veins of the antecubital fossa and forearm.
- **Heel Stick:** Capillary collection is normally recommended for pediatric patients, especially newborns and infants up to 12 months. Venipuncture is done in the area of the heel where there is little risk of puncturing the bone. According to CLSI the only safe areas of the heel are the plantar surface of the heel, medial to an imaginary line extending from the middle of the great toe to the heel or lateral to an imaginary line extending from between the fourth and fifth toes to the heel. Refer to Figure 7-15.
- **CLSI/NCCLS (2004) infant capillary puncture precautions include:**
  - Do not puncture earlobes.
  - Do not puncture deeper than 2.0 mm.
  - Do not puncture through previous puncture sites.
  - Do not puncture the area between the imaginary boundaries.
  - Do not puncture the posterior curvature of the heel.
  - Do not puncture in the area of the arch and any other areas of the foot.
  - Do not puncture severely bruised areas.

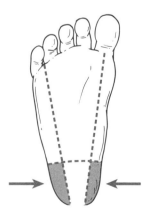

Figure 7-15 ■ Appropriate site for heel puncture on infant.

- Removal of large quantities of blood at once or even small quantities on a regular basis can lead to anemia. Removing more than 10% of an infant's blood volume at one time can lead to shock and cardiac arrest. Most facilities have limits on amount of blood that can be removed per draw. Many facilities do not allow more than 3% of a child's blood volume to be collected at one time, and no more than 10% in 1 month.

NOTE > CLSI (2003) recommends that procedures be in place to monitor amounts of blood drawn from pediatric, geriatric, and other vulnerable patients to avoid phlebotomy-induced anemia.

INS Standard For the pediatric patient the amount of blood obtained for laboratory assay should be documented in the patient's medical record. (INS, 2006a, 66)

- Interventions to ease pain include the use of EMLA cream, oral sucrose and pacifiers for infants and toddlers.

EBNP The use of 12%–24% solution of oral sucrose has been shown to reduce the pain of procedures such as heel puncture and venipuncture in infants up to 6 months of age. A 24% solution of sucrose can be administered by dropper, nipple, oral syringe, or on a pacifier, provided it will not interfere with the test to be collected. Sucrose nipples or pacifiers are available commercially. The sucrose must be given to the infant 2 minutes before the procedure (Gradin, Ericksson, Holmqvist, et al., 2002).

- Selecting the method of restraint is important in dealing with infants and children to ensure their safety. A newborn or young infant can be wrapped in a blanket but physical restraint is often required for older infants, toddlers, and younger children. Older children can sit by themselves in the blood drawing chair, but a parent or another phlebotomist should help steady the arm.

The Older Adult

Physical effects of aging, such as skin changes, hearing and vision problems; and mobility issues often related to a disease process require expert skills for a phlebotomist.

- Blood vessels lose elasticity, becoming more fragile and more likely to collapse, resulting in an increased change of bruising and failure to obtain blood.
- Hearing-impaired patients may strain to hear and have difficulty answering questions and understanding instructions.

- The phlebotomy area should have adequate lighting without glare. Assistance to drawing chair or escort to restroom may be needed. Provide instructions in large print.
- Slower nerve conduction may lead to slower learning, slower reaction times, and diminished perception of pain, which could lead to increase in injuries. Approach with a calm, professional manner.
- Effects of the disease process may affect blood collection. Patients who have coagulation disorders who take blood thinning medications are at risk for hematoma formation or uncontrolled bleeding at the blood collection site. Patients with Parkinson's disease may have difficulty with tremors and movement of the hands, which can make blood collection difficult.
- Poor nutrition can intensify the effects of aging on the skin, affect clotting ability, and contribute to anemia.
- If the patient is in a wheelchair and cannot be transported to the laboratory drawing chair, it is safest and easiest to draw blood with the patient in the wheelchair supporting the arm on a pillow or on a special padded board placed across the arms of the chair (McCall & Tankersley, 2008).

 Home Care Issues

A home care phlebotomist must have exceptional phlebotomy, interpersonal, and organizational skills; be able to function independently; and be comfortable working in varied situations. The physical setting can affect the collection of blood in the home care setting. If specimens are to be collected in homes, the procedures are similar and key points are listed.

- Obtain necessary supplies, including venipuncture supplies, blood collection tubes, a biohazard container for disposal and a specimen transport container, should be taken into the home.
- Perform hand hygiene: Wash hands before and after phlebotomy; most often, alcohol based hand gel is used.
- Identify the patient: Use at least two patient identifiers.
- Carefully inspect the area after the procedure to ensure that all trash and used supplies have been properly discarded before leaving the home environment.
- Label specimens and place in leakproof containers.
- Ensure that specimens are transported at appropriate temperatures.
- Reinforce patient education.

Patient Education

The first step and last steps of phlebotomy procedures is to prepare the patient for the procedure. Pretesting explanation to the patient or caregiver follows essentially the same pattern for all sites and types of studies and includes:

- Explain the purpose of the test.
- Describe the procedure, including site and method.
- Describe any sensations, including discomfort and pain that the patient may experience during the specimen collection procedure.

NOTE > Cultural and social issues, as well as concern for modesty, are important in providing psychological support.

- Instruct regarding pretesting preparations related to diet, liquids, medications, and activity as well as any restrictions.
- Identify any anxiety related to test results. Encourage the patient to ask questions and verbalize his or her concerns.
- Educate regarding any limitations of movement.
- Instruct the patient to notify the nurse if the puncture site begins to bleed after the pressure dressing is applied.
- Instruct the patient to notify the nurse if the puncture site becomes red, warm to touch, or pain develops (Van Leeuwen, Kranpitz, & Smith, 2006).

Nursing Process

The nursing process is a five- or six-step process for problem-solving to guide nursing action. Refer to Chapter 1 for details on the steps of the nursing process related to vascular access. The following table focuses on nursing diagnoses, nursing outcomes classification (NOC), and nursing interventions classification (NIC) for patients requiring laboratory analysis. The following table focuses on nursing diagnoses, NOC and NIC for patients requiring phlebotomy for laboratory analysis. Nursing diagnoses should be patient specific and outcomes and interventions individualized. The NOC and NIC presented here are suggested direction for development of specific outcomes and interventions.

Nursing Diagnoses Related to Management of Venipuncture for Laboratory Analysis	NOC: Nursing Outcomes Classification	NIC: Nursing Intervention Classification
Infection, risk for related to: Invasive procedure	Infection control, risk detection	Infection control, infection protection
Knowledge deficit related to: Information misinterpretation; lack of exposure; unfamiliarity with information resources (phlebotomy-lab analysis)	Health resources; knowledge of procedure	Teaching: Purpose of phlebotomy and laboratory tests
Skin integrity impaired related to: External: interruption in barrier protection—venipuncture	Skin integrity	Venipuncture site care; skin surveillance
Tissue integrity impaired related to: Mechanical factors—arterial puncture	Tissue integrity: skin and wound healing	Skin care; skin surveillance, wound care

Sources: *Ackley & Ladwig (2008); McCloskey-Dochterman &Bulechek (2004); Moorhead, Johnson, & Maas (2004); NANDA-I (2007).*

Chapter Highlights

- Specimens incorrectly acquired, labeled, or transported by the nurse can cause the laboratory tests to be useless or even cause harm to the patient.
- The nurse performing phlebotomy procedures must have the following knowledge base to perform blood withdrawal procedures safely: knowledge of basic anatomy and physiology, medical terminology, sources of error, safety measures and infection control practices, fundamental biology, quality control procedures, equipment and methods, sites for blood collection.
- A two-step process must identify the patient: ask name, and confirm the match among patient response, the test requisition, and ID bracelet.
- The vacuum (evacuated) tube system includes the evacuated sample tube, the double-pointed needle, and plastic holder.
- Vacuumized tubes for blood include those without additives and those with anticoagulant additives.
- Safety syringes should be used when the syringe method of blood collection is used.
- The antecubital area is the most frequently used area for blood collection. The dorsal side of hand or wrist should be used only if the arm veins are unsuitable.

- The tourniquet should be released once blood begins to flow into the tube (no longer than 1 minute) to prevent hemoconcentration of the blood specimen.
- The order of tube draw is: blood culture tubes (yellow), then plain tubes (nonadditives), coagulation tubes (light blue), additive tubes (green), EDTA (purple), and then oxalate/fluoride (gray top).

▬▬ Thinking Critically: Case Study

A 70-year-old Hmong, non–English-speaking woman was admitted to an acute care hospital, accompanied by her husband, who had limited English. On admission her physician had ordered a series of blood tests. When the healthcare worker arrived to collect blood for laboratory tests, she introduced herself and asked the patient her name. The patient did not respond and looked perplexed.
What should the healthcare worker do next?
What does The Joint Commission Patient Safety Goals state regarding patient identification?
What other factors need to be considered in this scenario (i.e., safety, ethics, legal)?

 Media Link: Answers to the case study and more critical thinking activities are provided on the CD-ROM.

Post-Test

1. Which of the following anticoagulants is found in a green-topped collection vacuum tube?

    a. EDTA
    b. Sodium citrate
    c. Sodium heparin
    d. Ammonium oxalate

2. The color coding for tubes indicates the:

    a. Length of needle needed to access the tube
    b. Manufacturer
    c. Additive contained within the tube
    d. Amount of blood necessary to fill the tube

3. From the following list of tubes, which would be the first tube to be used in the evacuated tube system?

    a. Lavender-topped tube
    b. Yellow-topped tube
    c. Light blue–topped tube
    d. Red-topped tube

4. What causes evacuated tubes to fill with blood automatically?

   a. Tube vacuum
   b. Pressure created by the application of the tourniquet
   c. Venous pressure
   d. Fist pumping by the patient

5. The most common site for venipuncture is in which of the following areas?

   a. The dorsal side of the wrist
   b. The antecubital fossa of the arm
   c. Hand veins
   d. The heel

6. Blood collection tubes are labeled:

   a. Before the collection
   b. Immediately after specimen collection
   c. After all draws are completed
   d. Whenever it is convenient for the phlebotomist.

7. Which of the following tubes contain an anticoagulant additive? (*Select all that apply.*)

   a. Lavender
   b. Pink
   c. Green
   d. Red

8. In which of the following situations may the use of a winged needle system be beneficial? (*Select all that apply.*)

   a. Heel puncture
   b. Veins in the hand
   c. Geriatric patients
   d. Central line blood collection

9. Which of the following solutions is used most frequently as a prep solution for venipuncture for lab collection of blood chemistry?

   a. 70% Isopropyl alcohol
   b. Povidone-iodine
   c. 2% Iodine
   d. Acetone

10. What is the minimum amount of time a pressure bandage should be left in place after a venipuncture for blood collection?

   a. 5 minutes
   b. 10 minutes
   c. 15 minutes
   d. 30 minutes

Media Link: Answers to the Chapter 7 Post-Test and more test questions together with rationales are provided on the CD-ROM.

▪ REFERENCES

Ackley, B.J., & Ladwig, G.B. (2008). *Nursing diagnosis handbook: An evidence-based guide to planning care* (8th ed.). St. Louis, MO: Elsevier Mosby.

Garza, D., & Becan-McBride, K. (2002). *Phlebotomy handbook* (6th ed.). Upper Saddle River, NJ: Prentice–Hall, pp. 183–271.

Gradin, M., Ericksson, M., Holmqvist, A., et al. (2002). Pain reduction at venipuncture in newborns; oral glucose compared with local anesthetic cream. *Pediatrics, 110,* 1053–1057.

Infusion Nurses Society (INS). (2006a). Infusion nursing standard of practice. *Journal of the Infusion Nursing, 29*(IS), S71–72.

Infusion Nurses Society (INS). (2006b). *Policies and procedures for infusion nursing* (3rd ed.). Norwood MA: Author

McCall, R.E., & Tankersley, C.M. (2008). *Phlebotomy essentials* (4th ed.). Philadelphia: Lippincott Williams & Wilkins.

McCloskey-Dochterman, J.C., & Bulechek, G.M. (2004). *Nursing interventions classification (NIC)* (4th ed.). St. Louis, MO: C.V. Mosby.

Moorhead, S., Johnson, M., & Maas, M. (2004). *Nursing outcomes classification (NOC)* (3rd ed.). St. Louis, MO: C.V. Mosby.

NANDA-I. (2007). *Nursing diagnoses: Definitions and classification, 2007–2008.* Philadelphia: Author.

National Committee for Clinical Laboratory Standards (NCCLS). (1992). Clinical laboratory improvement amendments of 1988: Final standard is published. *Clinical Chemistry News,* March.

National Committee for Clinical Laboratory Standards (NCCLS). (2003a). *Procedures for the collection of diagnostic blood specimens by venipuncture.* Approved Standard, H3-A5. Wayne, PA: Author.

National Committee for Clinical Laboratory Standards (NCCLS). (2003b). *Evacuated tubes and additives for blood specimen collection* (5th ed.). Approved Standard, H1-A5. Wayne, PA: Author.

National Committee for Clinical Laboratory Standards (NCCLS). (2004). *Procedures and devices for the collection of diagnostic capillary blood specimens* (5th ed.). Approved Standard, H1-A5. Wayne, PA: Author.

The Joint Commission (TJC). (2003). 2003 National patient safety goals. Retrieved from http://www.jointcommission.org/Patient Safety (Accessed September 16, 2008).

Van Leeuwen, A.M, Kranpitz, T.R., & Smith, L. (2006). *Davis's comprehensive handbook of laboratory and diagnostic tests with nursing implications* (2nd ed.). Philadelphia: F.A. Davis.

PROCEDURES DISPLAY 7-1

Collection of Blood in Evacuated Tube System

Equipment Needed
Gloves
Tourniquet
Sharps container
Waste receptacle
Collection vials or tubes
Vacutainer tube holder
ETS needle
Labels (bar coded) for tubes
Transport container
Site disinfectant (70% alcohol, or chlorhexidine gluconate, or povidone-iodine)
Gauze pads or cotton ball
Tape
Delegation:
This procedure can be delegated to phlebotomist.

Procedure	Rationale
1. Review the test request.	1. A test request is reviewed for completeness, date and time of collection, status, and priority. A written order is a legal requirement for blood analysis.
2. Approach, identify, and prepare the patient. Introduce yourself to the patient. Use two identifiers to verify patient identity. Place the patient in a position of comfort and safety, arm extended and in a dependent position if possible if in hospital bed. Use a draw chair in outpatient setting. Explain the procedure to the patient. Verify diet restrictions and latex sensitivity.	2. Establishes the nurse–patient relationship The Joint Commission (2003) safety goal recommendation. Explaining the procedure reduces anxiety Test results can be meaningless or misinterpreted and patient care compromised if diet requirements have not been followed. Exposure to latex can trigger a life-threatening reaction.

PROCEDURES DISPLAY 7-1

Collection of Blood in Evacuated Tube System—cont'd

Procedure	Rationale
3. Arrange all supplies in an accessible place so that reaching for equipment is minimized. Line up tubes in the order of draw.	3. Having all equipment at hand will save time and lessen patient anxiety.
4. Hand hygiene procedure/ don gloves; use alcohol-based product.	4. Good hand hygiene is the single most important means of preventing the spread of infection. According to OSHA BBP standard gloves must be worn.
5. Apply tourniquet, locate the vein, usually the antecubital fossa, usually the median cubital. Release the tourniquet.	5. A tourniquet is placed 3–4 inches above the antecubital area; it dilates veins and makes them easier to see, feel, and enter with a needle.
6. Cleanse the area with 70% alcohol or chlorhexidine, using a circular or back-and-forth technique. Allow the skin to air-dry or blot with sterile gauze.	6. Avoids contaminating the specimen with bacteria picked up by the needle. Letting the site dry naturally permits maximum antiseptic action.
7. Select the appropriate equipment for the size, condition, and location of the vein. Prepare while the site is drying. Attach a needle to an ETS holder. Put the first tube in the holder at step 7 or wait until after needle entry (step 10).	7. Ensure successful blood draw, make sure accuracy of test results.
8. Reapply the tourniquet.	8. Allows for dilation of vein.

Continued

PROCEDURES DISPLAY 7-1

Collection of Blood in Evacuated Tube System—cont'd

Procedure	Rationale
9. Apply traction to the skin of the forearm, below the intended venipuncture site, to stabilize the vein. Hold the vacuum tube assembly between the thumb and last three fingers of your dominant hand. Rest the backs of these fingers on the patient's arm. The free index finger rests against the hub of the needle and serves as a guide. With the needle held at an angle of 15–30 degrees to the arm and in line with the vein, insert the needle into the vein, with the bevel up.	9. Anchoring the skin so the needle enters easily and with less pain, and keeps vein from rolling.
10. Once you feel that you are in the vein, change your grip: the hand that was stabilizing the vein in place should now hold the hub firmly, while the index and third finger of the dominant hand grip the tube. This will prevent movement of the needle. Now use your thumb to gently but firmly push the tube onto the needle. This will allow the vacuum to pull blood into the tube.	10. Blood will not flow until the needle pierces the tube stopper.

PROCEDURES DISPLAY 7-1

Collection of Blood in Evacuated Tube System—cont'd

Procedure	Rationale
11. Fill the additive tubes until the vacuum is exhausted and mix them immediately on removal from the holder using 3–10 gentle inversions (depending on the type and manufacturer). Follow the order of draw. If more than one tube is to be drawn, pull the filled tube out of the hub very gently with the hand that pushed it in.	**11.** To ensure correct blood-to-additive ratio.
12. When the last tube of blood is drawn, remove it from the hub. Release the tourniquet, during filling of the last tube, then gently remove the needle from the arm and place a cotton ball or small gauze pad over the puncture site. Ask the patient to put pressure on the area if appropriate.	**12.** Prevent hematoma formation.
13. Activate the safety feature on the needle	**13.** OSHA standard.
14. Label all samples at the bedside.	**14.** Avoid mislabeling errors
15. Examine patient's arm to verify bleeding has stopped on the skin surface. If stopped, apply bandage and advise patient to keep it in place for a minimum of 15 minutes.	**15.** Prevent hematoma formation and bleeding.

Continued

PROCEDURES DISPLAY 7-1

Collection of Blood in Evacuated Tube System—cont'd

Procedure	Rationale
16. Dispose of used and contaminated materials in biohazard container and sharps container.	16. OSHA requirement
17. Remove gloves, sanitize hands.	17. Remove gloves in an aseptic manner and wash or decontaminate hands as infection control precaution.
18. Transport specimen to the laboratory.	18. Prompt delivery to the laboratory protects specimen integrity.

Sources: McCall & Tankersley (2008); INS (2006b).

PROCEDURES DISPLAY 7-2

Collection of Blood Using a Winged or Butterfly Collection Set

Equipment Needed
Gloves
Tourniquet
Sharps container
Waste receptacle
Butterfly (winged) needle with safety feature
ETS tube holder
Collection tubes
Labels (bar coded) for tubes or permanent marking pen
Transport container
Site disinfectant (70% alcohol, or chlorhexidine gluconate, or povidone-iodine)
Gauze pads or cotton ball
Tape
Delegation:
This procedure can be delegated to a phlebotomist.

PROCEDURES DISPLAY 7-2

Collection of Blood Using a Winged or Butterfly Collection Set—cont'd

Procedure	Rationale
1. Review the test request.	1. A test request is reviewed for completeness, date and time of collection, status, and priority. A written order is a legal requirement for blood analysis.
2. Approach, identify, and prepare the patient. Introduce yourself to the patient. Use two identifiers to verify patient identity. Place the patient in a position of comfort and safety, arm extended and in a dependent position if possible if in hospital bed. Use a draw chair in the outpatient setting. Explain the procedure to the patient. Verify diet restrictions and latex sensitivity.	2. Establishes the nurse–patient relationship. The Joint Commission (2003) safety goal recommendation. Explaining the procedure reduces anxiety. Test results can be meaningless or misinterpreted and patient care compromised if diet requirements have not been followed. Exposure to latex can trigger a life-threatening reaction.
3. Arrange all supplies in an accessible place so that reaching for equipment is minimized. Line up tubes in the order of draw.	3. Having all equipment at hand will save time and lessen patient anxiety.
4. Hand hygiene procedure/ don gloves; use an alcohol-based product.	4. Good hand hygiene is the single most important means of preventing the spread of infection. According to OSHA BBP standard gloves must be worn.
5. Apply tourniquet, locate the vein, usually the median antecubital fossa. Release the tourniquet.	5. A tourniquet is placed 3-4 inches above the antecubital area; it dilates veins and makes them easier to see, feel, and enter with a needle.

Continued

PROCEDURES DISPLAY 7-2

Collection of Blood Using a Winged or Butterfly Collection Set—cont'd

Procedure	Rationale
6. Cleanse the area with 70% alcohol or chlorhexidine, using a circular or back and forth technique. Allow the skin to air-dry or blot with sterile gauze.	6. Avoids contaminating the specimen with bacteria picked up by the needle. Letting the site dry naturally permits maximum antiseptic action.
7. Select the appropriate equipment for the size, condition, and location of the vein. Prepare while the site is drying. Attach the butterfly to an ETS holder. Grasp the tubing near the needle end and run your fingers down its length, stretching it slightly to help keep it from coiling back up. Position the first tube in the holder now or wait until vein entry.	7. Ensure successful blood draw, first step in accuracy of test results.
8. Reapply the tourniquet.	
9. Apply traction to the skin of the forearm, below the intended venipuncture site, to stabilize the vein. Hold the wing portion of the butterfly between your thumb and index finger or fold the wings upright and grasp them together. Cradle the tubing and holder in the palm of your dominant hand or lay it next to the patient's hand. Uncap and inspect the needle for defects, and discard if flawed.	9. Anchoring the skin so the needle enters easily and with less pain, and keeps the vein from rolling.

PROCEDURES DISPLAY 7-2

Collection of Blood Using a Winged or Butterfly Collection Set—cont'd

Procedure	Rationale
10. Insert the needle into the vein at a shallow angle between 10 and 15 degrees. A flash or small amount of blood will appear in the tubing when the needle is in the vein. Slightly thread within the lumen of the vein.	10. Winged needles can pierce the vein, causing a hematoma. Thread the needle carefully in the vein. Flash of blood indicates vein entry.
11. Establish blood flow, by placing the tube in the holder and push it part way onto the needle with a clockwise twist. Grasp the holder flange with your middle and index fingers, pulling back slightly to keep the holder from moving, and push the tube onto the needle with your thumb. Release the tourniquet.	11. Blood will not flow until the needle pierces a tube stopper. Release of tourniquet allows blood flow to normalize.
12. Maintain the tubing and holder below the site and positioned so that the tubes fill from the bottom up to prevent reflux. Fill additive tubes. Immediately upon removal use 3–10 gentle inversions (depending on type and manufacturer) to prevent clot formation. Follow CLSI Order of Draw.	12. To ensure correct blood-to-additive ratio.

Continued

PROCEDURES DISPLAY 7-2

Collection of Blood Using a Winged or Butterfly Collection Set—cont'd

Procedure	Rationale
13. Place a clean gauze over the site—apply pressure after the needle is removed from the hub. Ask the patient to put pressure on the area if appropriate.	13. Prevent hematoma formation.
14. Activate the safety feature on the needle.	14. OSHA standard to prevent needlestick injuries.
15. Label all samples at the bedside.	15. Avoid mislabeling errors
16. Examine the patient's arm to verify that bleeding on the skin surface has stopped. If stopped, apply bandage and advise patient to keep it in place for a minimum of 15 minutes.	16. Prevent hematoma formation and bleeding.
17. Dispose of used and contaminated materials in a biohazard container and sharps container.	17. OSHA requirement
18. Remove gloves; sanitize hands using alcohol-based product for 15 seconds.	18. Remove gloves in an aseptic manner and hands washed or decontaminated as infection control precaution.
19. Transport the specimen to the laboratory.	19. Prompt delivery to the laboratory protects specimen integrity.

Sources: INS (2006b); McCall & Tankersley (2008).

PROCEDURES DISPLAY 7-3

Collection of Blood Using the Syringe Method

Equipment Needed
Gloves
Tourniquet
Sharps container
Waste receptacle
Syringe
Syringe needle
ETS tubes
Labels (bar coded) for tubes or permanent marking pen
Transport container
Site disinfectant (70% alcohol, or chlorhexidine gluconate, or povidone-iodine)
Gauze pads
Tape
Delegation:
This procedure can be delegated to a phlebotomist.

Procedure	Rationale
1. Review the test request.	1. A test request is reviewed for completeness, date and time of collection, status, and priority. A written order is a legal requirement for blood analysis.
2. Approach, identify, and prepare the patient. Introduce yourself to the patient. Use two identifiers to verify patient identity. Place the patient in a position of comfort and safety, arm extended and in a dependent position if possible if in hospital bed. Use a draw chair in outpatient setting. Explain the procedure to the patient. Verify diet restrictions and latex sensitivity	2. Establishes the nurse–patient relationship The Joint Commission (2003) safety goal recommendation. Explaining the procedure reduces anxiety. Test results can be meaningless or misinterpreted and patient care compromised if diet requirements have not been followed. Exposure to latex can trigger a life-threatening reaction.

Continued

PROCEDURES DISPLAY 7-3

Collection of Blood Using the Syringe Method—cont'd

Procedure	Rationale
3. Arrange all supplies in an accessible place so that reaching for equipment is minimized. Line up tubes in the order of draw.	3. Having all equipment at hand will save time and lessen patient anxiety.
4. Hand hygiene procedure/ don gloves; use an alcohol-based product.	4. Good hand hygiene is the single most important means of preventing the spread of infection. According to OSHA BBP standard gloves must be worn.
5. Apply the tourniquet, locate the vein, release tourniquet. Note: The vein used most frequently is the median antecubital fossa	5. A tourniquet is placed 3–4 inches above the antecubital area; it dilates the veins and makes them easier to see, feel, and enter with a needle.
6. Cleanse the area with 70% alcohol or chlorhexidine, using a circular or back–and-forth technique. Allow the skin to air-dry or blot with sterile gauze.	6. Avoids contaminating the specimen with bacteria picked up by the needle. Letting the site dry naturally permits maximum antiseptic action.
7. Select the appropriate equipment for the size, condition, and location of the vein. Prepare while site is drying. Select a syringe needle according to the size and location of the vein; select the appropriate size syringe and tube size. Attach the needle to the syringe; do not remove the cap at this time. Hold the syringe as you would an ETS tube holder.	7. Ensure accuracy of test results. First step in accuracy of test results.
8. Reapply the tourniquet.	8. A tourniquet aids in dilation of vein.

PROCEDURES DISPLAY 7-3

Collection of Blood Using the Syringe Method—cont'd

Procedure	Rationale
9. Apply traction to the skin of the forearm, below the intended venipuncture site, to stabilize the vein. Hold the syringe in your dominant hand as you would an ETS holder. Place your thumb on top near the needle end, and fingers underneath. Uncap and inspect the needle for defects and discard if flawed.	9. Facilitates venipuncture and placement of the needle correctly in the vein.
10. Ask the patient to make a fist, line the needle up with the vein, and insert it into the skin using a smooth forward motion. Stop when you feel a decrease in resistance, often described as a "pop," and press your fingers into the arm to anchor the holder.	10. Anchoring stretches the skin so the needle enters smoothly with less pain.
11. Establishment of blood flow is normally indicated by blood in the hub of the syringe. Release the tourniquet and have the patient open his or her fist.	11. Allows blood flow to return to normal and helps prevent hemoconcentration. (According to CLSI Standard H3-A5, the tourniquet should be released as soon as possible after blood begins to flow and should not be left on longer than 1 minute.)
12. Fill the syringe.	12. Venous blood will not automatically flow into a syringe. It must be filled by slowly pulling back on the plunger with your free hand.

Continued

PROCEDURES DISPLAY 7-3

Collection of Blood Using the Syringe Method—cont'd

Procedure	Rationale
13. Place a folded gauze square over the site or cotton ball and apply pressure immediately after the needle is removed.	13. Prevent damage to vein and hematoma formation.
14. Discard the needle, fill the tubes, discard the syringe, and add the transfer device. An ETS tube is placed in the transfer device in the order of draw and pushed onto the internal needle until the stopper is pierced. Blood from the syringe is then safely drawn into the tube. Several tubes can be filled as long as there is enough blood in the syringe.	14. The needle must be removed and discarded in a sharps container so that a transfer device for filling the tubes can be attached to the syringe. A transfer device greatly reduces the chance of accidental needlesticks and confines any aerosol or spraying that may be generated as the tube is removed.
15. After use, the syringe and transfer device unit is discarded in the sharps container.	15. OSHA standard to prevent needlestick injuries.
16. Label all samples at the bedside.	16. Avoids mislabeling errors.
17. Examine the patient's arm to verify bleeding has stopped on the skin surface. If stopped, apply bandage and advise the patient to keep it in place for a minimum of 15 minutes.	17. Prevents hematoma formation and bleeding.

PROCEDURES DISPLAY 7-3

Collection of Blood Using the Syringe Method—cont'd

Procedure	Rationale
18. Dispose of used and contaminated materials in a biohazard container and a sharps container.	18. OSHA requirement
19. Remove gloves and sanitize hands.	19. Remove gloves in an aseptic manner and wash or decontaminate hands as infection control precaution.
20. Transport the specimen to the laboratory.	20. Prompt delivery to the laboratory protects specimen integrity.

Sources: INS (2006); McCall & Tankersley (2008b).

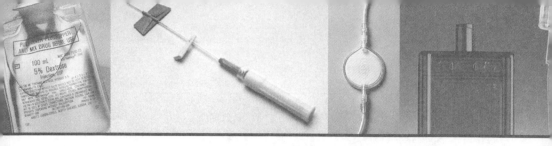

Chapter **8**

Techniques for Initiation and Maintenance of Central Venous Access

The expert nurse, with an enormous background of experience, now has an intuitive grasp of each situation and zeros in on the accurate region of the problem without wasteful consideration of a large range of unfruitful, alternative diagnoses and solutions.

—*Patricia Benner*

LEARNING OBJECTIVES

On completion of this chapter, the reader will be able to:

1. Define the glossary of terms as related to nursing care of the patient with a central venous access device.

2. Discuss evidence-based practices related to care and maintenance of central venous access devices (CVADs).

3. Assess risk and benefits for central venous catheter (CVC) placement.

4. Identify tip location for a properly placed central venous access device.

5. Explore the impact of federal and professional nursing guidelines when articulating policy and procedures for care of CVADs.

6. Identify advantages and disadvantages of different types of CVCs.

7. List the steps for dressing management of CVCs, with an emphasis on aseptic technique.

8. Compare and contrast advantages and disadvantages of nontunneled CVCs, peripherally inserted central catheters (PICCs), tunneled catheters, and implanted ports.

9. Explore the impact on catheter integrity and syringe size when maintaining patency of a CVC.

10. Identify care and maintenance of central venous catheters.

GLOSSARY

Anthropometric measurement   Measurement of the size, weight, and proportions of the human body

Biocompatibility   The quality of not having toxic or injurious effect on biological systems

Broviac catheter   Tunneled venous catheter with one Dacron cuff with an outer diameter of 1.0; useful for infusion of nutrient solutions, commonly used in the pediatric patient population

Central venous catheter (CVC)   Catheter inserted into the central circulation for infusion therapy, the tip located in the superior vena cava. All central lines are central venous catheters.

Central venous tunneled catheter (CVTC)   Catheter inserted into a centrally located vein with tip residing in the vena cava via tunneling subcutaneously from the site between sternum and nipple on chest wall to subclavian vein

Distal   Farthest from the heart; farthest from the point of attachment; below previous site of cannulation

External jugular   The vein located on the exterior aspect of the neck

Groshong® valve   Flaplike structure resembling a valve that retards or prevents a reflux of fluid or blood

Hickman catheter   Long-term tunneled Silastic catheter inserted surgically

Implanted port   Catheter surgically placed into a vessel, body cavity, or organ and attached to a reservoir, which is placed under the skin

Infraclavicular   Situated below a clavicle

Lymphedema   Swelling of an extremity caused by obstruction of lymphatic vessels

Peripherally inserted central venous catheter (PICC)   Catheter inserted into the superior vena cava through a peripheral vein; usually cephalic or basilic at the median cubital area

Polyurethane   Medical grade resins, widely varying in flexibility, used in chemical-resistant coatings and adhesives used to make catheters for venous access

Ports Distal: Lumen located farther from the catheter tip. **Medial:** The center lumen of a triple lumen catheter. **Proximal:** Lumen nearest the tip

Pulsatile flushing   Rapid succession of pulsatile push-pause–push-pause movements that create turbulence within the catheter lumen that causes a swirling effect to move any debris.

Silicone elastomer   A polymer of organic silicone oxides, which may be a liquid, gel, or solid depending on the extent of polymerization; used in surgical implants, a coating on the inside of glass vessels for blood collection. Some VADs are made of silicone elastomer.

Thrombogenicity   Generation or production of thrombosis

Trendelenburg position   Position in which the head is lower than the feet; used to increase venous distention

Tunneled catheter   A central catheter designed to have a portion lie within a subcutaneous passage before exiting the body

Valsalva maneuver   The process of making a forceful attempt at expiration with the mouth, nostrils, and glottis closed

Vascular access device (VAD)   Venous access device inserted into a main vein or artery, or bone marrow and used primarily to administer fluids and medication, monitor pressure, and collect blood.

◼ Anatomy of the Vascular System

The background of the anatomy and physiology of the upper extremity venous system, arm, and axilla is important for the infusion nurse to understand before placement of **central venous catheters (CVCs)**. These structures impact successful placement and tip location and ultimately the successful dwell time of the CVC. The important veins include the basilic, cephalic, axillary, subclavian, internal and external jugular, right and left innominate (brachiocephalic) veins, and superior vena cava (SVC). It is also imperative that registered nurses caring for CVCs are fully aware of the anatomic position and structures of the arm and axilla venous system.

Venous Structures of the Arm

The superficial veins of the upper extremities lie in the superficial fascia and are visible and palpable. Superficial veins include the cephalic and the basilic veins. The cephalic vein ascends along the outer border of the biceps muscle to the upper third of the arm. It passes in the space between the pectoralis major and deltoid muscles. The vein decreases in size just a few inches above the antecubital fossa and may terminate in the axillary vein or pass above or through the clavicle in a descending curve. Normally, the cephalic vein turns sharply (90 degrees) as it pierces the clavipectoral fascia and passes beneath the clavicle. Near its termination, the cephalic vein may bifurcate into two small veins, one joining the external jugular vein and one joining the axillary vein. Valves are located along the cephalic vein's course (Standing, 2004).

The basilic vein is larger than the cephalic vein. From the posterior–medial aspect of the forearm, it passes upward in a smooth path along the inner side of the biceps muscle and terminates in the axillary vein. The origins of these veins in the lower arm are most often used for short-term peripheral devices. At and above the antecubital fossa, these veins are appropriate for the placement of **PICCs** and arm ports.

Valves are present in the venous system until approximately 1 inch before the formation of the brachiocephalic vein. The presence of valves within veins helps to prevent the reflux of blood and is especially important in the lower extremities, where venous return is working against gravity (Fig. 8-1).

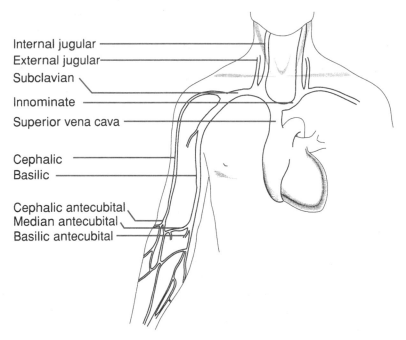

Internal jugular
External jugular
Subclavian
Innominate
Superior vena cava
Cephalic
Basilic
Cephalic antecubital
Median antecubital
Basilic antecubital

Figure 8-1 ■ Anatomic venous structures of the arm and chest. (From Markel, S., & Reynan, K. [1980]. Impact on patient care: 2652 PIC catheter days. *Journal of Intravenous Nursing*, 13[6], 349. Copyright 1990 by the *Journal of Intravenous Nursing*.)

Venous Structures of the Chest

The main venous structures of the chest include the subclavian, the internal and external jugular, and brachiocephalic veins (formerly called the innominate veins), and the SVC. Large veins in the head, neck and chest do not have valves. Gravity helps blood to flow properly from the head and neck, and negative intrathoracic pressure promotes flow from the head and neck and the inferior vena cava.

The subclavian vein extends from the outer border of the first rib to the sternal end of the clavicle and measures about 4 to 5 cm in length; the right brachiocephalic vein measures about 2.5 cm and the left brachiocephalic vein measures about 6 to 6.5 cm. The external jugular lies on the side of the neck and follows a descending inward path to join the subclavian vein along the middle of the clavicle. The internal jugular vein descends first behind and then to the outer side of the internal and common carotid arteries; it joins the subclavian vein at the root of the neck.

The right brachiocephalic (innominate) vein is about 1 inch long and passes almost vertically downward to join the left brachiocephalic (innominate) vein just below the cartilage of the first rib. The left brachiocephalic vein is about 2.5 inches long and is larger than the right vein. It passes from left to right in a downward slant across the upper front of the chest. It joins the right brachiocephalic vein to form the SVC. The SVC receives all blood from the upper half of the body. It is composed of a short trunk 2.5 to 3.0 inches long in an average adult. It begins below the first rib close to the sternum on the right side, descends vertically slightly to the right, and empties into the right atrium of the heart. The right atrium receives blood from the upper body via the SVC and from the lower body via the inferior vena cava. The vena cava are referred to as the great veins. Table 8-1 summarizes the **anthropometric measurements** of the upper extremity veins.

 NURSING FAST FACT!

> ■ *Blood flow in the SVC in the average adult is approximately 1.5–2.5 L/min. Poiseuille's law (fourth power law) states that flow through a single vessel is most affected by the vessel diameter, and as vessel diameter increases, the flow rate increases by a factor of 4. For example, when the diameter doubles, flow rate increases 16 times; when the diameter increases by 4, the flow rate increases 256 times The amount of blood flow in the veins follows this law:*
> *Cephalic and basilic veins: 45–95 mL/min*
> *Subclavian veins: 150–300 mL/min*
> *Superior vena cava: 2000 mL/min*

■ General Overview of Central Vascular Access Devices

Choosing the most appropriate **vascular access device (VAD)** for a patient is a collaborative process involving the patient, the practitioner placing the device, and the patient's referring physician. Knowledge of venous anatomy and physiology, VAD technology, and the patient's current health status and infusion plan are important aspects in this process. The goal of VAD selection and placement should be to deliver safe, efficient therapy that maximizes the patient's quality of life, with minimal risk of complication.

> Table 8-1	ANTHROPOMETRIC MEASUREMENTS OF VENOUS ANATOMY	
Vein	**Length, cm**	**Diameter, mm**
Cephalic	38	6
Basilic	24	8
Axillary	13	16
Subclavian	6	19
Right brachiocephalic	2.5	19
SVC	7	20

SVC = *superior vena cava.*

There are two types of central vascular access devices (CVADs): short-term and long-term devices. Short-term devices include nontunneled percutaneous catheters and peripherally inserted central catheters. Long-term devices include tunneled catheters and implanted ports.

The nontunneled percutaneous catheter, which is intended for use up to 7 to 10 days, is usually placed at the bedside, there is not a cuff; therefore the device is held in place by sutures or a securement device (Hamilton, 2006). The **peripherally inserted central catheter (PICC)** is a short-term device usually inserted in patients who require intravenous access from a few weeks to several months. It is inserted into the antecubital fossa or upper arm vein and advanced until the catheter reaches the superior vena cava.

The long-term CVADs are used when long-term access for infusion is needed. The external tunneled catheters are placed in the chest region via the subclavian or jugular vein. The term "tunneled" is derived from the insertion technique, which involves tunneling the **proximal** end subcutaneously from the insertion site and bringing it out through the skin at an exit site (INS, 2008). Embedded in the catheter is a cuff, which is a silver-impregnated tissue barrier. The purpose of the cuff is twofold: after about 2 to 3 weeks, the skin forms scar tissue around the cuff, thus fixing the catheter within the subcutaneous tunnel to prevent dislodgement. The cuff also acts as a barrier against the entry of microorganisms (Massorli & Angeles, 2002).

The implanted port contains a reservoir or port housing with a catheter attached to the reservoir. The port is located within a subcutaneous pocket under the skin. Locations can include the chest, abdomen, or inner aspect of the forearm. The port housing is made of titanium or plastic and encases a self-sealing septum made of **silicone**.

The port housing can be either single- or multilumen. Access is obtained by inserting a special noncoring needle through the skin and into the septum using sterile technique. The noncoring needle can remain in place up to 7 days (INS, 2006a, 45).

Assessment and Device Selection

There are multiple factors to consider in a comprehensive client assessment before initiation of central infusion therapy. Assessment parameters that must be considered before device selection and placement include prescribed therapy, expected duration of therapy, health history (including the client's vascular integrity), device availability, and client preferences (Higuchi, Edwards, Danseco, et al., 2007).

According to INS (2006a), correct VAD choice is based on the patient's history, physical exam, diagnosis, type and length of therapy, and available nursing skills to place and maintain the device. This is the first step in assessing for positive outcomes.

Physical factors need to be considered during assessment including the suitability of target vessels that should be evaluated for size and patency, inspection of skin for breaks in integrity, implanted pacemaker or cardioverter defibrillator, and assess for a VAD already in place (Ludeman, 2007). The vein must be large enough to accommodate the selected VAD to minimize the risk of phlebitis and thrombosis. The smallest device in the largest vein allows for maximal hemodilution of the infusate. Patients who are very thin may benefit from the newer "low-profile" port devices.

Patient preference and lifestyle should be evaluated, including the nondominant arm for ease of self-care should be considered if appropriate. The patient's lifestyle is an important consideration in choosing an implanted versus an external device. Take into consideration activity restrictions, maintenance requirements, body image distortion, and ease of use. The patient's usual occupational and recreational activities need to be included in the assessment process.

The ability of the patient or designated caregiver to manage day-to-day VAD care and infusions should be assessed before device selection and placement. Important considerations include the ability to see, hear, perform fine motor tasks, read and understand written instructions, and emotionally cope with the demands of site care and therapy. In addition, the home environment and caregiver support for patients who will transition from acute care to home care should be evaluated. The decision to place a CVC should be made after considering the risks and benefits to each patient.

Documentation supports evidence of nursing process related to initial assessment, action plan, communication of the plan, and ongoing monitoring of the patient. Documentation that can be retrieved for chart audits includes:
- Thorough, systematic assessment of:
  - Patient health problems
  - Previous I.V. complications
  - Purpose, nature, and duration of I.V. therapy
  - Patient needs/preferences
- Thorough information of planned action
  - Discussion of recommendation and planned action with patient and family
  - Discussion of multidisciplinary plan
- Clear evidence of communication of decision to healthcare team
- Evidence of consistent monitoring during each drug administration or nursing
- Intervention (Higuchi, Edwards, Danseco, et al., 2007).

Therapeutic indications include:
- Administration of chemotherapy
- Administration of total parenteral nutrition
- Administration of blood products
- Administration of medications
- Intravenous fluid administration

■ Performance of plasmapheresis
■ Performance of hemodialyis

Diagnostic indications include:
■ To establish or confirm a diagnosis
■ To establish a prognosis
■ To monitor response to treatment
■ For repeated blood sampling

Factors that need to be considered (assessed) before commitment to a CVC include coagulopathy, venous stenosis, acute thrombosis, and local skin infection at the insertion site. These abnormalities should be corrected, or considered as part of the risk/benefit ratio prior to cannulation (Lewis, Allen, Burke, et al., 2003).

Conditions that Limit VAD Placement

Conditions that may limit VAD site placement are listed in Table 8-2. These challenges can be overcome with careful device selection and placement.

> Table 8-2	CONDITIONS AFFECTING VASCULAR ACCESS DEVICE SITE PLACEMENT
Previous Surgical Interventions	Lymph node dissections Subclavian vein stenting or resection Vena cava filters Myocutaneous flap reconstruction Skin grafts Previous vein harvesting Presence of A–V grafts and hemodialysis fistulas Presence of intravascular stents
Cutaneous Lesions in Proximity to VAD Exit or Puncture Site	Herpes zoster and skin tears Malignant cutaneous lesions Bacterial or fungal lesions and non-intact skin Burns Extensive scarring or keloids
Disease Process or Conditions	Severe thrombocytopenia (< 50,000 platelets) Other coagulopathy (i.e., hemophilia, idiopathic thrombocytopenia purpura, thrombotic thrombocytopenia purpura) Concurrent anticoagulation therapy Lymphedema Allergies Extremity paraplegia Preexisting vessel thrombosis or stenosis
Other Considerations	Site within current radiation port Infection near exit site (e.g., tracheostomy) Morbid obesity Patient inability to position desired site for placement Patient inability to tolerate insertion procedure

Knowledge of the type of therapy can help identify the desired VAD and the number of lumens that will be necessary to deliver safe infusions. The number of concurrent and intermittent infusions along with drug compatibility and stability need to be considered. Nutritional solutions with final concentrations of 10% dextrose or 5% protein (or both) should be infused through a central line with the tip placed in the superior vena cava (SVC) (INS, 2006a, 75). Continuous vesicant therapy, solutions with extremes of pH (less than 5 or greater than 9) or medications with osmolarity greater than 600 mOsmol/L also should be given through a CVC (INS, 2006a, S37). Infusion of caustic, hypertonic fluids without the benefit of hemodilution in the SVC can result in thrombosis and loss of the vessel for future use.

Selection of Device

Selection of a device is influenced by the cost, risk factors, and benefits of various VADs in relation to any conditions that could limit VAD access, as well as patient and therapy characteristics.

The least expensive and invasive device is not necessarily the most appropriate selection, depending on the risks associated with peripheral infusions of irritant or vesicant agents. Using a venous access device selection algorithm along with a thorough patient assessment can help with device selection (Fig. 8-2).

Central Venous Catheter Materials

Most VADs are made of silicone elastomers, or thermoplastic urethane (polyurethane) are the two basic materials used in the manufacturing of long-term (greater than 30 days implant) venous access cannulation devices. The most common engineering characteristics used to describe the properties of both polyurethanes and silicones are tensile strength, ultimate elongation, durometer, and flexural modulus (DiFiore, 2005).

Tensile strength according to governing equations for vascular access must be very strong but remain soft and pliable while indwelling. The tensile strength is measured in pounds force per square inch (psi) and allows the material to resist breaking under high loads.

Ultimate elongation is usually measured as the relative change in length of a catheter that has been placed under load, to the breaking point. Catheters possessing elongation psi of 400% to 700% are usually very pliable, making them ideal for vascular placement. Less pliable catheters are easier to insert; however, they can create intravascular irritation leading to phlebitis.

Durometer is a measure of the hardness of a material. Hardness does not relate to stiffness of a device but to resistance of the material to compression. A low-durometer material is more easily compressed and feels

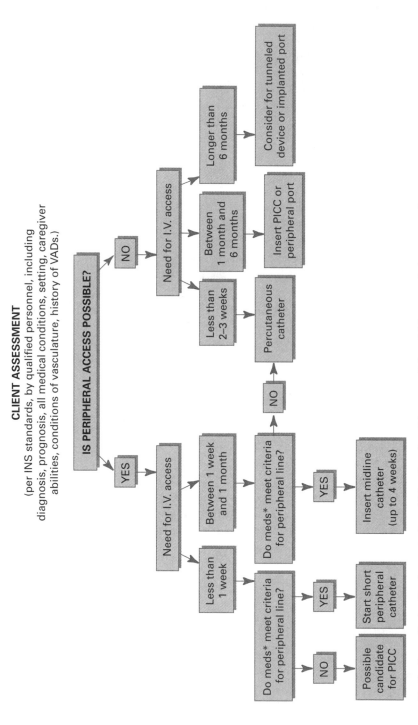

CLIENT ASSESSMENT

(per INS standards, by qualified personnel, including diagnosis, prognosis, all medical conditions, setting, caregiver abilities, conditions of vasculature, history of VADs.)

IS PERIPHERAL ACCESS POSSIBLE?

Medication criteria: Final osmolarity < 500 mOsm/L, pH between 5.0 and 9.0, not an irritant or vesicant.

Figure 8-2 ■ Venous access device selection algorithm.

softer than high-durometer material. Flexural modulus or its stiffness, is a way to describe the resistance of a material to events that would fatigue the catheter. Materials with high flexural moduli are much stiffer than those with low moduli and can be pushed easier through tissue and guidewires. Large-bore over-the-wire catheters tend to be stiffer than tunneled devices (DiFiore, 2005).

All catheters, whether they are used for short- or long-term access, should have a radiopaque lateral strip or a radiopaque distal end for visualization on radiography of tip location, and identification of a catheter fracture.

Silicone Elastomers

Silicone elastomers (Silastic®) are soft and pliable and cannot be inserted by the conventional over-the-needle technique. Catheters made of Silastic® require special insertion procedures with or without guidewires. Because of its soft, flexible nature, silicone is less likely to damage the intima of the vein wall and is reported to cause less fibrin adherence and thus decrease the risk of thrombosis or occlusion. Many PICCs are made of this biocompatible material. An additional advantage is decreased chance of catheter breakage. Silicone has a lower tensile strength and lower psi elongation than polyurethane; however, it has very good chemical resistance.

Polyurethane

Polyurethane catheters (Tecoflex®, Tecothane®, Carbothane®, Chronoflex®, Pellethane®) may be emerging as the most commonly used catheters because of the material's versatility, malleability (i.e., tensile strength and elongation characteristics), and **biocompatibility**. Polyurethane catheters do not have any plasticizers or other harmful additives that can be readily extracted. Polyurethane is a commonly used material for short-term percutaneously placed CVCs and is being used in long-term CVCs and PICCs. **Polyurethane** is stiffer than silicone, making threading of the catheter easier, and softens with increased temperature. Polyurethane catheters have thinner walls than silicone catheters owing to greater tensile strength and allow greater flow volume. Polyurethane is similar to silicone in biocompatibility and is thrombus resistant (DiFiore, 2005; Mayer & Wong, 2002).

Catheter Coatings

Certain catheters and cuffs are coated or impregnated with antimicrobial or antiseptic agents, which have been shown in multiple studies to decrease the risk for catheter-related bloodstream infection (CR-BSI). The coated catheters currently available include:

- Chlorhexidine/silver sulfadiazine: A combination of chlorhexidine/silver sulfadiazine on the external luminal surface, and a second-generation catheter with a coating on the internal surface extending into the extension set and hubs
- Minocycline/rifampin: Impregnated catheter on both the external and internal surfaces O'Grady, Alexander, Dellinger, et al., 2002)

NOTE > All studies involving antimicrobial/antiseptic impregnated catheters have been conducted using triple-lumen, noncuffed catheters in adults in place less than 30 days. All catheters that are impregnated currently are approved by FDA for patients weighing greater than 3 kg (O'Grady, Alexander, Dellinger, et al., 2002).

NOTE > Potential development of resistant organisms is a concern with these catheters (Sampath, Tambe, & Modak, 2001).

EBNP A multicenter, randomized, double-blind, controlled trial of 9 university-affiliated medical centers with 780 patients in ICU who required central venous catheterization was studied using two types of catheters (one with chlorhexidine/silver sulfadiazine and one without). The results demonstrated that the second-generation antiseptic catheter, coated with chlorhexidine and silver sulfadiazine on the internal and external surfaces, is effective in preventing microbial colonization (Rupp, Lisco, Lipsett, et al., 2005).

The VitaCuff® is a stand-alone add-on device made of silver ions in a biodegradable collagen matrix that is placed around the catheter (Fig. 8-3). The cuff works in conjunction with the Dacron cuff, an inherent component of some catheters, and is positioned beneath the skin surface during catheter placement. The device's collagen band is impregnated with silver ions that are released over several weeks, creating a physical barrier to bacteria. Silver ions have broad-spectrum activity against many of the bacteria and fungi that are related to catheter infections.

The CDC (2002) states that "the decision to used chlorhexidine/silver sulfadiazine– or minocycline/rifampin–impregnated catheters should be based on the need to enhance prevention of CR-BSI after standard procedures have been implemented (e.g., educating personnel, use of maximal sterile barrier precautions, and using 2% chlorhexidine skin antiseptics) and then balanced against the concern for the emergence for resistant pathogens and the cost implementing this strategy"(O'Grady, Alexander, Dellinger, et al., 2002).

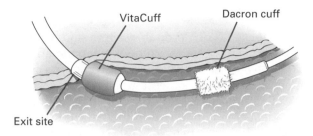

Proper VitaCuff positioning

Figure 8-3 ■ Positioning of VitaCuff® antimicrobial cuff. (Courtesy of Bard Access Systems, Salt Lake City, UT.)

Tip Configurations

Central venous access devices offer a range of tip configurations: open-ended and valved-tip devices. The open-ended catheters can be associated with more complications than valved devices including hemorrhage, air embolism, and occlusion from clots or fibrin. Open-ended CVADs should be clamped when not in use (Miller, 2006).

The valved-tip CVADs operate by a pressure-activated two- or three-way slit valve either at the distal end of the tip or located within the hub of the device (Fig. 8-4).

The smooth design and lack of rough edges on the tip decreases adherence of platelets or fibrin. Valved CVADs do not require clamping. Clamping can increase pressure, forcing the valves open and allowing blood to reflux up the lumen. Valved CVADs also require less frequent maintenance with flushing (Moorehead & Bergeron, 2007).

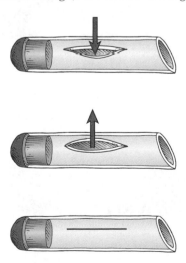

Figure 8-4 ■ Valved tip central venous catheter (Groshong tip). (Courtesy of Bard Access Systems, Salt Lake City, UT.)

Lumen Types

Catheters are available with single, double, triple, and quadruple lumens. The diameter of each lumen varies, allowing for the administration of hypertonic or viscous solutions. The lumens come in a wide variety of sizes, with an ample variety of lumen diameters, the selection of which depends on the clinical needs. Each lumen opens at a different point on the catheter for adequate dilution within the vessel. Refer to Figure 8-5. Refer to each particular manufacturer's information to ascertain which lumen is the largest if rapid administration is needed. A catheter with staggered lumens opens at different points on the catheter.

Multiple-lumen CVADs allow for a dedicated port for blood sampling. Refer to Figure 8-6. Port (lumen) protocols currently used are based on the following:

- **Distal port**: 16 gauge CVP monitoring and high-volume or viscous fluids, colloids, medications (distal port is the largest lumen), administration of blood or CVP monitor
- **Medial port 18 gauge:** Reserved exclusively for total parenteral nutrition (TPN). Medication only if TPN not ordered.
- **Proximal port 18 gauge**: Blood sampling, medications, or blood component administration
- **Fourth port 18 gauge:** Infusion of fluids or medications

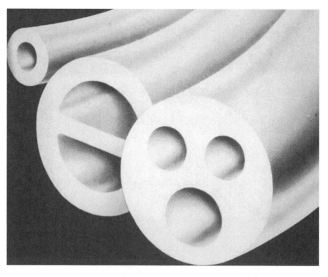

Figure 8-5 ■ Example of single, double, and triple lumens. (Courtesy of Bard Access Systems, Salt Lake City, UT.)

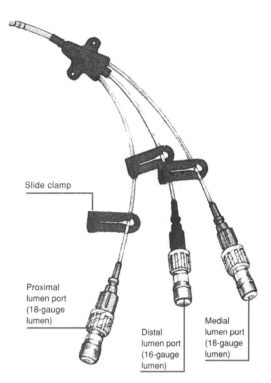

Slide clamp

Proximal
lumen port
(18-gauge
lumen)

Distal
lumen port
(16-gauge
lumen)

Medial
lumen port
(18-gauge
lumen)

Figure 8-6 ■ Injection ports of the triple-lumen catheter include the proximal lumen port, distal lumen port, and medial lumen port. The distal port *(middle line)* is usually the largest of the three lines.

Disadvantages of multi-lumen CVADs includes the small individual-lumen diameter and long catheter length, resistance to flow is high, making these catheters difficult to use for rapid fluid infusions. The multilumen catheter has a higher risk of infection due to more entry ports for microorganisms (Maki & Mermel, 2007). These catheters are more expensive and require more maintenance.

Catheter Length and Gauge

Length

The length of the CVAD can affect the ability to infuse solutions or medications. Multi-lumen catheters can range in length from 15 cm to 20 cm and PICC lines from 50 to 60 cm.

INS Standard The smallest size and shortest length that will accommodate the prescribed therapy. (INS, 2006a, 38)

Gauge and Flow

The gauge of a catheter influences flow rate. Gauge depends in part on the type of material from which the catheter is made. Ranges from 3 French to 7 French are available for single- and multi-lumen catheters. Silicone catheters tend to be smaller gauge than those made of polyurethane and have slower flow rates.

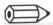 *NURSING FAST FACT!*

> *Equivalent gauge and French sizes of common central venous catheters are as follows:*
> *23 ga = 2.0 Fr*
> *20 ga = 3.0 Fr*
> *18 ga = 4.0 Fr*
> *16 ga = 5.0 Fr*
> *14 ga = 6.0 Fr*
> *(Gabriel, 2005)*
> *Manufacturers identify the flow rates for their catheters (INS, 2008a).*

NOTE > Flow rates of silicone vs. polyurethane:
4-Fr silicone on gravity 30 to 100 mL/hr; on a pump 125 to 250 mL/hr
4-Fr polyurethane on gravity 55 to 187 mL/hr; on a pump 545 to 965 mL/hr

Vascular Access Teams

Specially trained I.V. teams have demonstrated effectiveness in reducing complications associated with CVADs, especially infections, and have proven cost effective (O'Grady, Alexander, Dellinger, et al., 2002; Schelonka, Scruggs, Nichols, et al., 2006). The use of consistent, dedicated PICC teams have improved patient safety, decreases multiple insertion attempts, and improves outcomes (Burns, 2005). Early vascular access assessments are a multidisciplinary effort. Early assessment through a team concept may decrease the pain and suffering caused by short-term peripheral venous access. These teams may perform all PICC insertions, conduct daily surveillance of each catheter and dressing, perform dressing change, troubleshoot catheter problems, provide formal and informal staff education, and conduct outcome monitoring. A team concept further minimizes the use of inappropriate device selection and inappropriate catheter tip location (Pettit & Wyckoff, 2007).

Some I.V. teams today have one team responsible for PICC insertion and an additional educated team designated for care and maintenance, following standardized protocols (Linck et al., 2007). Advancing the team concept to include full responsibility for the CVC program is the ultimate goal, along with reduction of catheter-related bloodstream infections.

Quality improvement programs are an integral component of a hospital's PICC program.

Minimal criteria for outcome monitoring for PICCs as well as other CVADs should include as part of the documentation the following:

- Patient's weight at time of catheter insertion
- Indication for placement
- Catheter specifics (brand, composition, size, number of lumens)
- Complications occurring during insertion, dwell, or removal
- Length of catheter dwell
- Reason for removal

▪ Short-Term Access Devices

There are two short-term central venous access devices: nontunneled percutaneous catheters and peripherally inserted central catheters (PICCs). Short-term access devices are intended to be used for days to several months. These devices can be single- or multiple-lumen catheters made of silicone or polyurethane.

They are inserted by a percutaneous venipuncture and are not tunneled under the skin. The infraclavicular, jugular, or femoral veins are the sites if the insertion is performed by a physician, and the veins of the extremities are used if the insertion is performed by a registered nurse specially trained for peripheral central venous access. A recent position paper by the Infusion Nurses Society (INS) supports the external jugular peripherally inserted central catheters (EJPICCs) placement by qualified licensed proficient infusion therapy (INS, 2008b).

Nontunneled Percutaneous Catheters

The nontunneled CVADs are large-bore catheters inserted into the subclavian vein for fast access. In 1961, the first I.V. catheter for accessing the central circulation was introduced. Subclavian catheterization was initially inserted using surgical cutdown technique. However, percutaneous introduction into the subclavian vein using the Seldinger through-the-needle guidewire technique is now generally preferred. The percutaneous short-term catheter is secured by suturing, and the catheter is not tunneled. This catheter may remain in place for 7 to 10 days.

The most common site for insertion of percutaneous catheters is the **infraclavicular** approach to the subclavian vein. However, because of the need for preservation of the subclavian vasculature, it is important to avoid in certain patients. Subclavian vein catheterization for temporary access should be avoided in all patients with kidney failure and in patients with a history of renal failure or impending renal failure because of the risk of stenosis of the central veins. Use of central venous catheters is associated with a high degree of central venous stenosis, particularly in the subclavian vein, and placement of venous catheters may damage target vasculature necessary for dialysis access (National Kidney Foundation, 2002).

Insertion

CVADs are usually inserted by a physician. Strict aseptic technique is maintained during the procedure. During subclavian insertion, the patient is placed in the Trendelenburg position with a rolled bath blanket or towel between his or her shoulders. The patient should be instructed to perform a **Valsalva maneuver** during the venipuncture procedure to increase the size of the veins, and guard against air emboli. A 14-gauge needle is inserted into the subclavian vein, using the clavicle as a guide. When a venous blood return is obtained in the syringe, the syringe is disengaged from the needle and a guidewire is fed through the needle into the vein, then the needle is removed and discarded. The catheter is then fed over the wire into the subclavian vein, the tip rests in the superior vena cava. This exit site on the upper chest is well suited for many types of dressings, and care of the site is not complex.

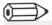 *NURSING FAST FACT!*

- *The infraclavicular approach site requires a well-hydrated patient.*
- *After insertion of the catheter, final verification by chest radiography must be obtained before any infusion. Chest x-ray confirmation should occur before the administration of vesicant chemotherapy and whenever tip location is questioned. After placement, the catheter can be maintained as a closed, patent device with an injection cap and heparinized while the catheter tip location is verified by radiologic examination. Do not infuse any solution before this radiographic confirmation.*
- *Central catheters should never be placed in the right atrium. When CVCs are placed in the right atrium, there is a risk of dysrhythmias, pericardial puncture, and fluid entry into the pericardial space, which can cause cardiac tamponade, a complication with a mortality rate of 78%–98%.*

The internal jugular vein is an accessible site for the physician; however, care of this site is more difficult. The motion of the neck, a beard on men, long hair, and close proximity of respiratory secretions prevent the adequate use of transparent occlusive dressings. The femoral veins are not recommended for this type of therapy because of the difficulty of placement of the catheter tip. It is also impossible to maintain an occlusive dressing on the femoral exit site.

Current patient safety recommendations advocate the use of ultrasound guidance in the placement of percutaneous and peripherally inserted central catheters. This technique is designed to help identify blood vessels and thereby avoid the inadvertent puncture of an artery before inserting a catheter. Ultrasound also allows for needle guidance and visual confirmation of catheter insertion within the selected vessel with greater success and fewer attempts (Anstett & Royer, 2003).

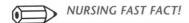 *NURSING FAST FACT!*

> *Of the four types of CVADs nontunneled catheters have the highest infection rate, so meticulous nursing care is demanded (Masoorli & Angeles, 2002).*

Peripherally Inserted Central Catheters

Peripherally inserted central catheters were introduced in the late 1970s as a means to administer infusates when traditional routes of venous access were unachievable. The PICC is a percutaneous I.V. line composed of silicone elastomers or polyurethane. It may have single or multiple lumens with ranges in lengths from 33 to 60 cm and diameters of 14 to 25 gauge (e.g., 3 Fr/20-gauge). Dual-lumen PICCs are the most commonly inserted PICC lines, allowing for multiple antibiotic or medication administration (Moureau, 2006). The dual-lumen PICCs have 18-gauge (4 Fr) to 20-gauge (3 Fr) lumens, whereas others are 20-gauge (3 Fr) and 23-gauge (2 Fr). Insertion is usually via the modified Seldinger micropuncture technique (MST), using a needle and guidewire. It is recommended that this PICC be placed in the upper arm. The placement of PICCs by registered professional nurses requires specialized education and demonstrated competency. PICCs are designed for delivery of therapies extending beyond 6 days to several months, with some PICCs having been documented with a dwell time of more than a year.

Indications for PICC Use

The following indications for PICC use include medical-based and specific prescribed therapies.

MEDICAL DIAGNOSES

Medical-based indications for PICC use include infectious diseases (e.g., osteomyelitis, endocarditis, delayed wound healing secondary to infection, meningitis, multiple abdominal fistulae), oncologic diseases, gastrointestinal (GI) diseases (e.g., pancreatitis, hyperemesis gravidarum, malabsorption syndromes), and low birth weight neonates. PICCs are also indicated when preexisting illness prevents the placement of a percutaneous device (low platelet count, neutropenia, inability to tolerate Trendelenburg position for placement of the device).

Therapies

Specific prescribed therapies for PICC use include drugs or infusates with extreme variations in osmolarity; parenteral nutrition formulations with dextrose contents greater than 10% or osmolarity greater than 50%; irritating anti-infective agents such as vancomycin, nafcillin, and amphotericin B; vesicant or irritant therapies; and prolonged duration of therapy (more than 6 days), such as with pain management or chronic vasopressor infusions.

Advantages

1. Peripheral insertion eliminates the potential complication of pneumothorax or hemothorax; significant reduction in risk of CR-BSI as compared to nontunneled catheters.
2. Decreases risk of air embolism owing to the ease of maintaining the insertion site below the heart and a small diameter.
3. Decreases pain and discomfort associated with frequent venipunctures for peripheral sites.
4. Preserves peripheral vascular system of upper extremities.
5. Is cost effective and time efficient.
6. Is appropriate for home placement and home I.V. therapy.
7. Risk of infiltration and phlebitis is reduced, especially with upper arm placement.
8. Appropriate for individuals of all ages.
9. May be used for laboratory draws if catheter diameter is appropriate (2 Fr not recommended).
10. Can be discontinued by an RN.
11. Carries a lower risk of infection 0.4 to 2.46/1000 catheter days (Moureau, Poole, Murdock, et al., 2002; Safdar & Maki, 2005).

Disadvantages/Risk

1. Possible bruising around the insertion site.
2. Special training is required to perform the procedure.
3. Forty-five minutes to 1 hour is needed to complete procedure.
4. Daily or weekly care is required.
5. Consistent flushing after infusions and blood draws are necessary to prevent clotting of the catheter.
6. Small-lumen PICCs may cause difficulty in obtaining blood samples because of fibrin buildup or partial withdrawal occlusion.
7. Contraindicated in patients whose lifestyles or occupations involve being in water; those with preexisting skin infections in the arm; those with anatomic distortions related to injury, surgical dissection, or trauma; and those with coagulopathies.
8. Requires chest radiography for placement verification before initiation of therapy as with all CVADs.
9. Potential for vein thrombosis and catheter occlusion.

Newer Technology: Power-Injectable PICCs

Power injection PICCs were developed to withstand higher psi during power injection of contrast media. Many manufacturers have developed the power-injectable PICCs. This catheter is engineered to tolerate injection pressures up to 240 psi and to accept a flow rate of 2 to 4 mL per second. The power injectable PICC is available in lumen 4 or 5 Fr single- and 6 Fr dual-lumen. An example of the power injection PICC is the Bard POWER PICC® (Bard, Salt Lake City, UT), which is purple and labeled on the hub for identification. Refer to Figure 8-7. Its insertion procedure, care and maintenance are the same as for any polyurethane catheter (C.R. Bard 2008; Pieger-Mooney, 2005).

NOTE > The FDA has issued a reminder to radiologists, radiologic technologists, radiologic nurses, and I.V. team nurses about the potential for serious patient injury involved in the improper usage of a power-injectable device. Be sure to follow the manufacturer's recommendations for use of device and know limit setting, maximum pressure, and flow rate of PICC.

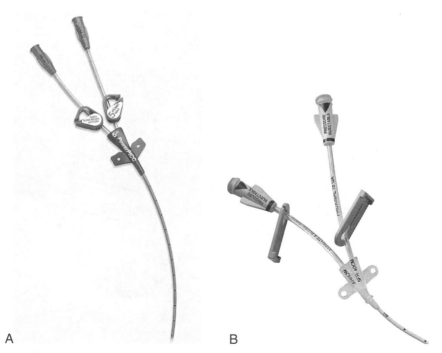

A   B

Figure 8-7 ■ *A*, Power PICC. (Courtesy of Bard Access Systems, Salt Lake City, UT.) *B*, Pressure injectable PICC. (Courtesy of Arrow International Teleflex Medical, Reading, PA.)

Vein Selection

The peripheral veins of the arm in adults and the arm and leg in children are the usual sites for PICC access (Fig. 8-8). Other veins that may be used include the basilic, cephalic, median–cephalic, brachial, and median–basilic veins and **external jugular.** The cephalic and median–cephalic veins are usually avoided if possible because of the higher incidence of tip malposition with placement. Brachial access requires ultrasound guidance to avoid arterial or nerve access.

 NURSING FAST FACT!

> All these sites are acceptable; however, the basilic vein is the primary preferred insertion site, and should be assessed immediately above and below the antecubital space by palpation and ultrasound before selection.

Selection of the external jugular site for PICC placement is indicated for emergent access when other veins cannot be accessed. This site can be used when high-pressure injection may be given through catheters rated for this use; and central venous pressure monitoring may be performed through these catheters (INS, 2008b).

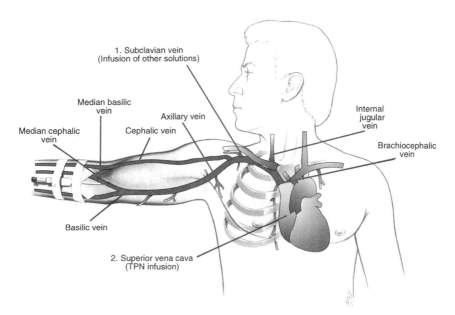

Figure 8-8 ■ Anatomical placement of peripherally placed central catheter. (Courtesy of Medivisuals, Dallas, TX.)

Placement

According to the recommendations in the INS Standards of Practice (2006a), PICCs should be placed in patients using maximum sterile barriers by a specially trained registered nurse in settings such as a patient's room, outpatient area, or the patient's home. Various PICC access designs are available for insertion, including the 21-gauge straight needle, intravenous cannula, break-away needle introducer, and the peel-away sheath, with guidewire. PICCs are commonly inserted with the aid of ultrasound guidance, allowing visual inspection of the vasculature and assessment of the size and location of the vessel.

INS Standard The nurse should consider using visualization technologies that aid in vein identification and selection. (INS, 2006a, 37)

 NURSING FAST FACT!

Central vascular access devices shall have the distal tip dwelling in the lower one third of the superior vena cava to the junction of the superior vena cava and the right atrium. Central catheter tip location shall be determined radiographically and documented prior to initiation of prescribed therapy (INS, 2006, S42).

Procedure

The insertion of a PICC is an advanced procedure requiring the nurse to have special training and competencies. The step-by-step procedure is not included in this textbook due to the requirement for specialized training. There are two methods of bedside PICC insertion: the peel-away cannula technique and the modified-Seldinger technique (MST). With the traditional peel-away cannula technique, access is established by inserting the cannula and stylet, much like a regular intravenous cannula, into a palpable vein in or near the antecubital fossa. The stylet is removed and the PICC is inserted through the cannula. The cannula is then pulled back and peeled away from the catheter. Refer to Figure 8-9 for an example of a peel-away catheter.

The modified-Seldinger technique (MST) uses a smaller needle or peripheral cannula for initial venipuncture, 21- or 22-gauge instead of a 16-gauge, in which a guidewire is threaded into the cannula several inches, then the cannula is removed, leaving the guidewire in place. The guidewire is not advanced. A nick is made in the skin beside the guidewire and an introducer/dilator unit is inserted over the guidewire. The guidewire is carefully removed along with the dilator, and the catheter is advanced through the introducer sheath, which is later pulled back and peeled away. Ultrasound is often used to locate and initially access the vein using the MST technique. Use of MST with ultrasound reduces the risk associated with larger needle access to deeper veins

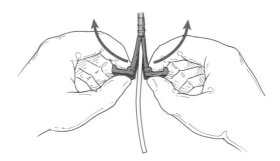

Figure 8-9 ■ Drawing of peel away catheter. (Courtesy of Bard Access Systems, Salt Lake City, UT.)

(Moureau, 2006). The actual procedure varies with different manufacturers' products.

Advantages to the MST insertion technique:
- Ability to access very small veins with a smaller gauge introducer
- Ability to perform access without visible veins
- Flexibility to employ ultrasound guidance
- Reduced risk of injury with small introducer
- Greater success

INS Standard Introducers for PICC should be equipped with a safety device with engineered sharps injury protection. (INS, 2006a, 38)

The length of time a PICC may indwell is dependent on factors related to the patient, clinical environment, skill of the inserter, skill of all caregivers, the composition of the infusate, and the VAD.

Use of Ultrasound Guidance

The use of diagnostic ultrasound to assist VAD placement dates back to the mid-1980s. Improvements in ultrasound portability and transducer ability, however, have greatly enhanced its viability for VAD placement. Creating a more convenient portable unit allows nurses to place PICC lines at the patient's bedside anywhere in the hospital. Evidence has demonstrated increased safety for central line insertions performed with ultrasound. This method is endorsed by the Agency for Healthcare Research and Quality (AHRQ). Utilization of ultrasound to help guide the insertion of vascular access devices increases the rate of successful insertions to more than 90% compared with about 80% with traditional, non-ultrasound PICC insertion. Ultrasound guidance for central line insertion is being implemented in all levels of practice for both nurses and physicians and is fast becoming the standard of care for all CVCs including PICCs. Refer to Figure 8-10.

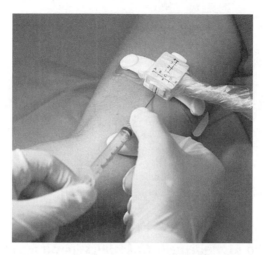

Figure 8-10 ■ Portable, hands free ultrasound technology to place PICC. (Courtesy of Inceptio Medical Technologies, Farmington, UT.)

Care and Maintenance of Short-Term Central Venous Access Devices

Owing to the concern regarding CR-BSI, investigators have recommended a hospital-specific or collaborative-based performance improvement initiative in which multifaceted strategies are "bundled" together to improve patient outcomes. Clinical decision-makers, healthcare payers, and patient safety advocates all emphasize the importance of implementing research findings into practice (O'Grady, Alexander, Dellinger, et al., 2002). A multifaceted approach in which strategies are "bundled" together to improve compliance with evidence-based guidelines includes:

1. Hand hygiene
2. Maximum barrier precautions
3. Central venous catheter cart that contained all necessary supplies
4. A checklist to ensure adherence to proper practices
5. Stoppage of procedures if evidence-based practices were not being followed (time out)
6. Prompt removal of central catheters during daily patient rounds if unnecessary
7. Feedback to the clinical teams regarding the number of CR-BSI episodes and overall rates
8. Buy-in from the chief executive officers.
9. Chlorhexidine gluconate site disinfection
10. Avoid femoral site. (Pronovost, Needham, Berenholtz, et al., 2006)

Refer to Evidence-Based Care Box 8-1 for a study reflecting evidence-based practice using a bundle approach.

EVIDENCE-BASED CARE BOX 8-1

Bundle Approach to Prevention of CR-BSI

Pronovost, P., Needham, D., Berenholts, S., et al. (2006). An intervention to decrease catheter-related bloodstream infections in ICU. New England Journal of Medicine, 355 (26), 2725–2732.

A collaborative cohort study of 108 Michigan targeted clinicians' use of five evidence-based practices: hand hygiene, maximum barrier precautions, chlorhexidine site disinfection, avoiding the femoral site, and removing unnecessary central venous catheters, and in addition educating clinicians about CR-BSI prevention and intervention.

Results: Using an interrupted time series design and multivariable regression, the investigators reported a statistically significant 66% decrease in CR-BSI rates approximately 18 months after the interventions began.

General Dressing Management Guidelines for Short-Term Devices

Nontunneled catheters can be dressed in one of two ways, depending on agency policy. An occlusive gauze or tape (preferred if the site is oozing or the patient is diaphoretic) or a transparent semipermeable membrane (TSM) dressing may be used. In today's practice, the TSM dressing has gained popularity because of its occlusive nature and ability to visualize the site. TSM dressings over a CVC should be replaced when it becomes damp, loosened, or soiled or at least every 7 days (O'Grady, Alexander, Dellinger, et al., 2002). When the dressing is changed, everything under the dressing is cleaned via sterile technique and replaced. Gauze dressings should be changed every 48 hours (2 days) or if the site requires visual inspection (INS, 2006a, S44; O'Grady, Alexander, Dellinger, et al., 2002).

INS Standard Gauze used in conjunction with a TSM should be considered a gauze dressing and changed every 48 hours. (INS, 2006a, 44)

The use of a chlorhexidine-impregnated sponge placed over the site of CVCs reduced the risk for catheter colonization and CR-BSI (Maki & Mermel, 2007). This dressing consists of a small foam disc impregnated with chlorhexidine gluconate. The dressing has a small slit, which allows it to be positioned under the vascular access device. Refer to Figure 8-11. The chlorhexidine-impregnated dressing is changed every 7 days.

A number of studies have demonstrated that the Biopatch (Ethicon, Inc.) has been effective in reducing the incidence of CR-BSI (Banton & Banning, 2002; Mermel, 2001).

EBNP In a randomized control trial using the chlorhexidine-impregnated sponge it was found that CR-BSIs were reduced in adults to 2.4% from 6.1% and local site infections reduced to 16.4% from 23.9% (Maki, Mermel, Kluger, et al., 2000).

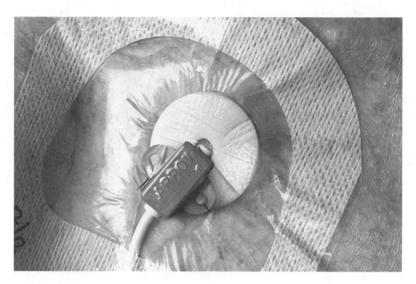

Figure 8-11 ■ Biopatch. (Courtesy of J & J Wound Management, Ethicon, Somerville, NJ.)

For PICC catheters two types of dressing are used for central venous access devices: the gauze and tape and the transparent semipermeable membrane dressing (TSM). Patients who are very active or perspire profusely will need more frequent dressing changes. PICCs are generally secured with manufactured stabilization devices, and tubing junctions must be secured with Luer locking connections and cleansed with an antiseptic agent before disconnecting or changing. Standards of practice (INS, 2006a, 44; O'Grady, Alexander, Dellinger, et al., 2002) include:

- Gauze dressing that prevents visualization of the insertion site should be changed routinely every 48 hours (2 days).
- If the patient is diaphoretic, or if the site is bleeding or oozing, a gauze dressing preferable.
- Do not use topical antibiotic ointment or creams on insertion sites (except when using dialysis catheters) due to potential of fungal infections and antimicrobial resistance.
- Gauze used in conjunction with a TSM dressing should be considered a gauze dressing and changed every 48 hours.
- Replace dressings used on tunneled or implanted CVCs no more than once per week, until the insertion site has healed.
- A TSM dressing for adults and adolescent patients at least weekly; however, the age and condition of the patient, infection control rate reported by the organization, and environmental conditions must be taken into consideration.

INS Standard   Catheter–skin junction sites should be visually inspected or palpated for tenderness daily through the intact dressing. (INS, 2006a, 44)

> *EBNP In 1988 Young, Alexeyeff, Russell, et al. (1988) conducted research to determine the most effective dressing materials and interval change time for patients with central venous access devices. The conclusion was that a sterile, transparent, occlusive dressing changed every 7 days was more effective when compared to sterile gauze and tape dressings.*

For PICC post-insertion, a small amount of bleeding from the insertion site occurs for the first 24 hours after insertion. After 24 hours, the original dressing should be replaced with a TSM that can remain in place up to 7 days. Dressings have two functions: (1) as a protective environment for the VAD and (2) to prevent catheter migration via stabilization. Dressing change is a sterile procedure. Refer to Procedures Display 8-1 at the end of the chapter. Refer to Figure 8-12 at PICC site at the basilic vein and Figure 8-13 dressing over external jugular PICC.

After removal of the catheter and dressing, the site should be assessed every 24 hours until the site is epithelialized. PICC dressing should be changed at intervals similar to those for other central line dressings. Transparent dressings are safe and effective up to 7 days (Maki & Mermel, 2007).

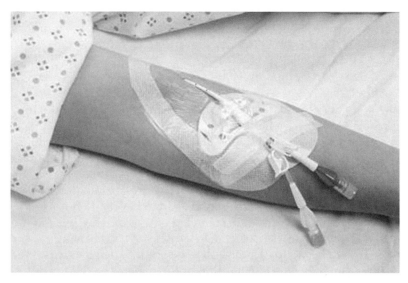

Figure 8-12   ■   Occlusive dressing over PICC placed in the basilic vein. (Courtesy of 3M Health Care Division, St. Paul, MN.)

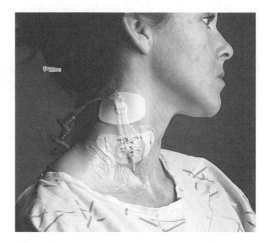

Figure 8-13 ■ Occlusive dressing over PICC placed in external jugular vein. (Courtesy of 3M Health Care Division, St. Paul, MN.)

 NURSING FAST FACT!

When removing the old PICC dressing lift it from the catheter hub toward the patient's head, taking care not to pull the catheter out of the insertion site (Ellenberger, 2002).

Infusion Set Changes

Administration set changes follow guidelines for sets specific to primary and secondary continuous, primary intermittent, parenteral nutrition, intravenous fat emulsion, and blood administration sets. Any administration set that is suspected of being contaminated or when the integrity of the product is in question should be changed. All administration sets should have Luer-Lok™ design. Aseptic technique should be used when changing any administration tubing.

INS Standard (2006a, S48) The following administration set changes:

- Primary and secondary continuous administration sets shall be changed no more frequently than every 72 hours.
- Primary intermittent administration sets shall be changed every 24 hours.
- Administration sets used for parenteral nutrition shall be changed every 72 hours.
- Administration sets used to deliver parenteral nutrition with fat emulsions shall be changed every 24 hours. If fat emulsion is piggybacked into administration sets that have been used for parenteral nutrition, the sets must be changed every 24 hours.

■ Intravenous fat emulsion administration sets shall be changed every 24 hours.

■ Administration sets and add-on filters that are used for blood and blood components shall be changed after administration of *each* unit or at the end of 4 hours, whichever comes first.

Flushing and Locking

The Infusion Nursing Standards of Practice (2006a, 50) state that VADs are flushed at established intervals to promote and maintain patency and to prevent mixing of incompatible solutions or medications.

For flushing of PICCs and nontunneled catheters the following is recommended (INS, 2008c). Flushing is to be done:

1. Whenever the line needs to be locked
2. After every blood draw
3. After intermittent medication administration
4. After blood or blood component administration
5. After TPN

Refer to Table 8-3 for flushing protocols from INS (2008c).

Heparin is used to maintain patency of some central venous catheters. Those with valves tend to not need heparin. When heparin is recommended a concentration that does not interfere with clotting factors should be used. Flushing techniques vary depending on the valve design.

The needleless injection system (NIS) or needleless access port (NAP) technology has changed. Four needleless injection systems are available and are divided by the type of fluid movement through them: split septum, negative-displacement, positive–displacement, and neutral-displacement valve types. It is important that nurses understand which system they are using in order to correctly maintain the NIS/NAP.

A negative-displacement needleless injection system will allow blood to reflux into the catheter lumen when the tubing or syringe is disconnected. The positive-pressure flushing technique is required when a negative-displacement device is used. The positive pressure technique recommends clamping the catheter while maintaining syringe pressure to minimize blood reflux while flushing (Hadaway, 2006).

Positive-displacement needleless injection systems will reserve a small amount of fluid to push toward the catheter tip at disconnection of the syringe or tubing, thus preventing blood from remaining inside the lumen. Recent technology has offered positive pressure valves that reduce or prevent blood reflux (CLC2000 Adapter Valve, ICU Medical; Ultrasite—B. Braun; Gorski & Czaplewiski, 2004). Positive-pressure flushing technique is not necessary because it is already provided by the positive displacement mechanism. Withdraw the syringe from the NIS, allow sufficient time for the positive fluid displacement, and then close the catheter clamp.

> Table 8-3   **FLUSHING PROTOCOLS**

Device	Intermittent Flushing	Flushing with no Therapy	Heparin Locking	Blood Draws	Blood Product Administration	Parenteral Nutrition Admin
Nontunneled	Minimum of 5 mL	Nonvalved: At least q 24 hours Valved: At least weekly	5 mL of 10 units/mL heparin	Predraw 5 mL Postdraw 10 mL	Preadmin 5 mL Postadmin 10 mL	Minimum of 5 mL
PICC	Minimum of 5 mL	Nonvalved: At least q 24 hours Valved: At least weekly	5 mL of 10 units/mL heparin	Predraw 5 mL Postdraw 10 mL	Preadmin 5 mL Postadmin 10 mL	Minimum of 5 mL
Tunneled	Minimum of 5 mL	Nonvalved: At least 1–2 times per week Valved: At least weekly	5 mL of 10 units/mL heparin	Predraw 5 mL Postdraw 10 mL	Preadmin 5 mL Postadmin 10 mL	Minimum of 5 mL
Port	Minimum of 5 mL	Accessed Nonvalved: At least 1–2 times per week Valved: At least weekly Deaccessed: At least monthly	3–5 mL of 100 units/mL heparin	Predraw 5 mL Postdraw 10 mL	Preadmin 5 mL Postadmin 10 mL	Minimum of 5 mL

NOTE: Always use a 10-mL syringe for all flushing of CVCs.
NOTE: Use single-use preservative-free 0.9% sodium chloride flushes.
Source: Infusion Nurses Society Flushing Protocols (2008c), with permission.

NOTE > Positive- and negative-displacement devices are dependent on the flushing technique.

Neutral-displacement needleless systems will not allow fluid to move in either direction when tubing or a syringe is disconnected. Function is not dependent on flushing technique (Hadaway, 2006).

NOTE > Refer to the manufacturer's guideline for specific device usage. Refer to Chapter 5 for a comparison of the three types of valves.

 NURSING FAST FACT!

Pulsatile (Push-Pause) Flushing
Using a rapid succession of pulsatile push-pause–push-pause movement exerted on the plunger of the syringe barrel creates a turbulence within the catheter lumen that causes a swirling effect to move residues of fibrin, medication, lipids, or other adherents attached to the catheter lumen.

Refer to Procedures Display 8-2 at the end of this chapter.

Use of Infusion Pumps

The PICC line has been used successfully with all types of infusion pumps. With 3.0-French and smaller PICCs, an infusion pump may be necessary to maintain the infusion and patency of the line. Gravity flow rates are slower with a PICC made of silicone, as compared to polyurethane. Silicone is softer with thicker catheter walls. When a positive pressure infusion pump is used for administration, potential flow rates increase to at least 400 mL/hr regardless of gauge or catheter material (Gorski & Czaplewski, 2004).

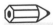 *NURSING FAST FACT!*

Pump manufacturers provide the maximum pressure limits of their pumps and catheter manufacturers provide pressure limits for their catheters.

NOTE > Maximum pressure of the infusion pump should not be greater than the upper limit of the catheter to prevent catheter rupture.

Blood Sampling

If blood sampling is needed from the PICC, a 4-French or larger catheter may improve aspiration success. The most common method to obtain blood is the discard method. The first aspirate of blood is discarded to reduce the risk of drug concentration or diluted specimen (Frey, 2003).

 NURSING FAST FACT!

> Be aware that withdrawal of blood through the PICC can contribute to thrombotic catheter occlusion when the PICC is not flushed adequately.

Key points in obtaining blood sampling from a PICC include:
- Stop the infusion before blood sampling
- Follow flushing protocol: 5 mL of saline before sample collection
- Withdraw 4 to 5 mL of blood to discard before drawing laboratory sample
- Flush with 10 mL of saline after the sample is collected using the pulsatile push–pause method.

Refer to Procedures Display 8-3 at the end of this chapter for steps in drawing blood sample from central vascular access device.

Blood Administration

Blood products may be administered through a 4-French or larger PICC. Care should be taken to flush the line thoroughly after administering a blood product. An infusion pump may be necessary to maintain the infusion if the pump is approved for the administration of blood.

Injection Cap Changes

The injection cap of nontunneled and PICCs are changed according to best practices of aseptic technique. It is important to disinfect the cap with either 70% alcohol or chlorhexidine/alcohol using a twisting friction for 15 seconds (10 twists) before any access (Kaler & Chinn, 2007). This technique for access prevents the entry of microorganisms into the vascular system, the injection or access port should be aseptically cleansed with an approved antiseptic solution immediately before use. The injection cap should be changed at least every 7 days.

> EBNP A study done to determine the effectiveness disinfection for needleless access ports to prevent CR-BSI was done in 2007. The ports of four models of needleless access ports were inoculated with bacteria. The ports were disinfected for 15 seconds with 70% alcohol alone or with 3.15% chlorhexidine/70% alcohol. Saline flush solutions were collected and cultured. Results indicated that no microorganisms were recovered from any of the access ports that were disinfected for 15 seconds. All models of needleless access ports were effectively disinfected using the two methods for 15 seconds of friction (Kaler & Chinn, 2007).

INS Standard Protocols for disinfection accessing and changing of injection and access caps shall be established in organizational policies and procedures. Injection access caps shall be of Luer-Lok design. The optimal interval for changing injection or access on peripherally inserted central catheters is unknown; however, it is recommended that they be changed at least every 7 days. (INS, 2006a, 35)

NOTE > Whenever an injection access cap/valve is removed from a catheter it should be discarded, and a new one attached.

Concerns have been raised over the relationship of needleless connectors to bacteremia. Controversy focuses on determining whether split septum or Luer-activated valve technology represents the safest approach to prevent CR-BSI. The impact of microbial biofilm is the accumulation of polymers excreted by bacterial cells adhering to a device surface. The accumulation of biofilm on medical devices, including injection caps, cannot be prevented and creates clinical management challenges (Ryder, 2005).

Repair

A PICC that is damaged externally can be repaired with a manufacturer-specific hub repair kit. If the catheter is damaged internally, consider referring the patient to interventional radiology for an over-the-wire exchange if applicable to preserve the access site, after considering the advantages, disadvantages, and infection risks. In many cases, the I.V. nurse must advocate for the patient's vascular access needs and create new techniques to preserve what may be the only access site available. A risk/benefit ratio must be considered with repair versus replacement.

The PICC can be repaired or replaced in one of three ways:
- Using the exchange-over-wire procedure using the Seldinger method
- Totally removing and replacing with another PICC
- Using the peel-away sheath introducer.

If the peripherally inserted central line is damaged, another catheter can be placed. An exchange-over-wire procedure can be used as a last resort for salvaging the line. The guidewires used for this procedure must be longer than the catheter; therefore, strict sterile technique with gowning and maximal sterile barrier is recommended. The guidewire is inserted into the catheter to be removed, and the catheter is pulled out over the wire. An introducer/dilator is advanced and the wire dilator removed. A new catheter is then threaded through the introducer. After the new catheter is in place, the guidewire can be removed.

Dual-lumen PICCs cannot be easily repaired. A sheath exchange allows for a damaged PICC to be removed and a new dual lumen to be placed. A chest radiograph should be taken to verify the placement of the new catheter tip of any exchanged or replaced catheter. This procedure should be performed only by experienced infusion nurses competent to insert a PICC (INS, 2006a, 59) and in accordance with the nursing practice acts. Specific manufacturers' recommendations are provided for this procedure.

Discontinuation of Short-Term Central Venous Devices

The discontinuation of a nontunneled catheter or a PICC can be performed by a qualified registered nurse with an order of a physician or authorized prescriber. Nontunneled and PICC devices should be removed immediately on suspected contamination, unresolved complication or therapy discontinuation in collaboration with the healthcare team. Caution should be used in the removal of a nontunneled central catheter, including precautions to prevent air embolism. Minimize the risk of air embolism by positioning the patient in a dorsal-recumbent position, and instruct the patient to perform the Valsalva maneuver while the catheter is being withdrawn. The recommended procedure is presented in Procedures Display 8-4 at the end of this chapter.

Digital pressure should be applied to the puncture site until hemostasis is achieved, then antiseptic ointment and sterile TSM dressing should be applied to the access site.

NOTE > A nontunneled or PICC should never be readvanced (INS, 2006a, 49). Documentation should be written in patient records of condition, and length of the catheter, along with interventions implemented as necessary with observations of the catheter removal site.

Difficulty with PICC withdrawal is an uncommon but not infrequent problem, with resistance encountered in 7% to 24% of removals (Macklin, 2000). Catheter removal may take several hours or more to achieve venous relaxation and total removal of cannula. The most common cause of "stuck" catheters is venospasm (Marx, 1995). Other causes include phlebitis, valve inflammation, and thrombophlebitis. Refer to Figure 8-14 for an algorithm for a "stuck" PICC catheter.

Techniques to aid in removal of catheter include:

- Never pull against resistance because catheter breakage or vein wall damage could occur.
- Apply warm moist compresses.
- Use mental relaxation exercises and distraction.
- Have the patient drink a warm beverage to increase vasomotor tone.
- Gently massage the area of the upper arm over the PICC to relax the vein.
- Re-attempt removal after a short (30 minutes) or an intermediate period of time (next day) (Gorski & Czaplewiski, 2004).

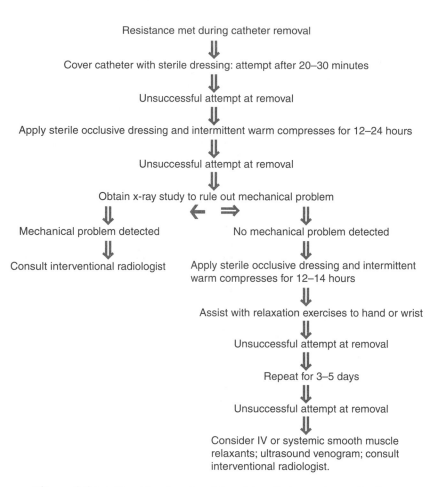

Figure 8-14 ■ Algorithm for a "stuck" peripherally inserted central catheter.

Risks and Complications: Short-Term CVCs

The risks and complications associated with short-term central venous access devices are covered in Chapter 9. With PICC catheters complications can also include arm edema, bleeding, tendon or nerve damage, cardiac dysrhythmias, malposition of the catheter, catheter embolism, phlebitis, catheter sepsis, thrombosis, air embolism, and Twiddler's syndrome. Nerve damage is related to the median nerve, which lies parallel and medial to the brachial artery in the antecubital space. On the lateral side, the lateral cutaneous nerve is proximal to the cephalic vein. Because of the close proximity to these nerves, damage is a risk for PICC insertion.

Cardiac dysrhythmias are related to irritation of the myocardial wall by an overinserted guidewire or catheter. Refer to Chapter 9 for detailed information on complications associated with central venous access devices.

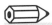

NURSING FAST FACT!

If the patient complains of pain in the shoulder, neck, or arm at insertion site, catheter placement should be checked by radiographic examination at any time during the course of therapy.

NURSING POINTS-OF-CARE
SHORT-TERM CVCs

Nursing Assessments
- Identify prescribed therapy, expected duration of therapy.
- Health history (including the client's vascular integrity)
- Identify client preferences.
- Assess for suitability of target vessels; evaluate for size (the vein must be large enough to accommodate the selected VAD to minimize the risk of phlebitis and thrombosis).
- Assess for skin lesions, implanted pacemaker, or cardioverted defibrillator.
- Discuss previous VAD placement.
- Obtain baseline vital signs.

Key Nursing Interventions
1. Implement bundle approach to catheter insertion and maintenance.
   a. Hand hygiene by catheter inserters
   b. Maximum barrier precautions (gowns, gloves, mask, cap)
   c. Chlorhexidine gluconate with alcohol skin antisepsis of catheter insertion site
   d. Trained catheter inserter
   e. Proper selection of type of catheter and insertion site
   f. Insert catheters only when medically necessary
   g. Have all materials needed for catheter insertion at the bedside before starting insertion
   h. Time-out called if proper procedures are not followed (then start again)
   i. Use of aseptic technique during catheter manipulation
   j. Remove catheters when no longer medically necessary
2. Document the following daily:
   a. Solution infusing and type of administration set
   b. Flow rate
   c. Use of electronic infusion device
   d. Location of insertion site
   e. Assessment of the catheter

Continued

    f. Inspection and description of the insertion site
    g. Condition of catheter tract and surrounding tissue
    h. Type of I.V. site dressing
    i. Patient response to catheter and patient education
 3. Avoid use of blood pressure cuffs or tourniquet over the site of the PICC but may be placed distal to the catheter's location.
 4. Follow standards of practice for dressing changes, flushing and locking, blood sampling, and administration set changes.
 5. Maintain occlusive dressing.
 6. Use an infusion pump for delivery of solutions when appropriate.
 7. Use a 10-mL syringe for all flushes to central line and to obtain blood samples.
 8. Follow guidelines for PICC placement, insertion, and follow-up care.
 9. Replace dressing on PICC after first 24 hours with occlusive dressing.
 10. Change TSM dressings every 7 days unless integrity compromised.

■ Long-Term Access Devices

Central Venous Tunneled Catheters

Devices designed for long-term use can be divided into two categories: tunneled catheters and implanted ports. The need for prolonged central venous access and a method to decrease potential infection from the skin exit site resulted in the development of central venous catheters **(CVTCs)**. They were originally developed by Broviac in 1973 and later modified by Hickman to meet the needs of patients undergoing bone marrow transplant. These long-term catheters can remain in place for many years (Massorli & Angeles, 2002).

CVTCs are intended to be used for months to years to provide long-term venous access for hypertonic solutions; obtaining blood samples; and for administering medications, blood products, and parenteral nutrition.

CVTCs are composed of polymeric silicone or thin polyurethane and have multiple lumens and varying diameters with a Dacron polyester cuff that anchors the catheter in place subcutaneously. All tunneled catheters have this synthetic cuff, which sits within the subcutaneous tunnel. This cuff is about 2 inches from the catheter's exit site, which becomes embedded with fibroblasts within 1 week to 10 days after insertion, reducing the chances for accidental removal and minimizing the risk of ascending bacterial infection. Within 7 to 10 days of catheter insertion, scar tissue grows onto the cuff, anchoring the catheter and preventing microorganisms from migrating up the tunnel. Once the cuff heals into place, the sutures can be removed and no dressing is required unless the patient is immunocompromised (Massorli & Angeles, 2002). The cuff provides an antimicrobial barrier between the skin and the vascular system (Arch, 2007).

An attachable cuff, VitaCuff™, is available for CVTCs. This cuff is made of biodegradable collagen impregnated with silver ion. Subcutaneous tissue grows to the cuff, providing a mechanical barrier, and the silver ion provides a chemical barrier against organisms. This cuff has proved to be cost effective in decreasing catheter-related septicemia (Maki & Mermel, 2007).

A development in CVTCs is the application of the Groshong® valve feature, which has been marketed since 1984. This catheter has a few unique features that set it apart from other CVTCs. The Groshong® catheter is made of soft, flexible silicone material. The outer diameter dimensions are small. The catheter is available with single, double, or triple lumens. The silicone material has a recoil memory that returns it to its original configuration if accidentally pulled. Another unique feature of the Groshong® catheter is the two-way valve placed near the distal end, which restricts backflow of blood, but can be purposefully overridden to obtain venous blood samples. This valve eliminates the need for flushing with heparin. The valve is open inward, minimizing the risks of blood backing up the catheter lumen. The Groshong® valve feature is now available on a variety of CVCs, including PICCs and ports.

ADVANTAGES

1. Can be repaired if it breaks or tears.
2. Can be used for many purposes including:
   a. Blood samples
   b. Monitoring central venous pressure
   c. Administering TPN
   d. Drug administration
3. Can be used for the patient with a chronic need for I.V. therapy.

DISADVANTAGES

1. Daily to weekly site care for first 10 days (tunneled catheter)
2. Cost of maintenance supplies (dressings, materials, and changes; frequency of flushing and cap changing)
3. Surgical catheter insertion procedure that requires maintenance
4. Can affect the patient's body image

Insertion of Tunneled Catheters

Central venous tunneled catheters are inserted with the patient under local or general anesthesia by percutaneous puncture, and the catheter is placed by locating the jugular, femoral, or subclavian vein by a physician, usually in the operating room or interventional radiology suite.

During insertion, the physician uses a needle to locate the subclavian vein and advances the catheter tip into the superior vena cava (Fig. 8-15).

With a blunt-ended trocar, he or she creates the subcutaneous tunnel from the subclavian vein down the chest wall; the exit site is usually at about the nipple line. The position is confirmed by fluoroscopy, adjusted if needed, and then the catheter is sutured to the skin or the incision is closed with Steri-Strips®. The catheter remains in place for 10 to 14 days (Fig. 8-16).

Initially after insertion of a tunneled catheter, an occlusive TSM dressing is in place and should be changed weekly or whenever the integrity of the dressing is compromised. If a gauze dressing is used, change the dressing every 48 hours (O'Grady, Alexander, Dellinger, et al., 2002). Once the cuff heals the dressing is not necessary.

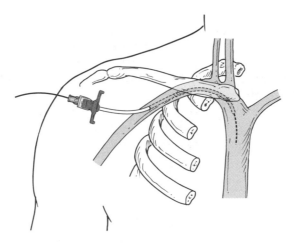

Figure 8-15 ■ Subclavian insertion site for a tunneled catheter.

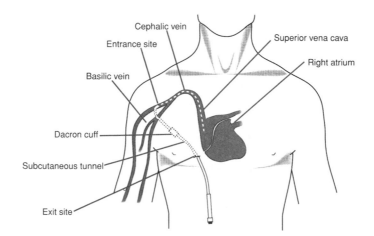

Figure 8-16 ■ Anatomic placement of tunneled catheter. (Courtesy of Bard Access Systems, Salt Lake City, UT.)

NURSING POINTS-OF-CARE
TUNNELED CATHETERS

- Be sure the catheter is clamped or capped at all times to prevent inadvertent air embolism. To maintain patency, follow the steps for flushing the catheter. Use Luer locking caps.
- Keep all sharp objects away from the catheter.
- Never use scissors or pins on or near the catheter.
- If the catheter leaks or breaks, take a nonserrated (without teeth) clamp and clamp the catheter between the broken area and the exit site. Cover the broken part with a sterile gauze bandage and tape it securely. Do not use the catheter. Notify the physician.
- Protect the catheter when showering or bathing by covering the entire catheter with transparent dressing or clear plastic wrap. Cover the connections and protect hub connections from water contamination.
- After a blood drawing, flush with 10 to 20 mL of 0.9% sodium chloride, using a pulsatile technique.
- Heparin is used to maintain the patency of the catheter, except for the closed-ended catheters such as Groshong® or PASV® catheter.
- Change the administration set for continuous infusions every 72 hours. If infusing blood, blood products, or lipids change within 24 hours of initiating therapy.

 NURSING FAST FACT!

The catheter should be clamped if malfunction is suspected or when catheter breakage occurs.

Avoid serrated clamps on the catheter. External clamps should not be used routinely; they are unnecessary and could damage the catheter.

Complications Associated with Tunneled Catheters

Refer to Chapter 9 for general complications associated with central venous access devices, both local and systemic. Common risks associated with CVTCs include exit site infections, sepsis, thrombosis, nonthrombotic occlusions, catheter migration, torn or leaking catheter, and air embolism (Moureau, 2001).

Implanted Ports

Totally implanted ports, another type of CVC, have been available for venous access since 1983. Originally, implanted ports were targeted to oncology patients who required frequent intermittent venous access. A port consists of a reservoir, silicone catheter, and central septum and has no external parts. Refer to Figure 8-17.

The implanted port vascular access system provides safe and reliable vascular access; the design provides patients with an improved body image, reduced maintenance, and improved quality of life. They are best used for cyclic therapies such as chemotherapy or antibiotics and for treatments for chronic or long term illnesses, such as cystic fibrosis. The port can accommodate bolus injections and continuous infusions (Massorli & Angeles, 2002).

Ports are composed of a metal (titanium) or plastic housing that surrounds a self-sealing silicone gel. A silicone catheter is attached to the port housing. The self-sealing septum of a regular profile can usually withstand up to 2000 needle punctures, with the lower profile ports withstanding about 500 needle punctures. The port has raised edges to facilitate puncture with a noncoring needle. Refer to Figure 8-18 for various port designs. The Huber Plus is an example of a noncoring needle with safety features built into the wings. Many types of implanted VADs are available today and are placed for venous, arterial, and epidural infusion. Figure 8-19 shows various locations for implanted ports.

ADVANTAGES

1. Less risk of infection and catheter-related complications when used intermittently
2. Less interference with daily activities
3. Minimal maintenance required—no dressing, usually monthly heparinization to maintain patency
4. May remain in place for months to years
5. Needs minimal flushing
6. Easy access for fluids, blood products, or medication administration
7. Less body image disturbance owing to the lack of an external catheter device
8. Few limitations on patient activity; ability to swim when not accessed

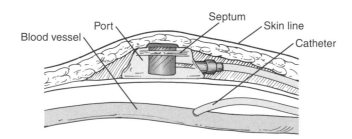

Figure 8-17 ■ Diagram of an implanted port. (Courtesy of Baxter Healthcare Corporation, Round Lake, IL.)

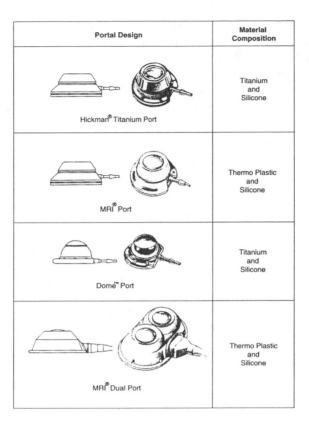

Figure 8-18 ■ Examples of types of port designs. (Courtesy of Bard Access Systems, Salt Lake City, UT.)

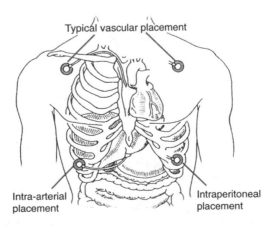

Figure 8-19 ■ Examples of placement sites for vascular access ports. (Courtesy of Bard Access Systems, Salt Lake City, UT.)

Disadvantages

1. Cost of insertion and removal is high (considerably greater than with other VADs).
2. Postoperative care is 7 to 10 days.
3. Repeated needlesticks cause discomfort.
4. Minor surgical procedure is necessary to remove the device.

Insertion

The port is usually inserted in the operating room or interventional radiology suite. The surgeon makes an incision in the upper to middle chest, usually near the collarbone, to form a pocket to house the port. The silicone catheter is inserted via cutdown into the SVC; the port is then placed in the subcutaneous fascia pocket. The port contains a reservoir leading to the catheter. The incision for the port pocket is sutured closed, and a sterile dressing is applied. The port requires a dressing until it heals. This area should be monitored until the incision has healed, about 10 days to 2 weeks after insertion.

The subcutaneous port system catheter can be placed in any of the following: SVC, hepatic artery, peritoneal space for intraperitoneal therapy, and epidural space.

Implanted ports are available in single- or dual-septum chambers. Ports designed for peripheral access are also available.

Accessing the Port

The access and maintenance of an implanted port or pump is performed by a nurse with validated competency. To access an implanted port, including how to inject a bolus and inject a continuous infusion, refer to Figure 8-20 and follow the guidelines listed in Procedures Display 8-5 at the end of this chapter.

It is important to follow hand hygiene procedures before donning sterile gloves and accessing the port. Accessing the port requires sterile technique with mask and gloves according to CDC (2002). While the port is accessed with a noncoring needle, an occlusive transparent dressing needs to be in place. The Huber needle and dressing should be changed every 7 days for continuous infusion. If gauze is used to stabilize the access needle but not obscure the catheter–skin junction, the dressing is not considered a gauze dressing and should be changed at least every 7 days (INS, 2006a, 44; O'Grady, Alexander, Dellinger, et al., 2002). If the port is not routinely used it can be flushed monthly using flushing protocol. Refer to Table 8-3 for flushing protocols.

INS Standard Specially designed noncoring safety needles shall be used to access an implanted port or pump and shall be changed at established interval. (INS, 2006a, 45)

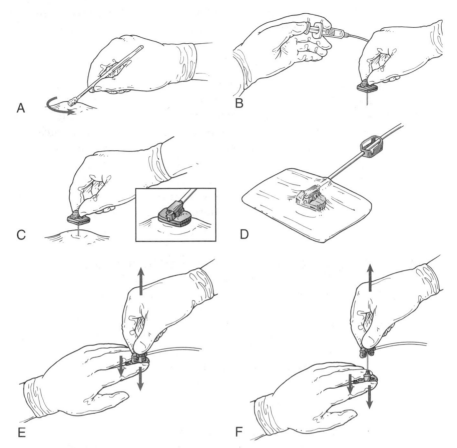

Figure 8-20 ■ Accessing the port wearing gloves: *A,* Prep the port site. *B,* Flush the port and extension tubing. *C,* Insert the noncoring needle into the port septum. *D,* Cover with transparent dressing. Deaccessing the port: *E,* Press down and pull straight up. *F,* Engage the safety device once removed.

Deaccessing an Implanted Port

To reduce the risk of infection transmission, wash hands before deaccessing the port. The use of sterile gloves for deaccessing a port is a controversial point. There is support in some of the literature for use of sterile gloves and technique when accessing and deaccessing a port (Arch, 2007; O'Grady, Alexander, Dellinger et al., 2002), whereas the Oncology Nursing Society (ONS) guidelines recommend aseptic technique (Camp-Sorrell, 2004).

> **INS Standard** Sterile technique shall be used when accessing an implanted port or pump. (INS, 2006a, 45)

Safety noncoring needle products are available on the market that are designed for use in implanted venous access devices to prevent inadvertent needlestick injury while deaccessing and should be used to ensure compliance to OSHA standards. Refer to Figure 8-21.

Refer to Procedures Display 8-6 at the end of this chapter for full instructions on deaccessing an implanted port.

Complications Associated with Implanted Ports

The same complications associated with all central venous access devices can occur with implanted ports. Refer to Chapter 9 for central venous access complications. Implanted ports can also develop site infection or skin breakdown and port migration. Extravasation of vesicant medications that are infusing into the port can occur if the needle is not in place through the septum of the port and the position is not confirmed. Fluid can extravasate and collect subcutaneously, resulting in burning or swelling around the port during infusion. Patients and nurses must always verify placement, secure the needle before initiating the infusion, and observe for signs of swelling or burning.

Care and Maintenance of Long-Term Access Devices

Dressing Management

The CVTC and ports do not routinely need a dressing after the insertion site is healed. A TSM dressing is usually used initially and is changed every 7 days for both ports and CVTC. The catheter–skin junction site should be visually inspected and palpated for tenderness daily through the intact dressing (INS, 2006a, 44). Dressing kits are available from manufacturers that include all the components for a sterile dressing change. Refer to Figure 8-21.

Transparent dressings reliably secure the device, permit continuous visual inspection of the catheter site, permit patients to bathe and shower without saturating the dressing, and require less frequent changes than do standard gauze dressings. If blood is oozing from the catheter insertion site, gauze dressing might be preferred (O'Grady, Alexander, Dellinger, et al., 2002). Refer to Figure 8-22.

> **INS Standard** Antiseptic solutions (2% chlorhexidine gluconate with ethyl of isopropyl alcohol (preferred) should be used for sterile cleansing of the catheter-skin junction during dressing changes along with a new stabilization device. (INS, 2006a, 51)

> **INS Standard** Labeling of the dressing should include type, size and length of catheter, date and time, and initials of the nurse performing dressing change. (INS, 2006a, 44)

NOTE > Acetone and acetone-based products should not be applied to the skin before insertion of a catheter or during dressing changes.

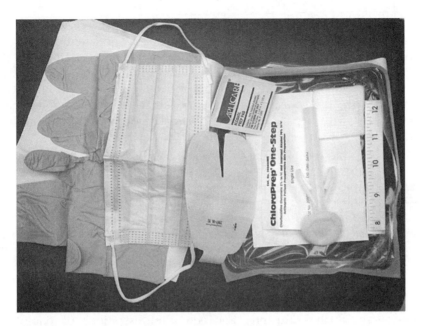

Figure 8-21 ■ Example of a dressing kit. (Courtesy of Baxter Healthcare Corporation, Round Lake, IL.)

EBNP In a meta-analysis chlorhexidine gluconate compared to povidone-iodine solution for vascular catheter-site care reduced CR-BSI and catheter colonization more than the use of povidone-iodine (Chaiyakunapruk, Veenstra, Lipsky, et al., 2002).

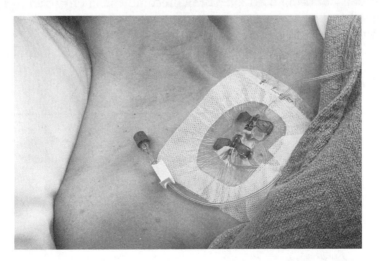

Figure 8-22 ■ Example of a dressing over a dual port. (Courtesy of 3M Health Care Division, St. Paul, MN.)

Flushing and Locking

Flushing procedures vary according to the agency and with the type of long-term device in use. Generally it is accepted practice to flush the CVCs with twice the catheter volume of heparinized saline for maintenance. After medication administration or daily maintenance, flush the catheter with 0.9% preservative-free sodium chloride single-use vials; then follow with heparinized saline. The use of heparinized saline is usually unnecessary in the Groshong® catheter. Refer to Procedures Display 8-3 at the end of this chapter.

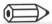 *NURSING FAST FACT!*

> When flushing the catheter, remember that different catheters require different amounts of heparin; always check the manufacturer's recommendations (Hadaway, 2000). Generally catheters have a volume of 1–3 mL (Massorli & Angeles, 2002).

For CVTCs, 5 mL of sodium chloride in a 10-mL syringe is used for intermittent flushes, flushing between administrations of parenteral nutrition. Before blood product administration, 5 mL of sodium chloride is used to clear the catheter, and post-administration a minimum of 10 mL of sodium chloride is recommended. If the CVTC is not being used and has a nonvalved cap the catheter should be flushed at least one or two times per week, and at least weekly if a valved cap is used. Refer to Table 8-3. To heparin lock the CVTC use 5 mL of 10 units/mL of heparin (INS, 2008c).

For ports, flushing procedures vary from institution to institution. If the port is not being used INS (2008c) recommends nonvalved cap ports be flushed at least one or two times per week, valved at least weekly, and ports not in use flushed with heparinized saline every 4 weeks with 3 to 5 mL of 100 units/mL of heparin. Blood administration requires pre-administration flush of 5 mL of sodium chloride and post-administration of 10 mL. Refer to Table 8-3.

NOTE > Typically the difference in concentrations of heparin between CVTC and ports is that CVTC use 10 units/mL, and ports 100 units/mL. However, the manufacturer's recommendations should be followed.

NOTE > The locking techniques of the three different locking devices (negative-displacement, positive-displacement, and neutral-displacement devices) discussed earlier in this chapter apply to long-term access devices.

Injection Cap Changes

The injection caps of tunneled catheters and ports are changed according to best practices. It is important to disinfect the cap with 70% alcohol or chlorhexidine using a twisting friction for 15 seconds (10 twists) before any access. This technique for access prevents the entry of microorganisms into the vascular system; the injection or access port should be aseptically cleansed with an approved antiseptic solution immediately before use (Kaler & Chinn, 2007). The injection cap should be changed at least every 7 days.

 NURSING FAST FACT!

If you have a multilumen catheter, remember to change all caps, even on unused lumens.

INS Standard Protocols for disinfection accessing and changing of injection and access caps shall be established in organizational policies and procedures. Injection access caps shall be of Luer-Lok design. The optimal interval for changing injection or access on peripherally inserted central catheters is unknown; however, it is recommended that they be changed at least every 7 days. (INS, 2006a, 35)

NOTE > Whenever an injection access cap/valve is removed from a catheter it should be discarded, and a new one attached.

Blood Draw from Long-Term Access Devices

The major method of blood draw from a VAD is the discard method. The purpose of the discard method is to remove from the catheter potential contaminants such as flush diluted venous blood or heparin to facilitate an accurate laboratory specimen. The rationale for discarding the first aspirate is based on an assumption that blood immediately beyond the hub is likely to be diluted by the I.V. or flush solution, and once diluted discard volume is removed, the vein will refill from the capillary bed with blood more representative of the total venous circulation (Frey, 2003).

For the steps in obtaining a blood sample from a CVTC or implanted port refer to Procedures Display 8-3 at the end of this chapter. Refer to Table 8-5 for a summary of care and maintenance of the four CVCs.

Repair of the Catheter

Repair of an external CVTC catheter might be indicated for one of the following reasons: repeated clamping; contact with a sharp object; rupture from an attempt to irrigate, and occluded catheter with a small syringe.

When catheter damage occurs, blood usually backs up and fluid leaks from the site (except with closed pressure-sensitive valves). Air can enter the catheter through the tear, causing an air embolism.

Keeping up to date on repair methods can be difficult. Several types of repair kits are available. CVTCs should always be repaired using the appropriate repair device, according to the manufacturer's instructions for use and after consideration of infection and safety risks to the patient.

Solutions to catheter repair:

- First clamp the catheter between the patient and the damaged area with a smooth-edged nontraumatic clamp.
- Determine the site of damage and the catheter size and type
- Refer to the appropriate catheter repair procedure to repair the damage. At least 2 inches of intact catheter beyond the skin exit site is needed to be able to repair the body of the catheter. Use appropriate size repair kit following the manufacturer's guidelines.
- Always use a 10-mL syringe or larger when accessing a central line.
- Repair is a sterile procedure.

INS Standard   Assessment of the patient's risk-to-benefit ratio should be performed prior to repair of the device. Access device repair should be considered for tunneled catheters, midline catheters and PICCs. (INS, 2006a, 57)

Discontinuation of Therapy

Removal of a tunneled catheter or implanted port is considered a surgical procedure and should be performed by a physician or advanced practice nurse. If a CR-BSI is suspected, consideration should be given to culturing the catheter and clinical assessment of the patient's condition with a possible treatment option for catheter salvage. If a catheter-related complication is suspected the catheter should be removed after patient assessment and collaboration with the healthcare team.

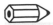 *NURSING FAST FACT!*

> *Removal of the tunneled catheter or port is a medical act. Care should be taken during removal of a tunneled catheter or implanted port to prevent air embolism. Digital pressure should be applied until hemostasis is achieved.*

INS Standard   After catheter removal, the dressing should be changed, and the access site assessed every 24 hours until the site is epithelialized. (INS, 2006a, 49)

Table 8-4 compares central venous catheters, with advantages and disadvantages of each. Table 8-5 summarizes the care and maintenance of the four types of CVCs.

> Table 8-4   COMPARISON OF CENTRAL VENOUS CATHETERS

Type and Use	Features	Advantages	Disadvantages
Short-Term			
Nontunneled Percutaneous Devices Intended for 7–10 days	Material: Polyurethane (most common), Silicone elastomer Length: 6–30 cm Gauge: 14–27 Available features: Heparin, hydromere, antibiotic and anti-septic coatings and antimicrobial cuff available Preattached exten-sions with clamps Multiple lumens	Inserted at bedside; cost effective, easy to remove, easy to exchange over guidewire	Placement time limited (usually 7–10 days) Requires sterile dressing changes; requires daily heparin flushes; catheter may break; requires activity restrictions. Higher rate of CR-BSI
Peripherally Inserted Central Catheter Several weeks up to one year	Material: Polyurethane (most common) Silicone elastomer Length: 33.5–60.0 cm Gauge: 14–25 Lumen: Double Groshong® valve	Insertion trays, spare needles, spare catheters, and repair kits available Preattached exten-sion with clamps Inserted at bedside by specially trained RN; cost effective; easy to remove; reliable for long-term use; eliminates risks associated with chest or neck insertion; pre-serves integrity of peripheral vascular system Low rate of CR-BSI Ultrasound guidance can increase success rate of insertion	Requires sterile dressing changes; requires routine heparin flushes except with Groshong® valve in place; catheter may break; requires activity restrictions; may experience restric-tions in blood sampling (i.e., small gauge, certain blood samples)
Long-Term			
External Tunneled Catheter Used for intermittent continuous or daily I.V access	Material: Silicone elastomer Length: 55–90 cm Gauge: 2.7–19.2 French Lumen: Multiple Valves: Open-ended and closed Detachable hub Antimicrobial collagen cuff	Can remain in place indefinitely; requires aseptic dressing changes; clean when site is healed; can be repaired exter-nally; self-care possible; lower rate of infection	May require routine heparin flushes, except with valves; catheter may break; daily to weekly site care; may be difficult to remove Surgical placement or placement in vascular interventional radiology

Continued

> Table 8-4 COMPARISON OF CENTRAL VENOUS CATHETERS—cont'd

Type and Use	Features	Advantages	Disadvantages
		Long-Term	
Implanted Ports Used for intermittent, continuous or daily I.V. access	Material: Silicone elastomer Catheter: Polyurethane Port: Titanium, stainless steel, plastic Average height: 9.8–17.0 mm Width of base: 24–50 mm (**Note:** Vary with manufacturer; low-profile ports available) Lumen: Dual Available with valved technology.	Can access dome port from any angle Preattached catheter or port or two-piece system Several catheter/ port locking devices available No dressing changes required, monthly heparin flushes, no activity restrictions, reduced risk of infection	Requires noncoring needle to access; expensive; requires minor surgery to remove

> Table 8-5 SUMMARY OF CARE AND MAINTENANCE FOR CENTRAL VENOUS ACCESS DEVICES

Care/Maintenance	Standards of Care
Dressings	Sterile dressings should be applied and replaced routinely. Gauze dressing should be replaced every 48 hours TSM dressings may stay in place up to 7 days If gauze is used in conjunction with a TSM dressing it is considered a gauze dressing and must be changed every 48 hours. **NOTE:** Initial PICC dressing needs to be changed after 24 hours
Administration Set Changes	Primary and secondary *continuous infusion* sets should be changed no more frequently than every 72 hours. Primary intermittent infusion sets should be changed every 24 hours Parenteral nutrition (PN) infusions: Change every 72 hours Sets used of PN containing I.V. fat emulsions change every 24 hours Sets used for PN with piggybacked I.V. fat emulsion change every 24 hours. Blood sets and add-on filters should be changed after administration of each unit or at the end of 4 hours.
Flushing and Locking	Refer to Tables 8-3 and 8-6 for specific flushing guidelines **NOTE:** Valved CVADs are designed to not require heparin locking Actual volume of flush or lock solution should follow catheter manufacturer's guidelines usually 2 times volume Positive pressure should be maintained on the flush syringe before it is disconnected to minimize reflux of blood. Refer to technique for positive or neutral displacement devices. Use a 10-mL syringe for all flushes **NOTE:** Ports when not in use do not require daily care.

> Table 8-5	SUMMARY OF CARE AND MAINTENANCE FOR CENTRAL VENOUS ACCESS DEVICES—cont'd
Care/Maintenance	**Standards of Care**
Injection Cap Changes	Disinfect with 70% alcohol with a twisting friction for 15 seconds (10 twists) before every access. Luer-Lok design Change cap every 7 days or at any time the cap/valve is removed.

Blood Sampling	Use discard method.
	Use a 10-mL syringe
	Flush the catheter with 5 mL of sodium chloride predraw.
	    Draw back 6 mL of blood and discard the sample. Attach a
	    new syringe or Vacutainer and collect samples.
	Label all samples at the bedside.
	Postdraw flush with 10 mL of sodium chloride using the
	    push–pause method.

NOTE: All add-on devices (extension tubing sets, injection caps, filters and syringes) should be Luer-Lok™ style.
Sources: Adapted from INS (2006a, 2008a).

NURSING POINTS-OF-CARE
LONG-TERM VENOUS ACCESS DEVICE

Nursing Assessments
■ Identify prescribed therapy, expected duration of therapy—months to years
■ Health history (including the client's vascular integrity)
■ Assess for skin lesions, implanted pacemaker, or cardioverted defibrillator.
■ Discuss with the patient previous VAD placement.
■ Obtain baseline vital signs.

Key Nursing Interventions
1. Implement the bundle approach to catheter insertion and maintenance:
   a. Hand hygiene by catheter inserters
   b. Maximum barrier precautions (gowns, gloves, mask, cap)
   c. Chlorhexidine gluconate with alcohol skin antisepsis of catheter insertion site
   d. Trained catheter inserter
   e. Proper selection of type of catheter and insertion site
   f. Insert catheters only when medically necessary
   g. Have all materials needed for catheter insertion at the bedside before starting insertion

Continued

    h. Time-out called if proper procedures are not followed (then start again)

    i. Use of aseptic technique during catheter manipulation

    j. Remove catheters when no longer medically necessary

2. Assist with insertion of central line when appropriate and enforce compliance with central line bundle.

3. Document the following daily:

    a. Solution infusing and type of administration set

    b. Flow rate

    c. Use of electronic infusion device

    d. Location of insertion site

    e. Assessment of the catheter and insertion site

    f. Inspection and description of the insertion site

    g. Condition of catheter tract and surrounding tissue

    h. Type of I.V. site dressing

    i. Patient response to catheter and patient education

4. Follow standards of practice for dressing changes, flushing and locking, blood sampling, and administration set changes.

5. Flushing procedures for ports vary from institution to institution. If the port is not being used nonvalved cap ports be flushed at least one or two times per week, valved at least weekly, and ports not in use flush with heparinized saline every 4 weeks with 3 to 5 mL of heparinized saline (except for closed-ended catheters).

6. Use a noncoring needle with appropriate port; change the needle and extension tubing every 7 days.

7. For ports with continuous infusion, change the dressing every 7 days.

8. For continuous infusion, change the tubing every 72 hours. Replace tubing used to administer blood, blood products, or lipids within 24 hours.

9. For CVTC be sure the catheter is clamped at all times.

10. Keep sharp objects away from the CVTC; never use scissors or pins on or near the CVTC catheter.

11. Protect the CVTC catheter when showering or bathing by covering the entire catheter with transparent dressing or clear plastic wrap. Cover the connections and protect hub connections from water contamination.

12. Use an infusion pump for delivery of solutions when appropriate.

13. Use a 10-mL syringe for all flushes to the central line and to obtain blood samples.

14. Change occlusive dressings every 7 days unless integrity is compromised.

15. Use active listening for patients who have a CVTC and express body image concerns.

AGE-RELATED CONSIDERATIONS ———————————————————————

Pediatric Central Venous Access

In addition to peripheral intravenous catheters and umbilical catheters, the use of surgically inserted tunneled central venous catheters (e.g., Broviac) and PICC catheters in neonates and pediatric clients have proven to be a realizable means of providing long-term access.

It is important to assess the infant early during hospital stay and to determine the most appropriate vascular access device. Selection criteria include:
• Length and type of anticipated therapies
• Age and weight of the infant
• Diagnoses
• Condition of the vasculature
• Current clinical condition of the infant

Long-term central venous access is an integral part of managing children with cancer, certain congenital malformations, and gastrointestinal (GI) malfunction as well as for those who need long-term access for medication or blood products.

Candidates for PICC insertion may include:
• Premature infants weighing less than 1500 g
• Infants requiring more than 6 days of intravenous therapy
• Limb anomalies (may limit the number of vascular sites)
• Infants requiring the infusion of fluids or medications with hyperosmolarity greater than 600 mOsm/kg and nonphysiologic pH less than 5 or greater than 9
• Infants with inadequate peripheral venous access (Pettit & Wyckoff, 2007)

After a decision is made to use a VAD, the device type must also be patient and disease specific. For children age 3 years and younger, totally implanted devices are used with the least frequency and most frequently in children older than age 15 years (Wiener & Albanese, 1998). The use of peripherally inserted central catheters has become accepted in the pediatric population. Typically, with diameters ranging from 20- to 28-gauge, they can be inserted to lengths ranging from 8 to 20 cm. Percutaneous midline catheters have been used in neonatal patients in 24- to 28-gauge and 8 cm in length, and are used to deliver fluids to the neonate (Dawson, 2002). Tunneled central venous catheters have been used but have disadvantages related to anesthesia and invasiveness of the insertion procedure along with risk of pneumothorax and hemothorax (Pettit & Wyckoff, 2007).

Guidelines for practices by the National Association of Neonatal Nurses (NANN) address educational competencies for nurses currently inserting and maintaining PICCs to promote infant safety (Pettit & Wyckoff, 2007).

Continued

PICC Insertion in the Infant

The following veins are used for PICC insertion in neonates and pediatric clients:

* Basilic and median cubital basilic vein
* Cephalic and median cubital cephalic vein
* Axillary vein
* External jugular (right sided approach is preferred)
* Temporal vein
* Posterior auricular vein
* Femoral vein (imaging technology is recommended while cannulating the femoral vein) (Rothschild, 2007).
* Greater saphenous: Multiple sites along the vein (reported higher incidence of phlebitis)
* Lesser saphenous
* Popliteal vein (premature infants) (Pettit & Wyckoff, 2007)

Infusion Nurses Standards of Practice (2006a, 2) has specific practice criteria for infusion in the pediatric patient. Some key standards are:

1. Assessment every hour
2. There shall be an informed consent for treatment of neonatal, pediatric, and adolescent patients.
3. The nurse providing infusion therapy for neonatal and pediatric patients shall have specific clinical knowledge and technical expertise.
4. The nurse providing infusion therapy should have validation of demonstrated competency in the areas of:
   a. Anatomy and physiology related to neonatal and pediatric patients
   b. Growth and development
   c. Competent in drug calculations with reference to age; height; weight or body surface area; dosage; metric conversions and calculations.
   d. Culturally, linguistically, and age-appropriate education and training for the patient; parents; significant other; caregiver; or legally authorized representative.
   e. Use of specialized neonatal and pediatric infusion related equipment, including care and maintenance procedures
   f. Obtaining consent from the school-age or adolescent patient as appropriate.

Pain Management

Pain management must be considered for children who will experience central venous access insertion and maintenance. There are many ways to identify and quantify pain in the pediatric setting. The use of pain scales is recommended such as the 0–10 numeric scale, Visual Analog Scale (VAS), and the Wong-Baker FACES Pain Rating Scale. For nonverbal children and infants observation scales have been used including Neonatal Pain, Agitation and Sedation Scale (NPASS), Face, Legs, Activity, Cry and Consolability (FLACC) and the CRIES (C: crying; R: requires oxygen to maintain saturation greater than 95%; I: increased vital signs; E: expression; S: sleepless) used for 32 to 60 weeks' gestational age.

Certain vascular procedures at times may need sedation or general anesthesia. Other products are available to assist with pain management of children with vascular access devices. They include the following:

• Sweet-Ease®
• Ethyl chloride
• Child life specialists
• Nitrous oxide
• Other conscious sedation (versed)
• EMLA/LM-X
• 1% Lidocaine subdermal/subcutaneous injection at the site.

All of the above require a physician or health professional's order (Heckler-Medina, 2006)

Care and Maintenance of Central Venous Access in Children

Blood Sampling

• Success in obtaining blood samples from PICC that range from 24- to 26-gauge or 1.9 Fr PICC are being reported but require further investigation
• Catheter lumens smaller than 26 gauge are too restrictive to allow blood samples. Evidence does support blood sampling through a 3 Fr PICC without a significant increase in occlusion (Knue, Doellman, Rabin, & Jacobs, 2005).

Flushing

• Maintaining patency of small-bore catheters requires meticulous care to prevent occlusion.
• Flush before and after administering potentially incompatible solutions and medications.
• Both sodium chloride and diluted heparinized saline solutions may be used.
• Use single-use vials (O'Grady, Alexander, Dellinger, et al., 2002).
• Syringes should be used one time and discarded.
• The volume of the flush should be twice the catheter volume and any add-on devices. Refer to Table 8-6 for current protocols on flushing central line catheters (INS, 2008c).

INS Standard All connectors must be Luer-Lok™ design. (INS, 2006a, S29)

Dressing Change

• No formal dressing-change practices have been done in neonates.
• Most NICUs change dressing only when dressing integrity is compromised.
• Weekly dressing changes are components of central venous catheter bundles.

Continued

> Table 8-6	NEONATAL AND PEDIATRIC FLUSHING PROTOCOLS		
Device	**Locked Device: Volume, Frequency and Solution**	**Medications: Pre- and Postadministration**	**Blood Product Administration and Sampling Withdrawal**
PICC	*2 Fr:* 1 mL NS + 10 units/mL heparin every 6 hours *2.6 Fr and larger:* 2–3 mL NS + 10 units/mL heparin every 12 hours	2 times administration tubing and add-on set volume	*2 Fr: Sampling and pre- and post-blood administration:* 1 mL to clear the catheter, then flush with 1 mL of NS followed by locking solution until clear. *2.6 Fr and larger: Sampling and pre- and post-blood administration:* 1–3 mL NS followed by locking solution or resume infusion *Withdrawal volume:* 3 times administration tubing and add-on set volume.
Tunneled and Nontunneled	*NICU patients:* 1–3 mL NS + 10 units/mL of heparin every 12–24 hours *Pediatrics:* 2 mL NS + 10 units/mL of heparin every 24 hours	2 times administration tubing and add-on set volume	*Pre- and post-blood administration:* 1 mL NS for NICU patients and 3 mL NS for all others followed by locking solution or resume infusion. *Withdrawal volume for sampling:* 3 times administration tubing and add-on set volume. **Note:** Variation in size makes it difficult to recommend one volume for all patients
Ports	*If used for more than 1 medication daily:* 3–5 mL NS + 10 units/ mL heparin *Monthly maintenance flush:* 3–5 mL NS + 100 units/mL of heparin	2 times administration tubing and add-on set volume	*Pre- and post-blood administration:* 3–5 mL NS followed by locking solution or resume infusion *Withdrawal volume for sampling:* 3 times administration tubing and add-on set volume. **Note:** Variation in size makes it difficult to recommend one volume for all patients.

NS = normal saline (sodium chloride); NICU = neonatal intensive care unit.
NOTE: Use single-use preservative-free 0.9% sodium chloride for flushes.
Source: INS (2008c), with permission.

- For gauze and tape every 48 hours (O'Grady, Alexander, Dellinger, et al., 2002)
- TSM dressings should be changed when they no longer adhere to the catheter or skin, or are damp or soiled (O'Grady, Alexander, Dellinger, et al., 2002)

> **INS Standard** The use of chlorhexidine gluconate in infants weighing < 1000 grams has been associated with contact dermatitis and should be used with caution. For neonates, isopropyl alcohol or products containing isopropyl alcohol are not recommended for access site prepartion. (INS, 2006a, 41)

The Older Adult
- When a central venous access device is placed in the older adult prehydration is often necessary, especially with PICC placement. Prehydration with a 22- or 24-gauge PIV, rehydration promotes venous dilation making the insertion of the larger venous access device easier.
- Evaluation of a short-term versus a long-term device should be evaluated, as should the older adult's ability to care for the device. The nontunneled short-term CVC may be appropriate for several weeks of therapy.
- The patient and/or caregiver may have difficulty maintaining and coping with dressing and flushing procedures.
- Implanted vascular access port may be a better alternative due to reduced cathter care requirements.

Home Care Issues

Central venous access devices are frequently used in the home for administering long-term antimicrobial medications, TPN, chemotherapy or biologic therapy, blood component therapy, and analgesics, and for frequent blood sampling. Home infusion is comprehensive, beginning with principles of asepsis, handwashing, and standard precautions.

It is essential to assess whether or not the patient being considered for using a central venous line at home is interested in and motivated to participate in self-care. This procedure requires a certain level of intellectual, emotional, and physical capacity and commitment to comply. Patients are generally expected to learn how to flush the CVC and perform site assessment and care of tunneled CVCs. Most often with PICCs, the home care nurse performs the dressing changes. All patients and / or caregivers must be instructed in potential complications of the CVC, what to look for, and what actions to take, for example, to call the home care nurse right away for signs of infection. For patients with implanted ports, self-care expectations are minimal unless there is a running infusion at home. If the patient is not physically or emotionally able to self-administer or monitor care, a reliable caregiver must be available.

Continued

Home Care Issues—cont'd

Factors affecting venous access device selection for the home care patient:
- Patient diagnosis and anticipated infusion therapy needs/infusate properties
- Anticipated length of therapy (midline catheter or PICC)
- Impaired immune status or bleeding disorders (avoid devices associated with a higher risk of infection; if low platelet count, avoid PICCs)
- Anomalies and other anatomic concerns: Previous chest surgery, wounds, infected areas or thrombosis in arm; PICCs are contraindicated in patients at risk for end-stage renal disease owing to need for vein preservation (Saad & Vesely, 2003)
(Gorski & Czaplewiski, 2004)

Pretreatment Assessment Includes:
1. Taking a health history, including issues relevant to planned therapy
2. Verifying the medication and dosage that the patient is to receive
3. Reviewing complications and side effects of drug therapy and central line management
4. Reviewing the patient's history and past experience, if appropriate, with central lines
5. Assessing the patient's current knowledge of managing central lines
6. Providing written instruction and diagrams of accessing line, site care, and flushing protocol
7. Verifying insurance coverage for home care

The patient and family should have full instructions on how central line devices function and the safety precautions associated with their use. The home infusion patient should have step-by-step written information regarding care and maintenance.

Pediatric Clients

The psychosocial and developmental needs of the child and family need to be addressed by the home infusion company along with education of child and family on therapy and equipment use.

Children are more mobile and active. The best infusion device is one that is lightweight and portable and that requires minimal programming.

When there are long-term and complex infusion therapy needs, alternative caregivers in the home should be identified early in the process to allow the parent respite periods.

Patient Education

Patient instructions for central line devices should include:
- Type of central venous access device, purpose, and length of catheter or port that will be inserted; signs and symptoms to report, such as increased temperature, discomfort, pain, and difficult breathing; site care of PICC, CVTC, or implanted port

Patient Education—cont'd

- Emergency measures for clamping the catheter if it breaks
- Flushing protocol
- Access line for administering medication, TPN, or fluids

Nurses are instrumental in educating patients and family members that the skin area over a subcutaneously implanted VAD should not be rubbed or manipulated in any way. Twiddler's syndrome, a condition in which a patient manipulates his or her ports by habit, can cause the internal catheter attached to the port to dislodge.

🔳 Nursing Process

The nursing process is a five- or six-step process for problem-solving to guide nursing action. Refer to Chapter 1 for details on the steps of the nursing process related to vascular access. The following table focuses on nursing diagnoses, nursing outcomes classification (NOC), and nursing intervention classification (NIC) for patients with central vascular access. Nursing diagnoses should be patient specific and outcomes and interventions individualized. The NOC and NIC presented here are suggested direction for development of specific outcomes and interventions.

Nursing Diagnoses Related to Central Venous Access	NOC: Nursing Outcomes Classification	NIC: Nursing Intervention Classification
Protection, ineffective related to: Treatments: Placement of central venous access device.	Health-promoting behavior	Injury protection
Risk for infection related to: Inadequate primary defenses (broken skin, traumatized tissue); inadequate secondary defenses (decreased hemoglobin, leukopenia); increased environmental exposure to pathogens through I.V. equipment.	Infection control, risk control, risk detection	Infection control practices and central line bundle implementation
Impaired skin integrity related to: VAD; irritation for I.V. solution; inflammation; infection	Tissue integrity: primary intention healing of VAD insertion site	Incision site care, skin surveillance

Continued

Nursing Diagnoses Related to Central Venous Access	NOC: Nursing Outcomes Classification	NIC: Nursing Intervention Classification
Body image disturbance related to: Illness treatment: central venous tunneled catheter	Psychosocial adjustment	Body image enhancement
Knowledge deficit related to: Unfamiliarity with central vascular access devices and information provided	Knowledge of treatment regimen	Teaching: Disease process and CVC care and maintenance
Interrupted family processes related to: Shift in health status of a family member	Family coping with ill child and life changes	Family process maintenance, family therapy, normalization promotion, role enhancement, support system enhancement
Anxiety (mild, moderate, and severe) related to: Threat to change in health status or misconception regarding therapy.	Anxiety level	Anxiety reduction

Sources: Ackley & Ladwig (2008); McCloskey-Dochterman & Bulechek (2004); Moorhead, Johnson, & Maas (2004); NANDA-I (2007).

Chapter Highlights

- Nurses must have knowledge of venous anatomy before initiation, care, and maintenance of central lines.
- Decision to place a CVC is based on a thorough assessment including patient health problems; device availability; the client's vascular integrity; previous I.V. problems; purpose, nature, and duration of I.V. therapy; and patient needs/preferences with lifestyle.
- The tip of central venous access devices should be in the SVC; the tip should reside within 3 to 4 cm of the right atrial SVC junction. It must be free floating and lie parallel to the vessel wall without any looping or kinking.
- Nurses should have knowledge of catheter materials, coatings, tip configurations, lumen types, and catheter length and gauges.
- Central venous access devices and the length of time they may remain include:
  - Nontunneled percutaneous catheters: 7 to 10 days
  - PICCs: 6 weeks to more than 1 year
  - CVTCs: 3 years
  - Implanted ports: 3 years

- The patient should be well hydrated if the infraclavicular approach to percutaneous catheterization is used.
- The basilic vein is the preferred insertion site for PICCs.
- After insertion of the central line, radiographic confirmation must be obtained before any infusion is administered.

Care and Maintenance Issues

- The optimum frequency for changing TSM dressing is unknown, but the dressing should be changed at established intervals (generally a minimum of 7 days) or immediately if the integrity of the dressing is compromised.
- Syringes with capacities of 10 mL or more must be used to access or irrigate central lines, as excessive pressure from smaller-barreled syringes can cause damage or rupture of the line.
- Nurses managing central lines must be trained in their use; follow manufacturer guidelines; comply with agency protocols and policies; and be fully competent in the assessment, planning, intervention, and evaluation of the patient.
- Use Luer-locking connections on all central lines.
- Use the "push–pause" method of flushing central lines.
- All CVCs must be maintained with flushing techniques and vary from device to device. INS (2008) flushing protocols are presented in tables in this chapter.
- The central line bundle approach is a new standard applicable to all central lines.
- Blood sampling from a PICC can be challenging if the size is less than 3 Fr.
- Due to biofilm from microorganisms, the caps must be maintained with diligent cleaning. Use alcohol for 15 seconds, twisting a minimum of 10 times to clean the cap/valve. This is to be done each and every time the cap is accessed.
- Competency needs to be demonstrated by the nurse for accessing and deaccessing ports.
- Injection caps and stabilization devices are changed every 7 days, or when the integrity of the device is compromised.

▪▪Thinking Critically: Case Study

As a new graduate, you have been asked to change a complicated abdominal dressing on a patient postoperatively. This patient is receiving chemotherapy via a tunneled catheter. As you are cutting the dressing off, you accidentally puncture the catheter.

What do you do?

How could this have been avoided?

Media Link: Answers to the case study and more critical thinking activities are provided on the CD-ROM.

Post-Test

1. Implanted ports, when not in use, can be flushed every:
   a. Week
   b. 2 Weeks
   c. 3 Weeks
   d. 4 Weeks

2. When tunneled catheters are used, an advantage to the patient is that they:
   a. Remain patent without flushing procedures
   b. Can be replaced easily
   c. Can be used for multiple purposes
   d. Have minimal associated body image change

3. The blunt catheter tip with a three-way valve is called a:
   a. PICC
   b. Dual-lumen catheter
   c. Groshong® tip
   d. Hickman® catheter

4. The nursing intervention most effective for removing a "stuck" PICC is to:
   a. Stretch the catheter and tape it to the arm for 2 to 4 hours, then remove.
   b. Leave it alone, gently massage or apply moist heat to the area of the upper arm, and reattempt removal in 20 to 30 minutes after the vein relaxes.
   c. Use the guidewire to assist in removal.
   d. Call the physician to remove the catheter under fluoroscopy.

5. The *best* nursing intervention for flushing a central line to prevent fibrin buildup in the catheter is the:
   a. Push–pause technique
   b. Use of positive pressure
   c. Gentle instillation of solution with no pressure or agitation
   d. Instillation of heparin with each flush

6. The choice of syringe barrel capacity for irrigating a central line would be:
   a. 1 cc
   b. 3 cc
   c. 5 cc
   d. 10 cc

7. Which of the following standards of practice are appropriate for dressing management? (*Select all that apply.*)
   a. Change gauze dressing after the first 24 hours on a PICC.
   b. Change gauze dressing every 48 hours
   c. Change TSM dressings every 7 days.
   d. Use a Biopatch under all dressings.

8. The assessments before consideration of placement of a CVC in a patient should include which of the following? (*Select all that apply.*)
   a. Vascular integrity
   b. Expected duration of the therapy
   c. Client preference related to lifestyle
   d. Health history

9. Which of the following is standard of practice for implanted port dressings? (*Select all that apply.*)
   a. Follow routine standards of practice for all CVCs
   b. After the site has healed dressing is not routinely needed
   c. After insertion by the physician no dressing is needed at any time.
   d. Apply a gauze or TSM dressing for 10 days after insertion.

10. Collection of a blood specimen from a central line that has parenteral nutrition infusing requires that the nurse *first*:
    a. Turn off the infusion 3 to 5 minutes before obtaining the blood sample.
    b. Flush the catheter with 10 mL of 0.9% sodium chloride.
    c. Use only a Vacutainer system.
    d. Withdraw 5 mL of blood and discard.

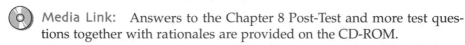 Media Link: Answers to the Chapter 8 Post-Test and more test questions together with rationales are provided on the CD-ROM.

▪ References

Ackley, B.J., & Ladwig, G.B. (2008). *Nursing diagnosis handbook: An evidence-based guide to planning care.* St. Louis, MO: Mosby Elsevier.

Anstett, M., & Royer, T. (2003). The impact of ultrasound on PICC placement. *JAVA, 8*(3), 24–28.

Arch, P. (2007). Port navigation: Let the journey begin. *Oncology Nursing 101, 11*(4), 485–488.

Banton, J., & Banning, V. (2002). Impact on catheter-related bloodstream infections with the use of the Biopatch dressing. *Journal of Vascular Access Devices, 7*(3), 27–32.

C.R. Bard Access Systems (2008). Product information on POWER PICC. Retrieved from www.bard.com (Accessed July 19, 2008).

Burns, D. (2005). The Vanderbilt PICC service: Program, procedural, and patient outcomes successes. *Journal of Association for Vascular Access, 10*, 183–192.

Camp-Sorrell, D. (2004). *Access device guidelines: Recommendations for nursing practice and education* (2nd ed.). Pittsburgh, PA: Oncology Nursing Society.

Chaiyakunapruk, H., Veenstra, D.L., Lipsky, B.A., et al. (2002). Chlorhexidine gluconate compared with povidone-iodine solution for vascular catheter-site care: A meta-analysis. *Annals of Internal Medicine, 136*(11), 792–801.

Dawson, D. (2002). Midline catheters in neonatal patients: Evaluating a change in practice. *Journal of Vascular Access Devices, 7*(2), 17–19.

DiFiore, A.E. (2005). Clinical and engineering considerations for the design of indwelling vascular access devices. *JAVA, 10*(1), 24–27.

Ellenberger, A. (2002). How to change a PICC dressing. *Nursing 2002, 32*(2), 50–52.

Frey, A.M. (2003). Drawing blood samples from vascular access devices: Evidence-based practice. *Journal of Infusion Nursing, 26*(5), 285–293.

Gabriel, J. (2003). PICC dressings. *JAVA, 8*(4), 41–43.

Gorski, L., & Czaplewski, L. (2004). Peripherally inserted central catheters and midline catheters for the homecare nurse. *Journal of Infusion Nursing, 27*(6), 399–409.

Hadaway, L.C. (2006). Technology of flushing vascular access devices. *JIN, 29*(3), 137–145.

Halerman, F. (2000). Selecting a vascular access device. *Nursing 2000, 30*(11), 59–61.

Hamilton, H.C. (2006). Complications associated with venous access devices: part one. *Nursing Standards, 20*(26), 43–50.

Heckler-Medina, G.A. (2006). The importance of child life and pain management during vascular access procedures in pediatrics. *JAVA, 2*(3), 144–151.

Higuchi, K.A., Edwards, N., Danseco, E., et al. (2007). Development of an evaluation tool for a clinical practice guideline on nursing assessment and device selection for vascular access. *Journal of Infusion Nursing, 30*(1), 45–51.

Infusion Nurses Society (INS). (2006a). *Infusion nursing standards of practice.* Philadelphia: Lippincott Williams & Wilkins.

Infusion Nurses Society (INS). (2006b). *Policies and procedures for infusion nursing* (3rd ed.). Norwood, MA: Author.

Infusion Nurses Society (INS). (2008a). Nursing practice management. Central vascular access devices: An overview. *Infusion Nurses Society, 1*(1), 4–11.

Infusion Nurses Society (INS). (2008b). Position Paper: The role of the registered nurse in the insertion of external jugular peripherally inserted central catheters (EJ PICC) and external jugular peripheral intravenous catheter (EJ PIV). Norwood, MA: Author.

Infusion Nurses Society (INS). (2008c). Flushing protocols. Norwood, MA: Author.

Kaler, W., & Chinn, R. (2007). Successful disinfection of needleless access ports: A matter of time and friction. *Journal of Association for Vascular Access, 12*(3), 140–142.

Knue, M., Doellman, D., Rabin, K., & Jacobs, B.R. (2005). The efficacy and safety of blood sampling through peripherally inserted central catheter devices in children. *Journal of Infusion Nursing, 28*(1), 3–35.

Lewis, C.A., Allen, T.E., Burke, D.R., et al. (2003). Quality improvement guidelines for central venous access. *Journal of Vascular and Interventional Radiology, 14*, S231–S235.

Linck, D.A., Donze, A., & Hamvas, A. (2007). Neonatal peripherally inserted central catheter team: Evolution and outcomes of a bedside-nurse-designed program. *Advances in Neonatal Care, 7*, 22–29.

Ludeman, K. (2007). Choosing the right vascular access device. *Nursing 2007.* Retrieved from www.nurisng2007.com (Accessed July 7, 2008).

Macklin, D. (2000). Removing a PICC. *American Journal of Nursing, 100*(1), 52–54.

Maki, D.G., & Mermel, L.A. (2007). Infections due to infusion therapy. In: W.R. Jarvis (Ed.), *Hospital infections* (5th ed.). Philadelphia: Lippincott, Williams & Wilkins.

Maki, D., Mermel, L.A., Klugar, D., et al. (2000). The efficacy of a chlorhexidine impregnated sponge (Biopatch) for the prevention of intravascular catheter-related infection – a prospective randomized controlled multicenter study (Abstract). Presented at the Interscience Conference on Antimicrobial Agents and Chemotherapy. American Society for Microbiology, Toronto. Canada, May.

Marx, M. (1995). The management of difficult peripherally inserted central venous catheter line removal. *Journal of Intravenous Nursing, 18*(5), 246–249.

Massorli, S., & Angeles, T. (2002). Getting a line on CVAD. Central vascular access devices. *Nursing 2002, 32*(4), 36–43.

Mayer, T., & Wong, D.G. (2002). The use of polyurethane PICCS an alternative to other catheter materials. *Journal of Vascular Access Devices, 7*(2), 26–30.

McCloskey-Dochterman, J.C., & Bulechek, G.M. (2004). *Nursing interventions classification (NIC)* (4th ed.). St. Louis, MO: C.V. Mosby.

Mermel, L.A. (2001). New technologies to prevent intravascular catheter-related bloodstream infections. *Emerging Infectious Diseases, 7*(2), 197–199.

Miller, P.A. (2006). Central venous access devices. *Radiologic Technology, 77*(4), 297–305.

Moorhead, H.R., & Bergeron, B.J. (2007). Valved catheters including high flow rate catheters. Retrieved from www.freepatientsonline (Accessed August 15, 2008).

Moorhead, S., Johnson, M., & Maas, M. (2004). *Nursing outcomes classification (NOC)* (3rd ed.). St. Louis, MO: C.V. Mosby.

Moureau, N. (2001). Preventing complications with vascular access devices. *Nursing 2001, 31*(7), 52–55.

Moureau, N. (2006). Vascular safety: It's all about PICCs. *Nursing Management, 37*(5), 22–27.

Moureau, N., Poole, S., Murdock, M.A., et al. (2002). Central venous catheters in home infusion care: Outcomes analysis 50,470 patients. *Journal of Vascular Interventional Radiology, 13*(10), 1009–1016.

The National Committee for Clinical Laboratory Standards (NCCLS). (1998). *Collection, transport, and processing of blood specimens for coagulation testing and general performance of coagulation assays; approved guidelines* (3rd ed.). NCCLS document H3–A4. Villanova, PA: NCCLS, June 1998.

NANDA-I (2007). *Nursing diagnoses: Definitions and classification, 2007–2008.* Philadelphia: Author.

National Kidney Foundation/Dialysis Outcomes Quality Initiative. (2002). Clinical practice guidelines for vascular access. *American Journal of Kidney Disease, 37*(Supplement 1), S137–S181.

O'Grady, N.P., Alexander, M., Dellinger, E.P., et al. (2002). Guidelines for the prevention of intravascular catheter-related infections. *Morbidity and Mortality Weekly Report MMWR 51*(RR-10).

Pettit, J., & Wyckoff, M.M. (2007). *Peripherally inserted central catheters* (2nd ed.). Glenview, IL: National Association of Neonatal Nurses.

Pieger-Mooney, S. (2005). Innovations in central vascular access device insertion. *Journal of Infusion Nursing, 28*(3S), S7–S12.

Pronovost, P., Needham, D., Berenholts, S., et al. (2006). An intervention to decrease catheter-related bloodstream infections in ICU. *New England Journal of Medicine, 355*(26), 2725–2732.

Rothschild, J.M. (2007). Ultrasound guidance of central vein catheterization. In: Wachter, R.M. (Director), Making healthcare safer: A critical analysis of patient safety principles—Agency for Healthcare Research and Quality. Retrieved from www.ahrq.gov/clinic/ptsafety/chapter 21.htm (Accessed February 22, 2010).

Rupp, M.E., Lisco, S.J., Lipsett, P.A., et al. (2005). Effect of a second-generation venous catheter impregnated with chlorhexidine and silver sulfadiazine on central catheter-related infections: A randomized, controlled trial. *Annals of Internal Medicine, 143*(8), 570–580.

Ryder, M. (2005). Catheter-related infections: It's all about biofilm. *Topics in Advanced Practice Nursing eJournal, 5*(3), 291–295.

Saad, T.F., & Vesely, T.M. (2003). Venous access for patients with chronic renal failure or end-stage renal disease: What is the role for peripherally inserted central catheters? *The Journal of Association for Vascular Access, 8*, 27–32.

Safdar, N., & Maki, D.R. (2005). Risk of catheter-related bloodstream infection in peripherally inserted central venous catheters used in hospitalized patients. *Chest, 128*(2), 489–495.

Sampath, L.A., Tambe, S., & Modak, S.M. (2001). In vitro and in vivo efficacy of catheters impregnated with antiseptics or antibiotics: Evaluation of the risk of bacterial resistance to antimicrobials in the catheters. *Infection Control & Hospital Epidemiology, 22*(10), 640–646.

Schelonka, R., Scruggs, S., Nichols, K., et al. (2006). Sustained reductions in neonatal nosocomial infection rates following a comprehensive infection control intervention. *Journal of Perinatology, 26*, 176–179.

Standing, S. (2004). *Gray's anatomy: The anatomical basis of clinical practice* (39th ed.). Philadelphia: Elsevier Churchill Livingston.

Wiener, E.S., & Albanese, C.T. (1998). Venous access in pediatric patients. *Journal of Intravenous Nursing* (Supplement), *21*(5S), S123–S131.

Young, G.P., Alexeyeff, M., Russell, D.M., et al. (1988). Catheter sepsis during parenteral nutrition: The safety of long-term OpSite dressings. *JPEN, 12*, 365–370.

PROCEDURES DISPLAY 8-1

Central Venous Catheter Dressing Change

Equipment Needed
(Custom-made or premade kits are available from manufacturers)
Sterile gloves and mask
Sterile drape or kit
Transparent semipermeable membrane (TSM) dressing
Stabilization device
Antiseptic solution: 70% alcohol swabs, 2% chlorhexidine gluconate
Labels

Delegation:
Do not delegate to an LPN/LVN or nursing assistive personnel
(NAP), unless there is part of state nursing practice for LPN/LVN,
and included in P& P for institution. The practitioner needs competency training for central venous access care and maintenance.

Procedure	Rationale
1. Review authorized pre-scriber's order or standing policy and procedure.	1. Policies and procedures provide a framework for standard of care at the institution.
2. Wash hands using friction for 15–20 seconds.	2. Good hand hygiene is the single most important means of preventing the spread of infection.
3. Introduce yourself to the patient.	3. Establishes the nurse–patient relationship
4. Verify patient's identity using two forms of ID (check ID bracelet and ask patient to state name).	4. The Joint Commission (2003) safety goal recommendation.
5. Wear powder-free gloves for the dressing removal.	5. Protects the nurse and patient from exposure to pathogens.
6. Remove the transparent dressing gently by pulling in an upward direction to prevent dislodging or pulling the catheter out. Stabilize the insertion site while removing the dressing to prevent inadvertent dislodgment of a nontunneled catheter or PICC. Remove the stabilization device.	6. Prevents accidental removal of catheters that are not tunneled or implanted. The stabilization device (e.g., StatLock®) must be changed every 7 days.

Continued

PROCEDURES DISPLAY 8-1

Central Venous Catheter Dressing Change—cont'd

Procedure	Rationale
7. Examine the dressing and site for drainage or foul odor.	7. These are signs of infection and may warrant a culture.
8. Inspect the catheter site for abnormalities: Catheter slippage, erythema, induration, loose or absent sutures, tenderness, redness, and edema, or if PICC, in addition, the arm and the track of the vein for redness. For PICC also measure the circumference of the upper arm and document.	8. Monitor for complications associated with central venous catheters.
9. Remove gloves and carry out proper hand hygiene.	9. To maintain aseptic technique
10. Prepare a sterile drape placing dressing and aseptically open supplies.	10. and 11. Maintain sterile barrier technique.
11. Don sterile gloves and mask.	
12. Clean the CVC site: Use friction back and forth to cleanse the site with alcohol for a minimum of 30 seconds.	12. To ensure proper and thorough cleaning and removal of debris
13. Use 2% chlorhexidine gluconate and alcohol prep using friction for a minimum of 30 seconds. *Allow to air dry.*	13. Studies have found chlorhexidine to aid in prevention of CR-BSIs.
NOTE: The prepped site will be approximately the size of the dressing (2–4 inches).	
14. Apply a new securement device.	14. Securement/stabilization devices must be changed every 7 days.

PROCEDURES DISPLAY 8-1

Central Venous Catheter Dressing Change—cont'd

Procedure	Rationale
15. Apply a new transparent dressing over the exposed catheter, including the hub. Avoid sealing the TSM dressing edges with tape.	15. Occlusive dressing required for CVC to inhibit the entry of microorganisms.
16. Remove the gloves and discard; dispose of all used materials in a biohazard container.	16. Reduces microbial contamination.
17. To the side of the dressing place the label with the nurse's initials and date, time.	17. To maintain proper documentation and communicate dressing change information to all who care for the patient
18. Document the procedure in the patient's permanent record, including assessment data, condition of the removed dressing, appropriate intervention data, and the evlauation of the patient's response to the procedure.	18. To maintain a legal record and communication with the healthcare team

Sources: INS (2006a,b).

PROCEDURES DISPLAY 8-2

Flushing a Central Venous Catheter

Equipment Needed
10-mL syringe
Preservative-free 0.9% sodium chloride: 1 10-mL vial (single use)
Gloves
Sharps container
Antiseptic solution
Prefilled air locked syringe with 5 mL of heparin, 10 U/mL, one 5-mL vial.
Sterile injection or access cap

Continued

PROCEDURES DISPLAY 8-2

Flushing a Central Venous Catheter—cont'd

Delegation:
This procedure cannot be delegated to an LPN/LVN or NAP. The practitioner needs competency training for central venous access care and maintenance.

Procedure	Rationale
1. Check the policy and procedure on flushing.	1. Policies and procedures provide a framework for standard of care at the institution.
2. Introduce yourself to the patient.	2. Promotes the nurse–patient relationship, and establishes communication.
3. Use two identifiers to verify patient identity: checking wrist band against the blood work order and asking patient his or her name (if conscious).	3. The Joint Commission (2003) safety goal recommendation.
4. Carry out proper hand hygiene.	4. Good hand hygiene is the single most important means of preventing the spread of infection.
5. Identify whether the needleless injection cap/valve is a negative-displacement device, a positive-displacement device or a neutral-displacement device.	5. Negative- and positive-displacement devices are dependent on flushing technique. A positive pressure technique is required with a negative-displacement device. With a positive-displacement device positive pressure flushing cannot be used. With neutral-displacement the function of the device is not dependent on the flushing technique.
6. Don gloves.	6. Prevents the spread of infection.
7. Cleanse the central venous catheter injection cap (port) with 70% isopropyl alcohol with a twisting motion for 15 seconds (10 twists). Allow to air-dry.	7. Prevents introduction of microorganisms into the system.

PROCEDURES DISPLAY 8-2

Flushing a Central Venous Catheter—cont'd

Procedure	Rationale
8. Attach a syringe containing 5 mL of 0.9% sodium chloride to the injection port via a needleless system.	8. To administer the irrigant and maintain patency of the catheter.
9. Open the CVC clamp.	9. Access to the length of the catheter.
10. Slowly aspirate until brisk positive blood return.	10. Confirms catheter patency.
11. Irrigate the line with 0.9% sodium chloride using the push–pause method.	11. Prevents the catheter from being the focus of microbial growth, cleans the lumen of the CVC, and prevents occlusion of the line.

Note: There are different types of NIS devices, be sure you know which devices are used in your facility. Negative and positive displacement devices are dependent on flushing technique.

12a. For negative-displacement devices (positive-pressure flushing required)	12a. Manufacturer requires positive-pressure flushing technique to prevent reflux of blood.

As the last 0.5–1 mL of solution is flushed inward, withdraw the syringe, allowing the last amount of flush solutions to fill the dead space.

Flush all solution into the catheter lumen; maintain force on the syringe plunger as a clamp on the catheter or extension set is closed; then disconnect the syringe.

Continued

PROCEDURES DISPLAY 8-2

Flushing a Central Venous Catheter—cont'd

Procedure	Rationale
12b. Positive-displacement device (Positive pressure flushing technique cannot be used because it will overcome the positive displacement mechanism.) Flush the catheter gently with solution, disconnect the syringe, and allow sufficient time for the positive fluid displacement; then close the catheter clamp.	**12b.** Manufacturer requires the catheter to be clamped before disconnection of the syringe. A positive pressure technique on this system will prevent proper function of a positive-displacement system.
12c. Neutral-displacement device (not dependent on flush technique)	
For CVC that require heparin Repeat steps 5 through 7.	
13. Disinfect the access cap with 70% alcohol for 15 seconds using a twisting motion (10 twists).	**13.** Prevents introduction of microorganisms into the system.
14. Attach the heparin-filled 10 mL syringe with the heparinized saline to the injection port indicated. Follow flush guidelines for the amount of heparin, 3–5 mL of 10 U/mL of heparin.	**14.** Maintains patency of the catheter and prevents occlusion.
15. Final irrigation of the line with heparinized saline solution: Use positive-pressure flushing following 12a or 12b depending on needleless injection system (NIS) used.	
16. Document the procedure on the patient record.	**16.** To maintain a legal record and communication with the healthcare team.

Sources: Hadaway (2006); INS (2006a,b).

PROCEDURES DISPLAY 8-3

Blood Sampling from a Central Venous Access Device (CVAD)

Equipment Needed
Prepping solution: 70% alcohol, 2% chlorhexidine gluconate
Vacuum tube sleeve
Vacuum tube adapters, single-ended needle for puncture of collecting tubes with reflux valve for use with needleless systems
Assorted blood collecting tubes
Appropriate number of empty 10-mL syringes (if vacuum system is not used)
Two or three 10-mL syringes with 10 mL of preservative-free 0.9% sodium chloride
5 mL of prefilled air-purged heparin 10 or 100 U/mL vials
Disposable gloves
Sharps container
Sterile injection cap (if applicable)
Delegation:
Most institutions do not have phlebotomists draw blood from a central line. This procedure cannot be delegated to an LPN/LVN or NAP. The practitioner needs competency training for central venous access care and maintenance.

Procedure	Rationale
1. Check orders to confirm laboratory work.	1. A physician's order is a legal requirement for blood collection.
2. Introduce yourself to the patient.	2. Promotes the nurse–patient relationship, and establishes communication.
3. Use two identifiers to verify patient identity: checking wrist band against the blood work order and ask the patient his or her name (if conscious).	3. The Joint Commission (2003) safety goal recommendation.
4. Carry out proper hand hygiene.	4. Good hand hygiene is the single most important means of preventing the spread of infection.
5. Set up equipment.	5. Saves time and prevents interruption during the blood draw. Verify the correct blood collection tubes.

Continued

PROCEDURES DISPLAY 8-3

Blood Sampling from a Central Venous Access Device (CVAD)—cont'd

Procedure	Rationale
6. Put on gloves.	6. Protects the nurse from potential blood contamination.
7. If CVAD is not in use: Prep the valved access port with alcohol for 15 seconds with a twisting motion; allow to dry. Follow with 2% chlorhexidine gluconate.	7. Prevents introduction of microorganisms into the system.
8. If CVAD is in use: a. Single-lumen: Close the slide clamp on the pigtail. Instruct patient to perform the Valsalva maneuver, then quickly disconnect the administration set tubing from the injection port, and cap the distal end of the administration set with the sterile cap.	8. To prevent air entry into the circulation and air embolism
b. Multi-lumen: Use the proximal lumen to draw blood and turn off all electrolyte- and glucose-containing infusates for a minimum of 1 full minute.	8b. So blood will be untainted
9. Prep the valved access port with alcohol; follow with 2% chlorhexidine gluconate and allow to dry.	9. To prevent contamination
10. Attach the 10-mL syringe prefilled with 5 mL of normal saline; open the slide clamp and vigorously irrigate with 5 mL of sodium chloride using the pulsatile, push–pause method. Clamp.	10. To maintain patency of the line and exert a flush

PROCEDURES DISPLAY 8-3

Blood Sampling from a Central Venous Access Device (CVAD)—cont'd

Procedure	Rationale
11. Attach the vacuum container to the injection cap. Unclamp.	
12. Hold the tube in place until blood flow ceases: this is considered the "discard." The volume should be 1.5–2 times the fill volume of the CVAD.	12. To obtain an accurate blood sample
13. Quickly insert and fill the required blood collection tubes, then close the slide clamp and remove the vacuum container collecting device.	13. To obtain all required specimens
14. Prep the injection cap again and attach a 10-mL syringe with normal saline (NS) and vigorously flush with at least 10 mL of NS using the pulsatile, push–pause method.	14. To clear the line and eliminate a site for microbial growth
15. Reconnect the infusion line and begin infusion; **OR** attach prefilled air-purged 3–5 mL heparinized saline, 10 U/mL for nontunneled, tunneled, and PICC, 100 U/mL for ports if access device is not going to be used.	15. To resume the ordered infusate or to prevent occlusion of the CVC line
16. Label the collection tubes and deliver the sample to the laboratory as soon as the integrity of the CVC is ensured.	16. To prevent clerical errors and ensure the right lab sample is for the correct patient
17. Dispose of used equipment in a sharps container.	17. To avoid needlestick injuries

Continued

PROCEDURES DISPLAY 8-3

Blood Sampling from a Central Venous Access Device (CVAD)—cont'd

Procedure	Rationale
18. Document the procedure in the patient's permanent record.	18. To maintain a legal record and communication with the healthcare team

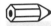 *NURSING FAST FACT!*

- *If total parenteral nutrition (TPN) is the infusion, stop the infusion for 3–5 minutes before obtaining a blood specimen.*
- *Consider obtaining a peripheral venipuncture for coagulation studies in a heparinized catheter with patients receiving aminoglycosides. Blood levels have been shown to be altered when drawn from silicone catheters when concomitant infusions of anticoagulants or aminoglycosides occur (The National Committee for Clinical Laboratory Standards, 1998).*

Sources: INS (2006b, 2008b).

PROCEDURES DISPLAY 8-4

Discontinuation of a Short-Term Vascular Access Device (Nontunneled Catheter or PICC)

Equipment Needed
10-mL syringe
Sodium chloride
Gloves
Suture removal set, if appropriate
Sterile dressing
Delegation:
This procedure **cannot** be delegated to an LPN/LVN or NAP. The practitioner needs competency training for central venous access care and maintenance.

PROCEDURES DISPLAY 8-4

Discontinuation of a Short-Term Vascular Access Device (Nontunneled Catheter or PICC)—cont'd

Procedure	Rationale
1. Verify the physician or authorized prescriber order for removal of the PICC or nontunneled catheter.	1. A physician's order is a legal requirement for discontinuation of a central venous access device.
2. Introduce yourself to the patient.	2. Promote nurse–patient relationship, and establish communication.
3. Verify the patient's identity using two forms (check ID bracelet and ask the patient to state his or her name).	3. The Joint Commission (2003) safety goal recommendation
4. Elevate the bed.	4. Conducive to a successful procedure and prevents back injury for the practitioner.
5. Position the patient in the dorsal recumbent position and abduct the patient's arm. (Some institutions recommend a Trendelenburg position.)	5. To raise intrathoracic pressure, which reduces the chance for air to enter into system and for embolism
6. Wash hands using friction for 15–20 seconds.	6. Good hand hygiene is the single most important means of preventing the spread of infection.
7. Don gloves.	7. Protects the nurse from potential blood contamination.
8. Clamp the infusion tubing and turn off the electronic infusion device (if appropriate).	8. The infusion must be discontinued before removal of the catheter.
9. Close the slide clamp on the CVC.	9. The CVC is no longer needed for therapy.
10. Remove the dressing and securement device.	10. Removal is to be done in a manner that will not compromise the skin and cannula exit site.

Continued

PROCEDURES DISPLAY 8-4

Discontinuation of a Short-Term Vascular Access Device (Nontunneled Catheter or PICC)—cont'd

Procedure	Rationale
11. Inspect the dressing for purulent drainage or foul odor.	11. Assessment for potential infection of site or catheter. Obtain culture per agency policy if abnormal drainage or odor is present.
12. Discard the dressing in the biohazard container.	12. To prevent contamination of patient's clothing and linens
13. Remove gloves and carry out proper hand hygiene.	13. To prevent cross-contamination
14. Place 4 × 4 inch gauze, skin antiseptics, a suture removal kit (if needed), and dressing materials in close proximity to the patient and open them using aseptic technique.	14. For efficiency of CVC removal, and to prevent contamination
15. Don sterile gloves, leaving the inside (sterile portion) of the wrapper at the bedside.	15. To place the CVC on once it is removed, so it can be inspected and placed in a culture tube if needed.
16. Inspect the site around the cannula insertion area.	16. To determine if a culture is needed before cleansing the site.
17. Cleanse the CVC insertion site and surrounding area, including the catheter and sutures in a concentric circle, starting at the catheter–skin junction. Clean first with the alcohol; repeat as needed (with fresh swab) to remove all debris. Follow with thorough cleansing with the 2% chlorhexidine gluconate. Allow to air dry. **NOTE:** Do not go back over the cleansed site with the same antiseptic swab.	17. This is necessary to remove any contaminants on or around the exit site that could migrate into the CVC removal site and cause contamination after the catheter is removed.

PROCEDURES DISPLAY 8-4

Discontinuation of a Short-Term Vascular Access Device (Nontunneled Catheter or PICC)—cont'd

Procedure	Rationale
18. Carefully clip and remove any sutures (if appropriate).	18. To prevent undue trauma to the skin
19. Place the 4 × 4 gauze over the CVC exit site, holding in place with the nondominant hand. Instruct the patient to perform the Valsalva maneuver.	19. To prevent air embolism
20. As the patient holds his or her breath, withdraw the CVC from the vein in one smooth, steady motion, continuing to hold the 4 × 4 over the site. (DO NOT STRETCH THE CATHETER.) Exert firm pressure over the exit site for 1–5 minutes after the catheter is removed.	20. The cannulation site must be held secure to prevent air entry into the vein. The CVC must be placed on a sterile field until it can be inspected.
21. Cover the site with a sterile 2 × 2 gauze pressure dressing with tape to make occlusive.	21. To prevent post-removal air embolism.
22. Leave the pressure dressing in place for 24 hours.	22. To prevent hematoma formation
23. Inspect the removed CVC and assess it for drainage, odor, integrity, and length. If a PICC, measure the length of the catheter and compare with the length recorded before insertion.	23. To assess for infection and catheter embolism
24. Assess the dressing site every 15 minutes for the first hour after the catheter is removed.	24. To ensure proper wound healing and assess for excess bleeding
25. Dispose of all equipment in biohazard or sharps containers, and carry out proper hand hygiene.	25. To prevent the spread of microorganisms

Continued

PROCEDURES DISPLAY 8-4

Discontinuation of a Short-Term Vascular Access Device (Nontunneled Catheter or PICC)—cont'd

Procedure	Rationale
26. Document the patient's response to CVC removal, the appearance of the site, dressing regimen, and the condition and length of the catheter as well as any interventions implemented.	26. To maintain a legal record and communication with the healthcare team

PROCEDURES DISPLAY 8-5

Accessing an Implanted Port

Equipment Needed
Sterile gloves (two pair) and mask
Sterile gauze 2 × 2 pads
Alcohol swabs
TSM dressing
Needleless injection cap
Chlorhexidine gluconate swabsticks
Noncoring needle with clamping extension set
Sterile barrier drape
Local anesthesia
Stabilization device
One or two 10-mL syringes
Flush solutions containing 0.9% sodium chloride and 5 mL of 100 U/mL heparin
Biopatch (depending on institutional policy)
Sharps container
General VAD dressing kit
Delegation:
This procedure **cannot** be delegated to an LPN/LVN or nursing assistive personnel (NAP). The practitioner needs competency training for central venous access care and maintenance.

PROCEDURES DISPLAY 8-5

Accessing an Implanted Port—cont'd

Procedure	Rationale
1. Verify the authorized prescriber's order or standardized policy and procedure.	1. An order and institutional guidelines are requirements for practitioners to access ports.
2. Introduce yourself to the patient.	2. Establishes the nurse–patient relationship.
3. Verify the patient's identity using two forms of ID (check ID bracelet and ask patient to state his or her name).	3. The Joint Commission (2003) safety goal recommendation.
4. Wash hands for 15–20 seconds using friction.	4. Good hand hygiene is the single most important means of preventing the spread of infection.
5. Don sterile gloves and mask.	5. Protects the nurse and patient from exposure to pathogens. Maintains sterile barrier technique.
6. Elevate the bed level.	6. Conducive to successful access and prevents back injury for the practitioner.
7. Position the patient either in a comfortable reclining position, or in a chair with pillow behind the shoulder.	7. Provide comfort for the patient and provide access to the port.
8. Palpate the site to locate the septum.	8. Ensure that the needle will be placed correctly.
9. Instruct the patient to turn head away from the port site.	9. Prevents the introduction of microorganisms, especially if the patient has a cough.
10. Set up a sterile field, and prime a noncoring needle and extension set with a 10-mL syringe of normal saline solution; purge out all of the air.	10. Flushing extension tubing and noncoring needle prevents air embolism.
11. Cleanse the port access with alcohol, rotating in a circular motion from inside out for a minimum of 15 seconds.	11. Promotes asepsis and prevents the spread of infection

Continued

PROCEDURES DISPLAY 8-5

Accessing an Implanted Port—cont'd

Procedure	Rationale
12. Repeat.	
13. Cleanse the access site with 2% chlorhexidine gluconate using friction. Repeat.	
14. Offer a local anesthetic if indicated.	14. Provides comfort during access of site through the skin
15. Remove and discard gloves.	15. Prevents cross-contamination.
16. Don a second pair of sterile gloves.	16. Maintains sterility
Single-Port Access:	
17. Relocate the port by palpation and immobilize the device with the nondominant hand.	17. To locate the correct position of the septum of the port.
18. Instruct the patient to perform the Valsalva maneuver.	18. To prevent air embolism.
19. Insert the noncoring needle perpendicular to the septum, pushing firmly through skin and septum until the needle tip contacts the back of the port (the gripper style device should lie flush with the skin)	19. To access the port correctly.
20. Aspirate for blood return to confirm patency; flush with the attached 10 mL of sodium chloride.	20. To verify correct needle placement and patency of the line.
21. Maintain positive pressure when removing the syringe from the port extension set by engaging the clamping device.	21. To maintain positive pressure to prevent reflux of blood.
22. If the port is to remain accessed: a. Place sterile gauze under device wing to prevent rocking motion of needle b. If Biopatch is used—apply now followed by Steri-Strips™ or sterile tape or stabilization device	22. To prevent trauma to the tissues.

PROCEDURES DISPLAY 8-5

Accessing an Implanted Port—cont'd

Procedure	Rationale
c. Anchor noncoring needle to skin using Steri-strips or sterile tape.	
d. Cover the needle and gauze with TSM dressing.	**22d.** Ensure a sterile occlusive site.
e. Initiate the prescribed therapy.	
23. If a port is to be used for intermittent infusion therapy, flush using heparin for final locking method.	
24. Document in the patient record the type of port and noncoring needle, assessment of the site, date and time of access, condition of the port, presence of blood return, ease of flushing, and topical analgesia used for insertion and patient tolerance of the procedure and dressing applied.	24. To maintain a legal record and communication with the healthcare team.

Sources: Arch (2007); INS (2006b).

PROCEDURES DISPLAY 8-6

Deaccessing an Implanted Port

Equipment Needed
Exam gloves
Sterile gloves
Sterile gauze dressing
Alcohol swabs
10 mL of sodium chloride
Two 10-mL prefilled saline syringes
10-mL syringe for 5 mL of 100 units/mL heparin
Occlusive dressing
Delegation:
This procedure **cannot** be delegated to LVN/LPN or NAP. The
practitioner needs competency training for central venous access
care and maintenance.

Procedure	Rationale
To deaccess the needle from the port:	
1. Introduce yourself to the patient.	1. Establishes the nurse–patient relationship.
2. Verify patient identity using two forms (check ID bracelet and ask patient to state his or her name).	2. The Joint Commission (2003) safety goal recommendation.
3. Wash hands using friction for 15–20 seconds.	3. Good hand hygiene is the single most important means of preventing the spread of infection.
4. Flush the port with 10 mL of sodium chloride using brisk push–pause method.	4. and 5. Maintains the integrity of the port and prevents occlusions.
5. Flush with 3–5 mL of heparin if appropriate—follow flushing guidelines for positive-displacement devices and negative-displacement devices.	
6. Don fresh nonsterile gloves and remove the dressing and inspect the port site.	6. Protects the nurse and patient from exposure to pathogens.

PROCEDURES DISPLAY 8-6

Deaccessing an Implanted Port—cont'd

Procedure	Rationale
7. Discard gloves, wash hands, and apply sterile gloves.	
8. Palpate the port edges with your nondominant hand and stabilize the port with your thumb and index finger.	8. To prevent damage to the port and afford patient comfort.
9. Have the patient perform the Valsalva maneuver, then gently but firmly remove the noncoring needle with a continuous upward pull, being careful to engage needle protection system.	9. To prevent air embolism.
10. Apply gauze pressure dressing to the site if needed	10. Cover the puncture site to prevent infection.
11. Discard the needle in the sharps container; remove gloves and perform hand hygiene procedure.	11. OSHA guidelines to prevent needlestick injuries, infection control procedure.
12. Document the procedure with date and time of deaccess, gauge and length of needle, needle intactness, presence of blood return, and resistance met with flushing, and skin condition at the port site.	12. To maintain a legal record and communication with the healthcare team.

Sources: Arch (2007); INS (2006b).

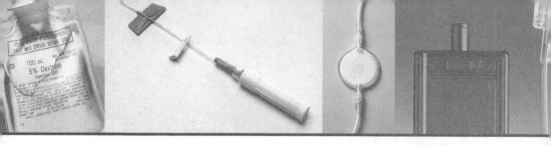

Chapter **9**

Complications of Infusion Therapy: Peripheral and Central Infusions

The most important practical lesson that can be given to nurses is to teach them what to observe—how to observe—what symptoms indicate improvement— what the reverse—which are of importance—which are of none—which are the evidence of neglect—and of what kind of neglect.
—Florence Nightingale, 1859

▪ **LEARNING**   *On completion of this chapter, the reader will be able to:*
OBJECTIVES

1. Define terms related to the hazards associated with infusion therapy.
2. Differentiate between local and systemic complications.
3. Describe the signs and symptoms of nine local complications.
4. Identify prompt treatment for local and systemic complications.
5. Identify the documentation criteria for each of the local and systemic complications.
6. Identify INS Standards of Practice for rating infiltration.
7. List three risk factors for phlebitis.
8. Use the INS phlebitis scale for identifying and rating postinfusion phlebitis.
9. Identify erratic flow rates as they relate to the hazards associated with I.V. therapy.
10. Identify organisms responsible for septicemia related to infusion therapy.
11. Identify prevention techniques for the six systemic complications.
12. Identify complications and risks of central venous access devices.

⑧ GLOSSARY

Air embolism (venous air embolis [VAE])   A sudden obstruction of a blood vessel caused by air introduced into the circulation

Catheter malposition   Position of the central line catheter outside the superior vena cava

Catheter occlusion   The state of being occluded; the inability to infuse or inject fluid into a catheter; the inability to aspirate blood from a catheter

Circulatory overload   Increased blood volume, usually caused by transfusions or excessive fluid infusions that increase the venous pressure

Ecchymosis   A bruise; a "black and blue spot" on the skin caused by escape of blood from injured vessels

Embolism   A sudden obstruction of a blood vessel by a clot or foreign material formed or introduced elsewhere in the circulatory system and carried to the point of obstruction by the bloodstream

Extravasation   Escape of fluid from its physiologic contained space in a vessel into the surrounding tissue

Fibrin sheath   Covering at the end of the catheter with a whitish, filamentous protein formed by the action of thrombin on fibrinogen. The fibrin is deposited as fine interlacing filaments that entangle red and white blood cells and platelets forming a clot

Hematoma   A swelling comprising a mass of extravasated blood confined to subcutaneous tissue caused by break in a blood vessel

Hemothorax   Blood in the pleural cavity caused by rupture of blood vessels

Infiltration   The accumulation of an external substance within tissue. Process of seepage or diffusion of infusates into tissue

Phlebitis   Inflammation of the intima of a vein associated with chemical irritation (i.e., chemical phlebitis), mechanical irritation (i.e., mechanical phlebitis), or bacterial infection (i.e., bacterial phlebitis); postinfusion inflammation of the intima of a vein within 48 to 96 hours after cannula removal

Pinch-off syndrome   Central venous catheter compressed by the clavicle and the first rib; results in mechanical occlusion

Pneumothorax   The presence of air or gas in the pleural cavity between the lung and chest wall

Pulmonary edema   Accumulation of extravascular fluid in lung tissues and alveoli.

Septicemia   The presence of pathogenic microorganisms in the blood.

Speed shock   A severe disturbance of hemodynamics in which the circulatory system fails to maintain adequate perfusion of vital organs due to sudden flooding of vital organs with medications

Superior vena cava syndrome   Obstruction of the superior vena cava or its main tributaries causing edema and engorgement of the vessels

Thrombophlebitis   Venous inflammation with thrombus (clot) formation

Thrombosis   Formation or presence of a blood clot; clotting within a blood vessel that may cause interruption of blood flow

Venous spasm   Sudden constriction of the vein

Vesicant   Any agent that produces blisters

Complications associated with peripheral and central infusion therapy are classified according to their location. A local complication is usually seen at or near the insertion site or occurs as a result of mechanical failure. These complications are more common than systemic complications. Systemic complications are those occurring within the vascular system, usually remote from the infusion site. Although not as common as local complications, they are very serious and can be life threatening.

Local Complications

Local complications of infusion therapy occur as adverse reactions or trauma to the surrounding venipuncture site. They can be recognized early by objective assessment. Assessing and monitoring are the key components in early intervention. Good venipuncture technique is the main factor related to the prevention of most local complications associated with infusion therapy. Local complications include hematoma, thrombosis, phlebitis, postinfusion phlebitis, thrombophlebitis, infiltration, extravasation, local infection, and venous spasm.

Hematoma

The terms **hematoma** and **ecchymosis** are used to denote formations resulting from the infiltration of blood into the tissues at the venipuncture site. Loss of integrity in a vessel wall due to disease or trauma allows the escape of blood into the surrounding area. Often this complication is related to nursing venipuncture technique. Patients who bruise easily can develop a hematoma when large cannulae are used to initiate intravenous therapy, owing to trauma to the vein during insertion. Patients receiving anticoagulant therapy and long-term steroid therapy are at particular risk of bleeding from vein trauma (Fig. 9-1).

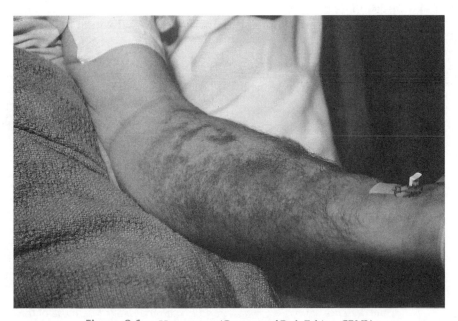

Figure 9-1 ■ Hematoma. (Courtesy of Beth Fabian, CRNI.)

Although not dangerous by itself, this complication can be a starting point for other complications such as thrombophlebitis and infection. Hematoma more often is caused by incorrect manipulation technique and rarely by spontaneous rupture of the vein.

Hematomas are most often related to:

- Faulty venipuncture technique in which the cannula passes through the distal vein wall
- Opening of the flow clamp for the infusion before the tourniquet is removed
- Too large a cannula to accommodate the vessel, resulting in rupture of the vein
- Pressure of the tourniquet to fragile skin

NOTE > For dilation of veins in elderly patients, use a blood pressure cuff or other techniques described in Chapter 6.

Signs and Symptoms

Signs and symptoms of hematoma include:

- Discoloration of the skin (i.e., **ecchymoses**) surrounding the venipuncture (immediate or slow)
- Site swelling and discomfort
- Inability to advance the cannula all the way into the vein during insertion
- Resistance to positive pressure during the lock flushing procedure

Prevention

Techniques for prevention of hematoma formation include:

1. Use of an indirect method rather than a direct approach for starting an I.V. This decreases the chance of piercing through the vein, which then causes seepage of blood into the subcutaneous tissue. (See Chapter 6 for venipuncture techniques.)
2. Apply the tourniquet just before venipuncture.
3. For elderly patients, patients taking corticosteroids, or patients with paper-thin skin, use a small needle or catheter, preferably 20- or 22-gauge. Use a blood pressure cuff rather than a tourniquet to fill the vein so you have better control of the pressure exerted on the vein.
4. Be very gentle when performing venipuncture.

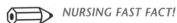 *NURSING FAST FACT!*

The presence of both ecchymoses and hematomas limits future use of the affected veins.

Treatment

1. Apply direct, light pressure using a sterile 2 × 2 inch gauze pad over the site after catheter or needle is removed for 2 to 3 minutes.
2. Have the patient elevate the extremity on a pillow to maximize venous return.
3. Ice may be applied to the area to prevent further enlargement of the hematoma.

Documentation

Document observable ecchymotic areas. Be sure to document the nursing interventions used for care of the site.

Peripheral Thrombosis

Catheter-related obstructions can be categorized as mechanical or non-thrombotic (42% of all obstructions) or thrombotic (58% of all obstructions) (Mayo, 2001). Trauma to the endothelial cells of the venous wall causes red blood cells to adhere to the vein wall, which may lead to the formation of a clot. This clot is referred to as a **thrombosis**, and usually occludes the circulation of blood. Thrombus formation is manifested by the flow of the I.V. solution: the drip rate slows, or the line does not flush easily and resistance is felt, especially in a lock device. The I.V. site may appear healthy. There are two areas of great concern in assessing for a thrombosis:

1. The potential for propelling the clot into the bloodstream with pressure from a syringe
2. Remember that a thrombus within a vein can trap bacteria

Thrombotic complications include the development of a thrombus either within or around the device or in the surrounding vessel. Thrombosis results when hemostasis occurs at an inappropriate time. Venous thrombi consist of fibrin and red blood cells, with tapering tails that extend into larger veins and are attached to the venous intima, usually at a valve or venous bifurcation.

Thrombosis formation is most often related to:

- Line is changed from an electronic infusion device (EID) to gravity flow (such as during showering or ambulation), slowing the infusion.
- Damage to the vein intima during cannulation, precipitating platelet attachment to the injured area and obstructing flow
- A low flow rate, which limits the fluid movement that is necessary to maintain patency

- The location of the I.V. cannula (e.g., a catheter placed in a flexor area may occlude when the position is changed)
- Obstruction of flow rate caused by the patient's compressing the administration set for an extended period of time
- Blood backing up in the system of a hypertensive patient.

NOTE > Thrombosis, along with thrombophlebitis, can lead to a systemic embolism.

 NURSING FAST FACT!

Nurses must avoid injuring the vein wall, performing multiple punctures, and performing through-and-through punctures.

Signs and Symptoms

Signs and symptoms of a thrombosis include:
- Fever and malaise
- Slowed or stopped infusion rate
- Inability to flush locking device
- Infusion site pain

Prevention

Techniques for the prevention of a thrombosis include:

1. Use EID for managing rate control. Rate control devices prevent blood from backing up in the tubing and produce an alarm when the solution container is dry.
2. Choose microdrip tubing (60 drops/mL) when I.V. gravity flow rates are below 50 mL/hr. Remember, more drops mean more movement.
3. Avoid placing an I.V. cannula in areas of flexion.
4. Use in-line filters.
5. Avoid cannulation of lower extremities.

Treatment

1. Never flush a cannula to remove an occlusion!
2. Discontinue the cannula and restart the I.V. infusion with a new catheter in a different site. Apply dry sterile 2 × 2 inch gauze dressing.
3. Notify the physician and assess the site for circulatory impairment if appropriate.

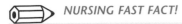 **NURSING FAST FACT!**

> *If an occlusion occurs, do not irrigate. Irrigation of an occluded line with saline can propel the clot into the circulatory system, causing an embolism. If there is any resistance when gentle pressure is exerted on the syringe plunger when you are attempting to flush an I.V. catheter, STOP! The application of force could dislodge the clot. Never use a syringe with a barrel size of 3, 5, or 10 mL to flush or aspirate clots in an I.V. line. Use a larger syringe barrel; a small syringe creates excess pressure that can damage the intima of the vein.*

Documentation

Document the change of infusion rate, the steps taken to solve the problem, and the end result. Be sure to chart the new I.V. site, its patency, and the size of the catheter used to restart the infusion. Document the appearance of the occluded site.

Phlebitis

Phlebitis is an inflammation of the vein in which the endothelial cells of the venous wall become irritated and cells roughen, allowing platelets to adhere and predispose the vein to inflammation-induced phlebitis. The site is tender to touch and can be very painful. At the first sign of redness or complaint of tenderness, the infusion site should be checked. The first indication of a potential problem is often when the patient reports pain. If treated early enough, the symptoms can resolve without further intervention (Lavery, 2005).

NOTE > Peripheral phlebitis can prolong hospitalization unless treated early.

> *EBNP Phlebitis is the most common complication associated with peripheral infusion therapy. A study by Panadero, Iohom, Taj, et al. (2002) demonstrated 20%–80% of patients receiving peripheral I.V. therapy develop phlebitis.*

The process of phlebitis formation involves an increase in capillary permeability, which allows proteins and fluids to leak into the interstitial space. The traumatized tissue continues to be susceptible to mechanical, chemical, or bacterial irritation (Table 9-1).

The immune system causes leukocytes to gather at the inflamed site. When leukocytes are released, pyrogens stimulate the hypothalamus to raise body temperature. Pyrogens also stimulate bone marrow to release more leukocytes. Redness and tenderness increase with each step of the

> Table 9-1   TYPES OF PHLEBITIS

Mechanical Phlebitis

Mechanical irritation causing a phlebitis or inflammation of the vein can be attributed to use of too large a cannula in a small vein. A large cannula placed in a vein with a smaller lumen than the cannula irritates the intima of the vein, causing inflammation and phlebitis. Large veins with thick walls hold up better during an infusion. In addition, veins higher on the forearm are less likely to develop phlebitis. The other cause of mechanical phlebitis is improper taping, in which the catheter tip rubs the vein wall, damaging the endothelial cell. Manipulation of the catheter during infusion causes irritation of vein wall. Securely affix the catheter hub and tubing using the Chevron method to prevent wiggling of the catheter.

Chemical Phlebitis

Chemical phlebitis occurs when a vein becomes inflamed by irritating or vesicant solutions or medication; medications improperly mixed or diluted; medications or solutions administered at a rapid rate; particulate matter and extended dwell time of catheters (Perruca, 2010). This is the result of contact with infusates with high or low osmolarities or pH or if very small veins are used for venous access.

Several factors contribute to chemical phlebitis.

The more acidic the I.V. solution, the greater is the risk of the patient's developing chemical phlebitis. I.V. solutions have a pH of 3–6, which helps to prevent them from caramelizing during sterilization and helps to maintain stability. Dextrose solutions have a pH of 3.5–6.5 or lower, whereas saline solutions have a pH of 5.5. The pH falls further with storage; pH values of 3.4 have been found in date-expired 5% dextrose solutions. Additives such as vitamin C, doxorubicin (Adriamycin), and cimetidine can further decrease the pH. Some drugs such as heparin, which has a pH of 5–7.5, can raise the pH. Hypertonic fluids such as 10% dextrose, which have a tonicity of greater than 375, increase the hazards of phlebitis. An increase in electrolytes also adds to the increased tonicity of the solution.

Additives such as potassium chloride (KCl), vancomycin hydrochloride, amphotericin B, most β-lactam antibiotics, benzodiazepines and many chemotherapeutic agents can produce severe venous inflammation.

Another factor contributing to chemical phlebitis is particulate matter in a solution, such as drug particles that do not fully dissolve during mixing and are not visible to the eye. The use of a 0.5- to 1.0-micron particulate matter filter eliminates this problem.

The use of catheters for peripheral I.V. therapy can predispose patients to phlebitis. Several different materials are used in the manufacture of catheters. Catheters made of silicone elastomer and polyurethane have a smoother microsurface, are thermoplastic, are more hydrophilic, become more flexible than polytetrafluoroethylene (Teflon) at body temperature, and induce less venous irritation. Maki and Ringer (1991) showed that the incidence of phlebitis increased progressively with increasing period of cannulation. Their study revealed the risk to be 30% by day 2 and 39%–40% by day 3.

Intermittent infusions cause less irritation to the vein wall over time than continuous infusions. The slower the rate of infusion, the less irritating the solution is to the vein wall because cells of the vein are exposed for a shorter period of time to solutions with less than normal pH. The fact that heparin is used to maintain the lock might have further significance in the reduction of phlebitis rates.

Continued

> Table 9-1   **TYPES OF PHLEBITIS—cont'd**

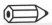 *NURSING FAST FACT!*

Examples of three common I.V. solutions and their pH and osmolarity:

Solution	pH	Osmolarity, mOsmol/L
5% dextrose in water	3–5	252
5% dextrose in water with 0.45% sodium chloride	4	406
5% dextrose in water with Ringer's lactate	5	524

Bacterial Phlebitis

Bacterial phlebitis, also referred to as septic phlebitis, is the least common type of phlebitis. It is an inflammation of the intima of a vein that is associated with a bacterial infection. Factors contributing to the development of bacterial phlebitis include poor aseptic technique, failure to detect breaks in the integrity of the equipment, poor cannula insertion technique, inadequately taped cannula, and failure to perform site assessments.

Bacterial phlebitis can be prevented by preparing solutions aseptically under a laminar flow hood. All solution containers should be inspected carefully before they are hung; in addition, handwashing and preparing skin carefully are necessary to prevent bacterial phlebitis.

 NURSING FAST FACT!

Handwashing is the most important procedure for preventing healthcare-associated infections and thus bacterial phlebitis. All equipment should be inspected for integrity, particulate matter, cloudiness, and any signs indicating a break in sterility. Shaving is not recommended because of the potential for microabrasion, which allows microorganisms to enter the vascular system.

Postinfusion Phlebitis

Postinfusion phlebitis is associated with inflammation of the vein that usually becomes evident within 48–96 hours after the cannula has been removed. Factors that contribute to its development are cannula insertion technique; condition of vein used; type, compatibility, and pH of solution or medication being infused; gauge, size, length, and material of cannula; and cannula indwelling time.

Postinfusion phlebitis can occur without the usual signs or symptoms. There is no way to anticipate this type of phlebitis; however, after it appears, the treatment is the same as for any other phlebitis

phlebitis (Maki & Ringer, 1991). When local inflammation is viewed under a microscope, histologic changes are marked, with loss of endothelial cells, edema, and presence of neutrophils in the vein wall. Inspection of the affected site reveals a similar appearance regardless of the underlying cause (Fig. 9-2).

Factors that influence the development of phlebitis include but are not limited to:

- Catheter material
- Large bore catheter
- Lack of experience of the person inserting the catheter
- Administration of solutions or medications with pH under 5 and over 9 and infusates with an osmolarity greater than 600 mOsmol/L through peripheral vein (INS, 2006a, 37)
- The insertion technique
- The gauge, size, length, and material composition of the cannula
- Duration of cannula placement (placement over 4 days)
- Frequent dressing changes
- Host factors, gender, age, underlying medical disease, and individual biologic vulnerability. (Refer to Table 9-2 for results of a study on factors affecting phlebitis formation.)

EBNP Maki and Ringer (1991) showed that the incidence of phlebitis increased progressively with increasing period of cannulation. Their studies revealed the risk to be 50% by the fourth day after catheterization.

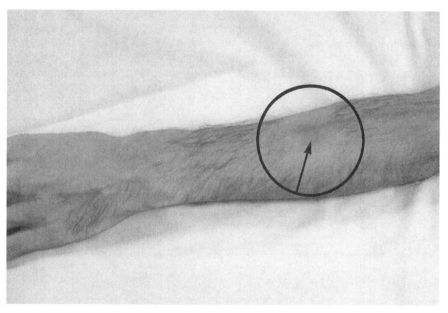

Figure 9-2 ■ Phlebitis. (Courtesy of Johnson & Johnson Medical [Ethicon], Somerville, NJ.)

> Table 9-2   **FACTORS AFFECTING PHLEBITIS FORMATION**

1. Catheter material
   Polypropylene > Teflon
   Silicone elastomer > polyurethane
   Teflon > polyurethane
   Teflon > steel needles
2. Catheter size
   Large bore > small bore
3. **Insertion in emergency room > inpatient unit**
4. **Increasing duration of catheter placement**
5. **Infusate**
   Low pH
   Potassium chloride
   Hypertonic glucose, amino acids, lipids
   Antibiotics (especially β-lactams, vancomycin, metronidazole)
   High flow rate of I.V. fluid (>90 mL/hr)
6. Daily I.V. dressing changes > dressing changes every 48 hours
7. Host factors
   Poor-quality peripheral veins
   Insertion in the upper arm or wrist > hand
8. Age
   Children: older > younger
   Adults: younger > older
   Women > men
   White > African American
9. **Individual biologic vulnerability**
   > denotes a significantly greater risk for phlebitis.
   Terms in **bold** print are significant predictors of risk in this study.

Source: Adapted from Maki, D.G., & Ringer, M. (1991). Risk factors for infusion-related phlebitis with small peripheral venous catheters: A randomized controlled trial. Annals of Internal Medicine, 114, 845–854.

INS Standard A peripheral-short catheter in the adult patient shall be removed every 72 hours and immediately upon suspected contamination, complication, or therapy discontinuation. (INS, 2006, 49)

Signs and Symptoms

Signs and symptoms associated with phlebitis include:

- Redness at the site
- Site warm to touch
- Local swelling
- Palpable cord along the vein
- Sluggish infusion rate
- Increase in basal temperature of 1°C or more

INS Standard The Phlebitis Scale should be standardized and used in documenting phlebitis; grade according to the most severe presenting indicator. (Table 9-3)

> Table 9-3	PHLEBITIS SCALE
Grade	**Clinical Criteria**
0	No clinical symptoms
1	Erythema at access site with or without pain
2	Pain at access site, with erythema and/or edema
3	Pain at access site with erythema and/or edema, streak formation, and palpable venous cord
4	Pain at access site with erythema and/or edema, streak formation, palpable venous cord >1 inch in length, purulent drainage

Source: Standards of Practice. (2006). Norwood, MA: Infusion Nurses Society; with permission.

Phlebitis always requires corrective action and documentation. The phlebitis rate is calculated according to a standard formula (INS, 2006a, 53):

$$\frac{\text{Number of phlebitis incidents} \times 100}{\text{Total number of peripheral I.V. lines}} = \text{Percent of peripheral phlebitis}$$

Prevention

Techniques for the prevention of phlebitis include:

1. Assess the patient before catheter placement to determine the length of infusion therapy and osmolality of the solution to be infused.
2. Consider midline for therapies of 7 days to 1 month; consider evaluation for peripherally inserted central catheter (PICC) or other central line for long term therapy.
3. Choose the smallest cannula appropriate for the infusate.
4. Rotate the infusion site every 72 to 96 hours (O'Grady, Alexander, Dellinger, et al., 2002).
5. Stabilize the catheter to prevent mechanical irritation.
6. Use a 0.22-micron inline final filter, which removes air, bacteria, and harmful particulate matter.
7. Catheter placement should be performed only by skilled professionals.
8. Observe good hand hygiene practices.
9. Add a buffer to known irritating medications and to hypertonic solutions.
10. Change solution containers every 24 hours.
11. Maintain peripheral-short catheter phlebitis rate of 5% or less in any patient population (INS, 2006a, 53).

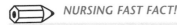 *NURSING FAST FACT!*

> *Be aware that:*
> ■ *Phlebitis risk factors increase after 24 hours.*
> ■ *All peripheral I.V.s should be changed every 72–96 hours.*
> ■ *A 3+ phlebitis (see Table 9-4) takes from 10 days to 3 weeks to heal.*
> ■ *Dextrose solutions, potassium chloride (KCl), antibiotics, and vitamin C have a lower pH and are associated with a higher risk of phlebitis.*

EBNP Two studies have supported the extension of peripheral I.V. catheter dwell time beyond 72 hours; however, this was dependent on type of medication administered. If the medication is irritating, then more frequent changes may be needed. In a study of 850 peripheral intravenous catheters (PIVs) over the indwelling life of the catheter, Gallant and Schultz, using the Visual Infusion Phlebitis scale as a measure to determine when an I.V. should be removed rather than routine removal at 72 hours, concluded there was decrease phlebitis (2.7%) for those with 1 PIV and 13.4% in those with PIVs that were restarted. Further studies need to support the practice of using assessment criteria for rotation of I.V. site over standard practice of 72–96 hours (Catney, Hillis, Wakefield, et al., 2001; Gallant & Schultz, 2006).

Treatment

1. Discontinue the infusion at the first sign of phlebitis.
2. Apply warm or cold compresses to the affected site. Cold significantly decreases intradermal skin toxicity for 45 minutes.
3. Consult the physician if the patient has a phlebitis rating of grade 2 or greater (INS, 2006a, 53).
4. Depending on agency policy, notify infection control.

Documentation

Documentation is critical when phlebitis has been detected. Document the site assessment, the phlebitis rating (1, 2, 3, or 4), whether the physician was notified, and the treatment provided. Document the discontinuation of the I.V. catheter and location of the new I.V. site.

Thrombophlebitis

Thrombophlebitis denotes a twofold injury: thrombosis and inflammation. A painful inflamed vein promptly develops from the point of thrombosis. Thrombophlebitis causes the patient unnecessary discomfort. Chemical or mechanical phlebitis can also precipitate thrombophlebitis.

Thrombophlebitis is related to:
- Use of veins in the legs for infusion therapy
- Use of hypertonic or highly acidic infusion solutions
- Causes similar to those leading to phlebitis (i.e., insertion technique; condition of patient; vein condition; compatibility [type and pH of medication or solution]; ineffective filtration; and the gauge, size, length, and material of the cannula)

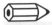 *NURSING FAST FACT!*

Thrombophlebitis is often the sequela of phlebitis.

Signs and Symptoms

Signs and symptoms of thrombophlebitis include:
- Sluggish flow rate
- Edema in the limbs
- Tender and cordlike vein
- Site warm to touch
- Visible red line above venipuncture site

 NURSING FAST FACT!

If the inflammation is the result of bacterial phlebitis, a much more serious condition may develop if the patient is not treated. Untreated bacterial phlebitis can lead to septicemia.

Prevention

Techniques used to prevent thrombophlebitis include:
1. Use the veins in the forearm rather than in the hands when infusing any medication.
2. Do not use veins in joint flexion areas.
3. Monitor the infusion site for signs and symptoms of redness, swelling, or pain at the site at least every 4 hours in adults and every 2 hours in children.
4. Anchor the cannula securely to prevent mobility of the catheter tip.
5. Infuse solutions at the prescribed rate. Do not attempt to catch up on delayed infusion time.
6. Use the smallest sized catheter that meets the needs of the patient.
7. Dilute irritating medications.

Septic thrombophlebitis can be prevented with:
- Appropriate skin preparation
- Use of aseptic technique in the maintenance of infusion
- Proper hand hygiene procedures

NURSING FAST FACT!

Thrombophlebitis can lead to a potential embolism owing to thrombus formation in the vein wall.

Treatment

1. Remove the entire I.V. catheter and restart the infusion in the opposite extremity, using all new equipment.
2. Consult the physician.
3. Provide comfort by applying warm, moist compresses to the area for 20 minutes.

NOTE > Discontinue the infusion, remove the cannula, and restart in a new site to prevent progression of thrombophlebitis.

Documentation

Document all observable symptoms and the patient's subjective complaints such as "feels tender to touch" and "it hurts." State your actions to resolve the problem and the time at which you notified the physician. Document the site in which you restarted the infusion.

Infiltration

Infusion Nurses Society (INS) Standards of Practice (2006a) define **infiltration** as the inadvertent administration of a nonvesicant solution into surrounding tissue. Infiltration occurs from the dislodgement of the cannula from the intima of a vein. It can also occur from phlebitis, causing the vein to become threadlike when the lumen along the cannula shaft narrows, so fluid leaks from the site where the cannula enters the vein wall. Infiltration is second to phlebitis as a cause of I.V. therapy morbidity.

Infiltration is related to:

- Puncture of the distal vein wall during venipuncture
- Puncture of any portion of the vein wall by mechanical friction from the catheter or needle
- Damage to the intima of the vein and subsequent swelling that prevents the infusate from flowing forward, with the infusion instead stopping or leaking out into the surrounding tissue (Rosenthal, 2007).
- Dislodgement of the catheter or needle from the intima of the vein
- Poorly secured infusion device
- High delivery rate or pressure (psi) from an electronic infusion device
- Overmanipulation of an I.V. device

Signs and Symptoms

Signs and symptoms of infiltration include:
- Coolness of skin around site
- Taut skin
- Edema at, above, or below the insertion site
- Absence of blood backflow
- A "pinkish" blood return
- Infusion rate slows but the fluid continues to infuse.

Complications associated with infiltration fall into three categories:

1. *Ulceration and possible tissue necrosis:* The severity of tissue damage depends on many variables, including the drug's vesicant potential, the amount of drug infiltrated, and the venipuncture site. Ulceration is not immediately apparent; the ulcer may actually take days or weeks to develop. See the section on extravasation later in this chapter.
2. *Compartment syndrome:* Muscles, nerves, and vessels are in compartments confined in inflexible spaces bound by skin, fascia, and bone. When fluid inside a compartment increases, the venous end of the capillary bed becomes compressed. If vessels cannot carry away the excessive fluid, hydrostatic pressure rises, leading to vascular spasm, pain, and muscle necrosis inside the compartment. Functional muscle changes can occur within 4 to 12 hours of injury. Within 24 hours, ischemic nerve damage can result in functional loss.
3. *Reflex sympathetic dystrophy syndrome:* This complication occurs when severe infiltration occurs, and a chronic and exaggerated inflammatory process begins, leaving the patient with limited function in the affected extremity (Hadaway, 2007).

Prevention

Prevention of infiltration includes performing adequate and continuous assessment of the site.

1. Site selection: avoid areas of joint flexion
2. Checking for blood return, or backflow of blood, is not a reliable method of determining the patency of a cannula. Blood return may be present when small veins are used because they may not permit blood flow around the cannula.
3. Do not use veins that have had previous punctures or veins that are very fragile due to seeping of fluid at the site above or below the vein cannula entry point; blood return may be present, yet an infiltration is occurring (Fig. 9-3).
4. Turn patients carefully. Infiltration and swelling below the I.V. site may occur as a result of placing hands underneath the patient during turning. Occlusion or restriction of blood flow causes fluid

to back up in the vessels, resulting in infiltration and dependent edema below the I.V. site rather than above.

5. Choose the smallest I.V. catheter that will safely deliver the infusion. This will allow blood flow to dilute the infusate and carry it away from the insertion site.

6. Stabilization: Using a manufactured catheter stabilization device, which has a mechanism that anchors the catheter and prevents unnecessary movement within the vein, is now the preferred method to secure an I.V. catheter.

The most accurate method of checking for infiltration is assessment of the site: With infusion running, apply pressure 3 inches above the catheter site in front of the catheter tip either with digital pressure or use of a tourniquet. If the infusion continues to run, suspect infiltration. When the vein is compressed and the catheter is in proper alignment in the vein, the

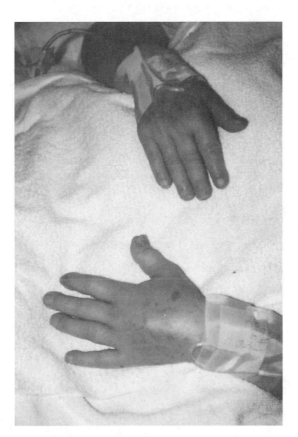

Figure 9-3 ■ Infiltration and swelling below the I.V. site occurring after hands were placed underneath the patient during turning. Occlusion or restriction of blood flow caused fluid to back up in the vessels, resulting in infiltration and dependent edema below the I.V. site rather than above. (Courtesy of Beth Fabian, CRNI.)

I.V. solution will stop because of occlusion. In addition, compare both of the patient's arms when assessing for infiltration (Fig. 9-4).

INS Standard Use Infusion Nurses Society infiltration classification for rating infiltration on a scale of 0 to 4. (INS, 2006a, 54) Refer to Table 9-4.

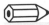 *NURSING FAST FACT!*

Immobilized patients and patients with muscular weakness or paralysis of an extremity may have edema of an extremity that is not related to infiltration of an I.V. site. Accurate assessment of the cannula and infusion site is the key to differentiation.

Treatment

1. Using warm or cold compresses as appropriate for the fluid or medication that has escaped into the tissue to treat infiltration has become controversial.

Refer to Table 9-7 for treatment options.

2. Elevation of the infiltrated extremity may be painful for the patient. Let the patient decide on the position of comfort in this situation.

3. Any incident of infiltration rating of grade 2 or greater should be reported as an unusual occurrence to the physician and other appropriate healthcare personnel.

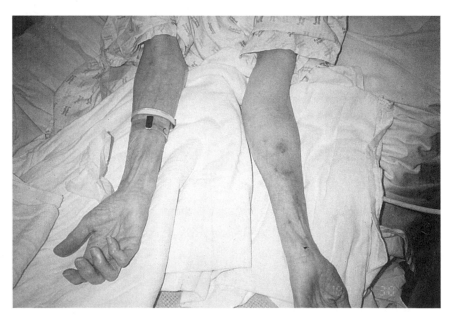

Figure 9-4 ■ Infiltration. Compare both arms when assessing for infiltration (note that the left arm is swollen compared with the right arm).

> Table 9-4	INFILTRATION SCALE
Grade	**Criteria**
0	No symptoms
1	Skin blanched Edema <1 inch Cool to touch With or without pain
2	Skin blanched Edema 1 to 6 inches Cool to touch With or without pain
3	Skin blanched and translucent Gross edema >6 inches Cool to touch Mild to moderate pain Possible numbness
4	Skin blanched and translucent Skin tight, leaking Gross edema >6 inches Deep, pitting tissue edema Circulatory impairment Moderate to severe pain Infiltration of any amount of blood product, irritant, or vesicant

Source: Standards of Practice. (2006). Norwood MA: Infusion Nurses Society; with permission.

4. The infiltration rate should be calculated according to a standard formula:

$$\frac{\text{Number of Infiltration Incidents}}{\text{Total Number of I.V. Catheters*}} \times 100 = \% \text{ infiltration}$$

*Total number of catheters: peripheral-short, ML, PICC, etc.

Documentation

The following is important to document for infiltrations: The fluid or medication that infiltrated; type of infusion method (syringe bolus; infusion pump); type, size, and length of catheter; complete description using INS Standards of Practice grading scale; all signs and symptoms; initial intervention; and patient education.

All infiltrations and extravasations, especially those that cause tissue damage, should be tracked for quality improvement purposes (Rosenthal, 2007a).

INS Standard Statistics on incidence, degree, cause and corrective action taken for infiltration shall be maintained and readily retrievable. (INS, 2006a, 54)

Extravasation

Extravasation, according to the Infusion Nurses Society, is the inadvertent administration of a vesicant solution into surrounding tissue. A **vesicant** solution is a fluid or medication that causes the formation of blisters, with subsequent sloughing of tissues occurring from the tissue necrosis (Figs. 9-5 and 9-6).

Patients who are at high risk for extravasation injury are presented in Table 9-5.

Risk factors for extravasation injury include:

■ Puncture of the distal vein wall during venipuncture and administration of irritating or vesicant medications or solutions
■ Puncture of any portion of the vein wall by mechanical friction from the catheter or needle while infusing irritating or vesicant solutions
■ Dislodgement of the catheter or needle from the intima of the vein
■ Poorly stabilized infusion device
■ High delivery rate or pressure from an electronic infusion device
■ Overmanipulation of the I.V. device
■ Thrombus or fibrin sheath formation at the vascular access device (VAD) catheter tip
■ Patient age, condition, acuity
■ Infusion prescription properties (infusate pH and osmolarity, rate of infusion) (Hadaway, 2007; INS, 2006)

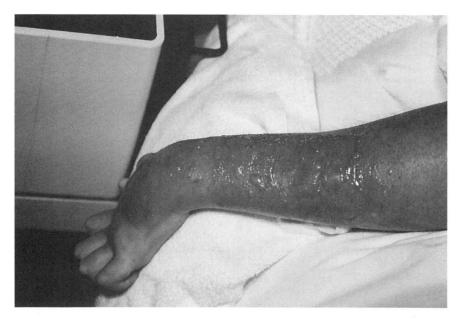

Figure 9-5 ■ Infiltration of vancomycin into subcutaneous tissue, causing blistering of skin. (Courtesy of Beth Fabian, CRNI.)

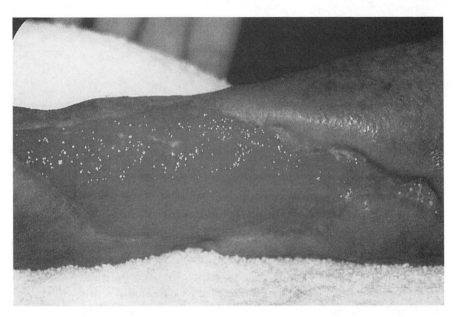

Figure 9-6 ■ Extravasation with tissue necrosis. (Courtesy of Johnson & Johnson [Ethicon], Somerville, NJ.)

Signs and Symptoms

Signs and symptoms of extravasation (Hadaway, 2007) include:
- Complaints of pain, tenderness, or discomfort
- Edema at, above, or below insertion site
- Blanching of the area around the insertion site
- Change in temperature of the skin at site
- Burning at the insertion site or along the venous pathway
- Feeling of tightness below the site
- Slow or stopped infusion

> Table 9-5	FACTORS AFFECTING RISK FOR EXTRAVASATION INJURY

Age

Neonate
Geriatric patient

Condition

Oncology patient
Comatose patient
Anesthetized patient
Patients with peripheral or cardiovascular disease
Diabetic patient

Equipment

High-pressure infusion pumps

- Fluid leaking from the insertion site
- Palpable cording of the vein

 NURSING FAST FACT!

Never increase the flow rate to determine the infiltration of a vesicant. Assessment of the site around the catheter tip is important, along with questioning the patient about discomfort at the access site. Once a vesicant site is suspected, discontinue the infusion immediately. Remember that extravasation is always rated a grade 4 on infiltration scale.

The severity of damage is directly related to the type, concentration, and volume of fluid infiltrated into the interstitial tissues. The endothelium is particularly sensitive to pH and osmolarity differences found in physiologic and nonphysiologic solutions. These fluids may induce cellular injury through irritation, stimulating the inflammatory process. The damaged tissue release precipitating proteins with an increase in capillary permeability, which allows fluid and protein shifts to interstitial space. Edema, ischemia, vasoconstriction, pain, and erythema are responses to these cellular changes and may lead to tissue necrosis (Hadaway, 2007).

Refer to Table 9-6 for a list of vesicant medications.

Prevention

To prevent vesicant extravasations, the following should be considered:

1. The use of skilled practitioners. Registered nurses specifically trained and supervised in chemotherapy administration should administer any medications that are irritating and vesicant. Practitioners should also be skillful in venipuncture and skillful and competent in using VADs.
2. The practitioner's knowledge of vesicants. The practitioner should have an understanding of the signs and symptoms of extravasation and be able to perform appropriate management.
3. The condition of the patient's vein. Patients with small, fragile veins; limited access; long-term therapy; and multiple vein sticks are prone to infiltration.
4. The drug administration technique.
   a. Give continuous vesicant administration into a long-term VAD.
   b. Avoid giving vesicant through a VAD without a good blood return.
   c. Use a free-flowing I.V. to give push medications, when possible.
   d. Avoid using a controlled infusion device for vesicants given peripherally.
   e. Assess for blood return frequently (such as every 2 to 5 mL or hourly).

> Table 9-6   VESICANT MEDICATIONS AND SOLUTIONS

Antimicrobials	Miscellaneous Agents	Antineoplastic Drugs	Vasodilators	Electrolyte Solutions	Vasopressors
Fluoroquinolones	Dextrose	Cisplatin (Platinol-AQ)	Nitroprusside sodium	Calcium chloride	Dopamine
Nafcillin	Fat emulsions	Dacarbazine (DTIC, imidazole)		Calcium gluconate	Epinephrine
Penicillin	Human immunoglobulin	Dactinomycin (Cosmegen)		Potassium chloride	Metaraminol
Gentamicin	Parenteral nutrition formulas, hypertonic	Daunorubicin (Cerubidine)		Sodium bicarbonate	Norepinephrine
Vancomycin	Phenytoin (Dilantin)	Doxorubicin (Adriamycin, Doxil)			Vasopressin (Pitressin)
		Epirubicin (Ellence)			
	Promethazine	Idarubicin (Idamycin PFS)			
	(Phenergan)	Mechlorethamine (Mustargen)			
	Radiographic contrast agents	Mitomycin (Mitomycin-C)			
		Paclitaxel (Taxol)			
	Vasopressin (Pitressin)	Plicamycin (Mithracin)			
	Propofol (Diprivan)	Streptozocin (Zanosar)			
		Vinblastine (Velban)			
		Vincristine (Oncovin)			
		Vinorelbine (Navelbine)			

5. The site of venous access. Avoid the large veins of the forearm, especially the posterior basilic vein, and the metacarpal veins of the dorsum of the hand. Avoid the use of the antecubital fossa and avoid using the lower extremity veins. Remove dressings to fully visualize the vein during administration.

6. The condition of the patient. Vomiting, coughing, or retching can cause excessive movement, resulting in a loss of access. Sedation from antiemetics or pain medications limits a patient's ability to report pain during infusion. Patients who are unable to communicate, such as infants and obtunded patients, also need to be observed closely (Schumeister, 2005).

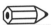 *NURSING FAST FACT!*

Restraints must be applied with extreme caution and within the guidelines established by The Joint Commission (TJC) and by the Food and Drug Administration (FDA). Immobilization devices should be well padded and applied so that they do not cause nerve damage, constrict circulation, or cause pressure areas; they should be removed at frequent intervals, and nurse-assisted range-of-motion exercises should be performed. Inadequate or improper use of immobilization devices can cause very serious complications; policies and procedures should be established to guide their use.

INS Standard Treatment of infiltration should be established in organizational policy and procedure. All extravasation injuries should be considered a Sentinel Event, with proper documentation and root cause analysis. (INS, 2006a, 55)

INS Standard The infiltration of any amount of blood product, irritant, or vesicant is classified as a grade 4. (INS, 2006, 54)

Treatment

The most effective treatment for extravasation is prevention. Conservative measures, including application of heat or cold and elevating the affected extremity, have been used. No data exist that supports withdrawal of vesicant from catheter or instilling antidotes to successfully treat extravastion (Schummer, Bayer, Muller, et al., 2005).

However, if extravasation is suspected:

1. Stop the I.V. flow, disconnect the administration set from the catheter hub, and attach an empty 3- or 5-mL syringe. Attempt to aspirate fluid from the catheter lumen.
2. Contact the physician.
3. Photograph the suspected area of extravasation according to institutional policy.

> **NOTE** > Do not apply excessive pressure to the area because it will disperse fluid further into surrounding tissues.

4. Discontinue the catheter using a dry gauze pad to control bleeding.
5. Apply thermal manipulation to alter the temperature in the superficial skin for 24 to 72 hours. Apply compresses for 15 to 30 minutes every 4 to 6 hours for 24 to 48 hours (Polovich, White, & Kelleher, 2005).
   ■ Cold topical applications are used for most extravasations except those of the vinca alkaloids, vincristine, and epipodophylotoxins.
   ■ Heat or cold can be used for hypotonic or isotonic solutions based on patient comfort.
6. Elevating the arm may be uncomfortable for some patients; the extremity may be slightly elevated based on patient comfort.
7. Provide written instructions on symptoms to report to the clinician, managing pain and any follow-up care.
8. Document all details of the incidence.
9. Compete unusual occurrence form, and sentinel event form as required by agency policy.
10. A plastic surgery consultation is recommended after large-volume vesicant extravasations, when the patient has severe pain, or if healing has not occurred 1 to 3 weeks after event (Wickham, Engelking, Sauerland, & Corbi, 2006).

Antidotes

In the most recent guidelines from the Oncology Nursing Society (Polovich, White, & Kelleher, 2005) antidotes are not generally recommended based on limited case reports and research. The use of antidotes is controversial. Data are limited regarding local antidotes except for sodium thiosulfate and hyaluronidase.

Antidotes for extravasation injury fall into four categories: (1) those that alter local pH, (2) those that alter DNA binding, (3) those that chemically neutralize, and (4) those that dilute extravasated drug. Common antidotes include:
■ Sodium bicarbonate has been used as an antidote, but due to its pH it can cause tissue destruction and has limited use.
■ Sodium thiosulfate 1/6 molar solution is indicated for extravasation of mechlortheamine or concentrated cisplatin (Polovich, White, & Kelleher, 2005).
■ Phentolamine (Regitine) is indicated for extravasation of vasopressors, because it reduces local vasoconstriction and ischemia. A disadvantage is the limited manufacturing of this drug (Deglin & Vallerand, 2009).

■ Hyaluronidase has been used for treatment of infiltration and extravasation of many drugs. This protein enzyme breaks down the cellular cement in the subcutaneous tissue (Schulmeister, 2005).

NOTE > If applicable, antidotes are administered within 1 hour of injury and can be given up to 12 hours post-injury. The goal is to lessen tissue injury.

Documentation

Comprehensive documentation of an extravasation event in the patient's medical record is vital for medicolegal purposes. Litigation rarely reaches a civil court until several years after the negative event. Medical record documentation is the key to understanding the events that occurred (Roth, 2003). Document assessments and interventions include:

■ Vascular access device type
■ Insertion site
■ Name of medication or solution
■ How it was infused (push or infusion, with or without pump).

Assess the status of circulation at, above, and below the insertion site, including skin color capillary refill and circumference of both the extremities at the site. Estimate how much solution entered the subcutaneous tissue by noting the time of the first complaint, the time the infusion was stopped, and the rate of the infusion.

Document the treatment of the infiltrated site, if an antidote is used, and the procedure for injection of the antidote. Document site checks and record the condition of the site before and after treatment. At the time of infiltration photo document for the chart according to facility policy. Notify the patient's primary care provider. File an unusual occurrence report according to facility policy (Hadaway, 2007). Table 9-7 summarizes key documentation criteria.

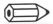 *NURSING FAST FACT!*

> *Soft tissue damage from extravasation can lead to prolonged healing, potential infections, necrosis, multiple débridement surgeries, cosmetic disfiguration, loss of limb function, and amputation.*

NOTE > There can be legal ramifications to venous extravasation events; the occurrence of extravasation does not of itself constitute negligence; rather it is the failure to take special precautions to minimize the potential for extravasation that may prove a successful cause of legal action (Roth, 2003).

> Table 9-7	KEY DOCUMENTATION CRITERIA FOR EXTRAVASATION

All extravasation injuries require thorough documentation and root cause analysis:
Date and time
All fluid and medications involved. Estimated volume of fluids and medications that
   escaped from the vein
The types of infusion methods used, such as manual injection from syringe, gravity infusion,
   or delivery by EID
The type, size, and length of the catheter in place
A complete description of the site, including anatomic location, size, color, and texture of
   the surrounding area. The Infusion Nurses Standards of Practice state that extravasation
   should always be rated Grade 4 on the Infiltration Scale.
All extravasation injuries are considered a Sentinel Event.
The methods used to assess the site before administering vesicant or irritant medications
All signs and symptoms
Initial interventions (such as aspiration, catheter removal, application of heat or cold)
Notification of the physician and other consultations
Use of antidotes, their dosages, and how they were administered
Photo documentation
Patient education regarding the event and follow-up care

Source: Hadaway, L. (2007); INS (2006a.)

Local Infections

Local infections related to infusion therapy consist of those related to microbial contamination of the cannula or infusate. One of the most serious forms of intravascular device–related infection occurs when intravascular thrombus surrounding the cannula becomes infected. This causes septic thrombophlebitis (suppurative phlebitis; Maki & Mermel, 2007).

INS Standard   Catheter-related infection shall include, but is not limited to, exit-site, tunnel, port pocket, or catheter-related bloodstream infection. (INS, 2006a, 56)

Local infections are preventable by maintaining aseptic technique and following guidelines established by the INS or Centers for Disease Control and Prevention for the duration of infusion, length of time of catheter placement, and tubing change criteria.

Local infections are related to:

- Lack of appropriate hand hygiene
- Inappropriate technique to swab needle-free valve (injection port) before access
- Catheters left in place for more than 72 hours
- Field sticks that are not changed after 48 hours
- Poor technique in maintaining and monitoring the peripheral site
- From patient's skin during introduction of catheter/poor skin prep technique

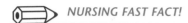 *NURSING FAST FACT!*

> *In any patient with an intravascular catheter who develops high-grade bloodstream infection that persists after an infected cannula has been removed, it is likely the patient has an infected thrombus in recently cannulated vein (Maki & Mermel, 2007).*

Signs and Symptoms

Signs and symptoms of local infection include:
- Redness, swelling, or induration at the site
- Temperature changes and drainage at the site.
- Possible exudate of purulent material
- Increased quantity of white blood cells
- Elevated temperature (chills are not associated with local infection)

Prevention

Techniques used to prevent local infections include:
1. Have the right designated specially trained I.V. therapy staff.
2. Perform hand hygiene with antiseptic-containing soap and water or waterless alcohol-based gel before and after palpating a catheter insertion site, and anytime you insert, replace, access, repair, or dress the site.
3. Choose the catheter type, insertion site, and technique based on which ones pose the lowest risk of infections for the type and duration of infusion therapy.
4. Disinfect your patient's skin with an appropriate antiseptic— 2% chlorhexidine is preferred.
5. Maintain aseptic technique during cannula insertion, during therapy, and catheter removal
6. Assess insertion site visually and document.
7. Maintain dressing. If the site is bleeding or oozing or the patient is diaphoretic, a gauze dressing is preferred.
8. Do not apply topical ointments to insertion site of a peripheral or central catheter.
9. Instruct the patient not to submerge the catheter in water.
10. Replace the catheter every 72 hours.
11. Replace administration sets at 72 hours with catheter change for primary infusions; change tubing for nutritional support or blood every 24 hours.
12. Use best practices in accessing the injection port (valve). Use alcohol with a twisting motion for twisting for 10 times; let dry before each access (Hadaway, 2003; Rosenthal, 2007b).

NOTE > See Chapter 2 for further information on infections at cannula sites.

INS Standard The infection rate should be calculated according to a standard formula. (INS, 2006a, 56)

Calculation:

$$\frac{\text{Number of Infections}}{\text{Total Number of I.V. Catheter Days}} \times 100 = \% \text{ of infections}$$

Treatment

1. Notify the physician or authorized prescriber immediately.
2. Obtain an order for site culture to verify the presence of a local infection.
3. Apply a sterile dressing over the site.
4. Apply warm moist compresses, if appropriate, as ordered.
5. Initate oral or parenteral anti-infective therapy, if appropriate, as ordered.
6. Monitor the site and document
   (INS, 2006a).

Documentation

Document the assessment of the site, culture technique, sources of culture, notification of the physician, and any treatment initiated.

NOTE > Culture technique procedure is presented in Chapter 2.

Venous Spasm

A spasm is a sudden, involuntary contraction of a vein or an artery resulting in temporary cessation of blood flow through a vessel. **Venous spasm** can occur suddenly and for a variety of reasons. The spasm usually results from the administration of a cold infusate, an irritating solution, or a too-rapid administration of I.V. solution or viscous solution such as a blood product.

Venous spasm is related to:
- Administration of cold infusates
- Mechanical or chemical irritation of the intima of the vein

Signs and Symptoms

Signs and symptoms of venous spasms include:
- Sharp pain at the I.V. site that travels up the arm, which is caused by a piercing stream of fluid that irritates or shocks the vein wall
- Slowing of the infusion

Prevention

Venous spasm can be prevented. Techniques used to prevent vasospasm include:

1. Dilute the medication additive adequately.
2. Keep the I.V. solution at room temperature, when appropriate.
3. Deliver the solution at the prescribed rate.
4. Use a fluid warmer for rapid transfusions of potent cold agglutinins.
5. Refrigerated medications and parenteral solutions should be allowed to reach room temperature before they are administered.

 NURSING FAST FACT!

If a rapid infusion rate is desired, use a larger cannula.

Treatment

1. Apply warm compresses to warm the extremity and decrease flow rate until the spasm subsides.
2. If spasm is not relieved, remove catheter, and restart with a new cannula.

Documentation

Document the patient complaints, duration of complaints, treatment, and length of time to resolve the problem. Also document whether the I.V. site needed to be rotated to resolve the problem.

Nerve Injuries

Nerves and veins lie close to each other in the arms; therefore a risk of inadvertently injuring a nerve during venipuncture could occur. Small nerve filaments are always contacted with the point of the needle during the catheter insertion procedure but do not result in nerve injury. When large nerves are penetrated by a needle point the patient is immediately symptomatic with sharp pain (Masoorli, 2007).

Nerve injury is related to:

1. Direct puncture of a nerve
2. Compression injury due to subcutaneous hematoma pressing on the nerve, infiltration of I.V. fluid, or tourniquet applied too tight.

Signs and Symptoms

Signs and symptoms of direct puncture nerve injury include:
- Immediate symptoms which include sharp acute pain at the venipuncture site.
- Sharp shooting pain up or down the arm

- Sensation of pain that changes in severity depending on needle position; "pins and needles" sensation or an "electric shock" feeling.
- Pain or tingling discomfort in the hand or fingertips

Signs and symptoms of compression injuries include:
- Pain radiating up or down the arm
- Compartment syndrome due to infiltrated solution
- Numbness or tingling in the arm or hand; typically appears 24 to 96 hours after the venipuncture

Prevention

1. Choose the most prominent of the acceptable veins (avoid inner surface of wrist and forearm; Arbique & Arbique, 2007).
2. Position the patient properly and anchor the vein securely.
3. Use a smaller needle angle (15 degrees) relative to vein depth. Do not exceed 30 degrees for deeper veins (CLSI, 2003).
4. Advance the needle into the vein lumen in the direction that the vein is running.
5. Avoid probing, which may nick the vein and cause subcutaneous bleeding.
6. Make only two attempts at venipuncture (INS, 2006a, 42).

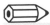 *NURSING FAST FACT!*

Avoid the wrist area. A simple landmarking technique involves placing the clinician's index, middle, and ring fingers at the crease of the wrist at the base of the thumb. This segment of the cephalic veins should be avoided! This is called the 3-finger test. Venipuncture should be 2 inches above the crease of the wrist and 1 inch above the crease of the wrist of a baby (Masoorli, 2007).

NOTE > Minor nerve injury results in scar tissue formation—neuroma—at the point of needle contact. The patient may require rehabilitation for up to 12 months. Major nerve injury, which occurs when the needle tears the nerve fibers, results in reflex sympathetic dystrophy (RSD) or complex regional pain syndrome (CRPS; Thrush & Belsole, 1995).

Treatment: Direct Pressure Injury

1. If at any time during the venipuncture procedure the patient complains of pain, electric shock, or pins and needles stop the venipuncture immediately and withdraw the I.V. device (Arbique & Arbique, 2007).
2. Apply pressure to the site to prevent a hematoma.
3. Document the incident.

Treatment: Compression Injury

1. Immediately notify the physician on recognizing compression nerve injury.
2. Discontinue the infusion.
3. Assess for swollen area becoming pale and pulseless: tissue necrosis and nerve compression injury are developing.
4. Do not elevate the extremity because it increases pressure.
5. Fasciotomy may be indicated.
6. Document and prepare Sentinel event report.

NOTE > Irreversible nerve damage begins after 6 hours of tissue hypertension (Paula, 2006).

Documentation

Document the patient complaints, duration of complaints, treatment, and length of time to resolve the problem. It is also important to document the time the physician was notified. Table 9-8 provides a summary of local and systemic complications.

■ Systemic Complications

Systemic complications can be life threatening. Such complications include erratic flow rate, circulatory overload, pulmonary edema, septicemia, air embolus, and speed shock.

Erratic Flow Rates

There are many factors to consider in determining flow rate (Table 9-8), including body size, fluid type, patient's age and condition, physiologic responses as reflected by urinary output, pulmonary status, and specific drugs being infused. The very young and the very old often need a slower rate of infusion and small volumes of solution. Patients with cardiac or renal diseases may also have problems tolerating large fluid volumes or fast rates. Situations in which flow rates have been poorly regulated can have serious consequences, especially with intravenous solutions containing medications.

Accurate flow rate is imperative when a drug level must be kept constant. If the rate is too slow:

■ The patient is not receiving the desired amount of drug or solution.
■ Can lead to a clogged I.V. needle or catheter and perhaps the loss of a premium vein.

> Table 9-8 **LOCAL AND SYSTEMIC COMPLICATIONS OF PERIPHERAL I.V. THERAPY**

Complication	Signs and Symptoms	Treatment	Prevention
		Local	
Hematoma	Ecchymoses Site swelling and discomfort Inability to advance catheter Resistance during flushing	Remove catheter if indicated. Apply pressure with 2 × 2 inch gauze. Elevate extremity. Cold compresses may be applied.	Use indirect method of venipuncture. Apply tourniquet just before venipuncture. Use BP cuff for patients with paper-thin skin.
Thrombosis	Slowed or stopped infusion Fever and malaise Inability to flush device Infusion site pain	Discontinue catheter. Apply cold compresses to the site. Assess for circulatory impairment. **Note:** Never flush a cannula to remove an occlusion.	Use EIDs. Choose microdrip sets with gravity flow if rate is below 50 mL/hr. Avoid flexion areas. Avoid cannulation of lower extremity
Phlebitis	Redness at site Site warm to touch Local swelling Palpable cord along vein Sluggish infusion rate Increase in basal temperature by 1°C or more	Discontinue catheter. Apply cold compresses initially, then warm. Consult the physician if grade 2 or greater. Notify infection control if appropriate.	Use larger veins for hypertonic solutions Choose smallest I.V. cannula that is appropriate for infusion Good handwashing practices Add buffer to irritating solutions Change solution containers every 24 hours Rotate infusion sites every 72 to 96 hours Stabilize catheter to prevent mechanical irritation. Monitor and maintain phlebitis rate using calculation formula.
Infiltration (extravasation)	Coolness of skin around site Taut skin Edema above or below insertion site. Backflow of blood absent Infusion rate slowing	Discontinue catheter. Apply cool compresses. Elevate extremity slightly. Follow guidelines if extravasation occurs.	Stabilize the catheter. Place the catheter in the appropriate site. Do not use veins that have a previous venipuncture. Avoid antecubital fossa.

> Table 9-8 | **LOCAL AND SYSTEMIC COMPLICATIONS OF PERIPHERAL I.V. THERAPY—cont'd**

Complication	Signs and Symptoms	Treatment	Prevention
	Local		
	For extravasation: Complaints of pain Blanching of area Burning at insertion site Blisters Palpable cord	Use antidote when appropriate. Any incident of infiltration grade 2 or greater needs unusual occurrence report.	Turn the patient carefully. Monitor and maintain infiltration rate using calculation formula.
Nerve Injury	Immediate sharp pain during venipuncture Shooting pain up arm Pain or tingling in hand or fingertips	Stop venipuncture. Apply pressure.	Choose prominent accessible veins. Position the patient properly and anchor the vein. Avoid probing. Make only two attempts.
Local Infection	Redness and swelling at site Possible exudate of purulent material Increased WBC count Elevated temperature	Discontinue catheter and culture site and cannula. Apply sterile dressing over the site. Administer antibiotics as ordered.	Inspect all solutions. Use good technique during venipuncture and site maintenance.
Venous Spasm	Sharp pain at I.V. site Slowing of infusion	Apply a warm compress to the site with infusion still running. Restart the infusion if spasm continues.	Dilute medications. Keep I.V. solution at room temperature.
	Systemic		
Septicemia	Fluctuating fever Profuse sweating Nausea and vomiting Diarrhea Abdominal pain Tachycardia Hypotension Evidence of decreased perfusion or dysfunction.	Restart new I.V. system. Obtain cultures. Notify the physician. Initiate antimicrobial therapy ordered. Monitor the patient closely.	Good hygiene technique Careful inspection of solutions Use Luer–Loks. Cover infusion sites with sterile dressings. Follow standards of practice related to rotation of sites and hang time of infusions. Use 2% chlorhexidine prepping solutions.

Continued

> Table 9-8   **LOCAL AND SYSTEMIC COMPLICATIONS OF PERIPHERAL I.V. THERAPY—cont'd**

Complication	Signs and Symptoms	Treatment	Prevention
	Systemic		
Circulatory Overload and Pulmonary Edema	Weight gain Puffy eyelids Edema Hypertension Changes in I & O Rise in CVP Shortness of breath Crackles in lungs Distended neck veins Restlessness and HA Increased pulse rate Cough Diagnostic tests: ABG, BUN, Creatinine	Decrease I.V. flow rate. Place the patient in a high Fowler position. Keep the patient warm. Monitor vital signs. Administer oxygen as ordered. Consider changing to microdrip set. Drug therapy Oxygen therapy	Monitor the infusion. Maintain flow at the prescribed rate. Monitor I & O. Know the patient's cardiovascular history. Do not "catch up" infusions; instead, recalibrate. Use EIDs that have dose-error reduction systems and anti-free flow administration sets.
Air Embolism (VAE)	Lightheadedness Dyspnea, cyanosis, tachypnea, expiratory wheezes, cough Mill wheel murmur, chest pain, hypotension Change in mental status, confusion coma, seizures	Call for help Place patient in Trendelenburg position Administer oxygen. Monitor vital signs. Notify the physician.	Remove all air from administration sets Use Luer-Loks Use 0.22-micron air eliminating filter. Follow protocol for dressing and tubing changes.
Speed Shock	Dizziness Facial flushing Headache Tightness in chest Hypotension Irregular pulse Progression of shock	Get help. Give antidote or resuscitation medications.	Reduce the size of drops by using a microdrip set. Use an electronic infusion device. Monitor the infusion rate. Dilute I.V. push medications if possible.

CVP = central venous pressure; I & O = intake and output.

If the rate is too fast:

- Hypotonic solutions can lead to the development of pulmonary edema or congestive heart failure.
- Rapid infusion of hypertonic glucose can result in osmotic diuresis, leading to dehydration.
- Hypertonic solutions are also irritating and phlebitis can result.
- Free-flow administration of drugs can cause serious cardiovascular and respiratory complications.

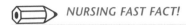 *NURSING FAST FACT!*

■ *A fast rate is considered more dangerous than a rate that is too slow.*
■ *In addition, notify the product evaluation committee or central services if the cause of erratic flow is an electronic infusion device.*
■ *Free flow infusions can lead to circulatory overload and pulmonary edema.*

Prevention

Measures to prevent erratic flow rates and the complications they cause include:

1. Allow only experienced nurses to set up, adjust, or remove I.V. administration sets.
2. Use pumps that provide free-flow protection; check with each manufacturer.
3. Properly closing clamps if removing the administration set from the pump.
4. Check or recalculate infusion rates.
5. Provide or attend staff development education on electronic infusion devices.
6. Report all free-flow incidents.

INS Standard The type of flow-control device selected shall be based on patient age, condition, prescribed infusion therapy, type of vascular access device and care setting.

Dose-error reduction systems shall be considered in the selection and use of electronic infusion devices.

Anti-free-flow administration sets shall be considered in the selection and use of administration delivery systems. (INS, 2006a, 33)

Treatment

Treatment techniques for erratic flow rates include the following:

1. Stop the flow and recalculate the drip rate.
2. Treat the patient symptomatically.
3. Consult the physician when necessary.
4. Recalculate the infusion rate.

Fluid Overload and Pulmonary Edema

Overloading the circulatory system with excessive intravenous fluids causes increased blood pressure and central venous pressure. **Circulatory overload** is caused by infusing excessive amounts of isotonic or hypertonic crystalloid solutions too rapidly, failure to monitor the I.V.

infusion, or too-rapid infusion of any fluid in a patient compromised by cardiopulmonary or renal disease.

Fluid overload can lead to pulmonary edema. Pulmonary edema is defined as clinical syndrome resulting in leakage of fluid from the pulmonary capillaries and veins into the interstitium and alveoli of the lungs (Dada & Sznajder, 2003).

Fluids infused too rapidly increase venous pressure and lead to pulmonary edema. In pulmonary edema, fluid leaks through the capillary wall and fills the interstitium and alveoli. "The pulmonary vascular bed has received more blood from the right ventricle than the left ventricle can accommodate and remove. The slightest imbalance between inflow on the right side and outflow on the left side may have drastic consequences" (Smeltzer, Bare, Hinkle, & Cheever, 2008).

Patients at risk for pulmonary edema are those with cardiovascular disease, those with renal disease, and elderly patients. It is important to identify patients at risk for pulmonary edema and provide nursing care that decreases the heart's workload. Sodium chloride given to correct profound sodium deficits can lead to pulmonary overload and must be monitored closely (Metheny, 2000).

Fluid overload and pulmonary edema are related to:
- Overzealous infusion of parenteral fluids, especially those that contain sodium
- Compromised cardiovascular or renal systems

Signs and Symptoms

Signs and symptoms of circulatory overload include:
- Restlessness, headache
- Increase in pulse rate
- Weight gain over a short period of time
- Cough
- Presence of edema (eyes, dependent, over sternum)
- Hypertension
- Hypoxia, with severe respiratory distress
- Oxygen saturation less than 90% on room air
- Wide variance between intake and output
- Rise in central venous pressure (CVP)
- Shortness of breath and crackles in lungs
- Distended neck veins
- Diagnostic tests: Arterial blood gases (ABGs), blood urea nitrogen (BUN), and creatinine to evaluate renal perfusion; natriuretic peptide levels may be increased; chest radiograph

As fluid builds in the pulmonary bed, later signs and symptoms include hypertension, severe dyspnea, gurgling respirations, coughing up frothy fluid, and moist crackles. If the condition is allowed to persist, congestive heart failure, shock, and cardiac arrest can result.

Prevention

Techniques used to prevent circulatory overload leading to pulmonary edema include:

1. Monitor the infusion, especially sodium chloride, and know the solution's physiologic effects on the circulatory system.
2. Maintain flow at the prescribed rate.
3. Do not "catch up" on I.V. solutions that are behind schedule; instead, recalculate all infusions that are not on time.
4. Monitor the intake and output on all patients receiving I.V. fluids.
5. Review the patient's cardiovascular history.
6. Use EIDs that have dose-error reduction systems, and anti-free flow administration sets.

Treatment

Consult the physician if you suspect circulatory overload. The goal of treatment is to decrease pulmonary venous and capillary pressure, improve cardiac output, and correct underlying pathology (Ezzone, 2007).

1. Drug therapy: Use loop diuretics to cause vasodilation and decrease pulmonary congestion; consider thiazide diuretic for treatment of congestive heart failure; consider vasodilators to decrease pulmonary vascular pressure (nitroprusside or nitroglycerin); morphine sulfate to cause venous dilation; aminophylline infusion for symptoms of wheezes.
2. Oxygen therapy that is dose titrated to patient response. (Intubation and mechanical ventilation may be necessary.)
3. A Swan–Ganz catheter may be placed to evaluate cause of pulmonary edema.
4. Position the patient in a semi-Fowler position.
5. Obtain daily weight to monitor fluid status.
6. Obtain frequent intake and output measurements.
7. Decrease flow rate; consider use of microdrip administration set for better control.
8. Keep the patient warm to promote peripheral circulation.
9. Monitor vital signs
   (Ezzone, 2007).

Documentation

Document patient assessment, notification of physician, and treatments instituted by physician order. Monitor the patient and record vital signs on an interval flow sheet.

Septicemia

Septicemia is a febrile disease process that results from the presence of microorganisms or their toxic products in the circulatory system. Health-care-associated intravascular device-related bloodstream infection is associated with a 12% to 28% attributed mortality. Intravascular device-related bloodstream infection is largely preventable (Maki & Mermel, 2007). The risks of bloodstream infection (BSI) are associated with various types of intravascular devices (IVDs; Maki, Kluger, & Crnich, 2006). An estimated 250,000 to 500,000 IVD-related BSIs occur each year (Crnch & Maki, 2005).

The microorganism most frequently implicated in healthcare-associated catheter-related bloodstream infections (CR-BSI) is coagulase-negative *Staphylococcus* and *Staphylococcus aureus* followed by *Candida* (Maki & Mermel, 2007). Prospective studies have shown strong concordance between organisms present on skin surrounding the catheter insertion site and organisms recovered from CVCs producing BSIs.

Nurses must be aware of risk factors, prevention techniques, and the presence of an infected catheter tip because bacteremia, fungemia, or septicemia could occur.

Risk factors associated with septicemia include:

- Patient factors: Age, alteration in host defense, underlying illness, presence of other infectious processes
- Infusion factors: Solution container, stopcocks, catheter material and structure, insertion site, hematogenous seeding, manipulation of the infusion system, certain transparent dressings, and duration of cannulation.
- Practitioner-related factors: Lack of handwashing, break in sterile technique, inexperience of the professional inserting the cannula, inadequately prepared or maintained insertion sites, repeated manipulation of infusion system

Refer to Evidence-Based Pratice Box 9-1.

Signs and Symptoms

Signs and symptoms of septicemia include:

- Fluctuating fever, tremors, chattering teeth
- Profuse, cold sweat
- Nausea and vomiting
- Diarrhea (sudden and explosive)
- Abdominal pain
- Tachycardia: Heart rate greater than 90 bpm
- Increased respirations or hyperventilation: More than 20 breaths/min
- Evidence of decreased perfusion or dysfunction of vital organs

- Change in mental status
- Hypoxemia—measured by ABGs
- Elevated lactate levels
- Urine output less than 30 mL/hr
- Elevated white blood cell count and the automated absolute neu-trophil count (better diagnostic tests for adults and most children for infection; Cornbleet, 2002)

Prevention

Techniques used to prevent septicemia include:

1. Perform good hand hygiene. Handwashing and sterile tech-nique are imperative to minimize the risk of technique-induced septicemia.
2. Carefully inspect solutions for abnormal cloudiness, cracks, and pinholes.
3. Use only freshly opened solutions.
4. Use protein solutions, such as albumin and protein hydrolysates, as soon as the seal is broken.
5. Use 2% chlorhexidine with alcohol as recommended in the central line bundles.
6. Use Luer-Lok™ connections.
7. Cover infusion sites with a sterile dressing.

EVIDENCE-BASED PRACTICE BOX 9-1

Risk of Bloodstream Infections in Adults with Different Intravascular Devices

Maki, D., Kluger, D.M., & Crnich, C.J. (2006). The risk of bloodstream infection in adults with different intravascular devices: A systematic review of 200 published prospective studies. Mayo Clinic Proceedings, 81(9), 1159–1171.

This study analyzed 200 published studies of adults in which every intravascular device in the study population was prospectively evaluated for evidence of associated infection.

Results: Rates of intravascular device-related BSI were lowest with peripheral intravenous catheters and midline catheters. Far higher rates were seen with short-term noncuffed and nonmedicated central venous catheters. Peripherally inserted central catheters posed risks approaching those seen with short-term conventional CVCs. Surgically implanted long-term central venous devices cuffed and tunneled and central venous ports appear to have high rate of infection when risk is expressed in BSIs per 100 IVDs, but actually pose much lower risk when rates are expressed per 1000 IVD days.

PRACTICE APPLICATION: Expressing risk of IVD-related BSI per 1000 IVD days rather than 100 IVDs allows for more meaningful estimates of risk. Since national effort to date to reduce the risk of IVD-related infection have focused on short-term CVCs used in ICUs, the researchers stated that infection control programs must begin to strive to consistently apply essential control measures and prevention technologies with *all* types of IVDs.

8. Limit use of add-on devices.
9. Inspect the site and assess the patient routinely to ensure early recognition of symptoms.
10. Change peripheral cannula according to the INS Standards of Practice.
11. Implement central venous catheter prevention bundle. Refer to Table 9-9.
12. Provide staff education.
13. Remove I.V. cannula at the fist sign of local inflammation.

 NURSING FAST FACT!

The key to prevention of septicemia is staff education.

EBNP A quasi-experimental pre- and post-test design was conducted in the ICU at a major pediatric hospital. A self-study module was distributed to all RNs working in ICU. Compliance with central line care policy was observed. Data collected on 47 patients over two months showed marked improvement in compliance with the policy after presentation of an educational module (East & Jacoby, 2005).

Treatment

It is sometimes difficult to differentiate between infusion-associated sepsis and septicemia from other causes, unless associated with phlebitis (Maki & Mermel, 2007).

The steps in treating suspected septicemia based on patient signs and symptoms are:

1. Consult the physician.
2. If a peripheral cannula is in place, restart a new I.V. system in the opposite extremity.
3. Obtain cultures from the administration set, container, and catheter tip site, as well as the patient's blood.
4. Administer antibiotics, fluid replacement, vasopressors, and oxygen as prescribed.
5. Monitor the patient closely.
6. Determine whether the patient's condition requires transfer to the ICU.

Documentation

Document the signs and symptoms assessed, the time the physician was notified, and all treatments instituted. Document the time of transfer to

> Table 9-9   **CENTRAL VENOUS CATHETER BLOODSTREAM INFECTION PREVENTION BUNDLE**

Hand hygiene by catheter inserters
Maximum barrier precautions (gowns, gloves, mask, cap)
Chlorhexidine with alcohol skin antisepsis of catheter insertion site
Trained catheter inserters
Proper selection of type of catheter and insertion site
Insertion of catheters only when medically necessary
Having all materials needed for catheter insertion at the bedside before starting insertion
Time-out called if proper procedures are not followed (then start again)
Use of aseptic technique during catheter manipulation (including hub disinfection)
Removal of catheters when no longer medially necessary.
Frequent monitoring of catheter-related infection rates, with feedback on bundle
   compliance and outcomes

ICU, the time the new I.V. infusion system was started, and how the patient is tolerating interventions.

Venous Air Embolism

Venous **air embolism** (VAE) is a rare but lethal complication, especially involving VADs. The problem is treatable with prompt recognition, but prevention is the key. The pathophysiologic consequences of air emboli are a result of air entering the central veins, which is quickly trapped in the blood as it flows forward. Trapped air is carried to the right ventricle, where it lodges against the pulmonary valve and blocks the flow of blood from the ventricle into the pulmonary arteries. Less blood is ejected from the right ventricle, and the right heart overfills. The force of right ventricular contractions increases in an attempt to eject blood past the occluding air pocket. These forceful contractions break small air bubbles loose from the air pocket. Minute air bubbles are subsequently pumped into the pulmonary circulation, causing even greater obstruction to the forward flow of blood as well as local pulmonary tissue hypoxia.

 NURSING FAST FACT!

   One-hundred milliliters of air can pass through a 14 gauge needle in 1 second (Kim, Gottesmann, Forero, et al., 1998).

Pulmonary hypoxia results in vasoconstriction in the lung tissue, which further increases the workload of the right ventricle and reduces blood flow out of the right heart. This leads to diminished cardiac output, shock, and death.

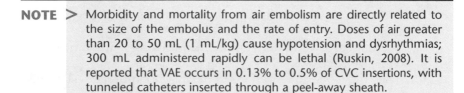

NOTE > Morbidity and mortality from air embolism are directly related to the size of the embolus and the rate of entry. Doses of air greater than 20 to 50 mL (1 mL/kg) cause hypotension and dysrhythmias; 300 mL administered rapidly can be lethal (Ruskin, 2008). It is reported that VAE occurs in 0.13% to 0.5% of CVC insertions, with tunneled catheters inserted through a peel-away sheath.

The same intrathoracic pressure changes that allow for pulmonary ventilation are responsible for air emboli associated with subclavian line removal. Pressure in the central veins decreases during inspiration and increases during expiration. If an opening into a central vein exposes the vessel to the atmosphere during the negative inspiratory cycle, air can be sucked into the central venous system in much the same manner that air is pulled into the lungs.

The causes of air embolism include:

- Allowing the solution container to run dry
- Superimposing a new I.V. bag to a line that has run dry without clearing the line of air
- Loose connections that allow air to enter the system
- Poor technique in dressing and tubing changes for central lines
- Presence of air in administration tubing cassettes of EIDs

Signs and Symptoms

Initial signs and symptoms of air embolism include:

- Patient complaints of palpitations
- Lightheadedness and weakness
- Pulmonary findings: Dyspnea, cyanosis, tachypnea, expiratory wheezes, cough, and pulmonary edema
- Cardiovascular findings: "Mill wheel" murmur; weak, thready pulse; tachycardia; substernal chest pain; hypotension; and jugular venous distention
- Neurologic findings: Change in mental status, confusion, coma, anxiousness, and seizures

If untreated, these signs and symptoms lead to hemiplegia, aphasia, generalized seizures, coma, and cardiac arrest.

Prevention

Techniques used to prevent air embolism include:

1. Vent all air from administration sets.
2. Vent air from port using a syringe attached to a needleless system.
3. Use a 0.22-micron air-eliminating filter.

4. Follow the protocol for dressing and tubing changes of central lines.
5. Superimpose I.V. solutions before the previous solution runs completely dry.
6. Attach piggyback medications to the injection port closest to the drip chamber so that the check valve will prevent air from being drawn into the line after the infusion of medication.
7. Use Luer-Lok™ connectors.
8. Do not bypass the "pump housing" of electric volumetric pumps.
9. Initial dressing should be occlusive.

NOTE > The second most frequent cause of VAE is iatrognic creation of a pressure gradient for air entry, such as with peripheral intravenous lines, central venous catheters, pulmonary artery catheter, and hemodialysis catheter. The first is surgical procedures performed in the upright position (neurosurgical; Wittenberg, 2006).

NOTE > A pressure difference of 5 cm of H_2O across a 14-gauge needle allows 100 mL of air per second to enter the venous system (Wittenberg, 2006).

Treatment

Treatment is largely supportive. If you suspect an air embolus, do the following:

1. Call for help and notify the physician.
2. Once VAE is suspected, any central line procedure in progress should be terminated immediately, and the line clamped.
3. Place the patient in the Trendelenburg position promptly on the left side (left lateral decubitus position) with the head down. This causes the air to rise in the right atrium, preventing it from entering the pulmonary artery.
4. Administer 100% oxygen, and intubate for significant respiratory distress or refractory hypoxemia.
5. Maintain systemic arterial pressure with fluid resuscitation and vasopressors/beta-adrenergic agents if necessary.
6. Monitor vital signs.
7. Call for emergency equipment.
8. If the patient experiences circulatory collapse, CPR should be started.
9. Consider transfer to a hyperbaric chamber.

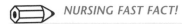 *NURSING FAST FACT!*

A pathognomonic indicator of an air embolism is a loud, churning, drum-like sound audible over the precordium, called a "mill wheel murmur." This symptom may be absent or transient.

Documentation

Document patient assessment, nursing interventions to correct the cause of embolism if apparent, notification of physician, and treatment. If emergency treatment was necessary, use an interval flow sheet to document the management of the air embolism, record interval vital signs, and indicate patient response.

Speed Shock

Speed shock occurs when a foreign substance, usually a medication, is rapidly introduced into the circulation. Rapid injection permits the concentration of medication in the plasma to reach toxic proportions, flooding the organs rich in blood—the heart and the brain. The vital organs, therefore, are "shocked" by a toxic dose. Syncope, shock, and cardiac arrest may result.

The causes of air embolism include:
- I.V. medications or solutions are administered at a rapid rate due to inadequate dilution with the circulating blood.
- The flow control clamp is inadvertently left completely open.
- The EID is programmed incorrectly.
- A bolus of medication is given too rapidly

Signs and Symptoms

Signs and symptoms of speed shock include:
- Dizziness
- Facial and neck flushing
- Patient complains of severe pounding headache ("brain freeze feeling")
- Tightness in the chest
- Hypotension
- Irregular pulse
- Progression of shock

Prevention

The best intervention is prevention. Techniques used to prevent speed shock include:

1. Reduce the size of drops by using microdrop sets for medication delivery.

2. Use an electronic flow control with free-flow high-risk drugs.
3. Monitor the infusion rate for accuracy before piggybacking in the medication.
4. Be careful not to manipulate the catheter; cannula movement may speed up the flow rate.
5. Administer bolus medication per the manufacturer's recommendations, but no faster than over 1 minute (e.g., morphine sulfate is recommended, as I.V. push over 5 min; Deglin & Vallerand, 2009).

 NURSING FAST FACT!

Prevention of speed shock is the key. When giving I.V. push drugs, give slowly and according to the manufacturer's recommendations.

Treatment

If you suspect speed shock, do the following:

1. Call for help.
2. Give an antidote or resuscitation medications as needed.
3. Have naloxone (Narcan) available on the unit if giving I.V. narcotics.
4. Begin CPR if cardiac arrest occurs.

NOTE > See Chapter 10 for appropriate steps in delivery of I.V. push medications.

Documentation

Document the medication or fluid administered and the signs and symptoms the patient reported and those assessed. Also document the physician notification, the treatment initiated, and the patient response.

NURSING POINTS-OF-CARE
PERIPHERAL INTRAVENOUS COMPLICATIONS

Nursing Assessments
■ Subjective complaints from patient regarding the I.V. site.
■ Inspect infusion site for signs and symptoms including redness, swelling, exudate, tenderness, dressing integrity.
■ Assess intake and output ratios.

- Assess cardiac and renal functions.
- Assess for age-related risks.
- Determine baseline weight.
- Assess vital signs, blood pressure, pulse, respirations and temperature, and pain.

Key Nursing Interventions
1. Maintain strict aseptic technique.
2. Follow CDC hand hygiene protocols.
3. Select and prepare an EID as indicated.
4. Administer fluids at room temperature.
5. Administer I.V. medications at prescribed rate and monitor for adverse effects.
6. Monitor the infusion site for:
   a. Flow rate
   b. Signs of phlebitis, infiltration, extravasation, or local infection
   c. Integrity of the dressing
   d. Stabilized catheter
7. Rotate the insertion site every 72 to 96 hours based on INS and CDC recommendations.
8. Use INS phlebitis scale and infiltration scale and document.
9. Maintain an occlusive dressing.
10. Determine if a drug or solution has vesicant or irritant qualities; maintain patency of infusion.
11. Perform site checks and document at regular intervals.

■ Central Venous Catheter Complications

Complications and risks related to central venous catheters (CVCs) include the local and systemic complications discussed so far in the chapter. Complications associated with central venous catheters fall into two groups: insertion-related complications and complications associated with indwelling CVCs. Insertion-related complications include pneumothorax, hemothorax, chylothorax, and extravascular and intravascular malposition. Complications associated with indwelling devices include thrombolytic and nonthrombolytic occlusions, pinch-off syndrome, vessel thrombosis, and superior vena cava syndrome (SVC syndrome). In addition, infections of CVCs have specific concerns related to central venous access.

Insertion-Related Complications

Pneumothorax/Hemothorax/Chylothorax

During insertion of the CVC the introducer may inadvertently cause trauma to the lung, veins, or thoracic duct due to the anatomical location of the subclavian vein and the lung during placement of a nontunneled or tunneled catheter and implanted ports. Complications related to the subclavian vein approach can cause a pneumothorax, hemothorax, or chylothorax.

A **pneumothorax** is created by the collection of air in the pleural space. It occurs because of the anatomic proximity of the lung to the subclavian veins. A **hemothorax** occurs when blood enters the pleural cavity as a result of trauma or transection of a vein during insertion. A chylothorax is a condition in which chyle (lymph) enters the pleural cavity as a result of transection of the thoracic duct on the left side.

Signs and Symptoms

Signs and symptoms of *pneumothorax* include:
■ Sudden onset of chest pain or shortness of breath during the procedure
■ On auscultation, a crunching sound is heard with heartbeat (caused by mediastinal air accumulation).
■ Dyspnea, persistent cough
■ Tachycardia

Signs and symptoms of *hemothorax* include:
■ Sudden onset of chest pain with mild to severe dyspnea
■ Bleeding into the pleural cavity
■ Tachycardia
■ Hypotension
■ Delayed symptoms: Dusky skin color, diaphoresis, and hemoptysis
■ Percussion may disclose dullness of affected side of chest.
■ Auscultation may detect decreased or absent breath sounds.

Signs and symptoms of *chylothorax* are similar to those of hemothorax and include:
■ Milk-like substance withdrawn during insertion into the needle or catheter

Prevention

1. Radiographic verification of placement of catheter before infusion of medication or solutions.
2. Highly skilled professional should insert CVC catheters.
3. Assess patient carefully for signs and symptoms during insertion.

Treatment

1. Oxygen is usually administered and a chest tube may be inserted for pneumothorax, hemothorax, or chylothorax.
2. Monitor vital signs.
3. Pressure should be applied over the vein entry site.
4. Remove the catheter.
5. Possible chest tube placement

Documentation

Document the insertion site, signs and symptoms, and all interventions. Document that radiographic verification was performed.

Catheter Malposition

Malposition results from erroneous insertion of the catheter into a small tributary of the SVC (i.e., internal mammary, azygous, or left brachio-cephalic), from migration of a correctly placed catheter into another vein, or from perforation of the SVC or endocardium by the catheter tip. During the insertion process the needle or introducer through which the catheter is passed may slip through the vessel wall.

Extravascular and Intravascular Malposition

The causes of malposition include:
- CVADs that terminate short of the SVC–right atrial junction
- Guidewire exchange process
- Cannulation of the left tortuous venous pathway
- Improper CVAD securement
- Changes in intrathoracic pressure (coughing, vomiting, sneezing)
- Incorrect measurement/trimming error of CVADs
- Port body flips due to "Twiddler's syndrome" if the port body not sutured adequately
- Introducer slips out of the vein during catheter insertion, or from migration.
- Improper positioning of the patient during insertion
- Stiff catheter material

SIGNS AND SYMPTOMS

Signs and symptoms of malposition include:
- Resistance on attempting to access device—unable to enter the port septum.
- Symptoms associated with pneumothorax or hemothorax if the pleural covering of the lung has been punctured.
- If fluid is infused through the catheter then the patient will experience hydrothorax as fluid is infused into the chest.
- Arm or neck swelling from fluid and adjacent to the tip of the catheter
- Can be noted when the catheter is first used with difficulty with aspiration or infusion through the catheter.
- Patient complains of discomfort or pain in the shoulder, neck, or arm.
- Catheters placed in internal jugular have been associated with annoyance called the "ear gurgling sign"; patient complains of the sound of a running stream rushing past the ear.

PREVENTION

1. Extreme care when using a break-away needle to remove the break-away introducer before threading the catheter.
2. Placement of the tip of ALL central venous catheters must have radiographic verification before use.
3. Well qualified, highly skilled professionals should place the CVC.
4. Use of silicone elastomer catheters.
5. Positioning of the patient: For PICCs inserted through the basilic vein, turn the patient's head toward the side of insertion. Place the patient in a slight Trendelenburg position with a rolled towel for placement of a catheter into subclavian vein.
6. Right-sided CVAD insertion is suggested.

TREATMENT

1. Surgical intervention to reopen a port pocket and reposition the port septum (Viale, 2003)
2. Medical interventions include removing the catheter and treating any associated complications.
3. Oxygen and chest tube may be necessary.
4. Monitor vital signs.
5. Not all malpositioned catheters are removed; some misplaced single-lumen silicone catheters can be repositioned with rapid flushing.
6. Catheters that loop back into the axillary or peripheral veins have a lower rate of successful repositioning, use of radiographic or direct fluoroscopic observation can be used to reposition catheters.
7. Catheters with simple looping into the subclavian, innominate, or internal jugular veins can often be repositioned by placing the patient in an ipsilateral position with the head of the bed slightly elevated.
8. Guidewire exchange has been used with success for placing a new catheter without repeated percutaneous cannulation.
9. Catheters placed in the right atrium or ventricle can be partially withdrawn.

DOCUMENTATION

Document the insertion site and positioning of patient, signs and symptoms, type of catheter used, and all interventions. Document that radiographic verification was performed.

 NURSING FAST FACT!

All central venous catheters must have radiographic documentation of tip placement in the superior vena cava before use.

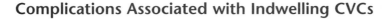

Complications Associated with Indwelling CVCs

Pinch-off Syndrome

Catheter **pinch-off syndrome** is the anatomical compression of the access device between the clavicle and the first rib. It occurs when the CVC enters the costoclavicular space medial to the subclavian vein and is positioned outside the lumen of the subclavian vein in the narrow area bounded by the clavicle, first rib, and costoclavicular ligament. This complication occurs when movement of the arm and shoulder further narrows the space, resulting in intermittent occlusion. Pinch-off syndrome is often unrecognized and underreported. It is recognized at times after the catheter fractures from the continuous compression between the first rib and the clavicle. Catheter pinch-off syndrome can result in catheter tearing, transection and catheter embolism. This syndrome occurs in 1% of the patients, and it is important to differentiate it from other causes of catheter obstruction (Mirza, Vanek, & Kupensky, 2004).

The causes of pinch-off syndrome include:
- Intravascular malposition of catheter
- Insertion technique using a percutaneous puncture medial to the midclavicular line
- Not placing the patient in the Trendelenburg position with a rolled towel or sheet between the shoulder blades to widen the angle between the clavicle and first rib.

SIGNS AND SYMPTOMS

Signs and symptoms of pinch-off syndrome include:
- Intermittent inability to aspirate blood or administer infusate unless the patient's position is altered
- The hallmark clinical sign is relief of occlusion during flushing by having the patient roll the shoulder backward or raise the arm on the ipsilateral side. The position change opens the angle of the costoclavicular space (Andris & Krzywda, 1997).

NOTE > Radiographic confirmation of the catheter with proper position of patient during radiography is crucial. It is important to note that because raising the arms or shrugging opens the costoclavicular angle, the films should be taken with the patient upright and with arms by the side (Mirza, Vanek, & Kupensky, 2004).

PREVENTION

1. Placement of the CVC with the patient in the Trendelenburg position with rolled towel can contribute to widening the clavicle and first rib. When procedure complete and patient returned to

upright position, the weight of the shoulder closes the angle and compress the catheter.

2. Placing the catheter lateral to the midclavicular line will decrease the risk of catheter pinch-off syndrome (Andris & Krzywda, 1997).

TREATMENT

1. Notify the physician immediately.
2. Remove the catheter if the patient has pinch-off syndrome and radiographic evidence of luminal narrowing of the catheter, even when it is functioning normally.

DOCUMENTATION

Intermittent positional flushing and infusion difficulties, radiographic confirmation performed, any signs and symptoms, and interventions.

Superior Vena Cava Syndrome

Superior vena cava syndrome (SVC syndrome) is impairment of blood flow through the SVC to the right atrium that significantly alters blood flow dynamics, resulting in extensive vein thrombosis.

The causes of SVC syndrome include:
- Traumatized endothelial lining of the vein predisposes the vein to clot formation.
- Any disease process that invades and internally obstructs the SVC

SIGNS AND SYMPTOMS

Signs and symptoms of SVC include:
- Progressive shortness of breath, dyspnea, cough
- Sensation of tightness in the chest
- Unilateral edema
- Cyanosis of the face, neck, shoulders, and arms
- Extensive edema of the upper body without edema in lower body parts (short cap edema)
- Jugular, temporal, and arm veins are engorged and distended.
- Prominent venous pattern usually is present over the chest from dilated thoracic vessels.
- Headache
- Potential for bronchial obstruction, cerebral anoxia (due to increased intracranial pressure), and death

PREVENTION

1. Avoid placing CVAD lines high in the SVC to decrease the risk of venous stasis and vessel injury.
2. Replace the DVAD with a smaller-caliber catheter.
3. Use alternative access sites not dependent on SVC patency.

4. Avoid placement of a CVAD over an area of scar tissue or stenosis.
5. Patient with hypercoagulable states such as atherosclerosis, diabetes mellitus, increased platelet levels, immobility.

NOTE > Hypercoagulability states increase the risk of clot or thrombus formation in either the arterial or venous circulations.

6. Well-trained, experienced professionals should place the catheter.

TREATMENT

1. Notify the physician immediately.
2. Diagnosis is confirmed by radiographic studies.
3. Removal of the catheter depends on the severity of symptoms, alternate I.V. route, and type of catheter in place.
4. Thrombolytic and/or anticoagulant therapy is prescribed and symptoms are treated.
5. Head of the bed is in the semi-Fowler's position.
6. Provide oxygen to facilitate breathing if needed.
7. Provide emotional support if the patient has the feeling of suffocating.
8. Monitor cardiovascular and neurological status.

DOCUMENTATION

Document all signs and symptoms, radiographic studies, and interventions.

Catheter Occlusion

LOSS OF PATENCY

Vascular access devices (VADs) can become occluded as a result of thrombotic occlusion (58%) or nonthrombotic occlusion (42% by lipid deposits, precipitates, or mechanical; McKnight; 2004). Loss of patency results from causes as simple as the patient's position to those as involved as combinations of complex clotting processes juxtaposed on the disease process.

Two criteria define CVC patency: the ability to infuse through the catheter and the ability to aspirate blood from the catheter. Withdrawal occlusion is a subset of **catheter occlusions** and describes the inability to freely aspirate blood from the catheter (Krzywda, 1999). The treatment must begin promptly; therefore, systematic evaluation of the catheter patency needs to be ongoing. If a VAD occlusion is left untreated, secondary complications can occur, such as loss of venous access, morbidity of recannulation, and risk of catheter infection because of a fibrin sheath for biofilm with bacterial or fungal colonization.

Preventive care of clot formation and subsequent occlusion includes careful catheter insertion, routine assessment of dressings, exit sites, tubing, pumps, infusion bags, and clamps; meticulous technique in blood sampling; and avoiding potential drug or solution incompatibilities. Table 9-10 presents a guide to troubleshooting occlusions. Catheter-related occlusions can be categorized as:

1. Complete occlusions: Total inability to withdraw blood and infuse fluids via the catheter
2. Partial occlusion: Difficulty in withdrawing and infusing fluids via the catheter
3. Withdrawal occlusion: Inability to withdraw blood via the catheter but with a capacity to infuse solutions without difficulty
4. Intraluminal obstruction: Obstruction within the catheter lumen that causes complete or partial occlusion
5. Extraluminal obstruction: Obstruction outside the lumen of the catheter, typically causing withdrawal occlusion

> Table 9-10 **TROUBLESHOOTING GUIDE FOR OCCLUDED CENTRAL VENOUS CATHETERS**

Purpose of Catheter (Agent Infused)	Cause of Occlusion	Treatment
Prolonged use of catheter	Fibrin sheath or thrombosis	Thrombolytic: rt-PA (alteplase)
Blood draw	Fibrin sheath or thrombosis	Thrombolytic: rt-PA (alteplase)
Transfusions	Fibrin sheath or thrombosis	Thrombolytic: rt-PA (alteplase)
Medication administration	Precipitate	$NaHCO_3$ or NaOH
Cold medications or solutions	Precipitate	$NaHCO_3$ or HCl
Stability (pH of medication)	Precipitate	$NaHCO_3$ or HCl
Medication with poor solubility (e.g., Dilantin)	Precipitate	$NaHCO_3$ or HCl
Time elapse since medication mixed	Precipitate	$NaHCO_3$ or HCl
Fat emulsions (or three-in-one TPN)	Lipid aggregation	70% ethyl alcohol

HCl = hydrochloric acid; $NaHCO_3$ = sodium bicarbonate.

6. Intravenous obstruction: An obstruction (usually a thrombus) in the vein that completely or partially stops blood flow; it may or may not affect the catheter's functionality.
7. Mechanical obstruction: An obstruction not related to precipitate or blood that partially or completely occludes the catheter (Mayo, 2001)

Nonthrombotic Occlusions

MECHANICAL OCCLUSION

Mechanical occlusions may result in partial or complete obstruction of VAD and are described as external and internal occlusions.

The causes of mechanical obstruction include:

External

■ External occlusion of flow may be caused by clogged injection cap, a clogged I.V. filter, an infusion pump that has been turned off, or an empty I.V. bag
■ Patient positioning (trapped in recliner, bed rails, or zippered pump pouches)
■ Occlusion can also occur at the catheter exit site or vein entry site if the suture used to secure the line constricts the catheter.

Internal

■ Malpositioned catheter tip as well as catheter kinking or compression
■ Pinch-off syndrome (often unrecognized)

Signs and Symptoms
■ Assess for signs of pinch-off syndrome.
■ Inability to infuse or withdraw fluids or sluggish flow
■ Frequent infusion pump alarms

Prevention
1. Make sure the catheter and tubing do not have kinks or closed clamps.
2. Assess suture placement; assess for tightness.
3. Follow prevention guidelines for pinch-off syndrome.

Treatment
1. First, determine whether the cause is internal or external.
2. Examine the I.V. setup for kinked tubing, closed clamps, an empty infusion bag, and readjustment of the I.V. delivery system.
3. Have the patient change position may correct the problem.
4. Radiography may help to confirm catheter tip placement and rule out migration. If pinch-off is documented on radiograph, medical intervention is needed to prevent catheter fracture.
5. Reposition the catheter, if possible.
6. Roll the patient's shoulder or raise the patient's arm on the ipsilateral side.

7. Thrombolytic agents are the only available drugs to lyse existing clots. They convert plasminogen to plasmin, which acts directly on the clot to dissolve the fibrin matrix.

DRUG PRECIPITATION AND LIPID RESIDUE

The nonthrombotic occlusion with drug precipitate or lipid residue occlusions may occur suddenly. Lipid residue can occur with the use of silicone catheters, as lipid emulsion tends to adhere to silicone.

The causes of drug precipitation include:
- Inadequate flushing between incompatible medications
- Simultaneous infusion of incompatible medications
- Infusion of medications with a low or high pH (usually under 5 and over 9)
- Infusion of parenteral nutrition, lipids, phenytoin, aminophylline, or gluconate (all known to cause precipitation; (Gorski, 2003)

Signs and Symptoms
- Inability to infuse or withdraw fluids
- Frequent pump alarms

Prevention
1. Adequate flushing of catheter with SASH sequence
2. Use of 1.2-micron filter for administration of lipid solutions.
3. Consult with infusion pharmacist to help identify causative agents and solutions and work collaboratively to identify the most common sources of nonthrombotic occlusions (INS, 2008).

Treatment
1. First determine the source of the occlusion (drug precipitate, lipids).
2. Determine catheter volume (refer to the specific catheter manufacturer for fill volume).
3. Obtain an order for a precipitate-clearing or thrombolytic agent.
4. Clamp the catheter and remove injection or access cap if in place
5. Disinfect the catheter hub, using 15-second friction prep.
6. Attach the stopcock to the catheter hub
7. Turn the stopcock to the "off" position.
8. Unclamp the catheter.
9. Connect the empty syringe to one port of the stopcock
10. Connect the syringe filled with precipitate-clearing or thrombolytic agent to the second port of the stopcock.
11. Open the stopcock port connected to the empty syringe.
12. Gently aspirate the empty syringe to 8 to 9 mL, then close the port, creating negative pressure within catheter lumen.
13. Open the stopcock connected to the syringe filled with precipitate-clearing or thrombolytic agent.
14. Gently instill the precipitate-clearing or thrombolytic agent into catheter. DO NOT FORCE.

15. Close the stopcock to the catheter.
16. Secure device to patient and label "DO NOT USE."
17. Allow the agent to dwell in catheter for the amount of time recommended by manufacturer.
18. Open the stopcock to the catheter, aspirate 3 to 5 mL of blood, and discard.
19. Flush the VAD. If unable to aspirate, repeat the procedure (INS, 2006b).

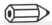 *NURSING FAST FACT!*

- *Drug precipitates are treated according to their pH, with the goal to increase the solubility of the precipitate by changing the pH within the catheter lumen.*
  a. Low-pH (1–5) drug: Hydrochloric acid (0.1 N)
  b. High-pH (9–12) drug: Sodium bicarbonate or 0.1 N sodium hydroxide (NaOH)
- *To restore patency in catheters occluded with crystallized calcium phosphate, use 0.1 N hydrochloric acid.*
- *Fat emulsions: 70% Ethanol*

NOTE > These agents should not be used with peripheral-short or midline catheters (Gorski, 2003; INS, 2008).

Thrombotic Occlusions

Thrombotic occlusions have a significant impact on the function of a central line. Deposits of fibrin and blood components within and around the CVC can impede or disrupt flow. Implanted devices can accumulate fibrin or precipitate within the portal reservoir. Thrombus formation can occur within the first 24 hours after insertion or over a period of time. A variety of thrombotic events can result in catheter occlusion (INS, 2008).

The causes of thrombotic occlusions include the following:
- Three factors play a significant role in the development of thrombotic occlusions, which is called Virchow's triad:
  1. A change in blood flow or venous stasis
  2. Hypercoagulability
  3. Trauma to the vessel wall (Andris & Krzywda, 1999)

When any of these three situations occurs, homeostasis is disturbed and the patient is at risk for thrombosis.
- Thrombotic occlusions are caused by intraluminal or extraluminal blood clots, a fibrin sheath totally or partially around the catheter tip, or catheter abutment against the vessel wall.
- Final tip position of the CVAD and the site of insertion

Signs and Symptoms

Intraluminal Thrombus Intraluminal occlusion occurs when the lumen of the catheter is obstructed by either clotted blood or an accumulation of fibrin.

- Frequently, the cause is blood remaining in the catheter after inadequate irrigation or retrograde flow (Fig. 9-7). Also, poor flushing technique after blood sampling may allow layers of fibrin to accumulate over time, narrowing or obstructing the lumen.

Mural Thrombus A mural thrombosis is caused by irritation of the catheter against the intima of the vessel wall causing accumulation of fibrin, and an aggregation of blood components that can lead to catheter adherence to the vein wall. This may develop into a venous thrombosis (Andris & Krzywda, 1999).

- Trauma to the vessel (catheter tip irritates the vessel wall) or prior injury to vessel wall.
- Frequent attempts at cannulation
- Use of rigid catheter

Fibrin Sheath and Fibrin Tail A fibrin sheath or (sleeve) forms when a layer of fibrin adheres to the external surface of the catheter. The thrombus may become trapped between the sheath and the catheter tip.

NOTE > Fibrin sheath is reported to occur in up to 47% of patients with CVADs (Boersma, Jie, & Verbon, 2007).

Platelet aggregation and fibrin deposition may completely encase the surface of the catheter and form a sac around the distal end of the catheter (Fig. 9-8).

- The sac causes retrograde flow of infusate up the catheter.
- The infusate may be observed on the skin (in nontunneled catheters), in the skin tunnel (in tunneled catheters), or in the subcutaneous pocket of implanted ports.
- A "tail" of fibrin extending off the catheter tip can occur owing to platelet aggregation and fibrin accumulation.

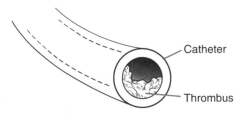

Figure 9-7 ■ Intraluminal occlusion.

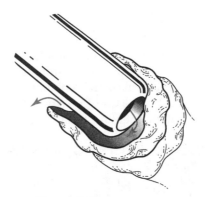

Figure 9-8 ■ Fibrin sleeve.

■ The tail usually does not interfere with infusion but may occlude the catheter on aspiration. This is commonly known as the "ball valve effect."

Portal Reservoir Occlusion Fluid viscosity or an improper flushing technique can produce fibrin or precipitate deposits within the reservoir of the port (Fig. 9-9). Accumulation of deposits leads to obstruction of the infusion.

PREVENTION OF THROMBUS OCCLUSIONS

■ Use adequate flushing protocols.
■ Use polyurethane and silicone catheters. Catheters made of polyvinylchloride and polyethylene have been reported to have a higher risk of thrombosis (Boersma, Jie, & Verbon, 2007).
■ Insert central catheters into the right side. Left-sided central line insertions have a higher incidence of thrombosis (Andris & Krzywda, 1999).
■ Place the tip in the distal superior vena cava/right atrial junction.

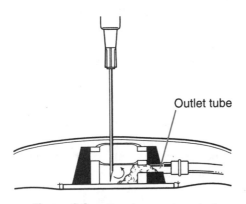

Outlet tube

Figure 9-9 ■ Portal reservoir occlusion.

TREATMENT

- Timely recognition and treatment can reduce complications.
- Catheter salvage is preferred over catheter replacement
- Once occlusion is confirmed, administration of a fibrinolytic agent may be appropriate. Alteplase (recombinant tissue plasminogen activator [rt-PA]; brand name Cathflo Activase®). It is the only FDA-approved thrombolytic agent for treatment of catheter occlusions.

> **EBNP** *A study by Ponec, Irwin, Haire, et al. (2001) demonstrated that one or two treatments with alteplase restored patency in 90% of the patients with occluded lines.*

THROMBOLYTIC ADMINISTRATION

Alteplase is a recombinant form of the naturally occurring tissue plasminogen activator (tPA) that enhances the conversion of plasminogen to plasmin in the presence of fibrin. When introduced into the systemic circulation, alteplase binds to the fibrin in a thrombus and converts the entrapped plasminogen to plasmin. This action initiates local fibrinolysis.

Cathflo Activase® (alteplase) is indicated for the restoration of function to central venous access devices as assessed by the ability to withdraw blood. Cathflo Activase® is a thrombolytic that works by targeting fibrin (the substance that causes blood to the clot), dissolving the thrombus (blood clot) and restoring function to the CVAD. Alteplase is packaged in 50- to 100-mg vials but only 2 mg is needed for catheter clearance. It is instilled into a dysfunctional catheter at a concentration of 1 mg/mL. For patients weighing more than 30 kg, instill 2 mg/2 mL into the occluded catheter. For patients weighing 10 to 29 kg, instill 110% of the internal lumen volume of the occluded catheter, not to exceed 2 mg/2 mL. Safety and effectiveness have not been established for patients weighing less than 10 kg (Deglin & Vallerand, 2009).

Contraindications to Thrombolytic Therapy Patients who have active internal bleeding, intracranial neoplasm, hypersensitivity to thrombolytic agents, liver disease, subacute bacterial endocarditis, or visceral malignancy or who have had a cerebrovascular accident within the past 2 months or intracranial or intraspinal surgery should not receive a thrombolytic agent.

COMPLICATIONS OF THROMBOLYTIC THERAPY

Bleeding The most frequent adverse reaction associated with all thrombolytics in all approved indications is bleeding. Caution should be exercised with patients who have active internal bleeding or who have had any of the following within 48 hours:

- Surgery
- Obstetrical delivery

- Percutaneous biopsy of viscera or deep tissues
- Puncture of noncompressible vessels

In addition, caution should be exercised with patients who have thrombocytopenia, other hemostatic defects (including those secondary to severe hepatic or renal disease), or any condition for which bleeding constitutes a significant hazard or would be particularly difficult to manage because of its location, or who are at high risk for embolic complications (e.g., venous thrombosis).

Catheter-Related Bloodstream Infections

A catheter-related bloodstream infection (CR-BSI) is defined as "bacteremia or fungemia in a patient who has an intravascular device with positive blood cultures." CR-BSI is a risk with the use of any vascular access device. Sepsis or septicemia was discussed previously in this chapter. An estimated 250,000 to 500,000 CR-BSIs occur each year in the United States (Crnich & Maki, 2005). In most hospitals, as now recommended by the CDC, The Joint Commission, and the Agency for Healthcare Research and Quality, risk of CVC-related BSI is expressed as catheter-associated BSIs per 1000 CVC days; therefore all healthcare-associated BSIs that cannot reasonably be linked to a site of local infection are attributed to patient's CVC (Maki, Kluger, & Crnich, 2006).

NOTE > Local infection was discussed previously in this chapter.

Biofilm

New research is challenging the well-known thought that "bacteria migrate from the skin down to the catheter surface and colonize the catheter." Current research is pointing to the development of a biofilm during insertion and dwell of intravascular devices. When the number of organisms exceeds a certain level, the patient develops a CR-BSI. Biofilm development occurs when, immediately after insertion, plasma proteins attach to the catheter. Within 5 minutes, the layer of proteins that are attached to the catheter surface and the proteins in the bloodstream have equalized. Platelets and white blood cells also adhere to the catheter surface. The coagulation cascade is initiated with vessel wall injury, and within a few hours, the catheter is coated with a fibrin sheath from all these substances. Microbes from the skin surface and dermal layers are introduced and flushed through the catheter. The microbes interact with the platelet–protein layer, and bacteria and fungi easily attach themselves to this protein layer. Some organisms produce a slimy matrix and encapsulate themselves loosely on the surface. The biofilm cell can naturally detach from shearing forces of blood flow, detach during flushing, and move to other sites for attachment and is generally resistant to host defense mechanisms of the immune system. Because of the presence and nature of biofilm adherence, aseptic technique during the insertion, care, and maintenance of the device is essential to prevent the morbidity and mortality associated with CR-BSIs (Hadaway, 2003).

Catheter Management to Prevent CR-BSIs

In 2008, the Healthcare Infection Control Practices Advisory Committee (HICPAC) revised guidelines for prevention of intravascular catheter-related infections. The following guidelines are for practitioners who insert catheters and for persons responsible for surveillance and control of infections in hospitals and outpatient and home healthcare settings:

1. Educate healthcare workers regarding the indications for intravascular catheter use and proper procedures for insertion and maintenance of intravascular catheters.
2. Surveillance: Hospital rates of catheter related infections
3. Special I.V. teams are desirable.
4. In adults, use an upper instead of lower extremity.
5. Select the catheter on the basis of the intended purpose and duration of use, and known complications.
6. Use a midline or PICC when the duration of I.V. therapy will likely exceed 6 days.
7. Weigh the risk versus the benefits of placing a device.
8. For nontunneled catheters use the subclavian site.
9. Promptly remove any intravascular device that is no longer essential.
10. Observe proper hand hygiene procedures
11. Maintain aseptic technique.
12. Wear clean or sterile gloves when inserting an intravascular catheter.
13. Use aseptic technique and maximal sterile barrier precautions, including the use of a cap, mask, sterile gown, sterile gloves, and large sterile sheet for insertion of CVCs, including PICC or guidewire exchanges.
14. Disinfect clean skin with an appropriate antiseptic before catheter insertion. A 2% chlorhexidine-based preparation is preferred. Allow the antiseptic to remain on the insertion site and to air dry.
15. Use sterile gauze or a transparent, semipermeable dressing to cover catheter site.
16. Do not use topical antibiotic ointments or creams on insertion sites.
17. Do not submerge the catheter under water.
18. Replace dressings used on short-term CVC sites every 2 days for gauze dressing; every 7 days for transparent dressings.

19. Use a sutureless securement device to reduce the risk of infection.
20. Use an antimicrobial or antiseptic-impregnated CVC in adults whose catheter is expected to remain in place for longer than 5 days.
21. Do not administer intranasal or systemic antimicrobial prophylaxis routinely before insertion or during use of an intravascular catheter.
22. Do not routinely use antibiotic lock solutions to prevent CR-BSI.
23. Do not use routine anticoagulant therapy to reduce CR-BSI.
24. Replace peripheral catheters every 72 to 96 hours.
25. Replace midline catheters only when there is a specific indication.
26. Do not remove CVCs or PICCs on the basis of fever alone. Use clinical judgment.
27. Do not use guidewire exchanges routinely for nontunneled catheters.
28. Only use guidewire exchanges to replace a malfunctioning nontunneled catheter if no evidence of infection is present.
29. Change the needleless components at least as frequently as the administration sets.
30. Minimize contamination risk by wiping the access port with an appropriate antiseptic (chlorhexidine is preferred).
31. Admixture of all routine parenteral fluids in the pharmacy under a laminar-flow hood.
32. Do not use any container of parenteral fluid that has visible turbidity, leaks, cracks, or particulate matter.
33. Use single-dose vials.
    (O'Grady, Alexander, Dellinger, et al., 2002).

According to Maki (2007) "well designed technologies for prevention of intravascular device related bloodstream infections (IVDR BSI) have been shown clearly to reduce rates of BSI substantially, to pose no risk of promoting resistance, and to be highly cost-effective." Those new technologies include the following:

1. Implementation of the bundle approach (Table 9-8)
2. Tunneling and subcutaneous cuffs
3. Antiseptic-impregnated dressings
4. Colonization-resistant polymers
   a. Heparin-bonded surfaces
   b. Antimicrobial coatings
   c. Antiseptic impregnation
   d. Ultrasmooth surfaces
   e. Use of anti-inflammatory drugs
5. Contamination-resistant hubs
6. Luminal antimicrobial flush/lock solutions
   (Maki, 2007).

Extraction Complications

Complications that occur during catheter extraction include air embolism, breakage, separation from the hub and knotting of the catheter. Accidental CVC removal is a serious problem because of the associated risks of hemorrhage and air embolism.

Venous air embolism can occur during insertion of a CVC but is more commonly seen as a complication of catheter extraction (Heckmann, Lang, Kindler, et al., 2000). It is reported to occur 0.13% to 0.5% of CVC insertions, with tunneled catheters inserted through a peel-away sheath the most common source. The associated mortality is substantial, ranging between 23% and 50% (Kim, Gottesman, Forero, et al., 1998). Technique standardization should include education about prevention of air embolism during CVC insertion and removal (Kusminsky, 2007). Additional complications during extraction of the CVC include breakage which is frequently a result of excessive traction force. At times, the catheter material can sometimes be faulty and ruptures or dilates (Fratino, Mazzola, Buffa, et al., 2001).

Table 9-11 provides a summary of the complications related to central venous access.

> Table 9-11   **SUMMARY OF COMPLICATIONS OF CENTRAL VENOUS ACCESS**

Complication and Cause	Signs and Symptoms	Treatment	Prevention
Pneumothorax Collection of air in the pleural space between the lung and chest wall; caused by puncture of the pleural covering of the lung	Shortness of breath during procedure, crunching sound on auscultation, dyspnea, cyanosis, subcutaneous emphysema Sudden chest pain	Administer oxygen. A chest tube may be inserted. May resolve slowly without evacuation of air. Monitor vital signs. Apply pressure over the site.	Radiographic verification of placement Highly skilled professional inserters Assess carefully during insertion.
Hemothorax Blood enters the pleural cavity as a result of trauma or transection of a vein	Sudden onset of chest pain, tachycardia, hypotension, dusky color, diaphoresis, hemoptysis	Usually noted during insertion of catheter (subclavian artery during infraclavicular placement). Remove the catheter and apply pressure to the site Monitor vital signs. Administer oxygen.	Same as for pneumothorax

> Table 9-11	SUMMARY OF COMPLICATIONS OF CENTRAL VENOUS ACCESS—cont'd		
Complication and Cause	Signs and Symptoms	Treatment	Prevention
Chylothorax Lymph (chyle) fluid enters the pleural cavity as a result of transection of the thoracic duct on the left side where it enters the subclavian vein; chyle is a milk-like substance.	Sudden onset of chest pain, dyspnea, with-drawal of a milk-like substance into the needle Large amounts of serous drainage from insertion site.	Remove the catheter. Monitor vital signs. Administer oxygen. Chest tube may be necessary.	Same as for pneumothorax
Intravascular Malposition	Difficulty with aspiration Complaints of discomfort or shoulder pain Edema of neck or shoulder "ear gurgling sign"	Not all are removed Rapid flush may sometimes correct malposi-tion with single-lumen reposition. Place patient in ipsilateral position. Guidewire exchange Partially withdraw into R atrium	Radiographic confirmation of tip before use Well qualified inserter Silicone elastomer Position of patient.
Extravascular Malposition Catheter penetrates the vessel and the tip lies outside the vascular system; occurs during threading a catheter or needle introducer	Symptoms of pneumothorax or hemothorax Resistance upon access of device Arm or neck swelling	Remove catheter. Monitor vital signs. Oxygen, chest tube may be necessary	Radiographic verification of catheter tip
Pinch-off Syndrome CVC inserted via the percutaneous subclavian site is compressed by the clavicle and the first rib; results in mechanical occlusion; can result in complete or partial catheter transection and embolization.	Frequently unrecognized, catheter is positional, weak points on the catheter balloon out, difficulty in aspiration of blood, resistance to flushing or infusion (often relieved by rolling the shoulder or raising the arm), infraclavicular pain or swelling	Remove the catheter. Retrieve the embolized segment if necessary.	Place CVC with patient in Trende-lenburg position.

Continued

> Table 9-11   SUMMARY OF COMPLICATIONS OF CENTRAL
                VENOUS ACCESS—cont'd

Complication and Cause	Signs and Symptoms	Treatment	Prevention
SVC Syndrome Condition caused by blood clot, fibrin formation, or both that occludes the SVC	Progressive shortness of breath; cough; sensation of skin tightness; unilateral edema; cyanosis of face, neck, shoulder, and arms; "short-cap edema" (edema of the upper extremities without edema of lower); jugular, temporal, and arm veins are engorged and distended; prominent venous pattern is present over chest	Notify the physician immediately. Radiographic confirmation of SVC syndrome Catheter may or may not be removed. Anticoagulant therapy Place the patient in semi-Fowler's position. Administer oxygen. Monitor fluid volume status. Monitor cardiac and neurological status.	Rare but serious Well-trained inserter Anticoagulant therapy for long-term catheters. High-risk patients
Nonthrombolytic Occlusion Crystallization of TPN admixtures and drug-to-drug or drug-to-solution incompatibilities	Sluggish flow rates, total occlusion, inability to flush or obtain blood withdrawal	Attempt to restore patency using appropriate solution (HCl or sodium bicarbonate, or ethanol).	
Thrombolytic Occlusions Deposits of fibrin and blood components within and around the CVC; intraluminal blood clot, fibrin sheath totally or partially; fibrin or precipitate accumulation can occur in portal reservoir in implanted devices.	Sluggish flow rates, total occlusion, inability to flush or obtain blood withdrawal (clinically silent), fibrin (may be able to infuse solutions), but unable to aspirate blood, "ball-valve-effect"	Attempt to aspirate the clot. Initiate appropriate fibrinolytic treatment with rt-PA.	Adequate flushing of catheter Use of 1.2 micron filter for lipids Consult pharmacist to identify possible sources.

NURSING POINTS-OF-CARE
COMPLICATIONS ASSOCIATED WITH CENTRAL VENOUS ACCESS

Nursing Assessments
- Obtain confirmation of tip placement in the SVC.
- Inspect the site for signs of infection.
- Obtain baseline vital signs.
- Examine PICC and tunneled catheters for line integrity.
- Review patient cardiovascular and neurological history.

Key Nursing Interventions
1. Assist with insertion where appropriate, including correct positioning of patient.
2. Maintain competency if performing PICC insertion.
3. Follow standard precautions
4. Maintain hand hygiene protocol.
5. Use best practice for care and maintenance of catheters.
6. Implement the bundle approach to prevent CR-BSI.
7. Maintain the integrity of the central line dressing.
8. Maintain sterile technique.
9. Use a 10-mL syringe to flush all central line catheters.
10. Administer oxygen as indicated.
11. Place patient in semi-Fowlers' position where appropriate
12. Provide emotional support.
13. Monitor cardiovascular and neurological status.
14. Do not use force when instilling a thrombolytic agent into a catheter; attempt to declot every 15 minutes after dwell time.
15. Monitor thrombin time, prothrombin time, or activated partial thromboplastin time.

AGE-RELATED CONSIDERATIONS
The Pediatric Client
It is important to assess the infant early during the hospital stay and to determine the most appropriate vascular access device for meeting an infant's ongoing needs. All complications discussed for the adult client can occur with the pediatric client. The following focus on the pediatric patient:
- Be aware that catheters inserted into the cephalic vein most commonly are malpositioned into the axillary and basilic veins.
- Catheters inserted through the saphenous or other leg veins (particularly on the left side) may enter the ascending lumbar vein (De & Imam, 2005).

Continued

• Catheters inserted into the scalp can enter intracranial veins or tissue and thoracic veins (Anderson, Graupman, Hall, et al., 2004).

• Sepsis appears to be the most consistently reported serious problem associated with PICCs in infants over PIV (Parellada, Moise, Hegemier, & Gest, 1999).

• The incidence of thrombosis varies due to the lack of a standardized method of diagnosis, but is higher in smaller children (Pettit & Wyckoff, 2007).

• Saphenous vein insertions may increase the risk for phlebitis.

The Older Adult

• Hematomas and ecchymoses are frequently seen in elderly persons. Fragile veins are easily injured.

• Elderly persons, particularly those older than 85 years with multiple comorbidities, multiple medications, and functional or cognitive impairment are at higher risk for adverse outcomes, including responses to medical or surgical events (Zwicker, 2003).

• The risk of fluid overload and subsequent pulmonary edema is especially increased in elderly patients with cardiac disease.

• Be alert to the potential presence of infection when even low-grade temperature elevations appear for short periods. In a majority of cases of acute confusion in the elderly, the etiology was multifactorial infections and dehydration was the most common cause (Cacchione, Culp, Laing, et al., 2003).

Home Care Issues

Home care practitioners must be aware of the potential danger that exists in I.V. drug administration and must be able to handle emergency situations. Adverse reactions, such as drowsiness, dizziness, nausea, diarrhea, and local and systemic complications, can occur with delivery of medications in the home setting.

Allergic reactions from hypersensitivity to a specific antigen can also occur. An emergency kit, including epinephrine, diphenhydramine (Benadryl), and dexamethasone (Decadron) or hydrocortisone (Solu-Cortef), should be available to clinicians delivering first doses of medications or medications with continuing risk for reactions (e.g., immune globulin infusions) in the home setting.

Home Care Issues—cont'd

NOTE > The actual incidence of anaphylaxis is very low in home care settings and is minimized by evaluating patients for risk factors and appropriateness of administering the prescribed drug in the home. If there is history of allergy, often the first dose should be administered in a setting with access to a full emergency cart. Potential problems and complications encountered in home infusion therapy include:

- Mechanical problems
- Nonrunning I.V. lines
- Inability to flush lines
- Malfunction of electronic infusion devices (EIDs)

Maintain strong infection control policies in the home setting, especially addressing such issues as storage and use of solutions.

 Patient Education

■ Instruct the patient to perform routine activities: bathing, movement in bed, and ambulation to maintain I.V. system.
■ Instruct the patient to report any signs or symptoms of common local complications (e.g., redness, swelling, pain at site).
■ Instruct the patient to report any interruption in flow rate.
■ Instruct the patient on the purpose of the EID.

Teach the client and family the symptoms of infection that should be promptly reported to the medical caregiver.

■ Nursing Process

The nursing process is a five- or six-step process for problem-solving to guide nursing action. Refer to Chapter 1 for details on the steps of the nursing process related to vascular access. The following table focuses on nursing diagnoses, nursing outcomes classification (NOC), and nursing intervention classification (NIC) for patients with local and systemic complications of infusion therapy. Nursing diagnoses should be patient specific and outcomes and interventions individualized. The NOC and NIC presented here are suggested direction for development of specific outcomes and interventions.

Nursing Diagnoses Related to Complications	NOC: Nursing Outcomes Classification	NIC: Nursing Intervention Classification
Anxiety (mild, moderate or severe) related to: Threat to change in health status or misconception regarding complications	Anxiety level	Anxiety reduction techniques
Fluid volume deficit related to: Vasodilation of peripheral vessels, leaking capillaries secondary to septicemia	Fluid balance, hydration	Fluid management, hypovolemia management, shock management
Gas exchange impaired related to: Alveolar-capillary membrane changes secondary to pneumothorax	Respiratory status, ventilation	Airway management
Pain, acute, related to: Peripheral vascular inflammation, edema, central malposition or occlusion, medication	Injuring agents: physical or chemical	Comfort level, pain control strategies
Infection risk of related to: Environmental exposure to pathogens; immunosuppression, invasive procedures	Infection control and risk detection	Infection control practices
Protection ineffective related to: Abnormal blood profiles, drug therapies (thrombolytics)	Blood coagulation	Bleeding precautions
Skin integrity, impaired, related to: VAD; irritation from I.V. solution, inflammation, infection	Tissue integrity: Skin	Skin surveillance, wound care
Thermoregulation, ineffective, related to: Infectious process, septic shock, septicemia	Thermoregulation	Temperature regulation strategies
Tissue perfusion, ineffective, (peripheral) related to: Infiltration or extravasation of fluid or medication	Tissue perfusion: Peripheral	Circulatory care: Peripheral
Tissue perfusion, altered cardiopulmonary, peripheral, related to: Arterial or venous blood flow exchange problems, hypovolemia, or decreased systemic vascular resistance related to sepsis	Circulatory status, fluid balance, hydration. Tissue perfusion: Peripheral	Circulatory care

Sources: Ackley & Ladwig (2008); Carpenito-Moyet (2008); McCloskey-Dochterman & Bulechek (2004); Moorhead, Johnson, & Maas (2004); NANDA-I (2007).

Chapter Highlights

◼ After reading this chapter, you have increased your awareness about the risks to patients receiving I.V. therapy. Remember, you have observation skills to assess for local complications, as well as cognitive skills to assess for systemic complications.

- There are two divisions of complications, local and systemic.
- Local complications can become dangerous systemic adverse processes.
- Prevention is the best intervention for avoiding complications of infusion therapy.
- Key tips for preventing local complications:
  - Maintain INS guidelines regarding tubing change, cannula change, and length of time I.V. solutions remain hanging.
  - Follow aseptic technique in skin preparation and venipuncture techniques.
  - Follow CDC hand hygiene guidelines.
  - Choose appropriate dressings.
  - Secure tubing and cannula with good taping technique.
  - Use a 0.22-micron inline filter as an extra safeguard.
  - Keep solutions at the prescribed rate.
  - Document the observed I.V. site every 4 hours for adults and every 2 hours for infants and children.
- Phlebitis (bacterial, chemical, or mechanical) is a frequently encountered problem associated with infusion therapy and can lead to cellulitis, thromboembolic complications, or sepsis.
- Key tips for preventing systemic complications:
  - Follow hand hygiene procedures.
  - Inspect solutions and equipment for breaks in integrity.
  - Use Luer-Lok™ connectors.
  - Limit the use of add-on devices.
  - Maintain flow rates at the prescribed rate.
  - Use a 0.22-micron filter when appropriate.
  - Use electronic infusion devices
  - Use bundle approach to prevent CR-BSI

Central Venous Catheter Complications

- Insertion-related complications
- Pneumothorax/hemothorax/chylothorax
- Catheter malposition: Extravascular and intravascular
- Indwelling complications
  - Pinch-off syndrome
  - Superior vena cava syndrome (SVC syndrome)
  - Catheter occlusion
    - Nonthrombotic occlusions
      Mechanical
      Drug precipitation and lipid residue
    - Thrombotic occlusions
      Intraluminal thrombus
      Mural thrombosis
      Portal reservoir occlusion

- Catheter-related bloodstream infections
  - Use bundle approach to prevent
- Extraction complications
  - Air embolism can occur during insertion and more commonly seen as a complicaiton of cathter extraction.
  - Breakage, separation from the hub and knotting of the catheter can result from excessive traciton force during removal.

■■ Thinking Critically: Case Study

A 40-year-old woman with insulin-dependent diabetes mellitus is familiar with her disease, but does not take care of herself. She is currently admitted with an infected plantar ulcer and had a transmetatarsal amputation. She was discharged home on a regimen of I.V. antibiotics via a PICC, with home care follow-up.

What potential complications would the home care nurse be alert for?
What documentation needs to be addressed at every visit?
What patient education needs to be reinforced at home?

 Media Link: Answers to the case study and more critical thinking activities are provided on the CD-ROM.

Post-Test

1. Which of the following are local complications associated with infusion therapy?

   a. Speed shock, septicemia, and venous spasm
   b. Phlebitis, venous spasm, and hematoma
   c. Septicemia, thrombophlebitis, and hematoma
   d. Phlebitis, pulmonary edema, and speed shock

2. Which of following are ways to prevent the formation of a thrombosis? (*Select all that apply.*)

   a. Use of pumps or controllers for managing rate control
   b. Avoiding placing the cannula in areas of flexion
   c. Use of needleless systems
   d. Good technique during vein cannulation.

3. A patient states that his I.V. site is sore. You assess the site and note redness and swelling but no signs of palpable cord or streak. Using the criteria for infusion phlebitis, what is the severity of this phlebitis?

   a. 3+
   b. 2+
   c. 1+
   d. 0

4. While a solution is infusing, which of the following is a treatment for venous spasm?

   a. Apply a cold pack to the site.
   b. Increase the flow rate of the solution.
   c. Apply a warm compress to the site.
   d. Administer pain medication.

5. You check an infusion site on a patient and find swelling and cool skin temperature. Also, the patient's skin appears blanched and feels rigid, and the infusion rate has slowed. These are signs of:

   a. Phlebitis
   b. Catheter embolus
   c. Hematoma
   d. Infiltration

6. You are performing a venipuncture and an ecchymosis forms over and around the insertion area, which has become raised and hardened. You are unable to advance the cannula into the vein. These are signs of:

   a. Phlebitis
   b. Infiltration
   c. Hematoma
   d. Occlusion

7. What is the one MOST important nursing intervention that is key to the prevention of many I.V.-related complications?

   a. Reading the policy and procedure manuals
   b. Hand hygiene procedures
   c. Using microdrip sets
   d. Competency testing

8. To prevent damage to the intima of the vein wall, which of the following syringe barrels should be used on a peripheral I.V. line?

   a. 1 mL or smaller
   b. 3 mL or smaller
   c. 3 mL or larger
   d. 10 mL or larger

9. Catheter occlusion may cause which of the following? (*Select all that apply.*)

   a. An inability to administer essential medications.
   b. Permanent loss of access through the device
   c. An increased risk of infection
   d. Tissue sloughing

10. Which of the following agents would be used to treat a non-thrombotic occlusion caused by lipids?

    a. 70% ethyl alcohol
    b. Sodium bicarbonate
    c. Hydrochloric acid
    d. Alteplase

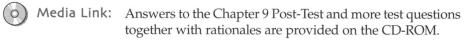 Media Link: Answers to the Chapter 9 Post-Test and more test questions together with rationales are provided on the CD-ROM.

▪ References

Ackley, B.J., & Ladwig, G.B. (2008). *Nursing diagnosis handbook: An evidence-based guide to planning care*. St. Louis, MO: Mosby Elsevier.

Anderson, D., Graupman, P.C., Hall, W.A., et al. (2004). Pediatric intracranial complications of central venous catheter placement. *Pediatric Neurosurgery, 40,* 28–31.

Andris, D.A., & Krzywda, E.A. (1997). Catheter pinch-off syndrome: Recognition and management. *Journal of Infusion Nursing, 20*(5), 233.

Andris, D.A., & Krzywda, E.A. (1999). Central venous catheter occlusions: Successful management strategies. *MEDSURG Nursing, 8,* 229–236.

Arbique, J., & Arbique, D. (2007). Reducing the risk of nerve injuries. *IV Rounds Nursing 2007, 20*–21.

Boersma, R.S., Jie, K.S., Verbon, A., et al. (2007). Thrombotic and infectious complications of central venous catheters in patients with hematological malignancies. *Annals of Oncology, 10,* 24.

Cacchione, P.Z., Culp, K., Laing, J., et al. (2003). Clinical profile of acute confusion in the long-term care setting. *Clinical Nursing Research, 12*(2), 145–158.

Catney, M., Hillis, S., Wakefield, B., et al. (2001). Relationship between peripheral intravenous catheter dwell time and the development of phlebitis and infiltration. *Journal of Infusion Nursing, 24*(5), 332–341.

Clinical Laboratory and Standards Institute (CLSI). (2003). *Procedure for the collection of diagnostic blood specimens by venipunctures* (5th ed.). Wayne, PA: Author.

Cornbleet, P.J. (2002). Clinical utility of the band count. *Clinical Laboratory Medicine, 22*(1), 101.

Crnich, C.J., & Maki, D.G. (2007). Infections caused by intravascular devices: Epidemiology, pathogenesis, diagnosis, prevention, and treatment. In: *APIC text of infection control and epidemiology,* Vol. 1 (2nd ed., pp. 21–24). Washington, DC: Association for Professionals in Infection Control and Epidemiology.

Dada, I.A., & Sznajder, J.I. (2003). Mechanisms of pulmonary edema clearance during acute hypoxemia respiratory failure: Role of the Na,K-ATPase. *Critical Care Medicine, 31*(Supplement), S248–S252.

De, A., & Imam, A. (2005). Long line complication: Accidental cannulation of ascending lumbar vein. *Archives of Disease in Childhood. Fetal and Neonatal Edition, 90,* F48.

Deglin, J., & Vallerand, A. (2009). *Davis's drug guide for nurses* (11th ed.). Philadelphia: F.A. Davis.

Doellman, D. (2007). The prevention and management of infiltration and extravasation injuries. INS Annual Meeting June 6, 2007.

East, D., & Jacoby, K. (2005). The effect of a nursing staff education program on compliance with central line care policy in the cardiac intensive care unit. *Pediatric Nursing, 31*(3), 182–194.

Ezzone, S.A. (2007). Pulmonary edema. *Clinical Journal of Oncology Nursing, 11*(3), 457–459.

Fratino, G., Mazzoal, C., Buffa, P., et al. (2001). Mechanical complications related to indwelling central venous catheter in pediatric hematology/oncology patients. *Pediatric Hematology Oncology, 18,* 317–324.

Gallant, P., & Schultz, A. (2006). Evaluation of a visual infusion phlebitis scale for determining appropriate discontinuation of peripheral intravenous catheters. *Journal of Infusion Nursing, 29*(6), 338–345.

Gorski, L.A. (2003). Central venous access device occlusions: Part 2: Nonthrombotic causes and treatment. *Home Healthcare Nurse, 21,* 168–171.

Hadaway, L. (2003). Infusing without infecting. *Nursing 2003, 33*(10), 58–63.

Hadaway, L. (2007). Infiltration and extravasation: Preventing a complication of IV catheterization. *American Journal of Nursing, 107*(8), 64–72.

Hastings-Tolsma, M.T., Yucha, C.B., Tompkins, J., et al. (1993). Effect of warm and cold applications on the resolution of I.V. infiltration. *Research in Nursing & Health, 16,* 171–178.

Heckmann, J.G., Lang, C.J.G., Kindler, K., et al. (2000). Neurologic manifestations of cerebral air embolism as a complication of central venous catheterization. *Critical Care Medicine, 28,* 1621–1625.

Infusion Nurses Society (INS). (2006a). *Infusion nursing standards of practice.* Supplement 1S. Philadelphia: Lippincott Williams & Wilkins.

Infusion Nurses Society (INS). (2006b). *Policies and procedures for infusion nursing* (3rd ed.). Norwood MA: Author.

Infusion Nurses Society (INS). (2008). New standards for catheter occlusion management. *Nursing practice management, 1*(2), 4–11.

Kim, D.K., Gottesman, M.H., Forero, A., et al. (1998). The CVC removal distress syndrome an unappreciated complication of central venous catheter removal. *Annals of Surgery, 64,* 344–347.

Kusminsky, R.E. (2007). Complications of central venous catheterization. *Journal of American College of Surgeons, 204*(4), 681–696.

Krzywda, E.A. (1999). Predisposing factors, prevention, and management of central venous catheter occlusions. *Journal of Intravenous Nursing, 22*(6S), S11–S17.

Lavery, I.P. (2005). Peripheral intravenous therapy: Key risks and implications for practice. *Nursing Standard, 19, 46,* 5564.

Maki, D.G. (2007). Novel approaches to catheter maintenance to prevent CR-BSI. INS Breakfast Symposium, November 11, 2007, Anaheim, CA.

Maki, D., Kluger, D.M., & Crnich, C.J. (2006). The risk of bloodstream infection in adults with different intravascular devices: A systematic review of 200 published prospective studies. *Mayo Clinic Proceedings 81*(9), 1159–1171.

Maki, D.G., & Mermel, L.A. (2007). Infections due to infusion therapy. In: W. Jarvis (Ed.), *Hospital infections* (5th ed.). Philadelphia: Lippincott Williams & Wilkins.

Maki, D.G., & Ringer, M. (1991). Risk factors for infusion-related phlebitis with small peripheral venous catheters. *Annals of Internal Medicine, 114,* 845–854.

Masoorli, S. (2007). Nerve injuries related to vascular access insertion and assessment. *Journal of Infusion Nursing, 30*(6), 346–350.

Mayo, D.J. (2001). Catheter-related thrombosis. *Journal of Intravenous Therapy, 24*(3S), S13–S21.

McCloskey-Dochterman, J.C., & Bulechek, G.M. (2004). *Nursing interventions classification (NIC)* (4th ed.). St. Louis, MO: C.V. Mosby.

McKnight, S. (2004). Nurse's guide to understanding and treating thrombotic occlusion of central venous access devices. *MEDSURG Nursing, 13,* 377–382.

Metheny, N.M. (2000). *Fluid and electrolyte balance: Nursing considerations* (4th ed.). Philadelphia: J.B. Lippincott.

Miza, B., Vanek, V.W., & Kupennsky, D.T. (2004). Pinch-off syndrome: Case report and collective review of the literature. *Annals of Surgery, 70,* 635–644.

Moorhead, S., Johnson, M., & Maas, M. (2004). *Nursing outcomes classification (NOC)* (3rd ed.). St. Louis, MO: C.V. Mosby.

NANDA-I (2007). *Nursing diagnoses: Definitions and classification, 2007–2008.* Philadelphia: Author.

Nightingale, F. (1859). *Notes on nursing: What it is, and what it is not.* London: Harrison, 59, Pall Mall, 59.

O'Grady, N.P., Alexander, M., Dellinger, E.P., et al. (2002). *Guidelines for prevention of intravascular infections. Morbidity and Mortality Weekly Report MMWR. 51* (RR-10).

Panadero, A., Iohom, G., Taj, J., et al. (2002). A dedicated intravenous cannula for postoperative use: Effect on incidence and severity of phlebitis. *Anaesthesia, 57*(9), 921–925.

Parellada, J.A., Moise, A.A., Hegemier, S., & Gest, A.L. (1999). Percutaneous central catheters and peripheral intravenous catheters have similar infection rates in very low birth weight infants. *Journal of Perinatology, 19*(4), 730–734.

Paula, R. (2006). Compartment syndrome. eMedicine. June.

Pettit, J., & Wyckoff, M. (2007). *Peripherally inserted central catheters: Guideline for practice* (2nd ed.) Glenview, IL: National Association of Neonatal Nurses.

Perruca, R. (2010). Peripheral venous access. In: M. Alexander, A. Corrigan, L. Gorski, J. Hankins, & R. Perucca (Eds.), *Infusion nursing: An evidence based approach* (3rd ed.). St. Louis, MO: Saunders Elsevier.

Polovich, M., White, J., & Kelleher, L. (2005). *Chemotherapy and biotherapy guidelines and recommendations for practice* (2nd ed.). Pittsburgh, PA: Oncology Nursing Society.

Rosenthal, K. (2007a). Reducing the risks of infiltration and extravasation. *Medical Surgical Insider,* Fall, 4–8.

Rosenthal, K. (2007b). *Infection prevention and needle-free devices: Educational poster series promoting best practices.* Bethlehem, PA: B. Braun.

Roth, D. (2003). Extravasation injuries of peripheral veins a basis for litigation? *JVAD, 8*(1), 21–24.

Ruskin, K. (2008). Venous air embolism. Retrieved from www.anestit.unipa.it/ gta/vae.html (Accessed July 2, 2008).

Schulmeister, L. (2005). Managing extravasation. *Clinical Journal of Oncology Nursing, 9*(4), 472–475.

Schummer, C., Bayer, O., Muller, A., et al. (2005). Extravasation injury in the perioperative setting. *Anesthesia and Analgesia, 100,* 722–727.

Smeltzer, S.C., Bare, B.G., Hinkle, J.L., & Cheever, K.H. (2008). *Brunner and Suddarth's textbook of medical-surgical nursing* (11th ed.). Philadelphia: Lippincott Williams & Wilkins.

Thrush, D., & Belsole, R. (1995). Radial nerve injury after routine peripheral vein cannulation. *Journal of Clinical Anesthesia, 7*(2), 160–162.

Viale, P.H. (2003). Complications associated with implantable vascular access devices in the patient with cancer. *Journal of Infusion Nursing, 26*, 97–102.

White, S.A. (2001). Peripheral intravenous therapy related phlebitis rates in an adult population. *Journal of Intravenous Nursing, 24*(1), 19–24.

Wickham, R., Engelking, C., Sauerland, C., & Corbi, D. (2006). Vesicant extravasation Part II: Evidence-based management and continuing controversies. *Oncology Nursing Forum, 33*(6), 1143–1150.

Wittenberg, A.G. (2006). Venous air embolism. Retrieved from www.emedicine.com/emerg/topic787.htm (Accessed July 2, 2008).

Zwicker, D. (2003). The elderly patient at risk. *Journal of Infusion of Nursing, 26(3)*, 137–143.

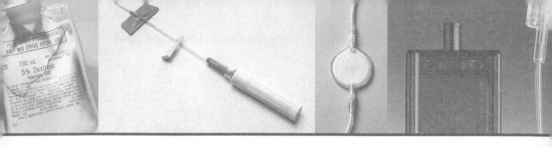

Chapter 10

Medication Infusion Modalities

In the future, which I shall not see, for I am old, may a better way be opened! May the methods by which every infant, every human being will have the best chance of health, the methods by which every sick person will have the best chance of recovery, be learned and practiced! Hospitals are only an intermediate state of civilization never intended, at all events, to take in the whole sick population.
—*Florence Nightingale, 1860*

Chapter Contents

▪ **LEARNING**   *On completion of this chapter, the reader will be able to:*
OBJECTIVES

1. Define the glossary terms related to nursing care of the patient receiving medications by infusion.
2. Identify strategies to prevent medication errors.
3. Identify the advantages and hazards of delivering medications by the intravenous route.
4. Compare three drug incompatibilities.
5. Describe the proper technique in delivery of a medication by the continuous, intermittent, and intravenous push routes.
6. Describe the treatment of adverse side effects of intravenous medications.
7. Describe the key nursing points-of-care for delivery of subcutaneous infusion.
8. State the precautions to be followed when medication is infused via the epidural route.
9. List the key steps in dressing management of an intraspinal catheter.
10. Describe the method of delivery and nursing considerations for intraperitoneal therapy.
11. Discuss the purpose of delivery of fluids and medications by the intraventricular route.
12. List the key points in delivery of fluids by the intraosseous route (IO)
13. Identify the candidates for IO fluid and medication administration.
14. Identify the three methods of insertion of an IO needle.
15. Identify common pediatric formulas.

⧉ GLOSSARY

Admixture   Combination of two or more medications

Adsorption   Attachment of one substance to the surface of another

Bolus   Concentrated medication or solution given rapidly over a short period of time; may be given by direct I.V. injection or I.V. drip

Chemical incompatibility   Change in the molecular structure or pharmacologic properties of a substance, which may or may not be visually observed

Compatibility   Capable of being mixed and administered without undergoing undesirable chemical or physical changes or loss of therapeutic action

Delivery system   A product that allows for the administration of medication

Distribution   Process of delivering a drug to the various tissues of the body

Drug interaction   An interaction between two drugs; also, a drug that causes an increase or decrease in another drug's pharmacologic effects

Epidural   Situated on or over the dura mater

Hypodermoclysis   The treatment of dehydration by injecting fluids into the subcutaneous tissues

Incompatibility   Chemical or physical reaction that occurs among two or more drugs or between a drug and the delivery device

Intermittent drug infusion   I.V. therapy administered at prescribed intervals

Intra-arterial (IA)   Route by which medication (usually chemotherapy) is delivered directly within the artery

Intraosseous (IO)   Route by which fluids and medications are delivered to the vascular system by percutaneous insertion of a needle into the marrow cavity of a bone

Intraperitoneal (IP)   Route by which medication is administered directly into the peritoneal cavity

Intraspinal   Spaces surrounding the spinal cord, including the epidural and intrathecal spaces

Intrathecal   Within a sheath, surrounded by the epidural space and separated from it by the dura mater; contains cerebrospinal fluid

Intravenous push   Manual administration of medication under pressure over 1 minute or as the manufacturer of the medication recommends

Intraventricular (IVt)   Route by which medication is delivered to the brain and spinal cord directly into the ventricles, using a reservoir

Patient-controlled analgesia (PCA)   A drug delivery system that dispenses a preset intravascular dose of a narcotic analgesic when the patient pushes a switch on an electric cord

Physical incompatibility   An undesirable change that is visually observed

Single-dose vial   Medication bottle that is hermetically sealed with a rubber stopper and is intended for one-time use; usually does not contain a preservative

Therapeutic incompatibility   Undesirable effect occurring within a patient as a result of two or more drugs being given concurrently

Volume control chamber (VCC)   A small inline container that is incorporated into the I.V. administration line. Used in pediatric infusions and with older adults in critical care areas to minimize risk of excess fluid delivery.

▪ Safe Delivery of Infusion Therapy

Standards of Practice

In 2006, The Infusion Nurses Society identified criteria for the safe administration of intravenous therapy by defining the Standards of Practice (2006) in infusion care. The following standards (INS, 2006) address the safe delivery of parenteral medications and solutions.

- The administration of parenteral medications and solutions shall be initiated by the order of a physician or an authorized prescriber.
- Protocols and procedures for administration of parenteral medications and solutions shall be established in organizational policies and procedures and practice guidelines.
- The validation of competency shall be documented in the knowledge and protocols for administration of medications and solutions.
- The nurse should verify the patient's identity by using at least two identifiers, including, but not limited to, date of birth or photographs, prior to initiation of therapy or procedure; neither identifier may be the patient's room number.
- Before administration of parenteral medications and solutions, the nurse shall appropriately label all containers, vials, and syringes; verify the patient's identity; and verify contents, dose, rate, route, expiration date, and integrity of the solutions.
- Documentation in the patient's permanent medical record shall include, but not be limited to, size and length of the access device, site, dressing, infusate, drug dose, volume and concentration, rate, complications, patient assessment, and response to therapy.
- Aseptic technique and Standard Precautions shall be observed.

Preventing Medication Errors

In July, 2006 the Institute of Medicine of the National Academies published a paper that addressed the consequences of medication errors and reported that overall, 1.5 million people are harmed annually from errors associated with medication administration at a cost of 3.5 billion dollars. Of these medication errors, 400,000 occur in acute care hospitals where medication dispensation and administration is managed by highly trained, licensed healthcare professionals (Aspden, 2006).

The concept of the "Six Rights" of medication administration (right drug, right dose, right route, right time, right patient, and right documentation) is one means of reducing medication errors. Omitting a medication, administering the wrong dose, administering an extra dose, administering a medication via the wrong route, and administering a medication at the wrong time are all examples of errors that may be prevented by a strict adherence to "the Six Rights of medication administration" (Broyles, Reiss, & Evans, 2007).

The ability to calculate dosages and rates of administration accurately is another factor in reducing medication errors. In high-risk medication administration scenarios, such as in pediatric and critical care, it is highly recommended, if not mandated by many hospital policies, that all calculations be double checked by two licensed staff for accuracy. The use of calculators is strongly recommended to ensure arithmetical accuracy. In addition, some key points in calculating solutions and medications accurately include:

1. Always place a zero before a decimal expression of less than 1. Example: 0.05
2. Do not place a decimal point and zero after a whole number, because the decimal may not be seen and result in a 10-fold overdose. Example: 2.0 mg read as 20 mg by mistake.
3. Avoid using decimals whenever whole numbers can be used as alternatives. Example: 0.5 g should be expressed as 500 mg.
4. Follow guidelines for use of correct abbreviations.

EBNP A retrospective study done in 2006 at Johns Hopkins Children's Center of 581 error reports containing 1010 medication errors reported between 2001 and 2003 found that administration errors are at least as common as prescribing errors in children. Findings suggest that 94% of the calculator-generated orders were correct, with an error rate of 6 per 100, while hand-written orders were 45 in 100 (Miller & Lehman, 2006).

"Error reporting is only as good as the actual changes that are made as a result of it" states Lehman (Miller & Lehman, 2006), coauthor of the retrospective study. Monitoring voluntary error reports has led to the creation of several programs that reduce and prevent medication errors. In the study, researchers found that errors occurred in every step of the medication process from prescribing to ordering to administering to the patient (Miller & Lehman, 2006). Suggestions for reducing medication errors include:

1. A computerized ordering tool for pediatric chemotherapy that reduces medication errors in children undergoing cancer treatment
2. An online infusion calculator that reduces mediation errors for I.V. infusion

NOTE > Online calculator and computerized drug ordering system has been developed at Johns Hopkins. Recommendations were made by Miller and Lehman (2006) that the adoption of digitalized systems for I.V. drug infusions, as well as chemotherapy orders, in high-risk clinical areas should be used.

▪ Principles of Intravenous Medication Administration

Advantages

The advantages of administration of fluids and medications via the **intravenous (I.V.)** route include (1) direct access to the circulatory system, (2) a route for administration of fluids and drugs to patients who cannot tolerate oral medications, (3) a method of instant drug action, and (4) a method of instant drug administration termination. This route offers pronounced advantages over the subcutaneous (SQ), intramuscular (IM), and oral routes in certain clinical situations (Table 10-1).

Drugs that cannot be absorbed by other routes because of the large molecular size of the drug or destruction of the drug by gastric juices can be administered directly to the site of **distribution**, the circulatory system, with I.V. infusion. Drugs with irritating properties that cause pain and trauma when given via the intramuscular or subcutaneous route can be given intravenously. When a drug is administered intravenously, there is instant drug action, which is an advantage in emergency situations. The I.V. route also provides instant drug termination if sensitivity or adverse reactions occur. This route provides for control over the rate at which drugs are administered; prolonged action can be controlled by administering a dilute medication infusion intermittently over a prolonged time period.

Intravenous medications are provided for rapid therapeutic or diagnostic responses or a delivery route for solutions or medications that

> Table 10-1	ADVANTAGES AND DISADVANTAGES OF INTRAVENOUS MEDICATION ADMINISTRATION

Advantages

1. Provides a direct access to the circulatory system
2. Provides a route for drugs that irritate the gastric mucosa
3. Provides a route for instant drug action
4. Provides a route for delivering high drug concentrations
5. Provides for instant drug termination if sensitivity or adverse reaction occurs
6. Provides for better control over the rate of drug administration
7. Provides a route of administration in patients in whom use of the gastrointestinal tract is limited

Disadvantages

1. Drug interaction because of incompatibilities
2. Adsorption of the drug is impaired, which is caused by leaching into I.V. container or administration set.
3. Errors in compounding (mixing) of medication
4. Speed shock
5. Extravasation of a vesicant drug
6. Chemical phlebitis

cannot be delivered by any other route. Nurses administering the solution or medication are accountable for achieving effective delivery of prescribed therapy and for evaluating and documenting deviations from an expected outcome, including the implementation of corrective action.

INS Standard The nurse administering parenteral medications and solutions should have knowledge of indications for therapy, side effects, potential adverse reactions, and appropriate interventions. (INS, 2006, 68)

Disadvantages

Despite the many advantages of I.V. medication, there are also disadvantages associated with this venous route; these disadvantages are not found with other drug therapies (refer to Table 10-1).

The number of drug combinations, along with the ever-increasing new drugs on the market, has compounded these disadvantages. The disadvantages specific to the administration of I.V. drugs include **drug interactions**; drug loss via **adsorption** of I.V. containers and administration sets; errors in mixing techniques; and the complications of speed shock, extravasation of vesicant drugs, and phlebitis.

Drug Interactions

Drug interactions are not always clear cut. Many factors affect drug interactions, including drug solubility and drug **compatibility**. Mixing of two drugs in a solution can cause an adverse interaction called drug **incompatibility**. Factors affecting drug solubility and compatibility include:

- Drug concentration
- I.V. fluid or drug
- Type of administration set
- Preparation technique, duration of drug–drug or drug–solution contact
- pH value
- Temperature of the room and light

Drugs can be compatible when mixed in certain solutions but incompatible when mixed with others. Mixing two incompatible drugs in solution in a particular order may be enough to avoid a potentially adverse interaction (Gahart & Nazareno, 2008).

The pH of both the solution and the drug must be considered when compounding medications. Drugs that are widely dissimilar in pH values are unlikely to be compatible in solution. For example, dextrose solutions are slightly acidic, with a pH of 4.5 to 5.5. Several antibiotics on the market have an acidic pH that is stable in dextrose; however, alkaline antibiotics, such as carbenicillin, are unstable when mixed with dextrose. Dextrose, with a pH of 4.5 to 5.5, should be used as a base for acidic drugs; sodium chloride solution, with a pH value of 6.8 to 8.5, should be used for alkaline medication dilution.

 NURSING FAST FACT!

> *To prevent I.V. drug incompatibilities, best practice is to flush the infusion device with sodium chloride before and after medications are infused.*

Adsorption

Adsorption is the attachment of one substance to the surface of another. Many drugs adsorb to glass or plastic. The disadvantage associated with adsorption is that the patient receives a smaller amount of the drug than was intended. The amount of adsorption is difficult to predict and is affected by the drug concentration, solution of the drug, amount of surface contacted by the drug, and temperature changes.

An example of adsorption is the binding of insulin to plastic and glass containers. The insulin rapidly adsorbs to I.V. containers and tubing until all potential adsorption sites are saturated. During the initial part of an infusion, very little insulin may reach the patient; later, after adsorption sites are saturated, more of the insulin in the solution is delivered to the patient. To prevent this from occurring, injecting the drug as close to the I.V. insertion site as possible will promote better therapeutic drug effects.

Polyvinyl chloride (PVC) in plastic flexible I.V. bags promotes drug adsorption. Di(2-ethylhexyl) phthalate [DEHP] is a plasticizer that is added to PVC that allows PVC to be flexible. Some drug formulations leach this plasticizer out of the plastic matrix and into the solution. DEHP is fat-soluble, I.V. fat emulsion products can extract the plasticizer from the PVC bags and tubing. DEHP is also leached from PVC bags by organic solvents and surfactants contained in some drugs, which may result in DEHP-induced toxicity. In the package inserts, many drug manufacturers recommend nonphthalate **delivery systems**. Many companies are manufacturing nonphthalate I.V. bags and tubing to prevent this problem. Chapter 5 provides further information on DEHP leaching.

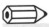 *NURSING FAST FACT!*

> - *When mixing medications into glass or plastic systems, refer to the manufacturer's guidelines to prevent adsorption.*
> - *A patient's complaint of burning at the I.V. site from a presumably dilute drug is a warning that the concentration of the drug is too high and needs to be diluted further.*
> - *Many hospitals allow only registered pharmacists to prepare admixtures.*

Errors in Mixing

Drug toxicity, subtherapeutic infusion, or erratic therapeutic effects can result from inadequate mixing of a drug into the infusion container. Inadequate mixing can contribute to a **bolus** of medication being delivered to the patient, which may cause adverse effects.

Factors that contribute to inadequate mixing include:

- Length of time required to adequately mix drugs in flexible bags
- Addition of a drug to a hanging flexible bag
- Additives injected at a slow rate into the primary bag (the turbulence of fast flow promotes mixing, especially in glass containers)
- Inadequate movement of the additive from the injection port (e.g., the long, narrow sleeve-type additive ports on some flexible bags, as opposed to the button type, hinder effective mixing)
- Tendency of very dense drugs to settle at the bottom of the infusion container

Ten key recommendations for adequate mixing of I.V. medications are presented in Table 10-2.

■ Drug Compatibility

Compatibility is required for a therapeutic response to prescribed therapy. Chemical, physical, and therapeutic compatibility must be identified before admixing and administering I.V. medications.

> Table 10-2	TEN KEY RECOMMENDATIONS FOR ADEQUATE MIXING OF I.V. MEDICATIONS

1. Gently invert the I.V. container several times to adequately mix the medication with the solution, taking care to avoid foaming the solution.
2. When inversion is impossible, gently swirl or rotate to mix to prevent the drug from settling to the bottom of the container.
3. When agitating an intermittent infusion set, clamp off the air vent; if the vent becomes wet, the solution will not infuse properly after mixing.
4. Vacuum devices can facilitate mixing in plastic flexible bags by creating a vacuum and drawing any drug left in the port into the body of the bag.
5. When possible, use premixed solutions from the manufacturer; for example, using premixed heparin or potassium chloride solutions can save time and avoid dose errors as well as preclude mixing problems.
6. Add one drug at a time to the primary I.V. solution. Mix and examine thoroughly before adding the next drug.
7. Add the most concentrated or most soluble drug to the solution first because some incompatibilities, such as precipitates, require a certain concentration or amount of time to develop. Mix well, and then add the dilute drugs.
8. Add colored additives last to avoid masking possible precipitate cloudiness.
9. Always visually inspect containers after adding and mixing drugs; hold the container against a light or a white surface and check for particulate matter, obvious layering, or foaming.
10. If you do not have a clear understanding of the compatibility or stability of the admixtures you are using, check the manufacturer's recommendation of consult a pharmacist.

An incompatibility results when two or more substances react or interact and change the normal activity of one or more components. Incompatibility may be manifested by harmful or undesirable effects and is likely to result in a loss of therapeutic effects. Incompatibility may occur when:

- Several drugs are added to a large volume of fluid to produce an **admixture**.
- Drugs in separate solutions are administered concurrently or in close succession via the same I.V. line.
- A single drug is reconstituted or diluted with the wrong solutions.
- One drug reacts with another drug's preservative.

Specific incompatibilities fall into three categories: physical, chemical, and therapeutic.

Physical Incompatibility

A **physical incompatibility** is also called a pharmaceutical incompatibility. Physical incompatibilities occur when one drug is mixed with other drugs or solutions to produce a product that is unsafe for administration.

Insolubility and absorption are the two types of physical incompatibility. Insolubility occurs when a drug is added to an inappropriate fluid solution, creating an incomplete solution or a precipitate. This risk occurs more frequently with multiple additives, which may interact to form an insoluble product. Signs of insolubility include visible precipitation, haze, gas bubbles, and cloudiness. Some precipitation may be microcrystalline (i.e., smaller than 50 microns) and not apparent to the eye. The use of micropore filters is intended to prevent such particles from entering the vein. The use of a 0.22-micron inline filter reduces the amount of microcrystalline precipitates.

The presence of calcium in a drug or solution usually indicates that a precipitate might form if mixed with another drug. Ringer's solution preparations contain calcium, so check carefully for incompatibility before adding any drug to this solution.

Other physical incompatibilities caused by insolubility include the increased degradation of drugs added to sodium bicarbonate and the formation of an insoluble precipitate when sodium bicarbonate is combined with other medications in emergency situations.

The following are important recommendations regarding physical drug incompatibilities:

- Never administer a drug that forms a precipitate.
- Do not mix drugs prepared in special diluents with other drugs.
- When administering a series of medications, prepare each drug in a separate syringe. This will lessen the possibility of precipitation. Insolubility may also result from the use of an incorrect solution to reconstitute a drug.
- Follow the manufacturer's directions for reconstituting drugs.

Chemical Incompatibility

A **chemical incompatibility** is a reaction of a drug with other drugs or solutions, which results in alterations of the integrity and potency of the active ingredient. The most common cause of chemical incompatibility is the reaction between acidic and alkaline drugs or solutions, resulting in a pH level that is unstable for one of the drugs. A specific pH or a narrow range of pH values is required for the solubility of a drug and for the maintenance of its stability after it has been mixed.

Therapeutic Incompatibility

A **therapeutic incompatibility** is an undesirable effect occurring in a patient as a result of two or more drugs being given concurrently. An increased therapeutic or a decreased therapeutic response is produced. This incompatibility often occurs when therapy dictates the use of two antibiotics. For example, in the use of chloramphenicol and penicillin, chloramphenicol has been reported to antagonize the bacterial activity of penicillin. If prescribed, penicillin should be administered at least 1 hour before the chloramphenicol to prevent therapeutic incompatibility.

Therapeutic incompatibility may go unnoticed until the patient fails to show the expected clinical response to the drug or until peak and trough levels of the drug show a lack of therapeutic levels. If an incompatibility is not suspected, the patient may be given increasingly higher doses of the drug to try to obtain the therapeutic effect. When more than one antibiotic is prescribed for intermittent infusion, stagger the time schedule so that each can be infused individually.

EBNP A descriptive study investigated 3170 hospitalized patients 0–12 years of age from January 2005 to December 2006, and 11,181 prescriptions were analyzed. The prescriptions presented 6857 drug interactions. The most frequent interaction was delayed therapeutic action. The probability of drug interaction increased with 10 or more drugs; 56% of the interactions indicated that treatment could have been impacted or the therapeutic response was different from the expected reaction. The analysis of interaction and incompatibility in prescribed drugs used the Micromedex Drug-Reax® program. (Martinbiancho, Zuckermann, Dos Santos, et al., 2007).

INS Standard The nurse shall verify chemical, physical and therapeutic compatibility and stability prior to compounding and administering prescribed infusion medications and solutions. (INS, 2006, 22)

CULTURAL AND ETHNIC CONSIDERATIONS: DRUG ADMINISTRATION

Data have been collected regarding differences in the effect some medications have on persons of diverse ethnic or cultural origins. Genetic predispositions to different rates of metabolism cause some patients to be prone to overdose reactions to the "normal dose" of medication, while other patients are likely to experience a greatly reduced benefit from the standard dose of the medication.

In ethnic and cultural groups (i.e., African Americans and Asian Americans) with a high incidence of glucose-6-phosphate dehydrogenase (G6PD) deficiency, some drugs may impair red blood cell metabolism, leading to anemia. Caffeine, a component of many drugs, is excreted more slowly by Asian-Americans. Asian Americans may require smaller doses of certain drugs (Giger & Davidhizar, 2004).

■ Medication Delivery Modalities

General Guidelines

Several methods are used to administer I.V. medications, including continuous, intermittent infusions, and I.V. push. Nursing responsibilities of I.V. drug administration include:

- Identifying whether a prescribed route (i.e., continuous, intermittent, or push) is appropriate
- Using aseptic technique and Standard Precautions when preparing an admixture
- Identifying the expiration date on solutions and medications
- Following the manufacturer's guidelines for the preparation and storage of the medication
- Monitoring the patient for therapeutic response to the medication

 NURSING FAST FACT!

> - *Be knowledgeable of the pharmacologic implications relative to patient clinical status and diagnosis.*
> - *Verify that all solution containers are free of cracks, leaks, and punctures.*

Guidelines for Infusion Medication Delivery

1. Check all labels (drugs, diluents, and solutions) to confirm appropriateness for I.V. use.
2. Use a filter needle when withdrawing I.V. medications from ampoules to eliminate possible pieces of glass.
3. Ensure adequate mixing of all drugs added to a solution.

4. Examine solutions for clarity and any possible leakage.
5. Double check with another RN prepackaged medication syringes for use in specific pumps.
6. Monitor room temperature. Controlled room temperature (CRT) is considered to be 25°C (77°F). Most medications tolerate variations in temperature from 15° to 30°C (59°–86°F) (Gahart & Nazareno, 2008).
7. Use only single-dose vials for parenteral additives or medications (O'Grady, Alexander, Dellinger, et al., 2002).

INS Standard   When preparing solutions or medications for administration, single-use medication vials or ampoules are recommended. (INS, 2006, 50)

▪ Methods of Administration

Continuous Infusions

Continuous infusion occurs when large-volume parenteral solutions of 250 to 1000 mL of infusate are administered over 2 to 24 hours. Medications added to these large-volume infusates are administered continuously. Continuous infusion is used when a medication must be highly diluted, constant plasma concentrations of the drug maintained, or large volumes of fluids and electrolytes administered. Electronic infusion devices are used to ensure an accurate flow rate.

ADVANTAGES

- Admixture and bag changes can be performed every 8 to 24 hours.
- Constant serum levels of the drug are maintained.

DISADVANTAGES

- Monitoring the drug rate can be erratic if not electronically controlled.
- There is a higher risk of drug incompatibility problems.
- Accidental bolus infusion can occur if the medication is not adequately mixed with the solution.

 NURSING FAST FACT!

> When adding medication to an infusion container, use single-dose vials instead of multiple-dose vials to decrease the potential for infection, complications, and medication errors.

INS Standard   After being added to an administration set, a parenteral medication or solution should be infused or discarded within 24 hours. (INS, 2006, 68)

Intermittent Infusions

Intermittent infusion is any administration of a medication or an infusion that is not continuous. A medication is added to a small volume of fluid (25–250 mL) and infused over 15 to 90 minutes. Types of intermittent infusions are piggybacked through the established pathway of the primary solution, simultaneous infusion, use of volume control set, and intermittent infusions through a locking device.

Secondary Infusion Through the Primary Pathway

A secondary I.V. line used intermittently to deliver medications is commonly called a piggyback set. Secondary infusion through an established pathway of the primary solution is the most common method for drug delivery by the intermittent route. A secondary set includes a small I.V. container, short administration set without ports, and a macrodrip system. The drug is diluted in 25 to 250 mL of 5% dextrose in water or 0.9% sodium chloride and administered over 15 to 90 minutes. When infusing medications with this method, the secondary infusion is administered via the Y port with the backcheck valve on the primary administration set. Refer to Figure 10-1A.

This Y port is located on the upper third of the primary line. Although the primary infusion is interrupted during the secondary infusion, the drug from the intermittent infusion container comes in contact with the primary solution below the injection port; therefore, the drug and the primary solution should be compatible. Electronic infusion devices may be used to maintain constant infusion rates and maintain accurate titration of drug dosages.

ADVANTAGES

- The risk of incompatibilities is reduced.
- A larger drug dose can be administered at a lower concentration per milliliter than with the I.V. push method.
- Peak flow concentrations occur at periodic intervals.
- The risk of fluid overload is decreased.

DISADVANTAGES

- The administration rate may not be accurate unless electronically monitored.
- The high concentration of drug in the intermittent solution may cause venous irritation.
- I.V. set changes can result in wasting a portion of the drug.
- If the patient is not properly monitored, fluid overload or speed shock may result.
- Drug incompatibility can occur if the administration set is not adequately flushed between medication administrations.

Secondary infusions can be infused concurrently with the primary solution. Rather than connecting the intermittent infusion at the piggyback

NURSING FAST FACT!

> Consider the volume of fluid delivered with a secondary infusion as part of the patient's overall intake when calculating intake.
> Simultaneous Infusion (Primary and Secondary)

port (closest to the primary infusion bag), it is attached to the lower Y site. Refer to Figure 10-1B. Disadvantages of administration of a secondary concurrent with a primary solution include the tendency for blood to back up into the tubing after the secondary infusion has been completed, causing occlusion of the venous access device and increased risk of drug incompatibility.

 NURSING FAST FACT!

> Drug incompatibility is a greater risk with the simultaneous infusion method.

NURSING POINTS-OF-CARE
INTERMITTENT DRUG DELIVERY

- Ensure the compatibility of the I.V. solution and medication, both the solution in the primary system and the diluent in the secondary system.
- Assess the I.V. site and the patency of the catheter.
- Calculate the amount of medication to add to the solution.
- Use the correct amount and type of diluent solution.
- Use the correct rate of administration.
- Determine the correct primary line port in which to infuse the medication
- Affix the correct label to the secondary bag, with start date and hour, discard date and hour, and your initials. (Wilkinson & Van Leuven, 2007).

Volume Control Chamber

The volume control chamber method of intermittent delivery of medication is used most frequently with pediatric patients or when a small amount of well-controlled drug needs to be administered to critical care patients. Medication is added to the volume control chamber and diluted with I.V. solution. The infusion is generally over 15 minutes to 1 hour. Volumes delivered vary from 25 to 150 mL per drug dose. Refer to Figure 10-2.

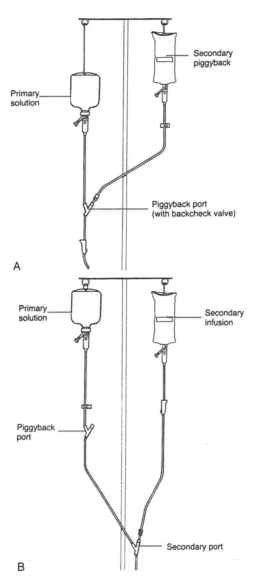

Figure 10-1 ■ Methods of delivery of secondary infusions. *A,* Secondary piggyback infusion. *B,* Simultaneous infusion.

ADVANTAGES

- ■ Runaway infusions are avoided without the use of electronic infusion devices (EIDs).
- ■ The volume of fluid in which the drug is diluted can be adjusted.

DISADVANTAGES

- ■ Medication must travel the length of the tubing before it reaches the patient, causing a significant time delay.

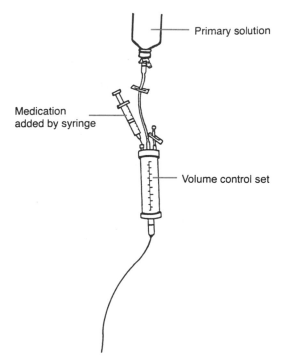

Figure 10-2 ■ Administration of medication via a volume control chamber.

- A portion of the medication can be left in the tubing after the chamber empties.
- Incompatibilities may develop when the chamber, which is usually within the primary line, is used for multiple drug deliveries.
- Labeling of the chamber must coincide with the drug being delivered. If multiple drugs are delivered, this could present a problem.

NURSING POINTS-OF-CARE
VOLUME CONTROL DRUG DELIVERY

- Calculate the amount of medication to be added to the volume-control set
- Use the correct amount and type of diluent solution, filling the volume control set first before adding the medication.
- Use the correct rate of administration.
- With pediatric patients always double check drug and dosage with another RN and document.

Direct Injection (I.V. Push)

Intravenous push administration of a medication provides a method of administering high concentrations of medication. Administration through this route can be accomplished by direct venipuncture, using a scalp vein infusion set or over-the-needle infusion device with needleless valve, or by access of a low-injection port of the primary administration set of the running I.V. The purpose is to achieve rapid serum concentrations. Refer to Procedures Display 10-1 at the end of this chapter.

Direct injection requires that the drug be drawn into a syringe before administration or that the drug be available in a prefilled syringe. Needle protector or needle-free systems can be connected to the venous access device or used with administration sets to deliver the medication. The use of multiple-dose vials increases the potential for infection, complications, and medication errors; use only single-use vials for mixing or diluting medication.

ADVANTAGES

- Barriers of drug absorption are bypassed.
- The drug response is rapid and usually predictable.
- The patient is closely monitored during the full administration of the medication.

DISADVANTAGES

- Adverse effects occur at the same time and rate as therapeutic effects.
- The I.V. push method has the greatest risk of adverse effects and toxicity because serum drug concentrations are sharply elevated.
- Speed shock is possible from too-rapid administration of medication.

Adverse effects that can occur during administration of a medication directly into a vein include changes in the patient's level of consciousness, vital functions, and reflex activity. There may be an increased risk of phlebitis if a medication that is irritating to the vein is injected.

NURSING POINTS-OF-CARE
DIRECT I.V. PUSH MEDICATIONS

- Wear clean gloves for infection control when administering push medications.
- Determine the type and amount of dilution needed for the medication.
- Determine the amount of time needed to administer the medication

Continued

- Flush the line with 0.9% sodium chloride (USP) before administration of medication.
- Maintain sterility.
- Use single-use vials for mixing and diluting medication.
- Administer all medication according to drug guidelines.
- Most medications are delivered slowly, between 1 and 5 minutes. (Example: Morphine I.V. push delivery is recommended over 5 minutes; Gahart & Nazareno, 2008).

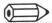 **NURSING FAST FACT!**

If adverse effects occur, supportive care is the basis for treatment of most symptoms, because specific antidotes are available only for certain drugs.

Intermittent Dosing (Patient-Controlled Analgesia)

The concept of patient-controlled analgesia (PCA) began in 1970. PCA is a pain management strategy that allows a patient to self-administer I.V. narcotic pain medication by pressing a button that is attached to a computerized pump. Patients may receive intermittent doses of narcotics when they state that the pain is episodic. It is desirable to treat pain only when experienced, with fast-acting narcotics that are effective for short periods. The goal of PCA is to provide the patient with a serum analgesia level for comfort with minimal sedation. Putting patients in charge of their own pain management makes sense because only the patient knows how much he or she is suffering. It is more desirable to use small doses of narcotics frequently than large doses of narcotics infrequently.

Criteria for PCA and nurse-controlled analgesia must be established. PCA can be used for a wide range of patients.

Candidates for whom PCA should be considered include:

1. Patients who are anticipating pain that is severe yet intermittent (e.g., patients suffering from kidney stones)
2. Patients who have constant pain that worsens with activity
3. Pediatric patients who are older than age 7 years who are capable of being taught to manage the PCA machine
4. Patients who are capable of manipulating the dose button
5. Patients who are motivated to use PCA
6. Home care patients with long-term pain control needs. Portable PCA pumps are available. Refer to Figure 10-3.

ADVANTAGES

- A pump infuser can be used to administer I.V. bolus doses of analgesics for the relief of acute pain.
- When patient-controlled analgesia is used, the nurse retains responsibility for assessing the patient's level of comfort and for

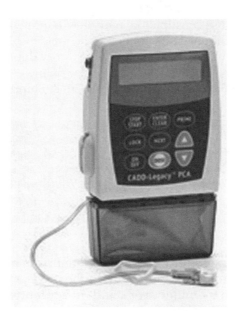

Figure 10-3 ■ Portable PCA pump. (Courtesy of Smith Medical, St. Paul, MN.)

addressing the deficient knowledge related to this method of pain relief.

- In the first 24 hours after surgery, the patient has the greatest need for pain control.
- PCA has been shown to be both safe and effective in relieving pain (Reiss & Evans, 2002).
- When patients are in control and know they can get more immediate pain relief by pushing a button, they are more relaxed.
- Analgesia is most effective when a therapeutic serum level is consistently maintained.
- Postoperative patients can easily titrate doses according to need and avoid peaks and troughs associated with conventional I.V. and intramuscular administration of an opioid.
- After abdominal surgery, patients ambulate sooner after surgery with a PCA.
- Patients whose pain is controlled are better able to cough and deep breathe.

DISADVANTAGES

- Opiates, even at therapeutic doses, can suppress respiration, heart rate, and blood pressure. Monitor carefully for the first 24 hours.
- Patients who are unsuitable candidates such as those whose level of consciousness, psychological reasons, or limited intellectual capacity cannot safely manage PCA.

- PCA can cause constipation, nausea, vomiting, and pruritus.
- Several studies have documented the incidence of respiratory depression with I.V. PCA. With respiratory depression the patient often had oxygen saturation per pulse oximeter readings between 85% and 90% (Hagle, Lehr, Brubakken, & Shippee, 2004).

> EBNP *In two studies, one with 6035 patients with I.V. PCA the incidence of respiratory depression was 0.19% and 1.08%, and in an additional study of 1466 patients the incidence of respiratory depression was 2.0%. The identified risk factors were basal infusion, family pushing PCA button inappropriately, large bolus dose, and elderly patients (Sidebotham, Dijkhuizen, & Schug, 1997; Tsui, Itwin, Wong, et al., 1997).*

- Misprogramming PCA concentration: Errors in initiating PCA infusion can occur at any point in the programming process. Use of a limited number of standard concentrations implementing smart PCA pumps with dose error reduction software and requiring double-check of the PCA programming can help reduce PCA doing errors (Institute of Medication Practice [ISMP], 2008).
- Risk of someone other than patient pushing the button on a PCA pump, even if the patient request is considered "by proxy." Place warning labels "For patient use only" on the PCA button. Remind patients and visitors that PCA is for patient use only (Marders, 2004; The Joint Commission [TJC], 2004).

Risk Factors for Respiratory Depression with I.V. PCA

- Patient older than 70 years of age
- Basal infusion with I.V. PCA
- Renal, hepatic, pulmonary, or cardiac impairment
- Sleep apnea
- Concurrent central nervous system depressants
- Obesity
- Upper abdominal or thoracic surgery
- I.V. PCA bolus greater than 1 mg morphine without basal (continuous) infusion

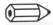 *NURSING FAST FACT!*

> *At no time should anyone but the patient push the PCA button.*

NURSING POINTS-OF-CARE
PCA ADMINISTRATION

- PCA is a philosophy of treatment, rather than a single method of drug administration.
- Determine the patient's baseline vital signs, cognitive status, and pain level.
- Determine the initial bolus (loading) dose, the lockout interval between each dose, and the 1-hour or 4-hour lockout dose limit. (Basal or continuous I.V. infusions are no longer recommended for patients receiving opioids via PCA; D'Arcy, 2008.)
- Validation by a second clinician or caregiver should be employed before initiation and administration of PCA, and when the syringe, solution container, or rate is changed (INS, 2006, 67).
- Current American Pain Society guidelines recommends the 6- to 8-minute dose interval and the 1-hour lockout.
- Insert the pump device containing the medication accurately.
- Set the pump for the loading dose (if ordered), basal rate, demand dose, lockout interval, and the 1-hour or 4-hour lockout dose limit.
- Put the button that controls dosing within reach of the patient (Wilkinson & Van Leuven, 2007).
- Anti-free flow administration sets shall be considered in the selection and use of PCA pumps. Dose-error reduction infusion systems shall also be considered when available (INS, 2006, 67 [33]).
- Mechanical monitoring such as pulse oximetry is needed to maintain pulse oxygen above 90% (Hagle, Lehr, Brubakken, & Shippee, 2004).
- Use a sedation scale to monitor patients with I.V. PCA. Refer to Table 10-3.

> Table 10-3	SEDATION SCALE TO MONITOR PATIENTS WITH I.V. PCA	
Sedation Scale	**Level of Sedation**	**Description and Assessment**
S—Asleep		
1	Fully awake, alert	Able to fully participate in recovery
2 Mild	Occasionally drowsy; easily aroused	Patient feels groggy; eyelids heavy Respiratory rate >10; able to participate in recovery.
3 Moderate	Frequently drowsy; easily aroused, drift off to sleep during conversation	Patient cannot complete sentence without falling asleep. Not able to perform activities of recovery. Respirations shallow, and/or irregular, rate may be <10
4 Severe	Somnolent; difficult to arouse, minimal or no response to stimuli	Shallow respirations and frequent apnea; rate <10. Pupils pinpoint.

Sources: D'Arcy (2008); Pasero & McCaffery (2002).

Ten Safe Practice Recommendations to Prevent Errors Associated with PCA Therapy

1. Limit choices.
   a. Limit the variety of medications used for PCA.
   b. Restrict fentanyl PCA administration to anesthesia or pain management team members only.
2. Improve access to information.
   a. Develop a quick reference sheet on PCA that includes programming tips as well as maximum dose warnings.
3. Improve label readability.
   a. Match the sequence of information that appears on PCA medication labels and order sets with the sequence of information that must be entered into the PCA pump.
4. Highlight the drug concentration on the label.
5. Program default settings.
6. Introduce new pumps slowly.
   a. Introduce a new pump in small controlled settings initially to ensure safety features are operational.
7. Consider the possibility of error.
   a. If the patient is not responding to the PCA doses, consider the possibility of an error, especially before administering a bolus dose. Re-verify the drug, concentration, pump settings, and line attachment.
8. Employ double-checks.
   a. Clearly define a manual independent double-check process for clinicians to follow when verifying PCA medications, pump settings via a confirmation screen, the patient, and line attachments.
   b. When possible use bar code technology; use smart PCA pumps that alert clinicians to potential programming errors.
9. Assess the proximity of the PCA pump to the general infusion pump.
   a. To decrease the potential for I.V. line mix-ups and possible medication errors
10. Educate the patient.
    a. Educate patients about the proper use of PCA before inititaion. (Vaida, Grissinger, Urbanski, & Mitchell, 2007)

NURSING POINTS-OF-CARE

DELIVERY OF INTRAVENOUS MEDICATION

Nursing Assessments
- Review the present illness.
- Review current drug therapy.
- Review previous drug therapy and side effects.
- Review lifestyle for home care.
- Note any allergies before starting the medication.
- Observe the patient's ability to ingest and retain fluids.
- Assess vital signs.
- Weigh the patient.
- Assess patient-related factors that may alter the patient's response to the drug, such as age or renal, liver, and cardiovascular function.
- Assess current medications for clues to drug interaction and incompatibility.

Key Nursing Interventions
1. Develop and use an environment that maximizes safe and efficient administration of medications.
2. Follow the six rights of medication administration.
3. Verify the prescription or medication order before administering the drug.
4. Determine the correct dilution, amount, and length of administration time as appropriate.
5. Use only single-use vials for dilution of medication.
6. Monitor for:
   a. Drug infusion at regular intervals
   b. Irritation, infiltration, and inflammation at the infusion site
   c. Therapeutic range of drug levels
   d. Therapeutic response
   e. Renal function for adequate excretion of drug through the kidneys
   f. Allergies, drug interactions, and drug incompatibilities
   g. Intake and output
   h. Need of pain relief medications, as needed
7. Maintain I.V. access.
8. Administer drugs at selected times.
9. Note the expiration date on the medication container.
10. Administer medications using the appropriate technique.
11. Dispose of unused or expired drugs according to agency policy.

Continued

12. Maintain strict aseptic technique.
13. Sign for opioids and other restricted drugs according to agency protocol.
14. For I.V. PCA monitor:
    a. Sedation level and respiratory rate every 1 to 2 hours for first 12–24 hours using a sedation scale
    b. Respiratory rate, depth, and rhythm with sedation assessment
    c. Oxygen saturation monitored for the first 6–8 hours
    d. For postoperative patients, I.V. PCA dose 1 mg morphine with 5-minute lockout; no basal infusion; titrate as needed.
    e. Increase by 25%–50% if pain not adequately controlled; reduce by 50% if sedation occurs (ISMP, 2002).
15. Document medication administration and patient responsiveness.

Continuous Subcutaneous Infusions

Subcutaneous infusion of fluids is an infusion modality to deliver fluids into subcutaneous tissues to provide hydration in patients with limited vascular access. Subcutaneous infusion, also referred to as **hypodermoclysis,** was first described in 1913 and was used widely until the 1950s, when complications from improper care related to poor patient selection, incorrect rates of administration, and poor choices of fluids led to the severe decline of this infusion modality. Hypodermoclysis provides an easy-to-use, safe, and cost-effective alternative to intravenous hydration for the elderly patient (Walsh, 2005). In addition, subcutaneous administration is an available route for some medications through a mechanical syringe driver device.

Different access devices can be used for hypodermoclysis. In the past the most common delivery method involved a Y-administration set attached to a fluid container with large-gauge 2- to 6-inch needles on each of the branches of the administration set. A more current method uses ordinary I.V. tubing spiked into a fluid container and smaller-gauge metal needles (butterfly needles). The needle is then placed into the subcutaneous tissue of one selected site. A special infusion set developed exclusively for hypodermoclysis provides infusion tubing with an integrated flow regulator spiked into a fluid container. The "clysis strip," which has two 25- to 27-gauge, 6 mm long needles placed 1½ inches apart on an adhesive vinyl strip, attaches to the end of the tubing (Walsh, 2005). Refer to Figure 10-4 showing an Aqua-C™ hydration set for hypodermoclysis.

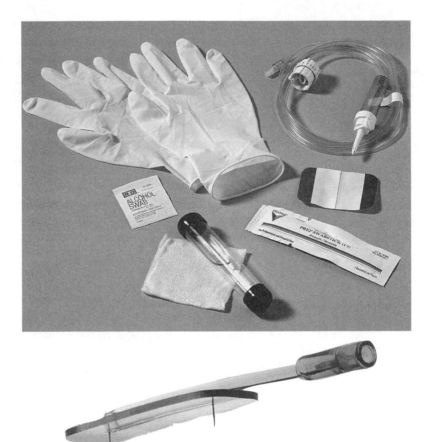

Figure 10-4 ◼ Aqua-C™ hydration set for hypodermoclysis. (Courtesy of Norfolk Medical, Skokie, IL.)

This infusion route is often associated with the delivery of palliative care therapy.

Candidates for continuous subcutaneous infusion:

- Patients unable to take medications by mouth
- Moderately dehydrated patients who are confused
- Patients with limited venous access
- To hydrate patients before placement of intravascular catheter.
- Continuous medication delivery

INS Standard An electronic infusion device should be used when administering medications via the continuous subcutaneous route; hydration fluids should be administered via a manual flow control device or an electronic infusion device. (INS, 2006, 64)

EBNP Walsh (2005) conducted a study of 30 long-term care residents from 24 to 90 years of age with a duration of subcutaneous infusions from 1 to 2 days. All were treatments for dehydration and all infusions were completed without adverse effects except for one incidence of local edema at the site.

EBNP Slesak, Schnurle, Kinzel, et al. (2003) conducted a randomized controlled trial of 96 patients, who received 5% dextrose and 0.9% sodium chloride by hypodermoclysis and found that the solution was well accepted by elderly patients and was comparable to the efficacy and safety of I.V. rehydration.

Advantages

- Ease of initiation and maintenance by registered nurse or LVN/LPN
- Reduction in transfers to acute care facilities from long-term care for intravenous access
- Fewer complications, less pain reported by patients, decreased cost
- Decreased number of times tissue is traumatized by repeated injections

Disadvantages

- Limited use during immediate fluid replacement of large volumes of fluid
- Local irritation at the infusion site
- The route is inappropriate for large volumes
- Edema
- Risk of infection
- Pain and inflammation at site
- Abscess
  (Younger, 2007).

INS Standard To reduce the risk of complications, the continuous subcutaneous access site used for medication administration should be rotated no more frequently than every 3 to 5 days and as clinically indicated; subcutaneous sites used for hypodermoclysis should be monitored frequently and the site rotated based upon the volume of fluid administered, patient comfort, and appearance of the infusion site. (INS, 2006, 64)

NURSING POINTS-OF-CARE
CONTINUOUS SUBCUTANEOUS INFUSIONS

- Most isotonic fluids are acceptable for infusion via the subcutaneous route.
- Medications are not routinely administered by hypodermoclysis.
- Consider using special infusion administration sets that have been developed exclusively for hypodermoclysis.
- Suitable sites for subcutaneous infusion include posterior upper arms, upper chest (avoiding breast tissue), abdomen at least 2 inches from the navel, anterior or lateral thighs, infraclavicular area and the flank areas in some patients (Walsh, 2005).
- Rotate the site every 3–5 days.
- Change the dressing every 3–5 days during site rotation.
- Monitor the access site and equipment:
  - Observe site for bleeding, bruising, inflammation, drainage, edema, or cellulitis.
  - Monitor the patient for complaints of burning or itching.

Intraperitoneal Infusions

Infusions via the **intraperitoneal (IP)** route involve the administration of therapeutic agents directly into the peritoneal cavity. The delivery of chemotherapeutic agents directly into the peritoneum has been practiced since the 1950s when nitrogen mustard was used for malignant ascites. Dedrick, Myers, Bungay, and De Vita (1978) are credited with using **IP** chemotherapy in ovarian cancer treatment. Early studies in the 1970s with IP infusions of cytotoxic agents for ovarian cancer or "belly baths" were conducted and demonstrated that IP drug delivery allowed for peritoneal exposure to higher cytotoxic drug concentrations than were achieved with systemic therapy. In the past cytotoxic agents were drained using mild suction or gravity after a specified dwell time, usually several hours (Swenson & Erikson, 1986). In current practice, drainage is no longer part of IP administration of chemotherapeutic agents because prolonged drug contact with the tumor provides a therapeutic advantage and the fraction of drug that is absorbed systemically is believed to be of benefit (Alhayki, Hopkins, & Le, 2006; Cannistra, 2006).

Many surgeons use the same vascular ports for IP chemotherapy as those used for I.V. chemotherapy. Ports should be placed below the bra line to avoid irritation (Markman & Walker, 2006). The port is sutured to the lower rib. The port placement can be done laparoscopically. This port is restricted only to IP chemotherapy and the catheter should not be used for I.V. administration of drugs or blood products (Potter & Held-Warmkessel, 2008). Once therapy has concluded, the port should be removed to prevent bowel and infection complications. Refer to Figure 10-5.

 NURSING FAST FACT!

- *Nursing staff must be well prepared to care for an IP catheter.*
- *The nurse and family must be familiar with the therapeutic effects of antineoplastic agents.*
- *When not in use, the IP port device is invisible, enhancing a positive body image.*

ADVANTAGES

- Hidden microscopic cancer cells are exposed, removing residual disease and increase in survival rate.
- Dose intensification is achieved in IP sites.
- IP chemotherapy diffuses into the peritoneal surface where it is absorbed systemically, prolonging exposure to the tumor via capillary flow.
- Lower systemic levels of agents can be used.

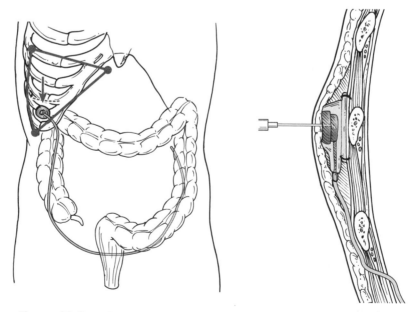

Figure 10-5 ■ Intraperitoneal port placement. (Courtesy of Ron Boisvert, RGB Medical Imagery, Inc., with permission.)

Disadvantages

- Catheter-related infections or complications:
  - Bowel perforation
  - Port rotation to the underside of the rib
  - Kinking or obstruction from the fibrin sheath or clot
  - Leaking fluid around the right-angled needle it if is dislodged
- Bowel obstruction, abdominal pain, or peritonitis
- The IP route is limited to select patients with minimal residual tumors.
- May not reach all tumor-bearing surfaces.
- Postinfusion rotation schedules may be difficult for patients with arthritis, spine or hip surgeries, or patients who cannot tolerate lying on the abdomen.
- IP chemotherapy can cause greater fatigue; pain; hematologic, gastrointestinal, and metabolic events; and neurologic toxicities.
- Healthcare providers have limited experience with IP delivery. (Alberts, Liu, Hannigan, et al., 2006; Potter & Held-Warmkessel, 2008).

NURSING POINTS-OF-CARE
INTRAPERITONEAL INFUSIONS

- Premedication is needed before IP chemotherapy infusion due to nausea and vomiting and continued for 3–4 post IP days (National Cancer Institute, 2006).
- Two liters of normal saline with chemotherapy added is warmed to 37°C (98.6°F) via an external warming device and flows by gravity **(do not use microwave)**. The large volume of normal saline facilitates intra-abdominal distribution.
- Infusion is as rapid as possible over 30–180 minutes.
- Infusion pumps are not used for IP chemotherapy because of the potential for high-volume pump pressure (Armstrong, Bund, Wenzel, et al., 2006).
- Use of a 19- to 20-gauge right-angle Huber needle 1–1.5 inches in length will facilitate flow and decrease administration time (Hydzik, 2007).
- Wound closure tapes over the Huber tubing with a stress loop and an occlusive dressing will help prevent dislodgement of needle (Marin, Oleszewski, Muehlbauer, 2007).
- Preflush with 10 mL of 0.9% sodium chloride to check patency.
- Because a small amount of systemic absorption is desirable, infused fluid does not need to be drained from the abdominal cavity.

Continued

- The turning protocol does not begin until the infusion is complete and the Huber needle has been removed.
- Heparinization of the IP port after the infusion currently is not standardized and varies among institutions. IP ports are not placed in the vascular system; therefore, there is no blood return. Flushing with 10–20 mL of 0.9% sodium chloride (USP) should be sufficient to maintain patency (Hydzik, 2007).
- The protocol for turning postinfusion is 15 minutes per position (left, right, supine, and prone) over 2 hours to distribute the solution (Armstrong, Bund, Wenzel, et al., 2006).
- Monitor for:
  - Presence of asymmetry around the port or leaking around the Huber needle
  - Respiratory rate or difficulty breathing due to fluid pressure on diaphragm (repositioning may be helpful)
  - Vital signs before and after the infusion

Intraosseous Infusions

The delivery of fluids and medications in a timely way can affect the morbidity and mortality of a patient in need of treatment for injuries or underlying disease. **Intraosseous (IO)** route technology has evolved to make it cost-effective and easily administered procedure for all age groups. Common routes for IO access include the proximal tibia, distal tibia, and sternum; however, the distal femur, clavicle, proximal humerus, and iliac crest are all potential sites in adults. In the pediatric patient, the first line choice site is the proximal tibia. Refer to Figure 10-6 for common adult and pediatric sites. The American Heart Association Guidelines for Cardiopulmonary Resuscitation and Emergency Cardiac Care (2005) supports IO cannulation access to a noncollapsible vascular plexus, enabling drug delivery similar to that achieved via central vascular access. The National Association of EMS Physicians (NAEMSP) position statement supports IO access to provide a significant time saving benefit to critically ill patients (NAEMSP, 2007).

The veins within the cancellous bone are held open by the rigid structure of the solid matrix. The blood pressure in the IO space is about 35/25 mm Hg, or approximately one third the systemic arterial pressure (Davidoff, Fowler, Gordon, et al., 2005). A bolus of approximately 10 mL of 0.9% sodium chloride must be rapidly given before starting of an infusion to establish a good IO flow rate (Landes, 2007). The medulla is richly supplied with pressure sensors that respond to the venous dilation caused by the bolus. This can be painful and the use of a small dose of Lidocaine should precede this bolus in all patients who are conscious at

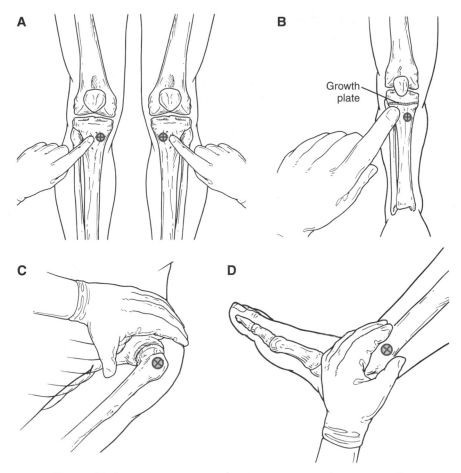

Figure 10-6 ■ Sites for intraosseous infusions. *A*, Tibia; *B*, pediatric tibia; *C*, proximal humerus; *D*, distal tibia.

the time of IO infusion. Any bolus given IO will appear in the arterial circulation in about 20 seconds for the sternal or humeral route and within 60 seconds from the tibial site (Landes, 2007). The flow rate of IO infusion is directly related to the pressure on the set:

1. Under normal gravity the maximum rates achievable are 30 mL/min (1800 mL/hr)
2. With a pressure bag at 300 mm Hg flow rates of 150 mL/min (9000 mL/hr) are possible.

There are three different methods for insertion of the IO needle: manual, impact driven and drill powered. Manual insertion has been available for some time; the needles are hollow with removable trocars. The manual method is dependent on the preparation and insertion time, patient's condition, and skill of the inserter. The steel needles are difficult to access in adult bones due to the density and hardness of the bone. The impact-driven device for sternal access is the FAST1((Pyng Medical, BC, Canada); it has several needle probes to accurately locate the depth of the sternum. Pressure is then applied and the central needle extends into the sternal medullary cavity. The second impact-driven device (Bone Injection Gun, B.I.G., WaisMed, TX) uses a spring-loaded injector mechanism to fire the IO needle into the medullary space of the tibia. Both impact-driven devices must be adequately stabilized to prevent patient or operator injury. The third type is drill based (EZ-IO®, Vidacare, TX); it is a hand-held battery-operated device to drill the IO needle into the IO space. (Walther, 2007). Insertion success rates of greater than 80% to 90% with the drill-type devices (de Caen, 2007). Refer to Figure 10-7.

Candidates for IO:

1. Severely dehydrated patients
2. To provide access in patients in whom peripheral I.V. access is difficult or impossible (e.g., those with cardiac arrest, trauma, obesity, diabetes)
3. First-line choice for pediatric patient resuscitation
4. Second-line choice in adults after failed I.V. attempts
5. Rapid and reliable prehospital emergency intravascular access by paramedic staff

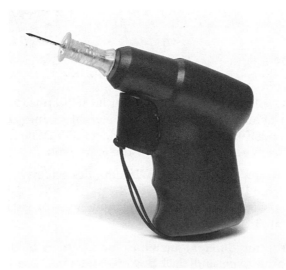

Figure 10-7 ■ EZ-IO® drill. (Courtesy of Vidacare, San Antonio, TX.)

6. Mass casualty scenarios due to natural disasters, major accidents, or terrorist incidents where very large numbers of patients may need rapid resuscitation in difficult physical environments (Dubick & Holcomb, 2000).
7. Premature infants (Ellemunter, Simma, Trawoger, et al., 1999).

EBNP Two prospective prehospital trials in adults have shown successful needle placement in 94%–97% of attempts with IO insertions. Time to insertion is short, approximately 10 seconds in 94% of cases, and flow rates of up to 150 mL/min were achieved (Davidoff, Fowler, Gordon, et al., 2005; Gillum & Kovar, 2005).

ADVANTAGES

- Provides immediate alternative to central line access
- Provides an immediate method of access in patients in whom peripheral I.V. access is difficult
- Provides immediate vascular access with minimal insertion pain when battery-powered drill is used
- Any fluid that can be given I.V. (colloid, crystalloid, or blood product) can be infused via the IO method.
- Normal blood samples can be taken IO for analysis.
- Only route during a nuclear, biological, or chemical incident that can be performed wearing protective clothing (Landes, 2007).

DISADVANTAGES

- Pain on insertion
- Compartment syndrome
- Osteomyelitis
- Cellulitis
- Possibility of fractures
- Cortical bone damage related to device design and poor choices of site location.
- Epiphyseal growth plate damage in children is avoidable by correct placement (Landes, 2007). Refer to Figure 10-6.

Contraindicated for patients with:
- Infection at the insertion site
- Prostheses in the access site
- Fracture in the same bone
- Recent orthopedic procedures in the area of insertion
- Local vascular compromise (Vidacarc, 2008)

NURSING POINTS-OF-CARE
INTRAOSSEOUS INFUSIONS

- Allows for rapid intravascular access within 1 minute (Vardi, Berkenstadt, Levin, et al., 2004)
- Mechanically easier to perform than I.V. access
- Any drug that is administered via the I.V. route may be administered via the IO route, without dosage adjustments.
- Pressure infusion into the IO space may cause significant pain in alert patients. This can be managed with the infusion of 2% preservative-free lidocaine. In adults infuse 40 mg of lidocaine slowly over 15 seconds, wait for 60 seconds, and then flush with 10 mL of 0.9% sodium chloride.
- In pediatric patients, infuse 0.5 mg/kg of Lidocaine slowly over 15 seconds, wait for 60 seconds, and then flush with 5 mL of 0.9% sodium chloride (Vidacare, 2008).
- Use of EZ-IO (Vidacare, San Antonio, TX) handheld battery-powered drill with detachable IO needle for IO insertion.

Refer to Figure 10-8 for EZ-IO steps.

Epidural and Intrathecal Medication Administration

Anatomy of the Epidural and Intrathecal Spaces

The spinal anatomy consists of two spaces, the **epidural** space and the **intrathecal** space. The term **intraspinal** is used to encompass both the epidural and intrathecal spaces surrounding the spinal cord. The intrathecal space is surrounded by the epidural space and separated from it by the dura mater; the intrathecal space contains cerebrospinal fluid (CSF), which bathes the spinal cord. The epidural and intrathecal spaces share a common center, the spinal cord. The epidural space surrounds the spinal cord and intrathecal space and lies between the ligamentum flavum and the dura mater. This is a potential space because the ligamentum flavum and the dura mater are not separated until medication or air is injected between them. This potential space contains a network of veins that are large and thin walled and has a strong leukocytic activity to reduce the risk of infection. Dividing epidural and intrathecal spaces is a tough, fatty membrane called the dura. The permeability of the dura is important in determining how fast epidural drugs cross into the intrathecal space and how long they remain there to be active. The epidural space also contains fat in proportion to a person's body fat. Opiate receptor sites are cells contained in the dorsal horn of the spinal cord, at which

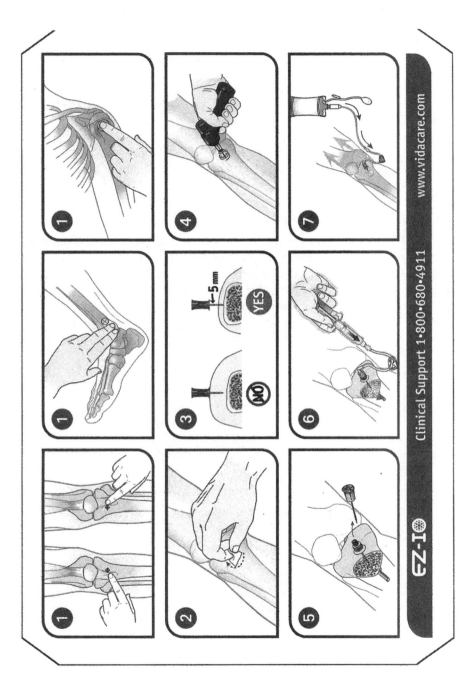

Figure 10-8 ■ EZ-IO steps. (Courtesy of Vidacare, San Antonio, TX.)

point opioids combine with their respective receptor site to generate analgesia (Berry, Bannister, & Standring, 1995).

Refer to Figure 10-9.

Local anesthetic agents are frequently used with opioids, and are instrumental in controlling pain and reducing postoperative complications. When a patient experiences acute pain, the sympathetic system (part of the autonomic nervous system) is activated, increasing the workload of the heart. When intraspinal local anesthetic agents are administered, a sympathetic block results, which produces a decrease in blood pressure, pulse, and respirations. The advantages of adding local anesthetic agents to an epidural opioid are that the sympathetic block decreases workload on the heart and decreases the incidence of thrombophlebitis and paralytic ileus.

Epidural Medication Administration

Epidural percutaneous catheters were used initially for surgical and obstetric anesthesia, and later for epidural opioid postoperative analgesia. Epidural anesthesia is a technique for relieving pain. To initiate epidural anesthesia, an anesthesia provider delivers one or more drugs (a local anesthetic, an opioid, a combination of both, or a steroidal compound) into the epidural space via a special needle or a microbore catheter. The medication diffuses through the dura mater, the arachnoid, and the pia

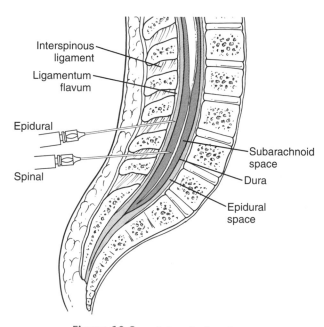

Figure 10-9 ■ Intraspinal anatomy.

mater to the spine. The spinal cord and nerve roots are bathed in the medication, which blocks pain impulses before they reach the brain. If a steroid is used, it reduces inflammation (Schwartz, 2006). Epidural pain control is applicable to patients of all ages. Refer to Table 10-4 for a list of epidural and intrathecal medications.

There are various approaches to the administration of narcotics and anesthetics via the epidural route: a single-bolus injection of opioid or local anesthetic, a continuous infusion of opioid with or without local anesthetics, or a continuous infusion of opioid with a patient-activated bolus. Dosages of medication can be titrated to effect the proper dermatome level; like filling a tube, the volume of medication given determines which dermatome level is affected. There are two types of epidural catheters: temporary and permanent. The temporary catheter is used in the periobstetric and perioperative period and is designed for short-term use with materials that easily pass into the epidural and intrathecal spaces. Teflon catheters allow visualization of aspirated fluid, but can become stiff and potentially migrate out of their original placement. These are external catheters. Temporary catheters are intended to be used for days to a few weeks. Use of the permanent catheters for weeks to months via the epidural route is supported by many pain specialists. The advantages of the permanent catheters are that they have a Dacron cuff to aid in the stabilization of the catheter to the tissues, and many have a second VitaCuff® impregnated with silver to reduce antimicrobial activity (DuPen, 2005). These are generally internal catheters.

A single injection of epidural opioid may be used for procedures that produce a short course of postoperative pain. This method may be appropriate for a patient having a cesarean section or vaginal hysterectomy, or after same-day surgical procedures. Care must be taken to avoid the inadvertent administration of additional opioids by another route that may oversedate the patient, causing respiratory depression. Continuous epidural infusion is administered for short or long periods of time. Patients with pain from surgery, trauma, and acute medical disorders creating severe pain may benefit from short-term continuous infusions. This

> Table 10-4	EPIDURAL AND INTRATHECAL MEDICATIONS

Baclofen
Bupivacaine hydrochloride
Clonidine
DepoDur
Fentanyl
Hydromorphone hydrochloride
Morphine sulfate
Sufentanil
Ziconotide

method can also be employed for the cancer patient with acute exacerbation of pain. The insertion of the epidural catheter is a sterile procedure and is a function performed by a physician or anesthesiologist. Administration of medication by a nurse through an epidural catheter must be in accordance with each state's Nurse Practice Act. Nursing responsibilities include: (1) patient and family education, (2) site and dressing management, (3) medication administration (depending on State Practice Acts), and (4) evaluation of pain relief. Most commonly epidural medication is administered by a certified registered nurse anesthetist or an anesthesiologist and the catheter is managed by the staff nurse (Schwartz, 2006).

Recent advances in drug delivery mechanisms have resulted in a formulation of extended-release epidural morphine, DepoDur® (SkyePharma), which is a lipid-encapsulated extended-release epidural morphine that provides up to 48 hours of analgesia (Keck, Glennon, & Ginsberg, 2007).

Refer to Evidence-Based Practice Box 10-1.

See Figure 10-10 for various methods of epidural administration.

 NURSING FAST FACT!

- *Epidural morphine as a single bolus dose has demonstrated analgesia that lasts up to 24–48 hours with DepoDur®.*
- *In clinical trials, 90% of respiratory depression occurred within the first 24 hours after administration.*
- *Patient monitoring requirements include pain score, respiratory rate, sedation scale score, every hour for 2 hours, then every 2 hours for the remainder of the 48 hours from the time of administration (Keck, Glennon, & Ginsberg, 2007).*

EVIDENCE-BASED PRACTICE BOX 10-1

Extended-Release Epidural Morphine

Viscusi, E.R., Martin, G., Harrick, C.T., et al., (2005). Forty-eight hours of postoperative pain relief after total hip arthroplasty with a novel, extended release epidural morphine formulation. Anesthesiology, 102(5)., 1014–1022.

In a multicenter randomized double-blind parallel-group dose-ranging study, 183 participants received the study drug or placebo when undergoing hip surgery. Participants were randomized to one of four groups: placebo or 15 mg, 20 mg, or 25 mg extended-release epidural morphine (EREM); all were given a fentanyl PCA pump for postoperative pain management. Pain intensity scores were measures at the first request for pain medication, with activity and at regular intervals.

Results: Median time to first dose of PCA fentanyl was prolonged for the ERME groups (21.3 hours), compared to 3.6 hours in the placebo group. Forty-six percent of the EREM participants did not require any fentanyl during the first 24 hours after DepoDur administration.

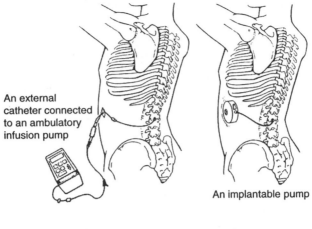

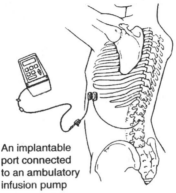

An external catheter connected to an ambulatory infusion pump

An implantable pump

An implantable port connected to an ambulatory infusion pump

Figure 10-10 ■ Methods of epidural administration. (Courtesy of Smith Medical, Inc., St. Paul, MN.)

Candidates for epidural anesthesia are patients with:

1. General surgeries of the thoracic or abdominal area.
2. Labor pains
3. Acute and chronic pain (chronic lumbar pain)
4. Cancer pain
5. Phantom limb pain
6. Pancreatic pain
7. Incisional pain

Epidurals are contraindicated in the following situations:

1. Active infection near the epidural catheter insertion site
2. Use of systemic anticoagulation and antiplatelet therapy
3. In patients on long-term use of aspirin products or nonsteroidal anti-inflammatory drugs
4. Hypovolemic shock

5. Identified allergy to drugs being used for epidural or intrathecal anesthesia
6. Heart failure or aortic stenosis
7. Patients who cannot understand the procedure well enough to give informed consent.
8. A scarred, distorted, or obliterated epidural space from previous thoracic or lumbar spinal surgery
9. A severe spinal curvature such as scoliosis

ADVANTAGES OF EPIDURAL MEDICATION ADMINISTRATION

- Permits control or alleviation of severe pain without the sedative effects
- Permits delivery of smaller doses of a narcotic to achieve the desired level of analgesia
- Prolongs the analgesia (average about 14 hours), or 24 to 48 hours for extended-release epidural morphine
- Allows for continuous infusion, if needed
- Allows terminal cancer patients treated with epidural narcotics to be more comfortable and mobile
- Can be used for short-term or long-term therapy
- Does not produce motor paralysis

DISADVANTAGES OF EPIDURAL MEDICATION ADMINISTRATION

- Nurses' lack of understanding of pharmacologic agents; nurses must be educated in the use of these agents.
- Only preservative-free opioids can be used.
- Complications such as paresthesia, urinary retention, and respiratory depression (greatest 6–10 hours after injection) can occur.
- Catheter-related risks (e.g., infection, dislodgement, and leaking) can occur.
- Pruritus can occur on the face, head, and neck or may be generalized.
- Unless the epidural catheter and medication **are clearly labeled**, an intravenous infusion could be inadvertently given via the intraspinal route, which could cause serious complications or death.

NOTE > A pain specialist will make sure the catheter is patent by aspirating to check for blood and checking the ability to administer medication throughout the catheter (Schwartz, 2006).

INS Standard　Medication shall be preservative free.

For intraspinal infusions, a 0.2-micron filter that is surfactant-free, particulate-retentive, and air-eliminating shall be used.

Sterile technique, including mask and sterile gloves should be used when accessing, caring for and maintaining an intraspinal access device. (INS, 2006, 62)

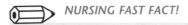

NURSING FAST FACT!

Ineffective pain control should be reported to the physician or anesthesiologist who is managing care of the epidural catheter.

MONITORING THE PATIENT WITH AN INTRASPINAL CATHETER

A flowsheet (Fig. 10-11) should be used to monitor the patient's response to epidural medication. This allows tracking of the patient's analgesia and any side effects.

ENLOE
MEDICAL CENTER

EPIDURAL FLOWSHEET
INTERMITTENT OR CONTINUOUS INFUSION

DATE _____ MEDICATION _____
EDUCATION: CHART ON BACK OF FLOW SHEET
1) INTERMITTENT INJECTIONS: VS Q 15" X 2 THEN Q 4 HOURS
2) CONTINUOUS INFUSION: VS Q 15" X 2 THEN Q 4 HOURS
    A) RESP., SEDATION LEVEL, MOTOR RESPONSE, DERMATOMES (ANESTHETICS) Q 1 HOUR X 4,
        THEN Q 2 HOURS X 24 HOURS. CONTINUE AT EVERY 4 HOURS.
FOR ANY INFUSION RATE CHANGE RETURN TO INITIAL ASSESSMENT FREQUENCIES

TIME														
TEMPERATURE														
BLOOD PRESSURE														
PULSE														
RESPIRATIONS: RATE DEPTH / QUALITY														
SEDATION LEVEL/RAP SCORE														
PAIN SCALE														
SITE ASSESS .Q8°														
MOTOR RESPONSE NO DEFICIT														
DERMATOMES LEVEL/RESPONSE														
PT C/O														
INTERVENTIONS														
INITIALS														

ASSESS PAIN Q 4 HOURS FOR ALL TYPES OF EPIDURAL ANALGESIA

RAP (Revised Aldrete Protocol): Add all 3 columns for total score

LOC	RESP	S & M
2 = Awake & oriented	Normal resp. & awake	Full function X 4
1.5 = Drowsy & oriented or awake	Normal respiration & asleep	Full motor return with nearly complete sensory return
1 = Responds to verbal stimuli	Labored respiration oral or nasal airway	Sensory & motor block with decreasing levels
.5 = Responds only to noxious stimuli	N/A	N/A
0 = Non-responsive	Apnea or ET tube	No spontaneous movement or sensory motor block with stable level

PT C/O
A. Circumoral tingling
B. Muscle twitching
C. "Metallic" taste/tinnitus
D. Nausea
E. Urinary Retention
F. Breakthrough Pain
G. Blurred Vision
H. Epidural Site Pain
I. Itching
J. Light Headedness
K. None

PAIN
0 – 10 scale
0 – no pain
10 – worst pain

RESPIRATIONS:
DEPTH / QUALITY
Regular
Unlabored
Deep
Irregular
Labored
Shallow

DERMATOMES
(Anesthetics only)

T4
T6
T8
T10
L1
L3
L4

INTERVENTIONS
1. Cont. Pulse Ox
2. Position Checked
3. Line and Bag Changed
4. Dressing Changed
5. Dose Increased
6. Dose Decreased
7. Med for Breakthrough Pain
8. See MAR
9. See Nurses Notes

Signatures

(07–15) _____

(15–23) _____

(23–07) _____

Addressograph

Figure 10-11 ■ Example of continuous or intermittent epidural flowsheet. (Courtesy of Enloe Medical Center, Chico, CA.)

Included on the flow sheet are the following assessments:
- Evaluate mental status, level of consciousness
- Assess respiratory rate and oxygen saturation of hemoglobin (SpO_2) using a pulse oximeter.
- Assess for any indication of numbness in the lower extremities.
- Assess for signs of infection at the catheter–skin junction site.
- Evaluate bowel function.
- Evaluate bladder function for urinary retention.
- Assess the integrity of the epidural system.
- Record the narcotic dose.
- Record the patient's pain rating.
- Document any site care.

DRESSING MANAGEMENT OF EPIDURAL CATHETERS

Temporary epidural catheters should be handled carefully during the site care because they are easily dislodged. Permanent external epidural catheters require dressing changes. Permanent epidural catheters have a Dacron cuff that acts as a protective barrier against bacterial migration and secures the catheter placement.

During the dressing change, the nurse must carefully stabilize the epidural catheter. This is a sterile procedure.

1. Wash hands with antimicrobial soap and water. Don gloves.
2. Secure the temporary catheter close to the exit site with a piece of tape. Remove the old dressing. Use a cotton ball soaked in sterile water to assist in lifting the edge of dressing if necessary.
3. Don sterile gloves. Apply antimicrobial solution **without alcohol** in a circular motion, starting at the exit site and working outward. Allow the solution to air dry.
4. Apply a new dressing, gauze or transparent, making sure that the catheter is well secured and cannot dislodge accidentally.
5. The catheter should be coiled near the insertion site to prevent accidental dislodgement.
6. Document the dressing change, reporting the inspection of the exit site and how the patient tolerated the procedure.

INS Standard The optimal time interval for changing dressings (of intraspinal catheter site) is dependent on the dressing material, age and condition of the patient, infection rate reported by the organization, environmental conditions, and manufacturer's labeled use(s) and directions for product use. (INS, 2006, 62)

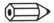 *NURSING FAST FACT!*

Do not use alcohol on skin or at dressing site because of the risk of migration of alcohol into the epidural space and the possibility of neural damage.

Intrathecal Medication Administration

Intrathecal opioid infusions can be considered for pain in malignancy. They can be used for patients with cancer; who do not receive adequate pain relief with systemic narcotics, tricyclic antidepressants, or nonsteroidal anti-inflammatory drugs (NSAIDs); and who have pain located below the midcervical dermatomes. In addition, patients who have experienced toxicity from systemic medications or have persistent, severe pain despite a multimodal treatment approach (Ghafoor, Epshteyn, Carlson, et al., 2007). Recently published multidisciplinary cancer pain management guidelines support the use of intrathecal therapy (Maiskowski, Cleary, Burney, et al., 2005).

Intrathecal narcotic infusions can be delivered via an implanted infusion pump, or tunneled epidural catheter. In a candidate who has a life expectancy of less than 3 months the initial cost of the implanted intrathecal pump is not cost effective. Long-term intrathecal therapy requires an implanted pump (Krames, 2002). The intrathecal injection of an opioid requires **less** medication than is needed in the epidural space. The intrathecal space, however, is associated with a greater risk for infection. Intrathecal opioids given as a single injection are commonly used for postoperative pain management, for cesarean surgeries, vaginal hysterectomies, and some orthopedic surgeries.

ADVANTAGES

- There is no external catheter creating a risk of dislodgement or infection.
- Prolonged analgesia is offered.
- The catheter is relatively simple to access.

DISADVANTAGES

- High levels of pain may be experienced as the opioid wears off.
- Respiratory depression may occur.
- The risk of infection is greater than that with epidural delivery because CSF is a good medium for bacterial growth.
- Spinal headache (for up to 3 days) may occur, especially in young women.

NOTE > Guidelines for monitoring, site care, and managing complications and side effects are the same as those for epidural infusions.

COMPLICATIONS ASSOCIATED WITH INTRASPINAL PAIN MANAGEMENT

Side effects of intraspinal opioids can include excessive somnolence and confusion, nausea, vomiting, urinary retention, and pruritus. Urinary retention is a common side effect and may occur 10 to 20 hours after the first injection of intraspinal narcotic. This may require either administration of bethanecol (Urecholine) or intermittent catheterization. Pruritus is caused by the opiate's interacting with the dorsal horn and not by a histamine release. This is best treated with an antagonist rather than with diphenhydramine (Benadryl). After an epidural injection, 8.5% of all patients experience pruritus; after an intrathecal injection, 46% experience pruritus.

Complications are not common; however, they may arise from several sources. Patients may have a reaction or side effect to the medication being administered or a problem resulting from the placement or displacement of the catheter.

NOTE > Hypotension is common in patients with epidural anesthesia, but it is a sign that the procedure is working. Epidural anesthesia blocks the autonomic sympathetic chain of nerves, which runs adjacent to the spinal cord. Monitor the patient and provide extra I.V. fluids, or the administration of vasoactive medications may be required (Schwartz, 2006).

Conditions requiring **immediate** physician notification include:

- Inadequate pain relief. This can occur for three reasons: epidural catheter migration, insufficient dosages of opioid and local anesthetics, and undetermined surgical complication.
- Respiratory depression from epidural or intrathecal narcotic administration. Vital signs should be assessed and naloxone should be available to reverse the depressant effects of a narcotic.
- Extreme dizziness as a result of inadequate orthostatic hypotension or excessive opioid effect
- New onset of paresthesia or paresis
- Difficulty or inability to infuse epidural medication
- Pain at the insertion site
- Displacement or migration of the epidural catheter. Catheter migration may occur in two ways: (1) the catheter may migrate through the dura mater into the intrathecal space, creating an overdose of opioid or (2) the catheter may migrate into an epidural vein or subcutaneous space, creating inadequate pain relief.
- Infections. These are rare from epidural catheters, but precautions should be instituted to keep the catheter insertion process and exit site sterile. If an infection develops elsewhere in the body, the patient should be evaluated for removal of the epidural catheter.
- Excessive drowsiness or confusion occurring when too much narcotic is being administered. This is usually improved by decreasing the amount of epidural narcotic infusion. Titrating an opioid antagonist, such as naloxone (Narcan) or an agonist/antagonist subcutaneously, may reverse side effects without eliminating the analgesia.

Other complications that may not warrant immediate physician notification but need to be reported at the earliest convenience include the inability to urinate and pruritus, which may be treated with parenterally administered medication while the epidural infusion continues.

 NURSING FAST FACT!

> *If catheter migration is suspected, the physician should be notified and the placement check should be verified by an anesthesiologist.*

NURSING POINTS-OF-CARE

ADMINISTRATION OF EPIDURAL AND INTRATHECAL PAIN CONTROL

- Nurses caring for intraspinal catheters need to demonstrate competency in maintenance, assessment of placement, and function of the access device and have an understanding of anatomy and physiology, neuropharmacology, and potential complications.
- Preservatives in narcotics or local anesthetics used in the epidural or intrathecal space need to be avoided to prevent nerve damage.
- Preservative-free morphine, which is water soluble and has a slower onset of action and longer duration of action, therefore is a better choice for patients who need more prolonged analgesia. Lipid-soluble fentanyl and sufentanil penetrate the dura mater faster than water-soluble opioids, providing a faster onset of action but a shorter duration of action.
- Sterile technique, including mask and gloves, should be used when accessing, caring for, and maintaining an intraspinal access device.
- Alcohol, disinfectants containing alcohol, or acetone **shall never** be used for site preparation or for cleansing the catheter hub due to potential for neurotoxic effects of the alcohol.
- For intraspinal infusions, a 0.2-micron filter that is surfactant-free, particulate-retentive, and air-eliminating must be in place.
- Epidural devices should be aspirated to ascertain the **absence** of spinal fluid and blood before medication administration.
- Intrathecal and ventricular devices should be aspirated to **ascertain the presence** of spinal fluid and the absence of blood prior to medication administration (INS, 2006, 62).
- Inspect the catheter–skin junction visually and palpate for tenderness daily through the intact dressing.

Continued

■ Catheter migration should be monitored by assessing for changes in external catheter length; ineffective internal length may result in changes in patient assessment, therapeutic effect, or loss of patency.

■ After insertion of the external catheter, lay the exposed catheter length cephalad along the spine and over the shoulder. Tape the entire length of the exposed catheter in place to provide stability and protection. The end of the catheter and the filter are generally placed on the patient's chest wall and taped securely in a position that allows the patient or family member to access the catheter for use.

■ Evaluate the effects of the drug on the patient's alertness; caregivers should also be taught to observe for levels of sedation.

■ Clearly label the epidural catheter after placement to prevent accidental infusion of fluids or medications. Use yellow striped tubing for epidural infusions only. DO NOT USE EPIDURAL TUBING FOR I.V. SOLUTIONS.

Intraventricular Infusions

Intraventricular (IVt) chemotherapy allows for the administration of antineoplastic agents into the CSF via an Ommaya reservoir (Fig. 10-12). A physician must place the ventricular reservoir. The nurse administering medications into the reservoir must follow the Nurse Practice Act for the state in which he or she practices. An Ommaya reservoir is a silicone rubber device that is implanted surgically under the scalp and provides access to CSF through a burr hole in the skull. Drugs are injected into the reservoir with a hypodermic syringe, and then the domed reservoir is depressed manually to mix drug with the CSF.

An intraventricular reservoir can be used to deliver chemotherapy or other medications to the brain directly. An Ommaya port or reservoir is used to deliver the medication. Medication is delivered following the Joint Commission (TJC, 2005) recommendations:

1. Prepare the IVt medication in the pharmacy as close to the administration time as possible; then deliver the drug to a separate designated area.

2. The IVt medications bag is wrapped in a sterile bag, then wrap again in a sterile towel or another bag labeled "FOR INTRAVENTRICULAR USE ONLY." Wraps or packages should be removed immediately before administration by the person administering the drug.

3. Before the start of the chemotherapy administration, conduct a final verification to confirm correct patient, procedure, site, and availability of appropriate documents. All medications must be labeled (Aiello-Laws & Rutledge, 2008; TJC, 2005).

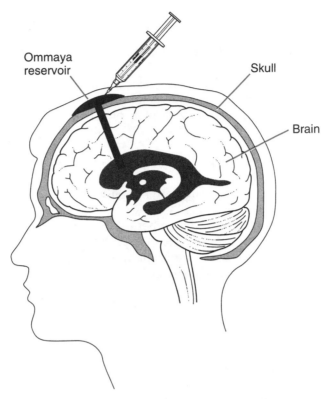

Figure 10-12 ■ Ommaya reservoir.

NOTE > IVt typically is administered by an oncologist. In some states, specially trained nurses can obtain privileges to administer such medications (Camp-Sorrel, 2004).

Candidates for intraventricular infusions include patient being treated for:

1. Fungal meningitis and brain abscesses
2. Chronic bacterial CNS infections
3. Meningeal leukemia and neoplastic infiltration of the CNS
4. Primary intraocular lymphoma with CNS spread
5. Intractable pain control with advanced head and neck cancer
6. Rapid increases in intracranial pressure
7. Unresectable tumors as a means to drain excessive fluid accumulation caused by cystic brain tumors
8. Conditions requiring antibiotic therapy to remove CSF, to monitor drug levels

ADVANTAGES

- Well tolerated
- Medication delivered directly into the CSF of the brain and spinal cord
- Can be used to obtain fluid sample to check for any abnormal cells
- Can be used to measure intracranial pressure
- Eliminates need for multiple lumbar punctures

DISADVANTAGES

- Increased risk of infection to the spinal cord and brain (iatrogenic meningitis) (Johnson & Sexton, 2006)
- Aseptic meningitis can affect 10% of patients.
- Catheter malposition
- Myelosuppression from chemotherapy
- Reversible posterior leukoencephalopathy syndrome (confusion, hallucinations, delusions, transient aphasia depression, suicidal ideation, irritability, and changes in mental status; Wen & Plotkin, 2006)
- Transverse myelopathy (inflammation of white and gray matter in the spinal cord) is more common among patients receiving IVt concurrent with radiation.

NURSING POINTS-OF-CARE
DELIVERY OF CHEMOTHERAPY VIA A VENTRICULAR RESERVOIR

- The patient should be taught the purpose of the reservoir.
- When accessing the IVt ventricular reservoir, wear sterile gloves, a gown, and a mask (Camp-Sorrell, 2004).
- Use only preservative-free medications.
- Aspirate to check placement before drug delivery; CSF should be present.
- Withdrawal of CSF for diagnostic purpose is a medical act.
- Due to controversial issues surrounding chlorhexidine gluconate with alcohol and neurotoxicity, and the FDA warning to "Avoid contact with meninges," it is prudent that 10% povidone-iodine be used to prepare skin before accessing the Ommaya reservoir (Hebl, 2006).
- Monitor for symptoms of neurotoxicity, confusion, disorientation, seizures, headache, and altered mental status.
- Monitor for changes in blood pressure and weight gain.
- Accurate placement of the IVt reservoir must be confirmed via a computed tomography (CT) scan.

Intra-Arterial Infusions

Chemotherapy administered through the **intra-arterial** (IA) route allows for high concentrations of antineoplastic agents to be delivered directly into tumor sites by means of arterial catheters or implanted devices. A temporary angiographical microcatheter is placed via percutaneous angiography for carotid, brachial, femoral, or specific limb artery for short-term therapies (from hours to 5 days). The catheter rests in the arterial vessel supplying the tumor and usually is placed by an interventional radiologist. This therapy is repeated by means of a new catheter insertion each time for 3 to 6 months of therapy.

An implantable arterial port is placed subcutaneously near the tumor site over a bony surface and sutured in place; the catheter is then threaded into the tumor artery site. The port is accessed via a noncoring needle, covered with a transparent dressing, and connected to a heparinized saline solution via an infusion pump.

Candidates for intra-arterial infusions are patients with:
- Advanced head and neck cancers
- Osteosarcoma (children and adults)

ADVANTAGES

- Allows for higher concentrations (two to five times higher) of the chemotherapeutic agent directly to the site (Teymoortash & Werner, 2003)
- Tumor-specific treatment
- Decreased systemic side effects

DISADVANTAGES

- Hematoma formation during insertion of catheter
- Occlusions in area of catheter insertion
- Chemotoxicity (gastrointestinal, hematological, and neurotoxic side effects) can occur.

NURSING POINTS-OF-CARE
INTRA-ARTERIAL INFUSIONS

- Administer I.V. prehydration before IA chemotherapy.
- Two RNs should verify the patient's height and weight.
- Consider insertion of a Foley catheter the morning of IA line placement due to bedrest for 4 hours after the procedure.
- Instruct on the importance of lying flat after line insertion.
- Strictly monitor intake and output.

Continued

■ IA drug infusion requires astute clinical observations and interventions.

■ The insertion site and the affected extremity should be observed every 2–4 hours.

■ Monitor vital signs.

■ Femoral catheter placement requires bedrest with log rolling to maintain catheter alignment.

■ Brachial catheter placement requires immobilizing the affected extremity.

■ All chemotherapy supplies should have Luer-Lok™ connections, and infusion pumps may require a higher psi (pounds per square inch) setting to overcome arterial flow resistance.

■ Implantable arterial ports must be flushed with heparin weekly to maintain catheter patency if a continuous infusion solution is not being administered.

AGE-RELATED CONSIDERATIONS

Older adults and pediatric patients require special consideration when delivering I.V. fluids and medications. Each poses special problems that must be carefully addressed to guarantee safe I.V. therapy. Medications may have many greater side effects and adverse consequences in these populations.

Pediatric Patients

• Continuous infusions in pediatric patients should have inline volume-control chambers and be controlled by infusion pumps. No more than 1 to 2 hours' worth of solution should be placed in the chamber at any one time.

• The diagnosis of pediatric cancer involves many members of the health-care team. New techniques to diagnose and stage cancers have facilitated the development of sophisticated plans of treatment.

• Intraosseous infusion for emergency situations is now used for children and adults.

• Pediatric patients also may have varying renal and hepatic functions and body water to fat ratios depending on age. In addition, weight variation as children mature varies tremendously. All pediatric drugs and fluid calculations should be checked for accuracy by two licensed care providers.

Calculations for Delivery of I.V. Medications and Solutions in Pediatric Patients

Assessment of Fluid Needs

There are three methods for assessment of 24-hour maintenance of fluids: meter square, caloric, and weight.

Meter Square Method

A nomogram, as discussed earlier, is used to determine the body surface area (BSA) of the patient in the **meter square method**.

The following are advantages of the meter square method:
- Provides calculation of body surface area to help determine the amount of fluid and electrolytes to be infused and assists with computing the rate of infusion.
- Helps to calculate adult and pediatric dosages of I.V. medications.
- Is simple to calculate.

The following is a disadvantage of the meter square method:
- Difficulty in accessibility to visual nomogram

To calculate the maintenance of fluid requirements, use the following:
Formula: 1500 mL/m² per 24 hours

Example: If the child's surface area is 0.5 m², then 1500 mL × 0.5 m² = 750 mL/24 hr.

WEIGHT METHOD

The weight method uses the child's weight in kilograms to estimate fluid needs. This method uses 100 to 150 mL/kg for estimating maintenance fluid requirements and is most useful in children weighing less than 10 kg. (Use of the square meter method is recommended for children weighing more than 10 kg.)

The following is an advantage of the weight method:
- Simple to use

The following is a disadvantage of the weight method:
- Inaccurate in children who weigh more than 10 kg

Example: For a child weighing 10 kg, 100 × 10 kg = 1000 mL in 24 hours.

CALORIC METHOD

The **caloric method** calculates the usual metabolic expenditure of fluid. It is based on the following metabolic expenditures:
- A child weighing 0 to 10 kg expends approximately 100 cal/kg per day.
- A child weighing 10 to 20 kg expends approximately 1000 calories plus 50 cal/kg for each kilogram over 10 kg.
- A child weighing 20 kg or more expends approximately 1500 calories, plus 20 cal/kg for each kilogram over 20 kg.

The following is an advantage of the caloric method:
- Simple to calculate

The following is a disadvantage of the caloric method:
- Not totally accurate unless actual calorie requirements and energy intake are continuously assessed

The formula for calculating fluid requirement is:
100 to 150 mL/100 calories metabolized

Example: If the weight of the child is 30 kg and the child expends 1700 cal/day, the fluid requirement is 1700 to 2550 mL/24 hr.

Formulas for Delivery of Pediatric Therapies

For many years, pediatric dosage calculations used formulas such as Fried's rule, Young's rule and Clark's rule. These formulas were based on the weight of the child in pounds, or on the age of the child in months, and the

Continued

normal adult dose of a specific drug. At the present time, the most accurate method of determining an appropriate pediatric dose is based on body weight. Body surface area is also used, especially in pediatric oncology and critical care (Olsen, Giangrasso, Shrimpton, & Dillon, 2008).

BODY WEIGHT

Doses of drugs based on kilograms of body weight require that nurses use the weight (in kg) of the child in dosage administration (1 kg = 2.2 lb). Many drugs are ordered as milligram per kilogram of body weight. Multiply the milligrams of the drug by the kilograms of body weight:

Formula:

$$mg \text{ of drug} \times kg \text{ of child's body weight} = \text{Child's dose}$$

BODY SURFACE AREA (BSA)

Doses of drugs based on BSA are determined by multiplying the child's BSA (m^2) times the recommended adult dose, divided by the adult's BSA (1.73 m^2). Drug manufacturers may recommend a pediatric dosage based on body surface area (BSA) (Olsen, Giangrasso, Shrimpton, & Dillon, 2008).

Formula:

$$\frac{\text{BSA of child } (m^3) \times \text{recommended adult dose}}{\text{BSA of adult } (1.73 \ m^2)} = \text{pediatric dose}$$

The Older Adult

The older adult may manifest several age-related changes that require consideration when calculating medication dosages. There is a decrease in total body water and a relative increase in body fat which may affect water and fat soluble medication bioavailability. Water-soluble drugs such as digoxin and the aminoglycoside antibiotics may have increased serum levels, and fat-soluble medications may have a reduced half-life. Liver blood flow is reduced by 0.5% to 1.5% per year after the age of 25; therefore, there is a decline in the body's ability to transform active drugs into inactive metabolites (Broyles, Reiss, & Evans, 2007). The older adult is more likely to experience drug toxicity due to decreased elimination related to decreased number of intact nephrons, along with glomerular filtration reduction due to decreased blood flow. All medications should be researched before administration to the older adult to determine if recommendations to reduce or increase the usual adult dosage are in effect.

Other factors may affect how intravenous drugs affect the older adult. There is some evidence that the number and possibly the nature of drug receptors change with age. The patient's homeostatic mechanisms are often impaired (e.g., cardiovascular, renal, endocrine), leading to an adverse response to drug therapy.

INS Standard The nurse providing infusion therapy to the older adult should have validation of demonstrated competency in the knowledge and technical expertise in performance of older adult nursing assessment and implementation of vascular and nonvascular access device insertion. Ethical, safety and environmental considerations related to older adults receiving infusion therapy and effective management of those considerations. (INS, 2006, S3)

- Almost 60% of older adults fear adverse drug reactions or overmedication, which leads to noncompliance in taking their medications. Drug side effects in elderly persons are often mistaken for signs of aging. Gender can have a profound effect on metabolism of drugs. For example, women have the potential for higher blood plasma levels. Women have a greater likelihood of adverse reactions to antipsychotic agents.

Home Care Issues

The rapidly growing home care infusion industry now provides many therapies in alternative settings. Therapies that are now being delivered in the home include antimicrobials, parenteral nutrition, hydration therapy, chemotherapy, pain management, cardiovascular medications, blood transfusions, chelation therapy, factor replacement for bleeding disorders, biological drugs, Prolastin therapy, and I.V. immunoglobulin (IVIG).

A number of methods exist for delivery of medication intravenously in the home environment: gravity, I.V. push, or ambulatory pump.

Safety and Effectiveness

Patients who are able to care for themselves are the best candidates for using ambulatory pumps and usually adjust quickly to home infusions. To ensure effective treatment, coordination of care among the patient, nurse, physician, and pharmacist is essential. Unless the patient understands the treatment, procedure, and administration regimen and accepts them into his or her lifestyle, home drug therapy will not be successful.

 NURSING FAST FACT!

As with any I.V. medication delivery, emergency drugs should be readily available and protocols established for their use in some home infusion therapy situations, for example, first doses of antimicrobial drugs or drugs/biologicals with ongoing potential for severe antibody/anaphylactic reactions. Clinical assessment of the home care patient on any infusion medication/fluids is based on the same standards as any other treatment setting. Patients are monitored for adverse reactions, disease processes, and laboratory test results.

Anti-Infectives

Administration methods for antimicrobial therapy in the home can include gravity drip, by elastomeric pump (which is common and easy to teach the

Continued

Home Care Issues—cont'd

patients and caregivers), syringe pumps with lower volume infusions, bedside electronic infusion pumps, I.V. push (certain antimicrobials), and by ambulatory electronic infusion pumps. When administering antimicrobials in the home, safety, effectiveness, acceptance, and cost need to be considered (Gorski, 2005).

Patient education is crucial to safe home infusion of medications. Home care situations vary in terms of the patient's ability to manage the infusion. Based on the type of infusion and the patient or caregiver's ability, the level of independence in home infusion therapy will vary. For example, drugs/fluids with a high risk for adverse reactions with every infusion, such as IVIG, are administered by the nurse while in most cases, self-administration of antimicrobial drugs is typically taught to the patient or caregiver (Gorski, 2005).

 NURSING FAST FACT!

> *To prevent medication errors home infusion pharmacy standards of practice state that the pharmacist is responsible for programming the pump and locking the program into the pump. The pump program is checked a second time before the pump is packed for delivery. The nurse must also review the program to verify that the program matches the medical order. There are some cases when a nurse will need to change a pump program, but this should be done by calling the pharmacy on the telephone and verifying the correct program together with the pharmacy.*

Pain Management

For home use, the subcutaneous, intravenous, and intraspinal (epidural/intrathecal) routes are used for pain management. Opioid drugs and anesthetic agents are typically infused via the intraspinal route (Gorski, 2005). An intraspinal catheter may be attached to a preprogrammed infusion pump containing a medication cassette that requires replacing on a regular basis. An implanted epidural infusion pump (e.g., Medtronic Synchromed) is used to deliver intrathecal medications and is refilled by specially trained home infusion nurses using a special computerized transponder and refill kits. Teach the patient and caregiver on how the intraspinal catheter works and the importance of keeping appointments for pump refills.

Subcutaneous infusions include both hydration of fluids or medications. A subcutaneous needle/catheter is placed into the subcutaneous tissue. The infusion volume per hour for medications delivered subcutaneously is generally less than 10 mL/hr and may be less depending on absorption of the drug. Typically, sites are rotated every 4 and 5 days, and sooner if there is irritation. Opioid drugs for pain management (morphine, hydromorphone) are the most common subcutaneously administered drugs in the home setting (Gorski, 2005).

Patient Education

- Patient education on I.V. medication administration is vital for the acute care and alternative settings. When possible, patient education should begin before a patient's discharge from the hospital to facilitate a smooth transition to home care.
- The education should begin with instructions outlining the insertion of the I.V. catheter and step-by-step details of the procedure for all peripheral, midline, and peripherally inserted central catheter (PICC) line insertions. All potential complications after insertion should be explained and the patient or responsible party should sign an informed consent.
- Routine maintenance care involved in central line management for medication infusions should be provided.
- Fully instruct the patient about the infusion pump; written step-by-step instructions with diagrams or pictures, and manufacturer manuals are excellent tools. Include troubleshooting instructions and telephone numbers to call for 24-hour assistance.
- Instructions on proper hand hygiene, setting up the infusion pump with medication, flushing the catheter, and self-administration of the medication must be included in patient training sessions.
- Instruct the patient on the expected actions and adverse effects of medication.
- The patient or caregiver must be taught the procedure of drug administration clearly and in simple terminology.
- Provide a checklist to help evaluate the steps in the learning process; this also provides a method of documenting the completion of self-drug administration.
- Instruct the patient on administration of anti-infectives around the clock to maintain blood levels

Patient Education Related to PCA
- Make sure the postoperative patient is alert enough to understand the directions for use of PCA. Make sure hearing aids or glasses are in place before instruction.
- Instruct on how to use patient-controlled analgesia.
- Instruct on when to push the bolus button.
- Instruct on when to communicate with the nurse (e.g., pain not controlled with PCA, feeling of sedation).
- Discuss fears (of addiction to medication, receiving too much medication)
- Discuss expected outcomes for the patient: Pain scale use, prevention of breakthrough pain and early ambulation.

■ Nursing Process

The nursing process is a five- or six-step process for problem-solving to guide nursing action. Refer to Chapter 1 for details on the steps of the nursing process related to vascular access. The following table focuses on nursing diagnoses, nursing outcomes classification (NOC), and nursing intervention classification (NIC) for patients with medication administration via intravenous and alternate modalities. Nursing diagnoses should be patient specific and outcomes and interventions individualized. The NOC and NIC presented here are suggested directions for development of specific outcomes and interventions.

Nursing Diagnoses Related to Central Venous Access	NOC: Nursing Outcomes Classification	NIC: Nursing Intervention Classification
Anxiety (mild, moderate, and severe) related to: Threat to or change in health status; misconceptions regarding therapy	Coping	Anxiety reduction strategies Teaching: Medication
Comfort impaired, pruritus	Comfort level	Pruritus management
Health maintenance ineffective, related to: Limited skills of family members in delivery of intravenous medications and fluids	Health beliefs, perceived resources, health-promoting behaviors	Health education, health systems guidance, support system enhancements
Injury, risk for related to: Toxic or effects of medications	Knowledge of medication, medication response	Health education Medication management Surveillance: Safety
Knowledge deficit, related to: Lack of motivation to learn and/or decreased energy available for learning	Knowledge of treatment regimen Participation in health-care decisions	Decision-making support Health system guidance Mutual goal setting Teaching: Procedure/ treatment
Mobility impaired (physical), related to: Pain and discomfort resulting from placement and maintenance of I.V. catheters	Activities of daily living, transfer performance	Exercise therapy, ambulation, joint mobility, positioning assistance.
Tissue integrity impaired, related to: Adverse reaction to medication	Wound healing, primary or secondary intention healing.	Skin care, skin surveillance, wound care management.

Sources: Ackerley & Ladwig (2008); Carpenito-Moyet (2008); McCloskey-Dochterman & Bulechek (2004); Moorhead, Johnson, & Maas (2004); NANDA-I (2007).

Chapter Highlights

- Advantages of I.V. medications include the fact that they provide a direct access to the circulatory system, a route for drugs that irritate the gastric mucosa, a route for instant drug action, a route for delivering high drug concentrations, instant drug termination if sensitivity or an adverse reaction occurs, and a route of administration in patients in whom use of the GI tract is limited.
- Disadvantages of I.V. medications include drug interaction because of incompatibilities, adsorption of the drug being impaired because of leaching into the I.V. container or administration set, errors in compounding of medication, speed shock, extravasation of a vesicant drug, and chemical phlebitis.
- Common errors in administering medications include lack of knowledge about drugs, errors in drug identity checking, mistakes in calculations, and improper use of pumps and controllers.
- Drug incompatibilities fall into three broad categories: physical, chemical, and therapeutic.
- I.V. medication can be delivered by continuous infusion, intermittent infusion, and I.V. push through a locking device.
- The subcutaneous infusion (hypodermoclysis) route is useful for hydration of patients, unable to take fluids by mouth or those who have poor venous access.
- The use of intraosseous infusions has expanded and can be used in adults and children and include: severely dehydrated patients, adults in whom PIV access is impossible, rapid and reliable prehospital emergency access.
- Intraosseous (IO) can be accessed in three ways: manual, impact-driven, and drill-powered.
- Disadvantages of IO include pain on insertion, compartment syndrome, osteomyelitis, or cellulitis.
- The intraventricular route via an Ommaya reservoir can be used for delivery of medications directly to the brain.
- There are two types of intraspinal catheters: epidural and intrathecal.
- Epidural and intrathecal administrations provide superior pain control, require small doses, and produce longer periods of relief between doses while preventing many systemic side effects.
- Alcohol must **NEVER** be used for site preparation or for accessing an intraspinal catheter. Only preservative-free medications can be delivered by the intraspinal routes.
- The intraperitoneal route is used when high concentrations of medication need to be delivered directly into the peritoneal cavity.

▄▄ Thinking Critically: Case Study

Mrs. Robertson is one day postoperative from an abdominal hysterectomy. She has an epidural catheter in place. Her baseline vital signs are: blood pressure, 110/80; respiration, 18 breaths/min; pulse, 72 bpm. Your assessment finds her difficult to arouse, but she does respond to simple commands. She is able to move her legs and squeezes your fingers. Her blood pressure is 90/60; pulse, 100 bpm; respirations, 14 breaths/min. She is moaning in pain, unable to rate her pain on the pain scale.

What further assessments need to be done?

What further actions should the nurse initiate?

What could be the reason for her change in status?

Media Link: Answers to the case study and more critical thinking activities are provided on the CD-ROM.

Post-Test

1. Which of the following are potential incompatibilities of medication admixtures?

   a. Intermittent, physical, and biotransformation
   b. Drug interaction, drug synergism, and drug tolerance
   c. Physical, chemical, and therapeutic

2. Which is the most common modality for delivery of I.V. medications to pediatric patients?

   a. Continuous infusion through a primary line
   b. Intermittent infusion using a volume control set
   c. Intermittent infusion using a intermittent vascular device
   d. Intermittent infusion using the piggy-back method

3. Several devices are available for placement of intraosseous needles, including the Bone Injection Gun (BIG), the EZ-IO, and the F.A.S.T.1 IO system. Overall, the success rate for insertion with theses drills is reported to be:

   a. >40%
   b. >50%
   c. >70%
   d. >80%

4. I.V. push medications should be administered according to the manufacturer's recommendations, but delivered over no less than:

   a. 10 minutes
   b. 5 minutes
   c. 1 minute
   d. 30 seconds

5. Advantages of the intraperitoneal modality include which of the following? (*Select all that apply*):
   a. Dose intensification is achieved in I.P. sites.
   b. I.P. chemotherapy diffuses into the peritoneal surface, where it is absorbed systemically.
   c. Lower system levels of agents
   d. Available to a wide variety of patients.

6. Safety precautions to prevent errors associated with PCA therapy include which of the following? (*Select all that apply.*)
   a. Employ double-checks
   b. Highlight the drug concentration on the label.
   c. Limit the variety of medications used for PCA.
   d. Develop a reference sheet on PCA that includes programming tips and maximum dose warnings.

7. Clear fluid in the syringe after aspiration of an epidural catheter is an indication of catheter:
   a. Patency
   b. Kinking
   c. Migration
   d. Damage

8. Which of the following are key points in the delivery of epidural infusions? (*Select all that apply.*)
   a. Use only alcohol swabs to prepare the site.
   b. Use only antimicrobial swabs to prepare the site.
   c. Use a 0.2-micron filter without surfactant for medication administration.
   d. Aspirate the catheter to ascertain the presence of spinal fluid.

9. Which of the following modalities are commonly used to deliver pain medication to postoperative patients? (*Select all that apply.*)
   a. Intravenous route
   b. Subcutaneous route
   c. Epidural route
   d. Intraperitoneal route

10. To reduce the hazards of vascular irritation with delivery of medication, nurses should:
    a. Use the largest cannula possible
    b. Use a cannula smaller than the lumen of a vessel
    c. Administer most medications via the intramuscular route
    d. Use electronic infusion devices with a psi of 10 or above

Media Link: Answers to the Chapter 10 Post-Test and more test questions together with rationales are provided on the CD-ROM.

■ References

Ackerly, B.J., & Ladwig, G.B. (2008). *Nursing diagnosis handbook: An evidence-based guide to planning care.* St. Louis, MO: Mosby Elsevier.

Aiello-Laws, L., & Rutledge, D.N. (2008). Management of adult patients receiving intraventricular chemotherapy for treatment of leptomeningeal metastasis. *Clinical Journal of Oncology Nursing, 12*(3), 429–435.

Alberts, D.S., Liu, P.Y., Hannigan, E.V., et al. (2006). Intraperitoneal cisplatin plus intravenous cyclophosphamide versus intravenous cisplatin plus intravenous cyclophosphamide for stage III ovarian cancer. *New England Journal of Medicine, 335*(26), 1950–1955.

Alhayki, M., Hopkins, L., & Le, T. (2006). Intraperitoneal chemotherapy for epithelial ovarian cancer. *Obstetrical and Gynecological Survey, 61*(8), 529–534.

American Heart Association. (2005). Advanced cardiac life support guidelines: management of cardiac arrest. *Circulation, 112-IV*, 57–66.

Armstrong, D.K., Bund, B.N., Wenzel, L., et al. (2006). Intraperitoneal cisplatin and paclitaxel in ovarian cancer. *New England Journal of Medicine, 345*(1), 34–43.

Aspden, P. (2006). Preventing medication errors: Quality chasm series. Institute of Medicine of the National Academies. Retrieved from www.iom.edu/en Reports/2006/Preventing-Medication Errors (Accessed October 10, 2009).

Berry, M., Bannister, L.H., & Standring, S.M. (1995). *Gray's anatomy* (38th ed., pp. 902–1397). New York: Churchill Livingtone.

Broyles, B.E., Reiss, B.S., & Evans, M.E., (2007). *Pharmacological aspects of nursing care* (7th ed.). Clifton Park, NY: Thomson Delmar Learning.

Camp-Sorrell, D. (2004). *Access device guidelines: Recommendations for nursing practice and education.* Pittsburgh, PA: Oncology Nursing Society.

Cannistra, S. (2006). Intraperitoneal chemotherapy comes of age. *New England Journal of Medicine, 354*(1), 77–79.

Carpenito-Moyet, L.J. (2008). *Nursing diagnosis: Application to clinical practice* (12th ed.). Philadelphia: Lippincott Williams & Wilkins.

D'Arcy, Y. (2008). Keep your patient safe during PCA. *Nursing 2008, 1*, 50–55.

Davidoff, J., Fowler, R., Gordon, D., et al. (2005). Clinical evaluation of a novel intraosseous device for adults: Prospective 250-patient, multi-center trial. *JEMS, 30*(Supplement 10), S20–S23.

de Caen, A. (2007). Venous access in the critically ill child when the peripheral intravenous fails! *Pediatric Emergency Care, 23*(6), 422–427.

Dedrick, R.L., Myers, C.E., Bungay, P.M., & DeVita, V.T., Jr. (1978). Pharmacokinetic rationale for peritoneal drug administration in the treatment of ovarian cancer. *Cancer Treatment Reports, 62*(1), 1–11.

DuPen, A. (2005). Care and management of intrathecal and epidural catheters. *Journal of Infusion Nursing, 28*(6), 377–381.

Dubick, M.A., & Holcomb, J.B. (2000). A review of intraosseous vascular access; current status and military applications. *Military Medicine, 165*, 552–559.

Ellemunter, H., Simma, B., & Trawoger, R., et al. (1999). Intraosseous lines in preterm and full term neonates. *Archives of Disease in Childhood Fetal Neonatal Edition, 80* (1), F74–F75.

Gahart, B.L., & Nazareno, A.R. (2008). *Intravenous medications* (20th ed.). St. Louis, MO: C.V. Mosby.

Giger, J.N., & Davidhizar, R.E. (2004). *Transcultural nursing: Assessment & intervention* (2nd ed.). St. Louis, MO: C.V. Mosby.

Gillum, L., & Kovar, J. (2005). Powered intraosseous access in the prehospital setting: MCHD EMS puts the EZ-IO to the test. *JEMS, 30*(Supplement 10), S24–S25.

Ghafoor, V.L., Epshteyn, M., Carlson, G.H., et al. (2007). Intrathecal drug therapy for long-term pain management. *American Journal of Health System Pharmacy, 64,* 2447–2460.

Gorski, L. (2005). *Pocket guide to home infusion therapy.* Sudbury, MA: Jones and Bartlett.

Hagle, M.E., Lehr, V., Brubakken, K., & Shippee, A. (2004). Respiratory depression in adult patients with intravenous patient-controlled analgesia. *Orthopedic Nursing, 23*(1), 18–27.

Hebl, J. (2006). The importance and implications of aseptic techniques during regional anesthesia. *Regional Anesthesia and Pain Medicine, 31*(4), 311–323.

Hydzik, C. (2007). Implementation of intraperitoneal chemotherapy for the treatment of ovarian cancer. *Clinical Journal of Oncology Nursing, 11*(2), 221–225.

Infusion Nurses Society (INS). (2006). Infusion nursing standards of practice. *Journal of Infusion Nursing, 29*(1S), S12–S78.

Institute of Medication Practices (ISMP). (2002). More on avoiding opiate toxicity with PCA by proxy. *Medication Safety Alert, 7*(15), 1–2.

Institute of Safe Medication Practices (ISMP). (2008). *Misprogramming PCA concentration leads to dosing errors.* Washington, DC: National Academy Press.

Johnson, K.S., & Sexton, D.J. (2006). Lumbar puncture: Technique, indications, contraindications and complications in adults. In: B.D. Rose (Ed.), *UpToDate Online 14.2.* Wellesley, MA: UpToDate.

Keck, S., Glennon, C., & Ginsberg, B. (2007). DepoDur extended-release epidural morphine: Reshaping postoperative care, what perioperative nurses need to know. *Orthopedic Nursing, 26*(2), 86–94.

Krames, E. (2002). Implantable devices for pain control: Spinal cord stimulation and intrathecal therapies. *Best Practice & Research Clinical Anaesthesiology, 16,* 619–649.

Landes, A.H. (2007). Intraosseous infusions: The current status. *The Journal for Critical Care Professionals, 23*(2), 53–57.

Maiskowski, C., Cleary, J., Burney, R., et al., (2005). *Guidelines for the management of cancer pain in adults and children.* APS Clinical Practice Guidelines Series, no. 3. Glenview, IL: American Pain Society.

Marders, J. (2004). PCA by proxy: Too much of a good thing. *Nursing 2004, 34*(4), 24.

Marin, K., Oleszewski, K., & Muehlbauer, P. (2007). Intraperitoneal chemotherapy: Implications beyond ovarian cancer. *Clinical Journal of Oncology Nursing, 11*(6), 8881–8889.

Markman, M., & Walker, J.M. (2006). Intraperitoneal chemotherapy of ovarian cancer: A review, with focus on practical aspects of treatment. *Journal of Clinical Oncology, 24*(6), 988–994.

Martinbiancho, J., Zuckermann, J., Dos Santos, L., & Silva, M.M. (2007). Profile of drug interactions in hospitalized children. *Pharmacy Practice, 5*(4), 157–161.

Miller, M., & Lehman, C. (2006). Computer based medication error reporting: Insights and implications. *Quality & Safety in HealthCare, 15*(3), 208–213.

McCloskey-Dochterman, J.C., & Bulechek, G.M. (2004). *Nursing interventions classification (NIC)* (4th ed.). St. Louis, MO: C.V. Mosby.

Moorhead, S., Johnson, M., & Maas, M. (2004). *Nursing outcomes classification (NOC)* (3rd ed.). St. Louis, MO: C.V. Mosby.

NANDA-I. (2007). *Nursing diagnoses: Definitions and classification, 2007–2008.* Philadelphia: Author

National Cancer Institute (NCI). (2006). NCI issues clinical announcement for preferred methods of treatment for advanced ovarian cancer. Retrieved from http://www.nih.gov/news/pr/jan2006/nci-04.htm (Accessed September 25, 2008).

National Association of EMS Physicians (NAEMSP). (2007). Position statement. Intraosseous vascular access in the out-of-hopsital setting. *Prehosptial Emergency Care, 11*(1), 62.

Nightingale, F. (1860). *Notes on nursing.* New York: Appleton & Co.

O'Grady, N.P., Alexander M. , Dellinger, E.P., et al. (2002). Guidelines for prevention of intravascular catheter-related infections. *Morbidity and Mortality Weekly Report MMWR, 51* (RR10).

Olsen, J., Giangrasso, A.P., Shrimpton, D.M. & Dillon, P.M. (2008). Medical dosage calculations (9th ed.). Upper Saddle River, NJ: Pearson Prentice Hall.

Potter, K.L., & Held-Warmkessel, J. (2007). Intraperitoneal chemotherapy for women with ovarian cancer: Nursing care and considerations. *Clinical Journal of Oncology Nursing, 12*(2), 265–271.

Reiss, B.S., & Evans, M. (2002). *Pharmacological aspects of nursing care* (pp. 236–239). Albany: Delmar.

Schwartz, A.J. (2006). Learning the essential of epidural anesthesia. *Nursing 2006, 36*(1), 44–49.

Sidebotham, D., Dijkhuizen, M., & Schug, S. (1997). The safety and utilization of patient-controlled analgesia. *Journal of Pain and Symptom Management, 14,* 202–209.

Slesak, G., Schnurle, J.W., Kinzel, E., et al. (2003). Comparison of subcutaneous and intravenous rehydration in geriatric patients: a randomized trial. *Journal of the American Geriatric Society, 51,* 155–160.

Swenson, K.K., & Erikson, J.H. (1986). Nursing management of intraperitoneal therapy. *Oncology Nursing Forum, 13*(5), 33–39.

The Joint Commission (TJC). (2004). Patient controlled analgesia by proxy. Sentinel Event Alert 33. Retrieved from http://www.jointcommision.org/Sentinel Events (Accessed September 27, 2008).

The Joint Commission (TJC). (2005). Preventing vincristine administration errors. Sentinel Event Alert 34. Retrieved from http://www.jointcommission.org/SentinelEvents/SentinelEventsAlert/sea_34.htm (Accessed September 26, 2008).

Teymoortash, A., & Werner, J.A. (2003). Selective intraarterial cisplatin chemotherapy in treatment of advanced malignant squamous cell carcinoma of the head and neck. *Cancer Therapy, 1,* 269–273.

Tsui, S., Irwin, M., Wong, C., et al. (1997). An audit of the safety of an acute pain service. *Anesthesia, 52,* 1042–1047.

Vaida, A.J., Grissinger, M., Urbanski, B., & Mitchell, J.F. (2007). *PCA drug libraries: Designing, implementing and analyzing CQI reports to optimize patient safety.*

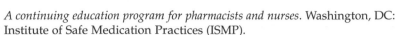

A continuing education program for pharmacists and nurses. Washington, DC: Institute of Safe Medication Practices (ISMP).

Vidacare Inc. (2008). Product information EZ-IO. San Antonio, TX: Vidacare Inc.

Vardi, A., Berkenstadt, H., Levin, I., et al. (2004). Intraosseous vascular access in the treatment of chemical warfare casualties assess by advanced simulation: Proposed alteration of treatment protocol. *Anesthesia and Analgesia, 98,* 1753–1758.

Walsh, G. (2005). Hypodermoclysis: An alternate method for rehydration in long-term care. *Journal of Infusion Nursing, 28*(2), 123–129.

Walther, K. (2007). Intraosseous vascular access. *Infusion Nurses Society Newsline, 29*(6), 9–10.

Wen, P., & Plotkin, S. (2006). Neurologic complications of cancer chemotherapy. In B.D. Rose (Ed.), *UpToDate Online 14.2.* Wellesley, MA: UpToDate.

Wilkinson, J.M., & Van Leuven, K. (2007). *Fundamentals of nursing: Theory, concepts & applications.* Philadelphia: F.A. Davis.

Younger, K. (2007). Promoting safe administration of subcutaneous infusions. *Nursing Standard, 21*(3), 50–56.

PROCEDURES DISPLAY 10-1

Administration of Medication by the Direct (I.V.) Push: Peripheral Catheter

Equipment Needed

General supplies:

Site disinfectant (alcohol, 2% chlorhexidine gluconate, or povidone-iodine)

Flush solution:

Preservative-free 0.9% sodium chloride, one 10-mL single-dose vial or prefilled saline syringes

Two or three 3-mL syringes (peripheral infusion)

Medication

Medication label

Filter needle (if drawing from glass vial)

Delegation:

This procedure **cannot** be delegated.

Procedure	Rationale
1. Check the authorized prescriber's order.	1. A written order is a legal requirement for infusion therapy.
2. Verify the allergy status of the patient.	2. This is a patient safety measure

Continued

PROCEDURES DISPLAY 10-1

Administration of Medication by The Direct (I.V.) Push: Peripheral Catheter—cont'd

Procedure	Rationale
3. Draw up sodium chloride/medication in syringes. ■ Draw up 2–3 mL of sodium chloride in each of two separate 3-mL syringes or use prefilled sodium chloride syringes. ■ Obtain medication from medication dispensing system. Dilute medication if appropriate with sodium chloride after checking compatibility. (Example: Morphine 5 mg/mL— dilute with 1 mL of NaCl to make a total volume of 2 mL) ■ Label syringes (medication syringe, each of two saline syringes) ■ Use a separate syringe for each medication if more than one is to be given. Label all.	3. Having all equipment at hand will save time and lessen patient anxiety. Prevention of medication errors (TJC, 2005)
NOTE: Pediatric doses must be verified by another RN before medication administration.	
4. Introduce yourself to the patient.	4. Establishes the nurse–patient relationship
5. Wash hands using friction for 15–20 seconds with an alcohol-based sanitizer	5. Good hand hygiene is the single most important means of preventing the spread of infection.

PROCEDURES DISPLAY 10-1

Administration of Medication by The Direct (I.V.) Push: Peripheral Catheter—cont'd

Procedure	Rationale
6. Verify patient identity using two forms (check ID bracelet and ask patient to state name).	6. The Joint Commission (2003) safety goal recommendation. Prepares the patient for procedure. Safety.
7. Explain the procedure to patient in terms the patient can understand. If pain medication is being delivered, assess pain level using scale and have patient describe pain. Assess the level of consciousness and vital signs if appropriate.	7. The patient has the right to know what medication is being administered and the right to refuse the medication. Establishes criteria for follow-up assessment and evaluation of drug response.
8. Don disposable gloves.	8. Barrier protection for the patient and the nurse
9. Cleanse the peripheral injection cap/valve with 70% isopropyl alcohol for 15 seconds using a twisting motion.	9. Assist in prevention of CR-BSI.
10. Insert the first syringe with sodium chloride and withdraw to check for brisk positive blood return to confirm patency. Slowly flush the solution. The catheter should not be forcibly flushed.	10. Clear the line of any medication, checks patency of the catheter and provides positve pressure in the line.
11. Disconnect the syringe from injection or access cap; discard.	11. Prepare to administer the medication
12. Disinfect the injection cap/valve with appropriate antiseptic solution using same technique as above. Insert medication syringe	12. Assist in prevention of CR-BSI

PROCEDURES DISPLAY 10-1

Administration of Medication by The Direct (I.V.) Push: Peripheral Catheter—cont'd

Procedure	Rationale
13. Slowly inject medication one-fourth volume at a time. Stop after every 0.5 mL and observe for reactions. Administration time should be a minimum of 1 minute. Some medicators require a longer administration time, check guidelines for all I.V. medications.	13. Slow injection provides time for the nurse to observe the patient for adverse effects. Always review medication guidelines for administration. (Example: Morphine 5 min by direct I.V. push)
NOTE: If administering medication with a running I.V. solution, the medication MUST be compatible with the I.V. solution, or the administration set needs to be clamped before the first flush.	
14. Disconnect the syringe from the injection or access cap; discard.	14. Prepares to perform final flush to remove any residual medication from the catheter and Luer-activated system (valve)
15. Disinfect the injection port again using the above technique and attach the second sodium chloride syringe. Slowly inject the sodium chloride after the medication administration to decrease the chance of a "bolus" of medication entering the patient's venous system. Depending on the type of access valve (positive displacement, negative displacement or neutral valve), use the appropriate technique for the last 0.5 mL of flush.	15. Positive pressure must be maintained within the lumen of the catheter during and following administration of a flush solution to prevent reflux of blood into the Luer-activated systems . Follow specific guidelines for postive displacement device.
	NOTE: The nurse MUST know which type of valve is being used.

PROCEDURES DISPLAY 10-1

Administration of Medication by The Direct (I.V.) Push: Peripheral Catheter—cont'd

Procedure	Rationale
15a. For negative-displacement devices (positive-pressure flushing required). As the last 0.5–1 mL of solution is flushed inward, withdraw the syringe, allowing the last amount of flush solutions to fill the dead space.	
15b. For Luer-activated systems negative displacement systems (positive-pressure flushing required). Flush all of the solution into the catheter lumen; maintain force on the syringe plunger as a clamp on the catheter or extension set is closed; then disconnect the syringe.	
NOTE: Negative- and positive-displacement devices are dependent on flushing technique.	
15c. Positive-displacement device (positive pressure flushing technique **cannot** be used—will overcome the positive displacement mechanism) Flush the catheter gently with solution, disconnect the syringe and allow sufficient time for the positive fluid displacement, then close the catheter clamp.	
16. Observe the patient for adverse effects.	**16.** Provides for patient safety

Continued

PROCEDURES DISPLAY 10-1

Administration of Medication by The Direct (I.V.) Push: Peripheral Catheter—cont'd

Procedure	Rationale
17. Discard all syringes in the appropriate biohazard container.	**17.** and **18.** OSHA standard, CDC guideline for prevention of infection.
18. Remove gloves and wash hands.	
19. Document the procedure.	**19.** Upholds the steps of the nursing process; provides a legal record.

PROCEDURES DISPLAY 10-2

Administration of Continuous Subcutaneous Infusion

Equipment Needed
Dressing materials—transparent semipermeable membrane (TSM)
Butterfly metal needle (21- to 25-gauge, ½ inch)
Syringe
Prepackaged dedicated subcutaneous set from manufacturer (if using instead of butterfly needles)
Antiseptic solution (chlorhexidine gluconate)
Prescribed fluids or prefilled medication container or cassette
Hyaluronidase or similar drug (to assist with absorption of medication if needed however is controversial)
Infusion pump
Delegation: This procedure can be delegated to LPN/LVN in some states that allow by nurse practice act to administer subcutaneous infusions for hypodermoclysis.

Procedure	Rationale
1. Check the authorized prescriber's order.	**1.** A written order is a legal requirement for infusion therapy.
2. Verify the allergy status of the patient.	**2.** This is a patient safety measure.

PROCEDURES DISPLAY 10-2

Administration of Continuous Subcutaneous Infusion—cont'd

Procedure	Rationale
3. Gather all equipment.	3. Having all equipment at hand will save time and lessen patient anxiety.
4. Introduce yourself to the patient.	4. Establishes the nurse–patient relationship.
5. Wash hands using friction for 15–20 seconds using an alcohol-based hand sanitizer.	5. Good hand hygiene is the single most important means of preventing the spread of infection.
6. Verify patient identity using two forms (check ID bracelet and ask patient to state name).	6. The Joint Commission (2003) safety goal recommendation. Prepares patient for procedure. Safety.
7. Explain the procedure to the patient in terms the patient can understand. Have the patient rate pain on scale of 1-10.	7. The patient has the right to know what medication is being administered and the right to refuse the medication. Establishes criteria for follow-up assessment and evaluation of drug response.
8. Select insertion site with adequate subcutaneous tissue: a fat fold of at least 1 inch (2.5 cm) when thumb and forefinger are pinched together. Site selection is also based on the patient's anticipated mobility and comfort.	8. Appropriate placement of access device for hypodermoclysis aids in delivery of solution and prevents complications.
NOTE: Avoid areas that are scarred, infected, irritated, edematous, bony, or highly vascularized.	
9. Don gloves.	9. Provides barrier protection for the patient and the nurse.

Continued

PROCEDURES DISPLAY 10-2

Administration of Continuous Subcutaneous Infusion—cont'd

Procedure	Rationale
10. Prime the administration tubing, or insert into pump.	10. Clear the line of any medication, checks patency of the catheter, and provides positve pressure in the line.
11. Wash the site with antiseptic soap and water as needed.	11. Assists in clean insertion site.
12. Disinfect the insertion site with chlorhexidine gluconate and let dry.	12. Assists in prevention of local infection or development of cellulitis.
13. Follow the manufacturer's labeled use and direction for access device placement.	
14. Lift the skin up into a small mound between the thumb and index finger.	
15. Insert the primed subcutaneous infusion system with attached access device into the skin at a 45-degree angle.	15. Ensure secure entry of the needle into the subcutaneous tissue and not deeper vascular tissue.
16. Check to make sure there is no blood present in set or cannula.	16. Indicates capillary has been punctured. The device should be removed and a new needle inserted into a new site.
17. Stabilize the access device, secure connection junctions, and apply TSM dressing over the site using transparent to allow for site observation and plapation.	17. Stabilize the catheter or needle to prevent dislocation, provide for site observation and moisture vapor permeability with TSM dressing.
18. Initiate therapy and adjust the rate.	18. To ensure timely and effective delivery of fluids or medications.
19. Do not flush subcutaneous infusion device postinfusion.	19. The needle or catheter is not in the vascular system. Flushing is not required postinfusion.

PROCEDURES DISPLAY 10-2

Administration of Continuous Subcutaneous Infusion—cont'd

Procedure	Rationale
20. Discard used equipment and supplies in the appropriate receptacle.	**20.** and **21.** OSHA standard
21. Remove gloves.	
22. Document in the patient's permanent medical record.	**22.** Upholds the steps of the nursing process; provides a legal record.

NOTE: Rotate the access site every 3–5 days. Change the dressing every 3–5 days. Monitor the access site and equipment; observe the site for bleeding, bruising, inflammation, drainage, edema or cellulitis. Monitor the patient for complaints of burning or itching.

Sources: INS (2006); Younger (2007).

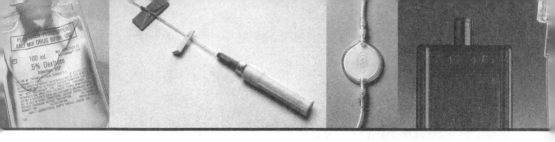

Chapter **11**

Transfusion Therapy

Blood—a gift of life
—Author Unknown

Chapter Contents

■ LEARNING
   OBJECTIVES

On completion of this chapter, the reader will be able to:

1. Define the glossary of terms as related to nursing care of patients receiving transfusion therapy.
2. Identify the antigens and antibodies in the blood system.
3. Identify the universal red blood cell donor type.
4. Identify the Rh antigens located on the red blood cells.
5. Identify the preservatives used in donor blood storage.
6. Summarize the tests used to screen donor blood.
7. Distinguish among homologous, autologous, and designated blood.
8. Describe each of the blood components, their indications, and key points in administration.
9. Describe the procedure for administration of blood components.
10. Establish a plan of action for a patient exhibiting symptoms of hemolytic transfusion, febrile transfusion, and mild allergic transfusion reactions.

▷ GLOSSARY

ABO system   Blood group of antigens that reside on structurally related carbohydrate molecules

ADSOL   Additive solution of 100 mL containing saline, dextrose, and adenine that is added to packed red blood cells

Agglutinin An antibody that causes clumping or agglutination of the cells that stimulated the formation of the agglutinin

Agglutinogen An antigenic substance that stimulates the formation of a particular agglutinin, that, under certain conditions, causes agglutination of the cells.

Allergic reaction Reaction from exposure to an antigen to which the person has become sensitized

Allogeneic Blood transfused to someone other than the donor

Alloimmunization Development of an immune response to alloantigens; occurs during pregnancy, blood transfusions, and organ transplantation

Antibody A substance produced by B lymphocytes in response to a unique antigen

Antigen A protein or oligosaccharide marker on the surface of cells that identifies the cell as self or non-self; identifies the type of cell and stimulates the production of antibodies by B lymphocytes

Autologous donation Originating within an individual, especially a factor present in tissues or fluids. Donation of a unit of blood to be reinfused if needed back to the original donor

Blood component Product made from a unit of whole blood such as platelet concentrate, red blood cells, fresh frozen plasma, or cryoprecipitate

Cryoprecipitate A plasma component rich in fibrinogen and other clotting factors.

Delayed transfusion reaction Adverse effect occurring after 48 hours and up to 180 days after transfusion

Directed/designated donation Use of blood or components from a specific donor for a specific patient

Febrile reaction Nonhemolytic reaction to antibodies formed against leukocytes

Fresh frozen plasma Collection of the fluid portion of the circulating blood by separation and freezing the plasma within 8 hours of collection

Hemoglobin Respiratory pigment of red blood cells having the reversible property of taking up oxygen or of releasing oxygen

Hemolysis Rupture of red blood cells, with the release of hemoglobin

Hemolytic transfusion reaction Blood transfusion reaction in which an antigen–antibody reaction in the recipient is caused by an incompatibility between red blood cell antigens and antibodies

Homologous donation Blood donation of serum or tissue derived from members of a single species

Human leukocyte antigen (HLA) Used for tissue typing and relevant for transplant histocompatibility

Hypothermia Abnormally low body temperature

Immunohematology Study of blood and blood reactions

Microaggregate   Microscopic collection of particles such as platelets, leukocytes, and fibrin that occurs in stored blood

Packed red cells   A blood product consisting of concentrated cells, most of the plasma having been removed

Pheresis   Derived from the Greek word *aphairesis*, meaning "to take away"; used to denote the removal of blood, the separation into component parts, the retention of only the parts needed, and the return of the rest to the donor (e.g., removal of plasma is plasmapheresis)

Plasma   Fluid portion of the blood, composed of a mixture of proteins in solution

Platelets   An irregularly shaped, disc-like cell that functions in clotting

Refractory   Not responsive or readily yielding to treatment

Rh system   Second most important system determining compatibility; Rh antigens are inherited and located on the surface of red blood cells; classified as positive or negative based on whether D antigen is present

Serum   Term used to describe plasma after fibrinogen has been removed

Thrombocytopenia   Abnormally small number of platelets in the blood

To ensure the delivery of safe transfusion therapy, nurses must possess a knowledge and understanding of the blood system as well as basic immunohematology. Nurses must also be knowledgeable about the theory and practical management of blood component therapy. The first part of this chapter presents fundamental concepts of immunohematology, blood grouping, and the criteria for donor blood, including homologous, designated, autologous, and donation. Fundamental concepts of blood component therapy, administration equipment, administration techniques for each blood component, and management of transfusion reactions are presented in the second part of the chapter.

> **INS Standard**   The RN administering transfusion therapy should have knowledge and understanding of immunohematology, blood grouping, blood and its components, administration equipment and techniques appropriate for each component, transfusion reactions and nursing interventions, and the risk to patient and the nurse. (INS, 2006, 70)

▪ Basic Immunohematology

Immunohematology is the science that deals with antigens of the blood and their antibodies. The antigens and antibodies are genetically inherited and determine each person's blood group. An **antigen** is a substance capable of stimulating the production of an antibody and then reacting with that antibody in a specific way. Antigens of the blood are called **agglutinogens**. Any substance that can elicit an immunologic response is an antigen, and is located on the cell membrane. Antigens are viewed as foreign substances when they enter the body (Cooling, 2008). The three antigens on the red blood cells (RBCs) that cause problems and are routinely tested for are A, B, and Rh D. The human leukocyte antigen (HLA) is located on most cells in the body except mature erythrocytes. Antibodies are found in the **plasma** or **serum**.

Antigens (Agglutinogens)

ABO System

The **ABO system** was developed in 1901 by Dr. Karl Landsteiner. The most significant antigens in the blood are the surface antigens A and B, which are located on the RBC membranes in the ABO system (Table 11-1). The name of the blood type is determined by the name of the antigen on the RBC. Individuals who have A antigen on the RBC membrane are classified as group A; B antigens, group B; A and B surface antigens, group AB; and neither A nor B antigens, group O. Table 11-2 provides an ABO compatibility chart.

Unique to the ABO system is the presence of antibody in the serum of persons who lack the corresponding antigen. That is to say, the antibody is present even when the body is not stimulated with the foreign antigen. These naturally occurring antibodies are responsible for the rapidity and

> Table 11-1 **ABO BLOOD GROUPING CHART**

Blood Groupings	Recipient Antigens on RBCs	Antibodies Present in Plasma
A	A	Anti-B
B	B	Anti-A
AB	A and B	None
O	None	Anti-A and Anti-B

> Table 11-2 **ABO COMPATIBILITIES FOR PACKED RED BLOOD CELL COMPONENTS**

Recipient	Donor Unit, First Choice	Donor Unit, Second Choice	Donor Unit, Third Choice
A+	A+	O+, A–	O–
B+	B+	O+, B–	O–
AB+	AB+	AB–, A+, B+	O+, A–, B–, O–
O+	O+	O–	—
A–	A–	O–	A+, O+
B–	B–	O–	B+, O+
AB–	AB–	A–, B–, O–	AB+, A+, B+, O+
O–	O–	O+	—

NOTE: The universal RBC donor is O negative; the universal recipient is AB positive.

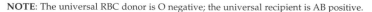

severity of reactions that occur when ABO-incompatible blood administered. This phenomenon occurs occasionally in other blood systems but
appears to be ubiquitous within the ABO system. As a result, if antigen A
is present on the RBC, then antibody to B (anti-B) is present in the serum.
If antigens A and B are present, no antibody exists in serum; conversely, if
no antigen is present, then both anti-A and anti-B are present in the
serum. Table 11-3 provides ABO compatibility for plasma.

CULTURAL AND ETHNIC CONSIDERATIONS: BLOOD TYPES AND RH FACTOR

Blood groups differentiate people in certain racial groups. A prevalence for type O blood has been found among Native Americans, with some
incidence of type A blood and virtually no incidence of type B blood. Almost
equal incidences of types A, B, and O blood occur in Japanese and Chinese
people while AB blood type occurs in only about 10% of this population.

African Americans and European Americans have been found to have
equal incidences of A, B, and O blood types, with predominant blood types
of A and O (Giger & Davidhizar, 2004).

Persons with type O blood are at a greater risk for duodenal ulcers, and
those with type A blood are more likely to develop cancer of the stomach.
The Rh-negative factor is most common in European Americans, much rarer
in other racial groups, and absent in Eskimos (Giger & Davidhizar, 2004).

Rh System

After A and B, the most significant RBC antigen is the D antigen, which
was discovered in 1940 by Drs. Landsteiner and Wiener. The **Rh system** is
so called because of its relationship to the substance in the RBCs of the
Rhesus monkey. There are approximately 50 Rh-related antigens; the five
principal antigens are D, C, E, c, and e. A person who has D antigen is
classified as Rh positive; one lacking D is Rh negative. A total of 85% of
the population is classified as D-Rh-positive (Westhoff, 2008). There are
no naturally occurring anti-D antibodies; however, D antibodies build up

> Table 11-3   **ABO COMPATIBILITY FOR FRESH FROZEN PLASMA**

Recipient	Donor Unit
A	A or AB
B	B or AB
AB	AB
O	O, A, B, or AB

easily in D-negative recipients when stimulated with D-positive blood. Therefore, typing is done to ensure that D-negative recipients receive D-negative blood. Because the Rh-antigen resides on the red cell, an Rh-negative recipient should receive Rh-negative blood if the components might contain RBCs. Table 11-4 lists the most common blood types.

HLA System

The HLA antigen was originally identified on leukocytes, but it has been established that **HLA** is present on most cells in the body. The HLA system includes a complex array of genes and their protein products. It is located on the surface of white blood cells (WBCs), platelets, and most tissue cells. HLA typing, or tissue typing, is important in patients with transplants or multiple transfusions and is used for identification in paternity testing. The HLA system is very complex and is involved in immune regulation and cellular differentiation.

The HLA system is important in transfusion therapy because HLA antigens and antibodies play a role in complications of transfusion therapy such as platelet refractoriness, febrile nonhemolytic transfusion reaction (FNHTRs), transfusion-related acute lung injury (TRALI), and post-transplant and post-transfusion graft-versus-host disease (GVHD). The HLA antigen of the donor unit can induce **alloimmunization** in the recipient. Methods used to decrease HLA alloimmunization include HLA matching and leukocyte depletion of the donor unit (Gebel, Pollack, & Bray, 2008).

The incidence of HLA alloimmunization and platelet refractoriness among patients receiving repeated transfusion ranges from 20% to 71% (AABB, 2008). In the refractory state platelet transfusions fail to increase the recipient's platelet count. HLA alloimmunization can be lessened with leukocyte-reduced blood components (Gebel, Pollock, & Bray, 2008). Blood may be depleted of leukocytes during three periods: (1) immediately after collection, (2) 6 to 24 hours after collection, and (3) at the time of infusion. The trend today is for prestorage leukocyte depletion of packed RBCs and

> Table 11-4   **MOST COMMON BLOOD TYPES**

Type	Percentage of U.S. Population
O Rh-positive	38
A Rh-positive	34
B Rh-positive	9
O Rh-negative	7
A Rh-negative	6
AB Rh-positive	3
B Rh-negative	2
AB Rh-negative	1

Source: AABB (2008).

platelets. Early removal of leukocytes reduces the development of cytokines that appear to be implicated in many transfusion reactions.

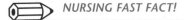 NURSING FAST FACT!

> Patients receiving multiple transfusions are at particular risk for developing complications related to leukocytes, such as sensitization to leukocyte antigens, nonhemolytic febrile reactions, transmission of leukocyte-mediated viruses, and graft-versus-host disease (Gebel, Pollack, & Bray, 2008).

Antibodies (Agglutinins)

An antibody is a protein that reacts with a specific antigen. Each blood **antibody** has the same name as the antigen with which it reacts. For example, anti-A reacts with antigen A. The antibodies anti-A and anti-B are produced spontaneously in the plasma after birth and usually mature in the first 3 months of life.

Antibodies of the blood system are **agglutinins**; that is, when stimulated by a specific antigen, they bind to the antigen to cause clumping. In the case of a red cell incompatibility, the interaction of the antibody with the like antigen (e.g., anti-B with antigen B) causes the red cells to clump together.

Antibodies, also known as **immunoglobulins** or immune antibodies, are a group of glycoproteins (i.e., complex molecules containing protein and sugar molecules) in the serum and tissues of mammals that have the ability to interact with foreign objects, such as bacteria or viruses, and neutralize them. There are five categories of immunoglobulin molecules in human blood: IgA, IgD, IgE, IgG, and IgM. These antibodies are classified as either complete or incomplete. The naturally occurring antibody in the blood, which occurs within the inherited blood group (ABO), is from the class of antibodies called immunoglobulin M (IgM). These antibodies have the ability to cause agglutination of blood cells even when suspended in saline. In vivo, these antibodies cause total cellular destruction and lead to intravascular hemolysis when stimulated by foreign antigen.

The other four antibody groups and some IgM antibodies are incomplete antibodies, meaning that they are not capable of causing agglutination in saline. These immunoglobulins are produced by the immune system in response to previous exposure to an antigen via previous transfusion or pregnancy; they are not genetically inherited. When these antibodies contact the corresponding antigen, the cells are affected but not destroyed in the intravascular system. The sensitized cells are removed intact by the reticuloendothelial system, primarily the spleen and liver (Porth & Martin, 2008).

Other Blood Group Systems

The International Society of Blood Transfusion (ISBT) recognized 29 blood group systems comprising a total of 302 specific genes. The ABO and Rh systems are best known and clinically most significant. The antigens of the H, Lewis, I, P, and globoside systems are carbohydrate structures that are biochemically closely related to ABO antigens. The most important aspect of blood groups in transfusion medicine is whether the antibodies are hemolytic and have potential to cause hemolytic transfusion reactions (HTRs) and hemolytic disease of the fetus and newborn. Other significant systems include the Lutheran, Kell, Duffy, Kidd, Diego, Scianna, Dombrock, Landsteiner-Wiener and Gerbick systems, to name a few (Daniels, 2008).

Pretransfusion Testing

At the time of donation, every unit of blood intended for **homologous (allogeneic) and directed** donation must undergo the following tests by the blood bank:

1. The ABO group must be determined by testing the RBCs with anti-A and anti-B serums and by testing the serum or plasma with A and B cells.
2. The Rh type must be determined with anti-D serum. Units that are D-positive must be labeled as Rh-positive.
3. Most blood banks test all donor blood for clinically significant antibodies. If all donors are not tested, then at least blood from donors with a history of previous transfusion or pregnancy should be tested for unexpected antibodies before the crossmatch.
4. All donor blood must be tested to detect transmissible disease. The blood component must not be used for transfusion unless the test results are nonreactive, negative, or within the normal range.
5. Each unit must be appropriately labeled. The label must include the following information: name of the component, type and amount of anticoagulant, volume of unit, required storage temperature, name and address of collecting facility, a reference to the circular of information, type of donor (i.e., volunteer, autologous), expiration date, and donor number (Fig. 11-1).

What anticoagulant used in PRBCs?

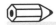 NURSING FAST FACT!

As of April 2006 the label must contain bar coded information about (1) the unique facility identifier (registration number), (2) the lot number relating to the donor, (3) the product code, and (4) the ABO group and Rh type of the donor. The four pieces of information must also be present in eye-readable format (FDA, 2006a).

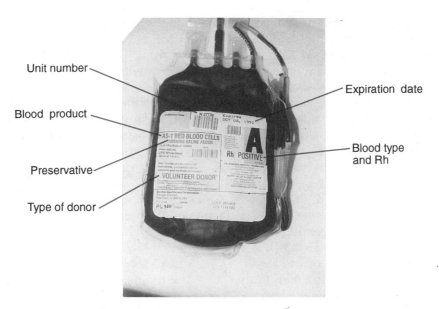

Unit number

Blood product

Preservative

Type of donor

Expiration date

Blood type and Rh

Figure 11-1 ■ Correct labeling of a unit of blood.

6. The facility performing the compatibility testing must do ABO and Rh grouping confirmation tests on a sample obtained from the originally attached segment of all units of whole blood or RBCs.

After blood is drawn from a donor, it is tested for ABO group (blood type) and Rh type (positive or negative), as well as for any unexpected RBC antibodies that may cause problems in the recipient. Screening tests are also performed for evidence of donor infection. The specific tests performed are:

Viruses:

■ Hepatitis B surface antigen (HBsAg)
■ Hepatitis B core antibody (anti-HBc)
■ Hepatitis C virus antibody (anti HCV)
■ HIV-1 and HIV-2 antibody (anti–HIV-1 and anti–HTVL-2)
■ Nucleic acid amplification testing (NAT) for HIV-1 and HCV
■ NAT for West Nile Virus (WNV)

Bacteria:

■ Serologic test for syphilis
■ Bacteria culture, isolation, and identification methods—all species (Fiebig & Busch, 2008)

Blood Preservatives

There are several available RBC preservatives. Understanding of the RBC preservative is necessary because adverse reactions may occur in some patients as a result of chemicals in the anticoagulant preservative solution. The solutions in the blood collection bag have a dual function: as anticoagulant and as RBC preservative. Citrate is used in all blood preservatives as an anticoagulant. Citrate binds with free calcium in the donor's plasma. Blood will not clot in the absence of free or ionized calcium. Citrate prevents coagulation by inhibiting the calcium-dependent steps of the coagulation cascade. Preservatives provide proper nutrients to maintain RBC viability, function, and metabolism. In addition, refrigeration at 1° to 6°C preserves RBCs and minimizes the proliferation of bacteria (Kakaiya, Aronson, & Julleis, 2008).

In 1971, citrate-phosphate-dextrose (CPD) became a common preservative for blood. Phosphate is added to buffer the decrease in pH. The compound in the RBC that facilitates the transport of oxygen is 2,3-diphosphoglycerate (2,3-DPG). When the pH of the blood drops, there is a decrease in 2,3-DPG and therefore a lowering of the oxygen-carrying capacity of the blood. The 2,3-DPG levels remain higher in blood stored in CPD than in that stored with adenine-citrate-dextrose preservative. The expiration of RBCs preserved in CPD is 21 days stored at 1° to 6°C. Additional approved anticoagulant preservatives include citrate-phosphate-dextrose-dextrose solution (CP2D) with a shelf life of 21 days and citrate-phosphate dextrose-adenine (CPDA-1), which was licensed in 1978 and contains 70 mL of anticoagulant-preservative in 500 mL of collected blood. This preservative contains adenine, which helps the RBCs synthesize adenosine triphosphate (ATP) during storage. Cells have improved viability in this anticoagulant preservative because the energy requirements of the cell are better preserved than with plain CPD. This preservative lengthens the shelf-life of the blood to 35 days at 1 to 6°C (Kakaiya, Aronson, & Julleis, 2008).

There are three forms of additive solution (AS) approved by the Food and Drug Administration (FDA): AS-1 **(ADSOL)**, AS-3 (Nutrice), and AS-5 (Optisol). The additive solution for red cell preservative system AS contains sodium chloride, dextrose, adenine, and other substances that support red cell survival and function up to 42 days. The volume of the AS in a 450-mL collection set is 100 mL. AS is added to the red cells remaining in the bag after most of the plasma has been removed (Kakaiya, Aronson, & Julleis, 2008).

NURSING FAST FACT!

RBCs prepared with AS-1, AS-3, and AS-5 have better flow rates and do not require dilution with saline. Hypocalcemia is an adverse reaction that can occur when large amounts of citrated blood are infused in a person with impaired liver function.

Blood Donor Collection Methods

Homologous/Allogeneic

The term **homologous** donation or allogeneic donors describes transfusion of any blood component that was donated by someone other than the recipient. Most transfusions depend on homologous sources and are provided by volunteer donors.

Guidelines for Homologous/Allogeneic Donation

Donor selection for homologous collection is based on a limited physical examination and a medical history to determine the safety of the donated unit. Strict criteria have been established for selection of prospective donors:

1. Donor History Questionnaire (DHQ). In October 2006, the FDA recognized the DHQ in a final guidance document that is currently used by the majority of blood centers in the United States (FDA, 2006b). An abbreviated donor history questionnaire is available for frequent donors.
2. Age: 17 years old without parenteral permission; some states allow 16 years old with parenteral permission.
3. Provisions must be made for donors not fluent in English or who are illiterate.

NOTE > Due to safety issues related to blood banking, the centers must consider interpreters during the donor interview. An interpreter could compromise the integrity of the health history due to misinterpretation of donor-sensitive information. The final authority for such decisions rests with the donor center's physician (AABB, 2008).

---

4. Provisions for donors who are hearing or vision impaired
5. Hemoglobin and hematocrit of at least 12.5 g/dL and 38%, respectively, in males and females
6. Weight (smaller volumes should be drawn from donors weighing less than 110 lbs.).
7. Vital signs: Blood pressure: systolic less than or equal to 180 mm Hg, diastolic less than or equal to 100 mm Hg and pulse 50 to 100 beats per minute
8. Temperature: Less than or equal to 37.5°C (99.5°F) measured orally
9. No evidence of skin lesions at site of venipuncture for blood collection
10. Has not donated blood or plasma within the last 8 weeks
11. Medications: The DHQ medication deferral list contains the required deferrals (Eder, 2008).

Figure 11-1 presents the necessary information on a unit of blood that is autologous donation.

Designated or Directed Donors

Directed donation refers to the donation of blood from selected friends or relatives of the patient. Most blood centers and hospitals provide this service. Designated donations have been requested more frequently because of the concern over the risk of transfusion-transmitted diseases. However, there is no evidence that directed donations are safer than blood provided by transfusion services (Eder, 2008). Relatives or friends who may be members of a risk group may feel forced into donating and hesitate to identify themselves as a risk group member. Figure 11-2 identifies the unit as designated or directed to a specific recipient.

Guidelines for Designated Donation

The selection and screening of directed donors are the same as for other homologous (allogeneic) donors, except that the units collected are labeled for a specific recipient. The designated donor must pass all the history and screening tests required, and the unit must be compatible with the intended recipient (Eder, 2008).

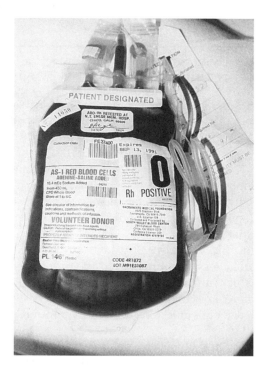

Figure 11-2 ■ Designated donor unit.

Autologous Donors

Autologous donation is the collection, storage, and delivery of a recipient's own blood. This option is considered for patients who are likely to receive a transfusion during elective surgery. In 2004, U.S. autologous collections comprised less than half a million units, or 2.0% of total blood collections. Decreased interest in autologous donations reflects the decline in viral risk associated with allogeneic blood transfusion and consequently the minimal medical benefit and increased cost of autologous blood (Schved, 2005). Patients may be able to donate their own blood up until 72 hours before surgery. The use of **autologous** blood avoids the possibility of alloimmunization because it does not contain foreign RBCs, platelets, and leukocyte antigens. The risk of exposure and disease transmission is also eliminated. Because of this, the use of autologous blood is regarded as safer than homologous transfusion. However, risks associated with labeling and documentation are still present. The same precautions used for preparing and administering a homologous **blood component** must be observed.

Donor Requirements

1. Age is the same as for allogeneic donor selection.
2. All blood collection shall be completed more than 72 hours before the time of surgery or transfusion.
3. Vital signs are the same as for allogeneic donor selection.
4. There is a deferral for conditions presenting risk of bacteremia.
5. Hemoglobin is greater than or equal to 11 g/dL or hematocrit value greater than or equal to 33%.
6. Must have a prescription or order from the patient's physician.
7. Candidates must be evaluated by the blood bank.
   (Eder, 2008)

ADVANTAGES

- Eliminates the risk of isoimmunization (sensitization to RBCs, platelets, and leukocyte antigens).
- Eliminates the risk of exposure to bloodborne infectious agents.
- Expands the blood resources.
- Reduces the need for homologous blood (decreases dependence on the volunteer donor supply).
- Provides an option for patients who find homologous transfusion unacceptable on religious grounds.
- Has a physiologic pH and higher levels of 2,3-DPG than does banked blood; 2,3-DPG increases the oxygen-carrying capacity of **hemoglobin**.
- Contains more viable RBCs than banked blood.

DISADVANTAGES

- Cost of predeposited autologous blood and increased paperwork due to special handling
- Used only For the donor-patient

Types

Three types of autologous blood donations are currently in use: (1) predeposit or preoperative (PAD), (2) intraoperative blood salvage (IBS), and (3) postoperative blood salvage (PBS).

PREOPERATIVE AUTOLOGOUS DONATION (PAD)

Predeposit or preoperative autologous blood donation is the collection and storage of the recipient's own blood for reinfusion during or after surgery several weeks before scheduled surgery. Patients need to receive erythropoietin to rebuild red cell mass before surgery. This blood is held for use for elective surgery. Intraoperative blood loss is unpredictable and half of the PD units are typically discarded. Donation without use presents a sizable waste of resources for many hospitals (Brecher & Goodnough, 2001).

Indication

- Elective surgical procedure with realistic possibility of transfusion

Typical Uses

- Hip or knee replacement surgery
- Elective cardiac surgery
- Spinal fusion
- Elective major vascular surgery
- Heart–lung transplant

Contraindications

- Hemoglobin less than 11 g/dL
- Bacterial infection
- Severe aortic stenosis
- Unstable angina
- Severe left main coronary artery disease

Disadvantages

- Relatively costly
- Risk of clerical error

INTRAOPERATIVE BLOOD SALVAGE (BLOOD RECOVERY)

Intraoperative blood salvage, or perioperative blood salvage or deposit, involves withdrawal of blood early in a procedure for use as a volume replacement later in the same procedure. Typically, two units of blood are collected early in the surgery from the surgical site. Shed blood can be readministered after concentrating and washing (washed recovered blood) with a blood recovery device, or it can be filtered and readministered (unwashed recovered blood). Unwashed recovered blood is usually reserved for the postoperative environment where small quantities of blood are collected and reinfused (Waters, 2008).

Indications
- Surgical procedure with anticipated major blood loss
- Patient unable to donate preoperatively

Typical Uses
- Cardiac surgery
- Major vascular surgery
- Revision hip replacement
- Spinal fusion
- Liver transplant
- Arteriovenous malfunction resection
- Trauma

Contraindications
- Malignancy at operative site
- Bacterial contamination at operative site
- Use of microfibrillar collagen materials

Advantages
- May be acceptable to patients opposed to transfusions for religious reasons.
- May eliminate need for allogeneic transfusion.
- Cost is approximately $150 for setup and technician time for processing.

Disadvantage
- Risk of air embolism and cell salvage syndrome

POSTOPERATIVE SALVAGE

Postoperative salvage involves the salvage of blood from the surgical field in a single-use, self-contained reservoir for immediate return and reinfusion to the patient. This technique is used most often after cardiac surgeries and, recently, with orthopedic surgeries.

Indication
- Substantial bleeding in postoperative period

Typical Uses
- Cardiac surgery
- Orthopedic surgery

Contraindication
- Same as for intraoperative blood collection

Advantage
- May decrease allogeneic transfusion in some clinical settings.

Disadvantages
- **Febrile reaction** to washed blood
- Cost increases if shed blood is washed
- Air embolism and cell salvage syndrome.

 NURSING FAST FACT!

Any autologous blood must be filtered during reinfusion to eliminate the possibility of microclots or debris being infused into the patient.

🗢 Blood Management

Blood management is an evidence-based, multidisciplinary process that is designed to promote the use of blood products throughout the hospital. The goal of blood management is to ensure the safe and efficient use of the many resources involved in the complex process of blood component therapy. Blood management includes nursing time, technician time, medical supplies, medical devices, laboratory tests, pharmaceuticals, hospital patients, and financial resources (Strategic Healthcare Group, 2008).

Transfusion of blood products is one of the most common interventions in the hospital setting. Twenty-nine million blood components are transfused each year, equating to nearly 80,000 blood components every day. Many blood components are not administered according to evidence-based practices, thereby consuming precious resources without benefit to patients (Boucher & Hannon, 2007). The following facts should be considered before transfusions:

- Transfusions are not risk free.
  Transfusions today are the safest in history; however, they can cause some degree of harm. The leading causes of transfusion-related morbidity and mortality are unrelated to viral transmission and include bacterial contamination of platelets, transfusion errors from patient misidentification, and transfusion-related acute lung injury. Blood transfusions can improve outcomes, but only when used in the right patient for the right indication and in the right dose (Boucher & Hannon, 2007).
- Blood is a liquid transplant.
  Infusing blood is not different from solid organ transplant. Blood transfusions can cause changes in the immune system function of patients, which presents a new set of immune challenges.

EBNP Based on controlled studies, the best evidence for transfusion therapy indicates that a more conservative approach to blood transfusion not only saves blood but also improves patient outcomes (Corwin, 2006).

- Transfusions can increase health-care–associated infections by 50% (Shorr, Duh, Kelly, et al., 2004).
- Transfusion education is limited. There are large gaps in education of physicians and nurses in ordering and administration of blood products (Corwin, 2006).
- Utilization of blood in the United States is significantly higher than in most other Western countries. Blood use in the United States increased by 16% over that in other Western countries from 1999 to 2004 (Wallis, Wells, & Chapman, 2006).
- Blood acquisition costs have more than doubled in the last few years and will continue to rise 5% to 10% per year as blood production costs increase and supply struggles to meet the increasing demand (Hannon & Paulson-Gjerde, 2005).
- The total cost of transfusing patients exceeds blood acquisition costs by five times (Hannon & Paulson-Gjerde, 2005).
- Emerging areas of medical-legal liability due to risk of exposure and potential liability relate to compliance with state, federal, The Joint Commission (TJC), and AABB regulations for blood component therapy. The Joint Commission National Patient Safety Goal no. 1 is to eliminate medication and transfusion errors. TJC included blood management performance measures as an element of hospital accreditation in 2009 (Boucher & Hannon, 2007).
- Financial penalties for poor clinical outcomes related to inappropriate transfusion practices are increasing. Beginning on October 1, 2008 Medicare and most commercial health insurance carriers will no longer pay for transfusion errors, bleeding complications in cardiac surgery, and a growing number of hospital-acquired infections that are increased two- to fivefold by blood transfusions.

Strategic Approach to Blood Management

Reduction in blood utilization with cost savings have been reported with use of Strategic Blood Management™ systems. The phases of blood management include:

1. Phase I: Strategic Blood Management Audit and Benchmarking
2. Phase II: Strategic Blood Management Program Development
3. Phase III: Strategic Blood Management Program Support

 Website:

Strategic Blood Management: www.bloodmanagement.com
Society for Advancement of Blood Management: www.sabm.org/ professionals

■ Blood Component Therapy

Blood is a "liquid organ" with functions as extraordinary and unique as those of any other body organ. Fifty-five (55) percent of blood is composed of plasma (fluid); the remaining cellular portion (45%) is made up of solids: RBCs, WBCs, and platelets.

Whole Blood

Whole blood is composed of RBCs, plasma, WBCs, and platelets. The volume of each unit is approximately 500 mL and consists of 200 mL of RBCs and 300 mL of plasma, with a minimum of 33% hematocrit. Whole blood is rarely available for allogeneic transfusion; RBCs and crystalloid solutions have become the standard for most cases of active bleeding in trauma and surgery with supplementation of hemostatic elements as needed.

Uses

Most whole blood units are now used to prepare separate RBC and plasma components to meet specific clinical needs. A whole blood unit can be centrifuged and separated into three components: RBCs, plasma, and platelet concentrates. By transfusing the patient with the specific component needed rather than with whole blood, the patient is not exposed to unnecessary portions of the blood product and valuable blood resources are conserved (Fig. 11-3).

Few conditions require transfusion of whole blood. A unit of whole blood increases RBC mass, which provides oxygen-carrying capacity and provides plasma for blood volume expansion. The major use of whole blood is for autologous transfusion.

 NURSING FAST FACT!

> *In an adult, 1 U of whole blood increases the hemoglobin by about 1 g/dL or the hematocrit by about 3%–4% (AuBuchon, 2008).*

Administration

- Amount: Volume of 500 mL
- Catheter size: 22- to 14-gauge with 20- to 18-gauge appropriate for general populations. With use of smaller gauge (22-gauge), blood dilution and a pump are helpful to administer the unit (AABB, 2008).
- Usual rate: 2 to 4 hours
- Administration set: Straight or Y type with 170- to 260-micron filter or microaggregate recipient set

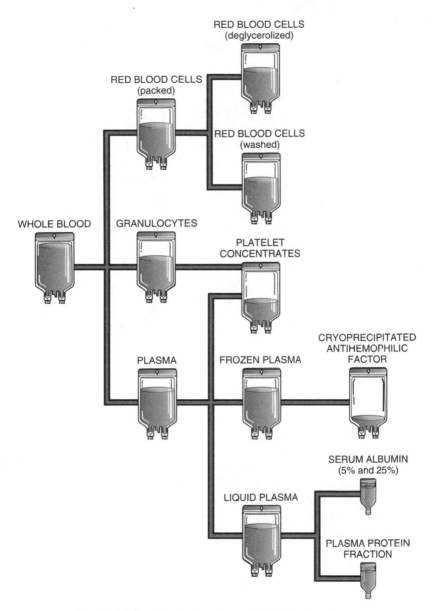

Figure 11-3 ■ Derivation of transfusible blood products.

Compatibility

Whole blood requires type and crossmatching and must be ABO identical.

Red Blood Cells

Red blood cell units are prepared by removing 200 to 250 mL of plasma from a whole blood unit. The remaining **packed red blood cells** (PRBCs) concentrate has a volume of approximately 300 mL. Each unit contains the same RBC mass as whole blood, as well as 20% to 30% of the original plasma, leukocytes, and some platelets. The advantages of RBCs over whole blood are decreased plasma volume and decreased risk of circulatory overload. Another advantage is that because most of the plasma has been removed, less citrate, potassium, ammonia, and other metabolic byproducts are transfused.

 NURSING FAST FACT!

> In a normal adult patient, 1 U of RBCs should raise the hemoglobin level approximately 1 g/dL and the hematocrit 3%, the same as with a unit of whole blood (AuBuchon, 2008).

Uses

Red blood cells are used to improve the oxygen-carrying capacity in patients with symptomatic anemia. The administration of RBCs should be considered only if improvement of the RBC count cannot be achieved through nutrition, drug therapy, or treatment of the underlying disease. A definitive **hemoglobin** and hematocrit threshold has not been established to determine when transfusion of RBCs is indicated or above which transfusion would be inappropriate. Criteria for transfusion are based on multiple variables, including hemoglobin and hematocrit levels, patient symptoms, amount and time frame of blood loss, and surgical procedures. Patients with chronic anemia should undergo transfusion only if they are symptomatic owing to a decrease in oxygen-carrying capacity: most patients adjust to the lower hemoglobin level and should not be exposed to transfusion-associated risks unless necessary. Even if large volumes of blood are lost, other components (e.g., platelets and plasma coagulation factors) can be provided rather than using whole blood (AuBuchon, 2008).

Administration of PRBC

- Acute anemia: Hypovolemia due to acute blood loss: hypotension and tachycardia not corrected by volume replacement
- Blood loss over 30% of blood volume for otherwise healthy patients

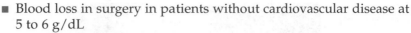

- Blood loss in surgery in patients without cardiovascular disease at 5 to 6 g/dL
- Hemoglobin of 7 g/dL in critically ill patients

> *EBNP A randomized controlled trial of 7 versus 10 g/dL hemoglobin triggers in critically ill patients showed that the lower trigger point reduced morbidity and mortality significantly overall. The conclusion was that a trigger of 7 g /dL hemoglobin was appropriate for critically ill patients except those with unstable cardiac situations (Vincent, Baron, Reinhart, et al., 2002).*

- Symptomatic anemia in a euvolemic patient (angina, syncope, congestive heart failure, transient ischemic attacks [TIAs], dyspnea, tachycardia)

Do not transfuse RBCs:
- For volume expansion
- In place of a hematinic (nonbiological compound for raising hemoglobin)
- To enhance wound healing
- To improve general well-being
  (AuBuchon, 2008).

ADMINISTRATION SUMMARY

- Amount of component: 250 to 300 mL
- Catheter size: 22- to 14-gauge with 20- to 18-gauge appropriate for general populations. With use of smaller gauge (22-gauge), blood dilution and a pump are helpful to administer the unit (AABB, 2008).
- Usual rate: 1½ to 2 hours per unit; maximum 4 hours. (If longer infusion times are required, the unit may be split and aliquots administered over 1.5–2 hours.)
- Administration set: Straight or Y type with 170- to 260-micron filter or microaggregate filter (Fig. 11-4)

Compatibility

RBCs must be ABO and Rh compatible.

Leukocyte-Reduced Red Blood Cells

Leukocyte-poor RBCs are grouped in a category referred to as modified blood products. A unit of whole blood contains more than 1 to 10×10^9 WBCs. Leukocyte-reduced PRBC are the result of removing the number of leukocytes in whole blood to 5×10^6. In the U.S., leukocyte reduction by filtration of RBCs must not result in a red cell loss greater than 15%; in addition, 40 g of hemoglobin must be present in each unit after leukocyte reduction.

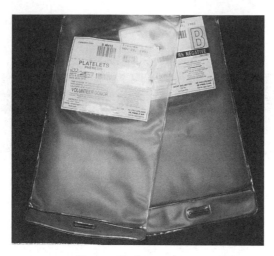

Figure 11-4 ■ Platelets.

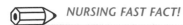 *NURSING FAST FACT!*

> *The leukocyte-reduced component will have therapeutic efficacy equal to at least 85% of that of the original component (Kakaiya, Aronson, & Julleis, 2008).*

Uses

Leukocyte-reduced components are indicated for patients who will receive multiple transfusions or patients requiring transplants. Leukocyte reduction as a means of preventing cytomegalovirus (CMV) transmission is well documented. These components may be beneficial in preventing HLA alloimmunization and in reducing transfusion-related immunomodulation but positive clinical effects from universal leukocyte reduction was not seen in the only large-scale, prospective, randomized trial of its implementation (Dzik, Anderson, O'Neill, et al., 2002).

> *EBNP A study by Preiksaitis (2000) demonstrated that leukocyte reduction prevented cytomegalovirus (CMV) transmission.*

Safety Concern: On rare occasions, patients may develop severe hypotension when leukocyte reduction is performed at the bedside. These reactions are due to the generation of bradykinin in the plasma as it passes over the filter medium. This reaction does not occur when leukocyte reduction is performed in the laboratory because bradykinin has a short half-life and is no longer active or present in the product by the time the patient receives it (Fitzpatrick, 2002).

Deglycerolized Red Blood Cells (Freezing RBCs)

Deglycerolized RBCs are prepared to allow for freezing of cells for long-term storage to increase the storage rate for rare units of RBCs (such as B negative) and autologous donor units. The RBCs are frozen after removal of the plasma and glycerol (a cryoprotective agent) is added. The RBCs are stored at –65°C. Glycerol enters the cell and protects the cell from damage caused by cellular dehydration and mechanical injury from ice formation. RBC units are usually placed in canisters to protect the polyolefin plastic bag during freezing, storage, and thawing.

To thaw the deglycerolized RBCs, the canister is placed in a 37°C dry heater or, after overwrapping, is placed in a 37°C waterbath. If the red cells have been frozen in the primary blood container then the container should be thawed at 42°C. Thawing should be complete within 40 minutes (Lockwood, Leonard, & Liles, 2008). The glycerol cryopreservative must be removed before the component is transfused. The removal is accomplished in a slow "deglycerolization" process to minimize hemolysis; it is performed using washing techniques. The manufacturer's instructions must be followed to ensure maximum red cell recovery and minimal hemolysis.

The shelf-life for thawed deglycerolized RBCs depends on the type of system used. Closed system devices allow storage for up to 14 days, but components prepared using open systems would expire within 24 hours of thawing.

Use: Special needs for rare donor antigen-negative units, autologous units

Irradiated Blood Products

Cellular components are required to be irradiated for certain patient populations to prevent transfusion-associated graft-versus-host disease. Irradiation is accomplished with the use of gamma irradiators, linear accelerators, ultraviolet-A irradiation, and other nonradioisotope equipment.

Uses

- Prevention of graft-versus-host disease (GVHD)
- Patients with acute leukemia and lymphoma (Hodgkin's disease and non-Hodgkin's disease)
- Bone marrow or stem cell transplant recipients
- Patients with immunodeficiency disorders
- Neonates and low-birthweight infants

 NURSING FAST FACT!

A label marked "irradiated" must be placed on the bag containing the product. Whole blood, red blood cells, platelets, or granulocytes can be irradiated.

■ **Safety Concern:** The shelf-life of irradiated red blood cells is limited to 28 days because irradiation damages the cells and reduces their viability (Lockwood, Leonard, & Liles, 2008). Platelets and granulocytes are not damaged, so their shelf-life is not affected.

RBC Rejuvenation

The use of an FDA-licensed solution of pyruvate-inosine-phosphate-adenine (PIPA) has been shown to restore the decreased levels of 2,3-DPG and adenosine triphosphate to normal in stored red cells. This solution has been licensed for use with citrate-phosphate-dextrose (CPD) and citrate-phosphate-dextrose-adenine-1 (CPDA-1) within 3 days after the expiration date of the original component, or at the 42-day expiration of CPD/AS-1 (Szymanski, Teno, Lockwood, et al., 2001).

Granulocytes

Granulocyte concentrations are prepared by leukopheresis from a single donor of whole blood. Each unit contains granulocytes and variable amounts of lymphocytes, platelets, and RBCs suspended in 200 to 300 mL of plasma. They are obtained for transfusion by the process of granulocytapheresis.

Hydroxyethyl starch (HES) may be used as a sediment agent; if used, residual HES will be present in the final component. Granulocyte infusions should be administered as soon after collection as possible because of the well-documented possibility of deterioration of granulocyte function during short-term storage. If stored, units should be maintained at 20 to 24°C without agitation and expire in 24 hours (Lockwood, Leonard, & Liles, 2008).

Uses

■ Patients with chronic granulomatous disease (CGD)

Compatibility

■ Neutropenic patients with absolute neutrophil counts <500
■ Neonates born prematurely or after prolonged premature rupture of membranes who are at increased risk for bacterial sepsis
■ Patients with severe infections who are unresponsive to conventional antibiotic therapy.

Administration of granulocytes is accompanied by a high frequency of nonhemolytic febrile reactions. These side effects can be managed with the use of diphenhydramine, steroids, and nonaspirin antipyretics and by slowing the transfusion rate. The transfusion should not be discontinued unless severe respiratory distress occurs (Kakaiya, Aronson, & Julleis, 2008).

Safety Concern: Granulocytes must be transfused before testing for infectious diseases can be completed. Authorization from the patient's physician is obtained to permit the transfusion before the testing of the current donation is completed.

Administration

There is no set standard regarding the amount or duration of granulocyte therapy, but generally transfusion therapy is delivered for at least 4 consecutive days.

- Amount: 300 to 400 mL suspended in 200 to 300 mL of plasma
- Catheter size: 22- to 14-gauge
- Usual rate: 1 to 2 hours; slower if reaction occurs (maximum of 4 hours)
- Administration set: Straight or Y type with 170-micron filter; microaggregate filter contraindicated
- Storage of unit is for the least time possible at room temperature without agitation

Compatibility

Must be compatible with the recipient's plasma.

Platelets

Platelets are normally suspended in plasma and are responsible for hemostasis. **Platelets** live up to 12 days in the blood, do not have nuclei, and are unable to reproduce. They contain no hemoglobin. Normal platelet counts are 150,000 to 300,000/µL. Platelets can be supplied as either random-donor concentrates or single-donor apheresis. Random-donor concentrates are prepared from individual units of whole blood by centrifuging the unit to separate the platelets. The platelets are stored at approximately room temperature, between 20 and 24°C for up to 7 days. To prevent agglutination of the cells, platelets must be continuously agitated during storage. The expiration date is 24 hours without agitation (Kakaiya, Aronson, & Jullieis, 2008). Single-donor platelet apheresis products are collected from a single donor. During **pheresis**, the platelets are harvested and all unneeded portions of the blood are returned back to the donor. A single pheresis unit is equivalent to 6 to 8 units of random donor platelets (Fig. 11-4).

The use of a single-donor unit has the obvious advantage of exposing the recipient to fewer donors and is ideal for treating patients who have developed HLA antibodies from previous transfusions and have become **refractory** (unresponsive) to random-donor platelets. HLA typing may be indicated when patients become refractory to platelets after multiple transfusions. Platelet crossmatch procedures are also being evaluated for their usefulness with refractory patients.

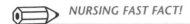 *NURSING FAST FACT!*

> *One platelet concentrate should raise the recipient's platelet count 5000–10,000/µL. The usual dose is 6–10 units of random or 1 unit of pheresis (AABB, 2008).*

Uses

Platelets are administered in the presence of **thrombocytopenia** to control or prevent bleeding from platelet deficiencies or to replace functionally abnormal platelets.

- 80% of platelet transfusions are given to patients with hypoproliferative thrombocytopenia.

Current prophylactic platelet transfusion triggers:

- Patients with acute thrombocytopenia: Platelet count less than 10,000/µL **OR**
- Stable patients with chronic thrombocytopenia: 5000/µL
- Patients with fever or recent hemorrhage (with bleeding controlled): 10,000/µL
- Patients with coagulopathy, on heparin, or with anatomic lesion likely to bleed: 20,000/µL

Platelet transfusions at higher platelet counts may be required for patients with systemic bleeding and for those at high risk for bleeding because of additional coagulation defects, sepsis, or platelet dysfunction related to medication or disease. Significant spontaneous bleeding with platelet counts above 20,000/µL is rare. Platelet transfusions are usually not effective in patients with conditions in which rapid platelet destruction occurs, such as those with idiopathic autoimmune thrombocytopenic purpura (ITP) and untreated disseminated intravascular coagulation (DIC). In patients with these conditions, platelet transfusions should be used only in the presence of active bleeding.

Do NOT transfuse platelets:

- To patients with ITP (unless there is life-threatening bleeding)
- Prophylactically with massive blood transfusions
- Prophylactically after cardiopulmonary bypass (AuBuchon, 2008)
- Transfusion in DIC remains controversial.

Administration

Single donor platelets are normally suspended in 40 to 70 mL of plasma, the volume of apheresed units is 350 to 500 mL total (plasma plus platelets). Platelets may be infused rapidly as the patient tolerates, with infusion rates ranging from 1 to 2 mL/min up to 5 min/single-donor bag. Platelets should be delivered to infants by means of a syringe-type device and can be transfused at a rate of 1 mL/min.

The effectiveness of platelet transfusions may be altered if fever, infection, or active bleeding is present. To determine the effectiveness of a transfusion, platelet counts may be checked at 1 hour and 24 hours after transfusion. Poor platelet count recovery may also indicate that the patient may be refractory to random donor platelets.

ADMINISTRATION SUMMARY

- Amount: 30 to 50 mL/unit; usual dose 6 to 8 units
- Catheter size: 22- to 14-gauge
- Usual rate: 1 unit in 5 to 10 minutes as tolerated
- Filter: 170-micron
- Administration set: Component syringe or Y drip set; tubing should be rubber free to prevent platelets from sticking; use 0.9% sodium chloride as primer

Platelet concentrates may be pooled before administration or infused individually; after they are pooled, platelets should be transfused within 4 hours

Safety Concern: HLA alloimmunization: Although patients receiving multiple platelet transfusions are usually immunosuppressed, they are still able to mount an immune response against antigens on platelets; antibodies to HLA antigens can occur (AuBuchon, 2008).

Compatibility

ABO-match is not required for the administration of platelets but is preferred. The amount of red cells and platelets harvested with the platelets is generally minimal but occasionally is sufficient to elicit an antigen–antibody response.

Plasma Derivatives

Plasma and Fresh Frozen Plasma

Plasma is the liquid portion of the blood in which nutrients are carried to body tissues and wastes are transported to areas of excretion. It is a colorless, thin, aqueous solution (91% water) that contains chemicals (bile pigments, bilirubin, electrolytes, enzymes, fats, and hormones), protein (7%), carbohydrates (2%), and clotting factors. When the clotting factors are removed, plasma is referred to as **serum**. Plasma does not contain any cellular portion of blood.

Fresh frozen plasma (FFP) is prepared from whole blood by separating and freezing the plasma within 8 hours of collection. FFP may be stored for up to 1 year at 18°C or lower. FFP stored at 65°C may be stored for up to 7 years. The volume of a typical unit is 200 to 250 mL. FFP does not provide platelets, and loss of factors V and VIII (i.e., the labile clotting factors) is minimal (Fig. 11-5).

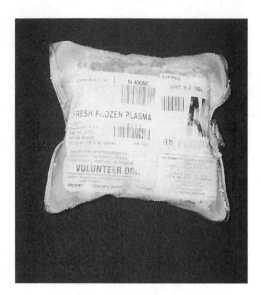

Figure 11-5 ▪ Plasma.

USES

- Limited to procoagulant deficiencies
- Disseminated intravascular coagulation (DIC)
- Massive transfusions in trauma

NOTE > The prothrombin time (PT) yields the most frequently abnormal results in patients with a potential coagulopathy and is the test most frequently consulted when deciding whether to transfuse plasma (AuBuchon, 2008).

 NURSING FAST FACT!

FFP contains optimal levels of all plasma clotting factors, with approximately 200 units of factor activity per bag and 200–400 mg of fibrinogen per bag (Kakaiya, Aronson, & Julleis, 2008).

ADMINISTRATION

Plasma must be frozen or administered within 8 hours of harvest to preserve labile coagulation factors. Plasma is administered at a rate of 200 mL/hr, unless there is a potential for fluid volume overload. Medications and diluents must never be added to plasma.

Fresh frozen plasma must be thawed in a 30 to 37°C water bath with gentle agitation or kneading. The thawing process takes up to 30 minutes, and the FFP should be transfused within 6 hours of thawing. FFP must be delivered through a standard blood filter. It can be infused as fast as the patient tolerates or condition indicates. The initial dose is 15 mL/kg. A rate of 4 to 10 mL/min has been suggested, and most units are generally completed within 1 to 2 hours.

Transfuse FFP:

- PT greater than 19
- To correct coagulation factor deficiencies in a bleeding patient with multiple coagulation factor deficits (e.g., liver disease, DIC, massive transfusion)
- Before an invasive procedure
- Warfarin overdose or vitamin K deficiency, when correction of coagulopathy is needed within 12 to 24 hours
- Replacement fluid in thrombotic thrombocytopenic purpura (TTP)

Do not transfuse FFP:

- For volume expansion
- As a nutritional supplement

Administration Summary

- Amount: 200 to 300 mL
- Catheter size: 22- to 18-gauge
- Usual rate: 1 to 2 hours
- Administration set: Straight or Y type with a 170-micron filter, primed with 0.9% sodium chloride

COMPATIBILITY

Must be compatible with the recipient's red cells.

Safety Concern: Not appropriate as volume expander (Stansworth, Brunsill, & Hyde, 2004). Acute allergic reactions are not uncommon, especially with rapid infusions.

Cryoprecipitate

Cryoprecipitate is the insoluble portion of plasma that remains as a white precipitate after FFP is thawed at 4°C under special conditions. The cold-insoluble precipitate is refrozen. Cryoprecipitate has a shelf life of 1 year and contains concentrated factor VIII: C; factor VIII: vWF (von Willebrand factor); fibrinogen; and factor XIII. It is the only concentrated source of fibrinogen and used for its fibrinogen content in today's practice. The frozen component is thawed in a protective plastic overwrap in a water bath at 30 to 37°C up to 15 minutes. It should not be used if there is evidence of container breakage or thawing during storage.

◁▭▷ *NURSING FAST FACT!*

- *Do not refreeze after thawing.*
- *Good patient management requires that the cryoprecipitate antihemophilic factor (AHF) treatment responses of factor VIII–deficient recipients be monitored with periodic plasma factor VIII: C assays*

USES

- Main use today: As a source of fibrinogen in acquired coagulopathies: DIC, massive hemorrhage
- As an alternative to factor VIII concentrate in the treatment of inherited deficiencies of:
  von Willebrand factor
  Factor VIII (Hemophilia A)
  Factor XIII

ADMINISTRATION

Cryoprecipitate is thawed before being transfused and must be used within 6 hours. It is usually supplied as a single donor pack or a pack of 6 or more single donor units that have been pooled. The inside of the bag should be rinsed with a small amount of saline to maximize recovery. Cryoprecipitate should be administered through a standard blood filter and, as with platelet administration sets, small priming volumes are recommended to decrease loss of the product in the set. Cryoprecipitate should be transfused as rapidly as the patient can tolerate. The cryoprecipitate units are usually pooled to simplify administration, but pooling of cryoprecipitate is not universally done.

Administration Summary
- Amount: 10 to 15 mL of diluent added to precipitate (3 to 5 mL) unit; usual dose 6 to 10 units
- Catheter size: 22- to 18-gauge
- Usual rate: 1 to 2 mL/min
- Administration set: Component syringe or standard blood component set, with 170-micron filter primed with 0.9% sodium chloride

COMPATIBILITY

Compatibility testing is not done, but the cryoprecipitate should be ABO compatible with the patient's RBCs because a very small volume of plasma is present. If the patient's blood group is not known, group AB is preferred, but any group can be given in an emergency because the plasma volume is small. Rh matching is not required.

Albumin

Albumin is a plasma protein that supplies 80% of the osmotic activity of plasma and is the principal product of fractionation (dividing plasma into its component parts). It is administered as plasma protein fraction (PPF) and as purified albumin. Both products (albumin and PPF) are derived from donor plasma, prepared by the cold alcohol fractionation process, and then subsequently heated. Both products do not transmit viral diseases because of the extended heating process. Normal serum albumin is composed of 96% albumin and 4% globulin and other proteins. It is available as a 5% or 25% solution.

NOTE > Additional information on albumin as a plasma expander is provided in Chapter 5.

Plasma Protein Fraction

Plasma protein fraction (PPF) is a similar product to albumin except that it is subjected to fewer purification steps in the fractionation process and contains about 83% albumin and 17% globulin. PPF is available only in a 5% solution.

USES

PPF and 5% albumin are isotonic solutions and therefore are osmotically equivalent to an equal volume of plasma. They cause a plasma volume increase, are used interchangeably, and share the same clinical uses. Both are used primarily to increase plasma volume resulting from sudden loss of intravascular volume as seen in patients with hypovolemic shock from trauma or surgery. Their use may also be indicated in individual cases to support blood pressure during hypotensive episodes or induce diuresis in those with fluid overload by assisting in fluid mobilization. The plasma derivatives lack clotting factors and other plasma proteins and therefore should not be considered plasma substitutes. Neither component (albumin or PPF) will correct nutritional deficits or chronic hypoalbuminemia.

Twenty-five percent albumin is hypertonic and is five times more concentrated than 5% albumin. This hyperosmotic product is used to draw fluids out of tissues and body cavities into intravascular spaces. This solution must be given with caution. Principal uses for 25% albumin include plasma volume expansion, hypovolemic shock, burns, and prevention or treatment of cerebral edema.

 NURSING FAST FACT!

Albumin 25% must not be used in dehydrated patients without supplemental fluids or in those at risk for circulatory overload.

ADMINISTRATION

Albumin and PPF are supplied in glass bottles. Depending on the brand, albumin in 5% concentrations is available in units of 50, 250, and 500 mL, and concentrations of 25% are supplied in units of 20, 50, and 100 mL. Manufacturers recommend that the solution be used within 4 hours of opening. Depending on the manufacturer, the solutions are sometimes supplied with an infusion set. If no I.V. set is provided, standard I.V. tubing without a filter is used. Blood transfusion sets and filters are not required for infusion of albumin.

Albumin, 5% and 25%, may be given as rapidly as the patient tolerates for reduced blood volumes. When the blood volume is normal or only slightly reduced, rates of 2 to 4 mL/min have been suggested for 5% albumin, and 1 mL/min for 25% albumin. More caution is used when infusing PPF because hypotension may occur with a rate greater than 10 mL/min (AABB, 2008).

Administration Summary
- Amount: 5% solution = 250 mL; 25% solution = 50 to 100 mL
- Catheter size: 22- to 18-gauge
- Usual rate: 5% solution: 2 to 4 mL/min; 25% solution: 1 mL/min
- Administration set: May come with administration set in package.

COMPATIBILITY

ABO or Rh matching and compatibility testing are not necessary for these components because antigens and antibodies are not present in these products.

A summary of blood components is listed in Table 11-5.

Clotting Factor Concentrates

Factor concentrates fall into two broad categories: plasma-derived and recombinant DNA technology–derived. The second generation of recombinant products provides smaller volume for patients with hemophilia, reducing the risk of fluid overload. Recombinant DNA technology–derived products are growing. Recombinant products are thought to have a safety and purity advantage because human plasma is not used in their manufacture, and DNA technology produces a specific coagulation replacement protein (Schaefer, 2002).

Administration

- Usually administered by bolus infusion in the home care environment.
- The package contains the vial of lyophilized (freeze dried) product and vial of diluent.
- Store in refrigerator or at room temperature (as directed by the manufacturer); shelf-life up to 2 years.

Safety Concern: A potential side effect of recombinant products includes any allergic reaction that would be typical of blood transfusion.

Factor VIIa

The production of the activated form of coagulation factor VIIA through recombinant technology has led to recombinant activated factor VII (rFVIIa) and has dramatically altered and improved the therapy of bleeding (AuBuchon, 2008). The use of a transfusion medicine specialist may be helpful in guiding the use of this product.

> Table 11-5   SUMMARY OF COMMON BLOOD COMPONENTS

Blood Component	Volume	Action and Use	Infusion Guide	Special Considerations
RBCs	250–300 mL	Improved oxygen-carrying capacity in patients with symptomatic anemia, aplastic anemia, bone marrow failure caused by malignancy, or chemotherapy	0.9% sodium chloride primer; transfuse in 4 hours; use standard 170-micron Y administration set. Recommend leukocyte reduction filter	AB and Rh compatible; 1 unit raises the hemoglobin 1 g and hematocrit 3%–4%
Irradiated RBCs	200–250 mL	Prevent graft-vs.-host disease in immunocompromised patients. Patients with immunodeficiencies, neonates and low birth weight infants.	Same as for RBCs	Same as for RBCs
Deglycerolized RBCs (frozen)	200–250 mL	Prolonged storage of blood for rare blood types and autologous donations; minimizes allergic reactions. Used for special needs antigen-negative donors.	Same as for whole blood; infuse within 4 hours	Must be used within 24 hours of being thawed and deglycerolized (open system), and 14 days in a closed system
Granulocytes	Prepared by leukapheresis 300–400 mL **Note:** Suspended in 200–250 mL of plasma	Patients with granulomatous disease. For neutropenia, fever, or significant infection unresponsive to antibiotics and for neonates	Usually administered for 4 consecutive days Standard blood filter; administer slowly over 1–2 hours, slower if reactions occur. As soon as collected or at least within 24 hours	ABO-/Rh-compatible; reactions common Check vital signs every 15 minutes **Note:** Febrile reactions occur in about two thirds of patients; chills, fever, and allergic reactions are common. Requires premedication to control reactions

Continued

> Table 11-5 SUMMARY OF COMMON BLOOD COMPONENTS—cont'd

Blood Component	Volume	Action and Use	Infusion Guide	Special Considerations
Platelets, Random Donor	40–70 mL/unit Usual dose: 6–10 units. Transfusions may be repeated every 1–3 days.	Control or prevent bleeding associated with platelet deficiencies, thrombocytopenia. Today 80% of platelet transfusions given to hypoproliferatiave thrombocytopenia.	Administer as rapidly as patient can tolerate: usually 1–2 mL/min Use blood filter, syringe push, or standard Y administration set; leukocyte depletion filter for platelets as ordered. **Note:** RBC leukocyte filters cannot be used with platelets.	Infuse individually or may be pooled; requires 20 minutes' pooling time by laboratory; ABO/Rh preferred but not necessary Prophylactic medication with antihistamines; antipyretics may be needed to decrease the incidence of chills, fever, and allergic reactions.
Platelets, Pheresis	Equivalent to 6 units from random donors	Same as for random donor; consider for patients anticipated to receive multiple long-term transfusions to limit exposure to multiple donors and reduce incidence of refractoriness.	Same as for random-donor platelets	Same as for random-donor platelets
Fresh Frozen Plasma (FFP)	Prepared from whole blood. 200–250 mL. Can be stored up to 1 year.	Replacement of clotting factors in patients with a demonstrated deficiency or for single-factor deficiency when concentrate not available. Transfuse FFP Prothrombin time >19 To correct coagulation deficiencies Before an invasive procedure Warfarin overdose.	Standard blood filter; may be infused rapidly: 20 mL over 3 minutes or more slowly within 4 hours	Does not provide platelets 1 unit (200 mL) raises the level of clotting factor 2%–3%; requires 20 minutes thawing time by laboratory Must be AB compatible

Cryoprecipitate	Each unit contains factor VIII, vWF, factor XIII, fibrinogen 15 mL plasma (5–10 mL/unit). Usual order is for 6–10 unit	Main use today as a source of fibrinogen in acquired coagulopathies: DIC, massive hemorrhage. As an alternative to factor VIII	Standard blood filter or component syringe; administer as fast as patient tolerates, 10–15 mL of diluent added to each unit. Rate 1–2 mL/min	ABO compatible with patient's RBCs; if blood group unknown, use AB blood; Rh matching not required. Infuse within 6 hours of thawing; saline may be added to bag to facilitate recovery of product.
Albumin (5% = 12.5 g/250 mL; 25% = 12.5 g/50 mL)	5% solution is in concentration of 250 mL or 500 mL; 25% solution is in 50–100 mL concentration	Plasma volume expander. For hypovolemic shock. Supports blood pressure during hypotensive episodes; induces diuresis in fluid overload	May be administered as rapidly as tolerated for reduced blood volume. Normal rates: 2–4 mL/min for 5% solution; 1 mL/min for 25% solution. Supplied in glass bottles with tubing for administration	25% albumin is hypertonic and is five times more concentrated than 5% solutions. Give with extreme caution; can cause circulatory overload. No type and crossmatching necessary; store at room temperature
Plasma Protein Fraction (PPF; 5% solution)	Glass 250-mL bottle with tubing (83% albumin, 17% globulin)	Same as for albumin. Osmotically equal to plasma	Equivalent to 5% albumin	Has fewer purification steps than albumin; no type and cross-matching necessary; has high sodium content

USES

- Life-threatening bleeding that is difficult to control
- Hemophilia or factor VII deficiency
- Counteracts the effect of warfarin
- Use in trauma, liver transplantation, and massive transfusion
- Liver biopsy

DISADVANTAGE

- Cost

Factor VIII

Factor VIII is partially purified factor VIII prepared from large pools of donor plasma. Patients have been maintained on regular prophylactic doses of factor VIII to reduce the risk of spontaneous hemorrhage and to preserve joint function, although the value of this practice has been difficult to prove due to small studies (Stobart, Iorio, & Wu, 2006).

USE

- Hemophilia A

Safety Concern: Development of antibodies against factor VIII

NOTE > The advent of recombinant factor VIIa has been used over factor VIII to improve the treatment of bleeding in hemophilia A (AuBuchon, 2008).

Factor IX Recombinant and Prothrombin Complex Concentrate

Procoagulants that require vitamin K for appropriate activity (factors II [prothrombin], VII, IX, and X) are called the vitamin K–dependent factors. Factor IX complex concentrate (recombinant) and prothrombin complex concentrate (PCC) are available.

USES

- Hemophilia B (Christmas disease)
- Immediate correction of prolonged prothrombin time

Safety Concern: Development of thrombosis. PCC is not advised in patients with liver disease or thrombotic tendency.

Immunoglobulins

Intravenous Immune Globulin

Concentrates of plasma immunoglobulins were developed in the early 1980s to treat congenital immunodeficiencies and certain viral exposures by the intravenous route. A variety of chemical modifications has allowed the development of IVIG preparations that have low proportions of aggregates. These preparations allow the administration of larger quantities over shorter intervals to achieve more pronounced clinical effects. Approximately 70% of patients receive treatment in a hospital inpatient/outpatient setting, and 20% in the home care setting. The administration of IVIG in a hospital usually takes longer because patients must be admitted, and the pharmacy does not mix the medication until I.V. access is achieved (Duff, 2006). Subcutaneous infusion of IgG products can be an alternative for patients who experience severe side effects from IVIG, have poor venous access, or have difficulty maintaining adequate trough levels throughout the interval treatment period (Kirmse, 2006). In January of 2006 the first subcutaneous IgG product, Vivaglobin 16% (ALB Behring), was approved for use in patients with primary immune deficiency diseases (PIDD).

Uses

- Reduce infections in immunodeficient patients
- Primary immune deficiencies
- Secondary (acquired) immune deficiencies (multiple myeloma, reduction of bacterial infection in pediatric AIDS)
- Immune cytopenias
- Presumed autoimmune disorders (Kawasaki's disease, Guillain-Barré syndrome, multiple sclerosis, myasthenia gravis, dermatomyositis, systemic vasculitides, factor VIII inhibitors)
- Prevention/treatment of infections
- Other immunologic conditions (graft-versus-host disease, asthma, myocarditis, inflammatory bowel disease, Stevens–Johnson syndrome)
- Other conditions: Alzheimer's disease, atherosclerosis, autism, chronic fatigue syndrome, multifocal motor neuropathy (AuBuchon, 2008)

Administration

- Assess for fluid status.
- Rotate I.V. sites if possible.
- Administer at room temperature.
- Administer through a dedicated I.V. line: Do not mix with other medications or piggyback into other infusions.
- Reconstitute medication only after I.V. access is established.
- Use I.V. tubing with product packaging if included. Some formulations will also require filtration.
- Premedications are sometimes ordered as a precaution.
- Use a large vein due to the relative concentration of the product.

- Most infusions are over 2 to 4 hours. Follow the manufacturer's recommendations for maximum rates.
- Monitor vital signs throughout the infusion.

NOTE > Not all IVIGs are the same, and each product must follow the manufacturer's recommendations for administration.

DISADVANTAGE

- Cost significantly higher than subcutaneous or intramuscular formulations (Kirmse, 2006)

Safety Concern: Infusion-associated allergic reactions (e.g., fever, chills, facial flushing, tachycardia, dyspnea, wheezing). Other associations: volume overload, stroke, venous thromboembolism, DICC, nephrotoxicity, neutropenia.

NOTE > Products contain a black box warning that fatal acute hemolysis may occur.

◾ Alternatives to Blood Transfusions

Alternatives to blood transfusion focuses on management of anemia and blood loss prevention. Many new strategies are now being used in blood management due to the shortages in the U.S. blood supply, risks associated with blood transfusions, and lack of evidence in efficacy of blood transfusions under certain conditions, along with blood product ordering practice inconsistencies. Interest in alternatives and adjuncts to transfusion therapy is incorporated into new dedicated blood management programs (Tolich, 2008). The following are some of the alternatives to blood transfusions or transfusion augmentations.

1. Augmentation of volume with colloid solutions
2. Autologous cell salvage
3. RBC substitutes
4. Modified hemoglobin or hemoglobin-based oxygen carriers (HBOCs) made from human, animal, or genetically engineered (recombinant) hemoglobin
5. Perfluorocarbons (PFCs)
6. Erythropoietic-stimulating agents (ESAs)
7. White cell growth factors
8. Hematinics

Augmentation of Volume with Colloid Solutions

Using allogenic blood to maintain blood volume is not appropriate; plasma expanders can be used for this purpose. Crystalloid and colloid volume expanders are discussed in Chapter 5.

Autologous Cell Salvage

Cell salvage refers to the collection of blood that would otherwise be lost during a surgical procedure. Collection systems remove debris and return the blood to the patient. The process rinses out clotting factors, which limits the usefulness of this procedure. However, autologous blood transfusion through cell salvage is an option. Collected blood cannot be stored for more than 6 hours (Kirschman, 2004).

RBC Substitutes

A variety of means have been explored to provide the oxygen-carrying capacity of hemoglobin without using red cells. Hemoglobin solutions in which the hemoglobin molecules have undergone one or more chemical modifications to optimize their oxygen and plasma retention characteristic are in clinical trials (AuBuchon, 2008).

Oxygen Therapeutics

Modified hemoglobin or hemoglobin-based oxygen carriers (HBOCs) are made from human, animal or genetically engineered (recombinant) hemoglobin.

Artificial blood is supposed to fulfill some functions of biological blood in humans. The term "oxygen therapeutic" is more accurate, as human blood performs other functions besides carrying oxygen. Hemoglobin is the main component of RBCs. Hemoglobin-based products are called HBOCs. However, pure hemoglobin separated from red cells cannot be used because it causes renal toxicity. Several HBOCs are in clinical trials. Hemopure (Biopure Corp.) is a chemically stabilized, cross-linked bovine hemoglobin suspended in saline solution. Hemopure™ molecules can be up to 1,000 times smaller than RBCs, facilitating oxygen transport. Additional HBOCs include PolyHeme™ (Northfield Laboratories, Inc.), Hemospan™ (Sangart), and HemoBiotech™ (Texas Tech) (Henkel-Hank & Oleck, 2007).

Perfluorocarbons

Perfluorocarbons (PFCs) will not mix with blood; therefore emulsions must be made by dispersing small drops of PFCs in water. PFC particles are about 40 times smaller than the diameter of a red blood cell. This small size can enable PFC particles to traverse capillaries. PFC solutions have oxygen-carrying capacity. The first PFC-based product was Fluosol-DA-20, approved by FDA in 1989 and withdrawn in 1994. Oxygent (Alliance Pharmaceuticals) and Oxycyte (Synthetic Blood International) are in clinical trials in the United States (Henkel-Hank & Oleck, 2007).

Erythropoietic Stimulating Agents

Erythropoietin is an endogenous hormone secreted by the kidneys that stimulates RBC production in the bone marrow. Recombinant human erythropoietin, which can be given intravenously or subcutaneously, is generally well tolerated and effective (Kirschman, 2004). Erythropoietin has been successfully used for dialysis patients who experience anemia due to kidney disease. It can increase a patient's hemoglobin before a surgical procedure where major blood loss is anticipated, and is used for patients receiving chemotherapy for malignancy. The FDA has recently alerted practitioners that erythropoietin should be used at the lowest possible dosage due to thromboembolic risks (Waters, 2008).

White Cell Growth Factors

Recombinant hematopoietic growth factor (G-CSF) is used to stimulate the production of granulocytes. Patients receiving chemotherapy have seen the greatest benefit of these medications. A dangerously decreased white cell count is a dose-limiting side effect of many cancer drugs. G-CSF products help maintain levels at near-normal levels, allowing patients to continue to receive scheduled doses of chemotherapy. Homologous or autologous donors can be stimulated to produce a higher yield of leukocytes, lymphocytes, and hematopoietic progenitor cells. When administered with oral dexamethasone or prednisone 12 hours before apheresis an optimal yield of granulocytes can be anticipated (Bishton & Chopra, 2004).

Hematinics

Hematinics are medications that are not biological products or substitutes but are able to increase cell efficiency by pharmacological means such as oral iron therapy. Some of these medications can raise a patient's hemoglobin level 2 g/dL over 3 weeks, reducing the need for transfusion in some cases (Kirschman, 2004).

 Websites

Synthetic Blood International, Inc.: www.sybd.com
Network for Advancement of Transfusion Alternative: www.nataonline.com

> Table 11-6	STEPS IN THE ADMINISTRATION OF A BLOOD COMPONENT

Step 1: Recipient consent
Step 2: Verify the authorized prescriber's order
Step 3: Pretransfusion
Step 4: Venous access, selecting and preparing the equipment
Step 5: Assessment and education of the patient
Step 6: Dispensing and transportation of the component
Step 7: Initiating the transfusion
Step 8: Monitoring the transfusion
Step 9: Completing the transfusion

■ Administration of Blood Components

The procedure for obtaining a blood component from a hospital blood bank varies from institution to institution. Regardless of the specific institutional procedure, certain essential guidelines must be followed (Table 11-6).

Step 1: Recipient Consent

Recipient consent for transfusion must be obtained from patients who are competent to make such decisions. Documents of informed consent must contain indications, risks, possible side effects, and alternatives to transfusion with allogeneic blood components.

INS Standard Informed consent of the patient or a legally authorized representative shall be obtained prior to the administration of transfusion therapy and shall be documented in the patient's permanent medical record. (INS, 2006, 70)

Step 2: Verifying the Authorized Prescriber's Order

An order for the blood component is required. The order should specify:
- The patient's name and other identifiers
- The component to transfuse
- Any special processing required for the component (e.g., washing, irradiation or filtration)
- The number of units or volume to be administered
- Date and time of infusion
- Flow rate or duration of the transfusion (up to 4 hours)

NOTE > When multiple types of components are transfused, the order should specify the sequence in which they are to be transfused. Orders must specify any premedications that are to be given before transfusion.

INS Standard The administration of transfusion therapy shall be initiated upon the order of a physician or an authorized prescriber by the rules and regulations promulgated by the state Board of Nursing. (INS, 2006, 70)

Step 3: Pretransfusion

Laboratory Testing

Once the order has been obtained, the transfusion service initiates a series of steps to ensure the provision of compatible components. The laboratory must have a sample of the patient's blood, which must be drawn within 3 days of the individual being transfused; the draw date is considered day 0 (AABB, 2008).

Identification Wristband

Most transfusion agencies require patients to be identified with an arm band that matches the recipient to the intended product. Bar-code–based ID systems are available for safety in transfusion.

Testing of Transfusion Recipient's Blood Specimen

ABO group and Rh type must be determined in order to transfuse ABO- and Rh-compatible components. The serum or plasma of the recipient must be tested for expected and unexpected antibodies before components containing red cells are issued for transfusion (AABB, 2008). ABO "forward typing" is the process in which the recipient RBCs are mixed with anti-A or anti-B. This process identifies the antigens present in the RBCs by visually apparent agglutination of the cells when the antibody combines with its corresponding antigen. ABO "reverse typing" is the testing of the recipient's serum for the presence of predicted ABO antibodies by adding RBCs of a known ABO type to it.

Rh typing of both recipient and donor blood is accomplished by testing the RBCs against anti-D serum. If agglutination occurs, the RBCs possess the D antigen and the blood is Rh-positive. If no agglutination is apparent, the RBCs must be tested further to rule out the presence of the weakly expressed D antigen, called weak D (formerly referred to as D). This antigen can be identified most reliably by indirect antiglobulin testing (IAT) after incubating the RBCs with anti-D sera. RBCs that possess the weak D are given to Rh-positive recipients (Downes & Shulman, 2008).

Compatibility testing is performed between the recipient's plasma and the donor's RBCs to ensure that the specific unit intended for transfusion to the recipient is not incompatible. Blood samples from the donor and recipient are mixed and incubated under a variety of conditions and suspending medium. If the recipient's blood does not agglutinate the donor cells, compatibility is indicated. Blood bank personnel are responsible for providing serologically compatible blood for transfusion.

When testing is complete, transfusion therapy can begin. The blood bank has two objectives: (1) to prevent antigen–antibody reactions in the body and (2) to identify an antibody that the recipient may have and supply blood from a donor who lacks the corresponding antigen. The testing of donor blood and recipient blood is intended to prevent adverse effects of transfusion therapy.

Labeling of Blood and Blood Components with the Recipient's Information

At the time of issue, the following must be in place:
- A tag or label indicating the recipient's two independent identifiers, the donor unit number, and the compatibility test interpretation, if performed, must be attached securely to the blood container.
- A final check of records maintained in the blood bank for each unit of blood or component
  - Two independent identifiers, one of which is usually the patient's name
  - The recipient's ABO group and Rh type
  - The donor unit or pool ID number
  - Donor's ABO group, and if required, Rh type
  - The interpretation of the crossmatch tests (if performed)
  - The date and time of issue
  - Special transfusion requirements (e.g., cytomegalovirus reduced risk, irradiated, or antigen-negative)
- A process must exist to confirm that the identifying information, the request, the records, and the blood or component are all in agreement, and that any and all discrepancies have been resolved before issue (Downes & Shulman, 2008).

Step 4: Venous Access; Selecting and Preparing the Equipment

It is important for the transfusionist to determine whether a central or peripheral intravenous line is in place and if it is acceptable for infusion of blood components. Selecting the proper equipment includes catheter and solution selection and obtaining administration sets, special filters, blood warmers, and electronic monitoring devices.

Venous Access

The recommendation for catheter size is dependent on how quickly the blood needs to be administered. A 20- to 18-gauge catheter is the catheter of choice for peripheral infusions in most situations. The use of PICC for administration of blood is dependent on the catheter gauge and the manufacturer's recommendations for use of infusion device. Sluggish flow rates with smaller PICCs have been documented (Houck & Whiteford, 2007).

NOTE > It is important that vascular access has been obtained before the component is received at the patient's bedside.

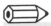 *NURSING FAST FACT!*

> Forcing blood through a tiny or damaged catheter may cause lysis of the cells.
> If the patient requires medication or solution administration while the blood component is being administered, a second I.V. site should be initiated.

Equipment

SOLUTION

No medication or solution other than 0.9% sodium chloride injection (USP) should be administered simultaneously with blood components through the same tubing (AABB, 2008). The use of dextrose in water or hypotonic solutions can cause RBC hemolysis due to cell swelling. Another concern with dextrose solutions is a condition known as Rouleaux syndrome, in which red cells adhere together like a stack of coins. Lactated Ringer's solution is not recommended because it contains enough ionized calcium to overcome the anticoagulant effect of CPDA-1 and allows small clots to develop.

INS Standard   No medications or solutions should be added to blood and blood components other than preservative-free 0.9% sodium chloride (USP). (INS, 2006, 70)

NOTE > AABB Standards (2008) allows exceptions to the above restrictions when
1. The drug or solution has been approved by the FDA for use with blood administration.
2. There is documentation in the literature to show that the addition is safe and does not adversely affect the blood components.

EBNP Yousef, Padmore, Neurah, & Rock (2006) studied the effect of patient-controlled analgesia on coadministered red blood cells and the literature supports the safe use of morphine and hydromorphone (Abbott Laboratories) as a bolus in the same tubing as red cells.

ADMINISTRATION SETS

Blood administration sets are available as a two-lead Y-type tubing or as single-lead tubing. Y-type administration sets allow for infusion of 0.9% sodium chloride before and after each blood component. A Y-type set also allows for dilution of RBCs that are too viscous to be transfused at an appropriate rate, by allowing for sterile transfer of saline into the unit. Platelets and cryoprecipitate should be infused through a filter similar to the standard blood filter but with a smaller drip chamber and shorter tubing so that less priming volume is needed. A syringe device designed specifically for platelets, and cryoprecipitate may also be used to administer these products.

Blood administration sets come with an inline filter. Most routine blood filters have a pore size of 170 to 260 microns designed to remove the debris that accumulates in stored blood. It is necessary to fill the filter chamber completely to use all the surface area. Red cell filters are designed to filter 1 unit of whole blood or packed red blood cells. Filters used for platelets and cryoprecipitate may be used to administer multiple units. Filters are changed for two reasons: debris in the blood clogs the filter pores, slowing the rate, and the risk of bacterial contamination increases when filter-trapped blood particles are maintained at room temperature.

INS Standard   Blood and blood components should be filtered. The maximum time for use of a blood filter is 4 hours.

Administration sets used for blood and blood components shall be changed immediately upon suspected contamination or when the integrity of the product or systems has been compromised. (INS, 2006, 48)

The Centers for Disease Control and Prevention (2002) recommends replacing tubing used to administer blood, blood products, or lipid emulsions (those combined with amino acids and glucose in a 3:1 admixture or infused separately) within 24 hours of initiating the infusion to prevent catheter-related bloodstream infections (O'Grady, Alexander, Dellinger, et al., 2002).

SPECIAL FILTERS

Microaggregate filters are second-generation filters used to help reduce adverse reactions. These filters come already incorporated into the tubing or may be added to a standard administration set. Microaggregate filters are designed to remove 20- to 40-micron particles, filtering out the microaggregates that develop in stored blood. Microaggregates consist primarily of degenerated platelets, leukocytes, and strands of fibrin and microaggregate filters are used for reinfusion of shed autologous blood collected during or after surgery which has a high risk of containing such debris. Refer to Figure 11-6.

Leukocyte-depleting filters are third-generation filters used for the delivery of RBCs and platelets. Refer to Figure 11-7. Filtration may occur immediately after blood collection in the blood bank or at the time of administration.

These filters are capable of removing more than 99.9% of the leukocytes present in the unit. They were developed in response to data supporting clinical benefits associated with the administration of leukocyte-poor blood products. HLA immunization (alloimmunization) is directly linked to the number of leukocytes present in a blood product. The benefits of leukocyte depletion include prevention of HLA alloimmunization, nonhemolytic transfusion reactions, and leukocyte-mediated viral transmission. However, prestorage removal of leukocytes eliminates the phagocytic property of blood. Since platelets are stored at room temperature, the risk of bacterial growth is increased. Nonetheless, leukocyte depletion is commonly performed on platelets and red cells 4 to 6 hours after donation. Leukocyte depletion is not performed on blood that will be stored as whole blood. If prestorage reduction is not performed it can be done at the bedside. These filters are more expensive than standard blood filters and require a physician's order before use. When using microaggregate- or leukocyte-removal filters, follow the manufacturer's recommendations regarding the number of units that can be filtered through one filter (Sink, 2008).

BLOOD WARMERS

Blood warmers are rarely needed during routine transfusion therapy. Warmers are useful when rapid transfusion of components is required, especially in trauma or surgery settings. They are also useful for transfusions to neonates or patients with cold agglutinin syndrome.

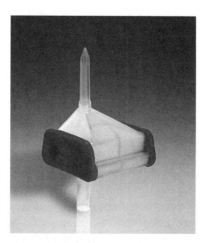

Figure 11-6 ■ SQ40S microaggregate blood filter for red cell transfusion. (Courtesy of Pall Medical, Ann Arbor, MI.)

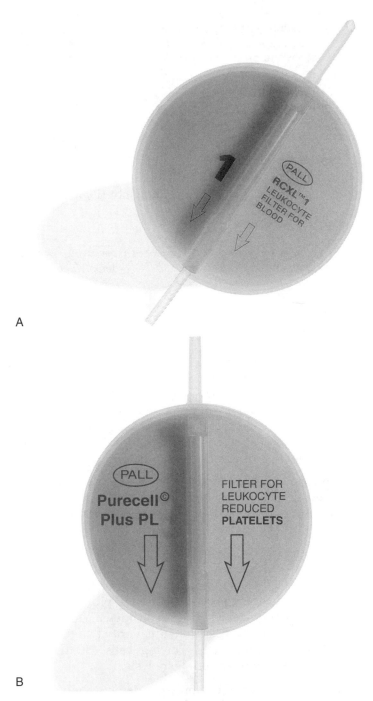

Figure 11-7 ■ *A*, RCXL™1 leukocyte reduction filter for red cell transfusion. *B*, Purecell Plus PL® leukocyte reduction filter for platelets. (Courtesy of Pall Medical, Ann Arbor, MI.)

NOTE > AABB (2008) states "warming devices shall be equipped with a temperature sensing device and a warning system to detect malfunctions and prevent hemolysis or other damage."

The manufacturer's guidelines should be adhered to when using any of the many types of blood and fluid warmers. The temperature control should not warm the blood or fluid above 42°C (AABB, 2008).

INS Standard   Blood warmers should be used for large volumes or rapid transfusions, exchange transfusions, and patients with clinically significant conditions requiring this modality. (INS, 2006, 2000, 7075)

 NURSING FAST FACT!

Blood components should NEVER be placed in microwave ovens or hot water baths because of damage to RBCs and the lack of temperature control, which may cause fatal complications for the patient.

ELECTRONIC INFUSION DEVICE

Some transfusions may require an electronic monitoring device to control the blood flow. Only pumps designed for the infusion of whole blood and RBCs may be used because other types of infusion pumps may cause hemolysis. Pumps require the use of pump-compatible tubing. Little if any increased hemolysis occurs secondary to the use of most infusion pumps. A pump's manufacturer should be consulted for detailed information on the pump's suitability for transfusing blood components.

INS Standard   The manufacturer's labeled use and directions should be followed in the use of positive-pressure electronic infusion devices for blood and blood component administration. (INS, 2006, 70)

PRESSURE DEVICES

The use of an externally applied pneumatic pressure device may achieve flow rates of 70 to 300 mL per minute depending on the pressure applied. The use of pressure devices has been reported to provide only a small increment in component flow rates. This is considered a safe practice in the majority of red cell transfusions. Before use, verify that the I.V. access device is functioning appropriately. Forcing cells through a damaged catheter may increase the risk of cell hemolysis.

INS Standard   External compression devices should be equipped with a pressure gauge and should exert uniform pressure against all parts of the blood container. (INS, 2006, 70)

> **NOTE** > When rapid infusion is desired, an increase in cannula size typically provides better results.

Step 5: Preparing the Patient

Patient preparation begins when the transfusion of a blood component is anticipated. Urgency factors related to the transfusion may affect the amount of time available to prepare the patient for the transfusion. The steps of the nursing process are activated, including assessment and the establishment of new goals and interventions related to the transfusion.

Patient/Family Education

The patient's and the patient's family's understanding of the need for blood, the procedure, and related concerns need to be assessed. Concerns are typically expressed regarding the risks of disease transmission; these need to be addressed.

The patient should be instructed regarding the length of time for the procedure and the need for monitoring his or her vital signs and physical condition. Signs and symptoms that may be associated with a complication of the component to be given should be explained to the patient and family members. It is not necessary to offer graphic explanations regarding symptoms; rather, a brief description of possible symptoms should be provided and the patient should be asked to report any different sensations after the transfusion has been started. Because transfusions typically take several hours, preparation also includes making the patient physically comfortable.

Assessment

Preparation includes a thorough assessment of the patient. Baseline vital signs should be taken before initiation of the transfusion. If the vital signs are abnormal, consult with the physician before initiating the transfusion. An elevated temperature may destroy cellular components at an increased rate and mask symptoms of a transfusion reaction (Klein & Anstee, 2005).

Assessment of the lungs and kidney function should be documented before transfusion. The nurse should review the laboratory data (hemoglobin [Hgb], hematocrit [Hct], platelets, clotting times) and anticipate how the component to be administered will affect these values over the next 24 hours. Premedication with diuretics, antihistamines, or antipyretics may be necessary to help keep the vital signs at an acceptable level. The patient should also be questioned regarding any symptoms he or she may be experiencing that could be confused with a transfusion reaction.

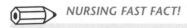

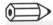 *NURSING FAST FACT!*

Patient education and assessment should be documented in the chart.

The patient should also be assessed for any symptoms that could later be confused as a transfusion reaction (e.g., rash, fever, shortness of breath, lower back pain). A transfusion record and report form are helpful for recording component specifics, vital signs, administration specifics, and reactions (Fig. 11-7).

Step 6: Dispensing and Transportation of the Component

As a rule, except in emergency situations, if blood is obtained from an on-site blood bank, only one product will be issued at a time and must be initiated within 30 minutes or returned to blood bank for proper storage (Sink, 2008). The blood component should not be obtained until the patient is ready to receive the component. If blood is obtained from an off-site blood bank, multiple units may be issued at one time. These units will be packaged to provide optimum storage conditions, and time limits for safe initiation will be detailed by the blood bank.

Placing a unit of blood in the nursing unit refrigerator is not acceptable practice. Most refrigerators cannot ensure the rigid temperature controls required to prevent storage lesions. Accidental freezing can destroy the unit. If the transfusion will be initiated within 30 minutes, the blood should be left at room temperature. If a longer period of time will pass (for alternate sites), the blood should be continued to be stored in the container in which it was sent.

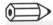 *NURSING FAST FACT!*

Refrigerators on the units may not be used to store blood products.

Proper identification is essential to ensure that the blood component is going to the intended recipient. Several items must always be verified and recorded before the transfusion is initiated.

- The order should always be verified before the component is picked up.
- When the blood is issued, the intended recipient's two independent identifiers should be verified (name, date of birth, or patient identification number and/or unique identifier given at the time the crossmatch sample is drawn).
- Verify the donor unit or pool identification number, donor ABO group, and, if required, the Rh type.

- The notation of ABO group and Rh type must be the same on the primary blood bag label as on the transfusion form. This information is to be recorded on the attached compatibility tag or label.
- The donor number must be identically recorded on the label of the blood bag, the transfusion form, and the attached compatibility tag.
- The color, appearance, and expiration date of the component must be checked.
- The name of the person issuing the blood, the name of the person to whom the blood is issued, and the date and time of issue must be recorded. Often this is in a book in the laboratory.

Step 7: Initiation of the Transfusion

The identification of the unit and the recipient must be verified by two licensed nurses before initiation of the transfusion. Refer to Figure 11-8.

INS Standard   Validation by a second clinician or caregiver shall be employed in the positive identification of the recipient and the blood product. (INS, 2006, 70)

The transfusion check between two nurses includes:
- *Prescriber's order*: Check the blood or component against the prescriber's written order to verify that the correct component and amount are being given.
- *Recipient identification:* The name and identification number on the patient's identification band must be identical with the name and number attached to the unit.
- *Unit identification:* The unit identification number on the blood container, the transfusion form, and the tag attached to the unit must agree.
- *ABO and Rh type:* The ABO and Rh type on the primary label of the donor unit must agree with those recorded on the transfusion form.
- *Expiration:* The expiration date and time of the donor unit should be verified as acceptable.
- *Compatibility:* The interpretation of compatibility testing must be recorded on the transfusion form and on the tag attached to the unit.

 NURSING FAST FACT!

> *It is helpful if one nurse reads the information for verification to the other nurse; errors can be made if both nurses look at the tags together.*
> *Unless the exact time is given, the component expires at midnight on the expiration date.*
> *Watch for any discrepancies during any part of the identification process; the transfusion should not be initiated until the blood bank is notified and any discrepancies are resolved.*

BLOOD TRANSFUSION RECORD

Resident's name: _____ ID #: _____

| Transfusion visit | Date: _____ Start time: _____ Completion time: _____ Nurse: _____

Blood component: Unit # _____ ABO type _____ Rh _____ Exp. date _____

Unit # _____ ABO type _____ Rh _____ Exp. date _____

Component: ❏ Intact ❏ not intact   Transport Temp: At Blood Bank ____ Time _____ At infusion site ____ Time _____

Unit(s) match order: ❏ Yes ❏ No _____

Unit(s) match Blood Bank tag: ❏ Yes ❏ No _____

Unit(s) match resident identification band: ❏ Yes ❏ No _____

Identification band on resident's wrist or ankle: ❏ Yes ❏ No _____

Pre-Medication ❏ Yes ❏ No   Drug   Dose   Route   Time

Anaphylaxis kit present: ❏ Yes   Exp. Date _____ ❏ No   Explain _____

Transfusion start: Unit # _____ Time _____ Unit # _____ Time _____

Vital signs (15 minute intervals recommended up to 30 minutes post-transfusion)

Time	BP	Temp	Pulse	Resp	Observations

Symptom	Pre-transfusion		During/Post	Time	Observation/Treatment
Fever	❏ Yes	❏ No	❏ Yes		
Chills	❏ Yes	❏ No	❏ Yes		
Hives/rash	❏ Yes	❏ No	❏ Yes		
Itching	❏ Yes	❏ No	❏ Yes		
Dyspnea/SOB	❏ Yes	❏ No	❏ Yes		
Chest pain	❏ Yes	❏ No	❏ Yes		
Hypotension	❏ Yes	❏ No	❏ Yes		
Tachycardia	❏ Yes	❏ No	❏ Yes		
Bradycardia	❏ Yes	❏ No	❏ Yes		
Other	❏ Yes	❏ No	❏ Yes		

Nurse Signature: _____ Date/Time: _____

| Post transfusion follow-up | Resident's response: ❏ Tolerated without complications ❏ Post-transfusion reaction noted

Remarks: _____

❏ Lab tests drawn

	Date	Time	Test	Result

Figure 11-8 ■ Transfusion record. (Courtesy of Lynda Cook, CRNI, and Linda Timmons, CRNI.)

Use good hand hygiene and follow Standard Precautions when administering blood components. Wear gloves! When using a Y-type blood set, spike one port with 0.9% sodium chloride and prime the tubing, being sure to saturate the filter. To administer whole blood or RBCs, spike the blood container on the second port and hang it up. Turn off the 0.9% sodium chloride and turn on the blood component. It is recommended that transfusions of RBCs be started at 5 mL/min for the first 15 minutes of the transfusion (AABB, 2008).

INS Standard The patient should be monitored for 15 minutes after initiation of transfusion therapy and at established intervals throughout the transfusion period in accordance with organizational policies and procedures and practice guidelines. (INS, 2006, 70)

This small amount is large enough to alert the nurse to a possible severe reaction but small enough that the reaction can probably be successfully treated. If the patient shows signs or symptoms of an adverse reaction, the transfusion can be stopped immediately and only a small amount of blood product will have been infused. After the first 15 minutes has safely passed, the rate of flow can be increased to complete the transfusion within the amount of time indicated by the physician or by policy. The rate of infusion should be based on the patient's blood volume, hemodynamic condition, and cardiac status (Fig. 11-9).

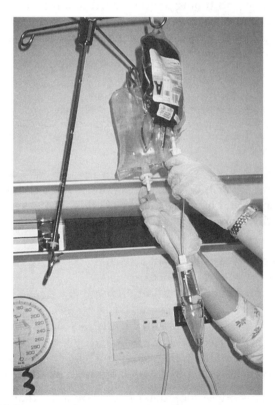

Figure 11-9 ▪ Hanging PRBCs with Y administration set. Always wear gloves when handling blood products.

Red cell products should be infused within a 4-hour period (AABB, 2008). When a longer transfusion time is clinically indicated, the unit may be divided by the blood bank and the portion not being transfused can be properly refrigerated.

Step 8: Monitoring the Transfusion

The patient's vital signs should be repeated at the end of the first 15 minutes and then periodically throughout the transfusion. The transfusion should be started slowly at a rate of approximately 2 mL/min except during urgent restoration of blood volume. Careful observation of the patient and the I.V. site during and after a blood transfusion is necessary to provide a more reliable assessment. Vital signs must be recorded before and after the transfusion (AABB, 2008).

Step 9: Completing the Transfusion

At the completion of the transfusion, the patient's vital signs should be obtained. The bag and tubing are discarded in a biohazard container. At this point, another unit may be infused, the unit and line may be discontinued, the line can be capped with a PRN adaptor, or a new infusion line and solution container may be added.

 NURSING FAST FACT!

Do not save previous solutions and tubing that were interrupted to give the blood component; they are considered contaminated. Restart with a fresh set and solution.

Documentation is an important part of the nursing intervention. The documentation should be made in the patient's medical record. At a minimum, the AABB Standards require the following:

1. Medical order for transfusion
2. Documentation of recipient consent
3. Name or type of component
4. Donor unit or pool identification number
5. Date and time of transfusion
6. Pre- and post-transfusion vital signs
7. Volume transfused
8. Identification of the transfusionist
9. Any adverse events possibly related to the transfusion.

Some transfusion service departments require that a copy of the completed transfusion form be returned to them. Returning the blood component after an uncomplicated transfusion is not required in all facilities. If disposal is allowed on the unit, use hospital standards in disposing the blood bag in contaminated trash.

NOTE > If an additional unit needs to be transfused, the institution's guidelines should be followed. A new blood administration set is to be used with each component. Blood unit administration must be completed within 4 hours.

NURSING POINTS-OF-CARE
DELIVERY OF BLOOD COMPONENT THERAPY

Nursing Assessments
- Interview the patient regarding his or her understanding of the need for the blood component
- Determine the patient's understanding of options: autologous, homologous, and directed donations.
- Assess vital signs (blood pressure, pulse, respiration, temperature)
- Assess renal and cardiovascular function.
- Assess and evaluate the I.V. site before requesting blood component from the blood bank.
- Assess the patient's level of consciousness.
- Review laboratory tests.
- Assess current intake and output ratios.

Key Nursing Interventions
1. Obtain the patient's written informed consent.
2. Monitor
   a. The I.V. site for signs and symptoms of infiltration, phlebitis, and local infection.
   b. Vital signs
   c. Fluid status
   d. Flow rate of the transfusion
3. Verify with another nurse that the blood product matches the patient's blood type.
4. Validate patient identification with two identifiers.
5. Administer blood products as set by AABB.
6. Prime the administration system with 0.9% sodium chloride.
7. Prepare an I.V. pump as indicated.
8. Refrain from administering I.V. medication into blood or blood product lines.

9. Change the blood administration set after every unit of red cells transfused or every 4 hours, whichever comes first.
10. Document the timeframe of the transfusion and volume infused.
11. Stop the transfusion if a reaction is suspected and follow policy and procedure for interventions related to the reaction.
12. Notify the laboratory immediately in the event of a blood reaction.
13. Maintain Standard Precautions.
14. Evaluate the effect of transfusion on laboratory tests at 24 hours.

■ Complications Associated with Blood Component Therapy

Despite its numerous and obvious benefits, there are also complications associated with blood component therapy (Table 11-7). The administration of any blood component carries with it the potential of adverse reactions. Most reactions are caused by biologic aspects of blood; however, nonimmune reactions can occur and may be linked to the collection, preparation, or administration of the blood. Table 11-8 lists the complications in a quick-guide format.

> Table 11-7   **RISKS OF TRANSFUSION THERAPY**

Viral Infection	Estimated Risks per Unit
HIV-1 and HIV-2	1:2,300,000
HTLV-1 and HTLV-2	1:2,993,000
HAV	1:1,000,000
HBV	1:220,000
HCV	1:1,800,000
Parvovirus B19	
Parasitic infections	1:20,000–50,000
Dengue virus	1:1000 blood donors in Puerto Rico
Acute Transfusion Reactions <24 hours	
Hemolytic transfusion reactions	ABO/Rh mismatch: 1:6000–1:20,000
	Fatal HTRs 1:100,000–1:600,000
Febrile nonhemolytic transfusion reaction	0.1–1% with universal leukocyte reduction
Minor allergic reaction	1%
Transfusion-related acute lung injury	1:5000–1:190,000
Transfusion-related sepsis	Dependent on clinical setting
Circulatory overload	<1%
Delayed Reactions	
Alloimmunization, HLA antigens	1:100
Delayed hemolytic	1:2500–11,000

Source: *AABB technical manual (2008).*

> Table 11-8   **SUMMARY OF TRANSFUSION REACTIONS**

Transfusion Reaction	Etiology	Signs and Symptoms	Key Interventions	Prevention
Acute Immediate (<24 hours)				
Acute hemolytic transfusion reaction (AHTR)	Hemolysis occurs when antibodies in plasma attach to antigens on the donor's RBCs. Cause: infusion of ABO-incompatible blood	Fever with or without chills Hypotension Burning sensation along vein Lumbar pain Flank pain, flushing of face and chest pain Bleeding Tachycardia, tachypnea, hemoglobinemia Hemoglobinuria, shock, vascular collapse, death	STOP THE TRANSFUSION! Get help immediately. Treat shock. Maintain blood pressure with colloidal solutions. Administer diuretics to maintain blood flow. Monitor for need for dialysis.	Extreme care during the entire identification process Start transfusion slowly and monitor for first 15 minutes.
Febrile nonhemolytic reaction	Occurs due to antibodies directed against leukocytes or platelets. Febrile reactions occur immediately or 1–2 hours after transfusion completed.	Fever rise of 1° in association with transfusion Chills Headache Nausea and vomiting Chest pain Nonproductive cough Malaise	Stop the transfusion, and start the normal saline. Notify the physician. Monitor vital signs Anticipate order for antipyretic agents. If ordered, restart transfusion slowly	Use of leukocyte-reduced blood component. Filter. HLA compatible products may also be helpful
Allergic reactions (mild)	Caused by recipient sensitivity to the donor's foreign plasma proteins	Itching Hives (local) Rash, urticaria Facial flushing Runny eyes Anxiety Dyspnea Wheezing	Stop the transfusion. Keep vein open with normal saline. Notify the physician. Monitor vital signs. Anticipate antihistamine order. If ordered, restart transfusion slowly. Mild reactions can precede severe allergic reactions. Monitor.	If known mild allergic reaction occur with blood transfusion may receive diphenhydramine (Benadryl) 30 minutes before the transfusion.

Continued

> Table 11-8   SUMMARY OF TRANSFUSION REACTIONS—cont'd

Acute Immediate (<24 hours)

Transfusion Reaction	Etiology	Signs and Symptoms	Key Interventions	Prevention
Severe allergic reactions: Anaphylaxis	Caused when donor blood with IgA proteins is transfused into an IgA-deficient recipient who has developed IgA antibody.	Anxiety Urticaria Wheezing Hypotension GI distress Shock Cardiac distress Death	Discontinue the transfusion. Keep the vein open with normal saline. Administer CPR if necessary. Anticipate order for steroids. Maintain BP.	Use of autologous blood Using blood from donors who are IgA deficient or by administering only well-washed RBCs in which all plasma has been extracted.
Transfusion-related acute lung injury (TRALI)	Infrequent Related to antibodies to leukocyte antigens and the infusion sequence of events damage basement membrane. Pulmonary edema occurs: **Leading cause of transfusion-related deaths**	Severe respiratory distress Chills Fever Cyanosis Increase in BP followed by hypotension	Discontinue the infusion. Provide respiratory support. Administer oxygen. May need mechanical vent. Corticosteroids Pressor agents	Frequent monitoring of patient. Reduced flow rate in high-risk patients. Monitor intake & output.
Transfusion-related circulatory overload (TACO)	Administration of blood faster than the recipient's cardiac output.	Hypervolemia Headache Dyspnea Constriction of chest Coughing Cyanosis JVD Pedal edema Increased BP	Stop the transfusion. Elevate the head of the bed. Notify the physician. Diuretics Oxygen Therapeutic phlebotomy may be indicated.	Frequent monitoring of patient. Reduced flow rate in high-risk patients. Monitor intake & output.

Complications of Massive Transfusions

Citrate toxicity	Infrequent High-rate infusions, liver unable to keep up with the rapid administration and cannot metabolize the citrate (which chelates calcium), reducing the ionized calcium concentration in the recipient's blood.	Hypocalcemia-induced cardiac dysrhythmias Tingling of fingers Muscular cramps Confusions Hypotension Cardiac arrest	Slowing rate of infusion Administration of calcium chloride or calcium gluconate Do not add calcium to infusing blood!	Administer fresh blood. Monitor calcium levels. Monitor patients with liver impairment closer for hypocalcemia.
Potassium toxicity Hyperkalemia	Administration of blood that has been stored. Related to release of potassium from the RBCs as they go through lysis. Occurs most frequently in multiple transfusions.	Elevated potassium levels Slow, irregular heart rate Nausea Muscle weakness ECG changes Diarrhea Renal failure	Stop or slow the transfusion. Monitor the ECG. Notify the physician. Remove excess potassium: concurrently administer hypertonic dextrose and insulin or administer polystyrene sulfonate orally or by enema.	In patients receiving multiple transfusions—use only the freshest blood.
Hemostatic abnormalities in massive transfusions	Coagulopathy related to massive transfusions. Caused by dilution of platelets and clotting factors.	Occurs after replacement of 2–3 blood volumes Clinical evidence of bleeding Platelet count <50,000 Shock and DIC	Intraoperative laboratory testing. Use of recombinant factor VIIA	Prophylactic replacement of hemostatic components. Frequent monitoring of prothrombin time and activated partial thromboplastin time

Continued

> Table 11-8   SUMMARY OF TRANSFUSION REACTIONS—cont'd

Delayed Transfusion Reactions

Transfusion Reaction	Etiology	Signs and Symptoms	Key Interventions	Prevention
Delayed hemolytic reaction	Result of RBC antigen incompatibility other than the ABO group. Occur due to destruction of transfused RBCs by alloantibodies not discovered during the process of crossmatching	Decreased hematocrit and hemoglobin Fever (continual, low grade) Jaundice (mild) Malaise Indirect hyperbilirubinemia	No acute treatment required. Monitor hematocrit level. Renal function Coagulation profile Notify physician and transfusion services.	Strict attention to crossmatching protocols
Transfusion-associated graft-versus-host disease (TA-GVHD)	Delayed reaction associated with donor lymphocytes–leukocyte reaction Highest risk in the immunocompetent patient. **High mortality rate**	Fever Rash Hepatitis Bone marrow suppression Overwhelming infection	No effective therapy Treatment of symptoms	Irradiation of blood products used in immunocompromised patients Use leukocyte reducing filter.
Iron overload	Multiple units of RBC chronically transfused. Excretion of iron from 1 unit slow.	Development of organ failure, tissue damage Heart failure Diabetes		Use of iron chelators

Infection-Related Complications

Bacterial contamination	Occurs at the time of donation or in preparing the component for infusion. Cold-resistant gram-negative bacteria such as *Pseudomonas* species, *Citrobacter freundii,* and *Escherichia coli* are potential causes – release endotoxin	Septic reaction, includes high fever Flushing of skin "Warm" shock Hemoglobinuria Renal failure DIC	Discontinue the transfusion. Aggressively treat shock and anticipate order of steroids and antibiotics. Culture patient's blood, component, and all I.V. solutions.	Preventable Bedside transfusion errors Inspection of the unit before administration: Observe for any discoloration of the blood or plasma. Report obvious clots. Ensure the integrity of the system before administration.
Human immuno-deficiency virus (HIV-1)	Viral infection transmitted via bodily secretions from HIV-positive individual.	Six stages by Walter Reed Classification System Positive HIV-flulike syndrome to total anergy with chronic fungal and viral infections	No cure Treatment is symptomatic.	Donor screening Nucleic acid amplification test (NAT)
Hepatitis-B	Viral infection, spread by blood and serum derived fluids and by direct contact with body fluids Average incubation is 90 days.	Elevated liver enzymes Fever Jaundice Malaise Nausea Pharyngitis Dark urine	No specific treatment – nursing care revolves around sympto-matic treatment.	Hepatitis B vaccine Pretransfusion testing of donor blood No vaccine for hepatitis C

Continued

> Table 11-8   SUMMARY OF TRANSFUSION REACTIONS—cont'd

Transfusion Reaction	Etiology	Signs and Symptoms	Key Interventions	Prevention
Cytomegalovirus	Viral infection, most at risk are low-birthweight neonates, immunosuppressed patients, and recipients of bone marrow and solid organ transplants	Systemic CMV infection (pneumonia, hepatitis, and retinitis)	No specific treatment	Reduce CMV exposure in specific patient populations; use blood from CMV-seronegative donors or depleted leukocytes.
West Nile virus (WNV)	Viral infection spread by infected mosquito. Incubation period 2–14 days	Fever and headache Eye pain Body aches GI complaints	Minimal data available at this time	FDA developing investigation nucleic acid tests to screen blood for WNV. Screening of donors
Variant Creutzfeldt-Jakob disease (vCJD)	Rare degenerative and fatal nervous system disorder. Occurs when humans eat beef contaminated with bovine spongiform encephalopathy	There has been no evidence at this time that vCJD has been transmitted through blood transfusion.	Precautions are taken in screening donors.	No screening test currently FDA required deferral policies for anyone who potentially could have been exposed to the disease by eating contaminated beef products.

INS Standard Transfusion reactions shall require immediate nursing and medical intervention, and shall be reported according to organizational policies and procedures and practice guidelines. (INS, 2006, 70)

Interventions include but are not limited to:
- Terminating the transfusion
- Maintaining patency of the catheter with 0.9% sodium chloride
- Notifying the physician and hospital blood bank or transfusion services
- Implementing other interventions as indicated

Patient-Focused Interventions

1. Stop the transfusion immediately but keep the line open with saline. Because the blood setup contains a significant amount of blood, it may be advantageous that a new I.V. set and fluid be added.
2. Reconfirm that the unit of blood is being administered to the intended recipient; document this recheck of identification. The labels on the component, patient records, and patient identification should be examined to detect any identification errors. Transfusion facilities may require repeat ABO and Rh typing of the patient on a new sample.
3. Contact the treating physician immediately for instructions for patient care.

Component-Focused Interventions

1. Contact the transfusion service for directions for investigation.
2. Obtain instructions concerning the return of the remaining component and complete I.V. setup (fluid and tubing).
3. Determine appropriate samples (blood and urine) to be sent to the laboratory.
4. The transfusion service determines whether the blood provider should be notified (Mazzei, Popovsky, & Kopko, 2008).

Acute or Immediate Transfusion Reactions

Acute or immediate adverse reactions to blood or blood products occur within 24 hours of transfusion, and may occur during the transfusion. The clinical significance of an acute reaction often cannot be determined via clinical history or signs and symptoms alone but requires laboratory evaluation.

Acute Hemolytic Transfusion Reactions

The most serious and potentially life-threatening reaction is **acute hemolytic transfusion reaction (AHTR)**. The transfusion of red cell components to the wrong patient occurs in 1:12,000 to 1:19,000 transfusions. ABO/Rh mismatches have been estimated to occur in 1:6000 to 1:20,000 transfusions. Death from AHTRs is estimated to occur in 1:500,000 to 1:1,000,000 transfusions (Spiess, 2004). This type of reaction occurs after infusion of incompatible RBCs. There are two classifications of hemolytic reactions. Intravascular hemolysis is usually associated with ABO-incompatible RBCs; complete hemolysis of cells occurs directly in the bloodstream. Extravascular hemolysis is seen in Rh incompatibility; cells are coated with the antibody and subsequently removed by the reticuloendothelial system. These incompatibilities may lead to an activation of the coagulation system and release of vasoactive enzymes, which can result in vasomotor instability, cardiorespiratory collapse, or DIC. Intravascular hemolysis is the most serious and is usually fatal.

Incompatibilities involving other RBC antigens and IgG antibodies can result in fever, anemia, hyperbilirubinemia, and a positive direct antibody test result. The severity of the reaction can be dose related but can occur with less than 30 mL of blood administered. Most hemolytic reactions are a result of clerical errors, such as incorrect labeling of the blood specimen or errors in identifying the recipient.

SIGNS AND SYMPTOMS

Many of the symptoms of immune-mediated AHTR are common to other acute transfusion reactions:
- Fever with or without chills
- Hypotension

Symptoms more unique to AHTR include:
- Lumbar pain, flank pain, flushing of the face, and chest pain

If infusion is allowed to continue, symptoms include hemoglobinemia, oozing of blood at the injection site, shock, and DIC.

INTERVENTIONS

Prompt recognition of AHTR is critical to successful outcome.
- Stop the transfusion.
- Disconnect the tubing from the I.V. catheter and infuse fresh saline not contaminated by the blood.

 NURSING FAST FACT!

In acute hemolytic transfusion reaction, you must not give the recipient another drop of donor blood.

- Notify the physician and blood bank or transfusion service *immediately*. Monitor vital signs and maintain intravascular volume with fluids to prevent renal constriction. In addition, diuretics, mannitol, and dopamine can support the renal and vascular systems. This is an emergency situation. The patient's respiratory status may have to be supported.

Interventions that can be anticipated by the nurse include:
- Continuation of saline initially will help with hypotension.
- Dopamine 1 to 5 mcg/kg per minute may be ordered to increase blood pressure and improve renal blood flow.
- Diuretics, such as 40 to 100 mg of furosemide given via I.V. push, may be ordered to maintain urine output above 100 mL/hr to decrease the risk of renal damage.
- Other therapies, such as heparin to prevent DIC or mannitol to produce an osmotic diuresis, are controversial but are sometimes used cautiously (Mazzei, Popovsky, & Kopko, 2008).

Extreme care during the entire identification process is the first step in prevention. Clerical and human error involving proper patient, sample, and blood unit identification are the most common causes of mistransfusion AHTR. The transfusion must be started slowly, and evaluation of the patient for reactions during the first 15 minutes is needed to monitor for initial AHTR.

Febrile Nonhemolytic Febrile Reactions

Nonhemolytic febrile reactions are defined as a temperature rise of 1°C or more occurring in association with transfusion and not having any other explanation. These are usually reactions to antibodies directed against leukocytes or platelets. Febrile reactions occur in only 1% of transfusions; repeat reactions are uncommon. These reactions can occur immediately or within 1 to 2 hours after transfusion is completed. Fever is the most common symptom associated with this type of transfusion reaction (Mazzei, Popovsky, & Kopko, 2008).

SIGNS AND SYMPTOMS

- Fever, greater than 1° chills
- Headache
- Nausea and vomiting
- Hypotension
- Chest pain, dyspnea, and nonproductive cough

INTERVENTIONS

- Discontinue the transfusion and initiate transfusion reaction workup.
- Keep the vein open with normal saline and notify the physician.
- Monitor vital signs.

- Administer antipyretic agents.
- Another transfusion unit may be safely infused once symptoms subside.

NOTE ▷ The remainder of the implicated component should not be transfused.

 NURSING FAST FACT!

In a nonhemolytic febrile reaction, you may turn off the blood and turn on the sodium chloride primer and infuse slowly. Do not take down the blood until notified by the physician; leave the blood hanging but clamp the Y connector to the blood unit.

PREVENTION

This type of reaction can be prevented or reduced by the use of leukocyte-reduced blood components. HLA-compatible products may also be indicated.

Allergic Reactions: Mild

In its mild form, **allergic reactions** constitute the second most common type of reaction and are probably caused by antibodies against plasma proteins. The patient may experience mild localized urticaria or full systemic anaphylactic reaction. This can occur immediately or within 1 hour after infusion. Most reactions are mild and respond to antihistamines.

SIGNS AND SYMPTOMS

- Itching, hives (local erythema), rash, urticaria
- Runny eyes
- Anxiety
- Dyspnea and wheezing

INTERVENTIONS

- Pause the transfusion.
- Keep the vein open with normal saline.
- Notify the physician.
- Monitor the vital signs.
- For a mild reaction, administer antihistamines per physician order.

 NURSING FAST FACT!

Urticaria is the only transfusion reaction in which the administration of the component may be routinely resumed after treatment (Mazzei, Popovsky, & Kopko, 2008).

Prevention

For mild reactions, the patient may be premedicated with 25 to 50 mg of diphenhydramine (Benadryl) 30 minutes before the transfusion. For patients whose reactions are severe, washing red cells or platelets may be considered. Administration of deglycerolized rejuvenated RBCs has met with some success (Mazzei, Popovsky, & Kopko, 2008).

Transfusion-Related Acute Lung Injury

There are three main conditions that need to be distinguished from transfusion-related acute lung injury (TRALI): (1) anaphylactic transfusion reactions, (2) transfusion-associated circulatory overload (TACO), and (3) transfusion-related sepsis. TRALI has been associated with the infusion of antibodies to leukocyte antigens and the infusion of biological response modifiers. Infusion of either is thought to initiate a sequence of events that results in cellular activation and damage of the basement membrane. Antibodies to HLA class I antigens and human neutrophil antigens (HNA) have been associated with TRALI. These antibodies are formed after exposure to foreign antigens via pregnancy, transfusion, or transplantation. Pulmonary edema occurs secondary to leakage of protein-rich fluid into the alveolar space (Mazzei, Popovsky, & Kopko, 2008). TRALI is the leading cause of transfusion-related mortality reported to the U.S. Food and Drug Administration, with 20 cases reported per year (Kopko & Popovsky, 2007).

Signs and Symptoms

- Fever and chills
- Dyspnea, cyanosis
- Hypotension
- New onset of bilateral pulmonary edema
- Increase in blood pressure followed by hypotension

NOTE > TRALI is life-threatening or fatal.

Treatment

- Respiratory and volume support
- Oxygen therapy with or without mechanical ventilation
- Pressor agents—support blood pressure
- Diuretics are not indicated; TRALI is not related to fluid overload.
- Corticosteroids

Prevention

Strategies to reduce the risk of TRALI are complicated. Multiple strategies to reduce the risk have been explored. Potential solutions include deferring donors implicated in a TRALI reaction, deferring multiparous women testing for HLA and HNA antibodies, and using male-donor plasma exclusively.

Transfusion-Related Circulatory Overload

The rapid administration of any blood product can lead to transfusion-related circulatory overload (TACO). RBC products, plasma products, and 25% albumin are the blood components most commonly associated with overload. Patients at risk for circulatory overload are those of small stature, infants and young children, and adults older than 60 years of age. Individuals with compromised cardiac or pulmonary function are also at risk.

SIGNS AND SYMPTOMS

- Dyspnea
- Engorged neck veins
- Orthopnea
- Cyanosis
- Tachycardia
- Jugular venous distension
- Pedal edema
- Increased blood pressure and widening pulse pressure
- Tightness in chest, dry cough (Mazzei, Popovsky, & Kopko, 2008)

INTERVENTIONS

- As soon as symptoms appear, suggest TACO and stop the transfusion.
- Place the patient in a sitting position.
- Administer oxygen therapy.
- Administer diuretics.
- Therapeutic phlebotomy (250-mL increments) may be considered (Mazzei, Popovsky, & Kopko, 2008).

PREVENTION

Patients identified as at-risk for TACO should have blood infused at a reduced rate. Recommendations are to administer blood at a rate of 1 mL/kg body weight/hr, which is about 4 hours per unit to prevent overload. Consider administration of a diuretic when beginning the transfusion in at-risk recipients. Monitor vital signs and intake and output throughout the transfusion (Mazzei, Popovsky, & Kopko, 2008).

Complications of Massive Transfusions

Citrate Toxicity

A reaction to toxic proportions of citrate, which is used as a preservative in blood, can cause hypocalcemia. The citrate ion can combine with the recipient's serum calcium, causing a calcium deficiency, or normal citrate metabolism is hindered by the presence of liver disease. Patients at risk for development of citrate toxicity or a calcium deficit are those who receive infusions of blood products at rates exceeding 100/mL per minute, or lower rates in patients who have liver disease. The liver, unable to keep up with the rapid administration, cannot metabolize the citrate, which chelates calcium, reducing the ionized calcium concentration. Hypocalcemia may induce cardiac dysrhythmias. Slow the infusion rate and, based on symptoms and blood values of calcium, administer calcium chloride or calcium gluconate solution. Do not administer calcium via the administration set infusing the blood.

SIGNS AND SYMPTOMS

- Perioral and peripheral tingling
- Shivering
- Lightheadedness
- Muscle cramps
- Fasciculations and spasm
- Nausea

INTERVENTIONS

- Slow the infusion.
- Replace calcium.

PREVENTION

Massively transfused patients may benefit from calcium replacement. Slowing the transfusion rate may prevent the occurrence of hypocalcemia unless the patient has a predisposing condition that hinders citrate metabolism.

Potassium Toxicity (Hyperkalemia)

Potassium toxicity is a rare complication. As blood ages during storage, potassium is released from the cells into the plasma during RBC lysis. When RBCs have been stored at 1° to 6°C, biochemical changes, known as storage lesions, develop. During the first few weeks of storage, extracellular potassium in the unit may increase by as much as 1 mEq daily. As a result of this storage lesion, the recipient receives excessive potassium. Single-unit transfusion is generally not a problem, but individuals who receive multiple units of aged blood may experience this reaction. Patients with renal failure and premature infants and newborns receiving large transfusions are at risk.

SIGNS AND SYMPTOMS

- Hyperkalemia
- Slow, irregular heartbeat
- Nausea
- Muscle weakness
- Electrocardiographic changes.

Intervention

■ Treat the underlying cause.

Prevention

■ Use fresh blood.

Hemostatic Abnormalities in Massive Transfusions

Coagulopathy can be observed when massive transfusion is required for severe blood loss, especially when the lost blood is initially replaced with red cells. It is caused by the dilution of platelets and clotting factors, which occurs as the patient loses hemostatically active blood, and by reduction of enzymatic activity.

Signs and Symptoms

■ Occurs after replacement of two to three blood volumes
■ Clinical evidence of bleeding
■ Platelet counts 50,000/μL with alteration in other coagulation factors.
■ Shock and DIC

Treatment and Prevention

The possible prophylactic replacement of hemostatic components based on volume of red cells transfused may prevent occurrence; however, no specific regimen has proven to be superior in prospective studies. Another consideration is anticipation of specific component needs— avoid aggravated dilutional coagulopathy. Frequently monitor prothrombin time (PT) and activated partial thromboplastin time (aPTT) when using platelets and plasma products to avoid overuse. Intraoperative laboratory testing such as thromboelastography may be useful (Mazzei, Popovsky, & Kopko, 2008). Use of recombinant factor VIIA in massive transfusions for treatment of bleeding in trauma and surgery works by targeting the site of tissue damage, where it binds to tissue factor; this is an off-label use (Dutton, Hess, & Scalen, 2003).

Delayed Transfusion Reactions

Delayed Hemolytic Transfusion Reaction

Delayed hemolytic transfusion reactions are a result of RBC antigen incompatibility other than the ABO group. Rapid production of RBC antibody occurs shortly after transfusion of the corresponding antigen as a result of sensitization during previous transfusions or pregnancies. Destruction of the transfused RBCs gradually occurs over 2 or more days or up to several weeks after the transfusion. Reactions are common but frequently go unnoticed.

SIGNS AND SYMPTOMS

- Fever and anemia occurring days to weeks after transfusion of red cell component
- Decrease in hemoglobin and hematocrit levels
- Persistent low-grade fever, malaise
- Indirect hyperbilirubinemia
- Possible development of jaundice and leukocytosis

INTERVENTIONS

- Usually no acute treatment is required.
- Monitor hematocrit level, renal function, and coagulation profile routinely for all patients receiving transfusions.
- Notify the physician and transfusion services if delayed reaction is suspected.

PREVENTION

Reactions can be prevented by transfusion of antigen-negative red cells. Past transfusion records should be reviewed because alloantibodies may have been identified.

Transfusion-Associated Graft-versus-Host Disease

Transfusion-associated graft-versus-host disease (TA-GVHD) occurs when a recipient is immunocompromised, a fresh blood component containing a sufficient number of viable T lymphocytes is transfused, and the recipient reacts to one of the donor HLA cells. The T lymphocytes become activated, engraft, and proliferate, and begin to attack host tissue cells. The patient will experience tissue dysfunction as the epithelium of various organs such as the liver, gastrointestinal tract, and bone marrow is destroyed. Death due to bleeding or infection normally occurs within 3 weeks. There is no cure for TA-GVHD. Gamma irradiation of all cellular components is the only way to prevent TA-GVHD. Leukoreduction of the products will not prevent TA-GVHD, but it reduces the number of white blood cells requiring irradiation (Harris, 2002).

 NURSING FAST FACT!

Immunoincompetent recipients are at risk for TA-GVHD.

 CULTURAL AND ETHNIC CONSIDERATIONS: ⎯⎯⎯⎯⎯⎯⎯
RISK FOR TA-GVHD

The degree of genetic diversity in populations affects the risk of developing TA-GVHD; in Japan the range is 1:874 whereas in France it is 1:16,835. The difference is related to a decreased diversity in HLSA antigen expression in the Japanese population (Alyea & Anderson, 2007).

SIGNS AND SYMPTOMS

- Begins 8 to 10 days after transfusion
- Maculopapular rash
- Fever
- Enterocolitis with watery diarrhea
- Elevated liver function tests
- Pancytopenia
- Leads to profound marrow aplasia with the mortality rate of 90% (Mazzei, Popovsky, & Kopko, 2008).

INTERVENTIONS

- Use of a variety of immunosuppressive agents
- Almost universally fatal

PREVENTION

TA-GVHD may be prevented by irradiation of cellular blood components. AABB standards require a minimum dose of 25 Gy delivered to the central portion of the container and minimum of 15 Gy dose elsewhere (AABB, 2008).

Iron Overload

A unit of RBCs contains approximately 250 mg of iron. The average rate of excretion of iron is approximately 1 mg per day. As red cells are destroyed, the majority of the released iron cannot be excreted and is stored in the body as hemosiderin and ferritin. As iron accumulates the reticuloendothelial system, liver, heart, spleen, and endocrine organs, tissue damage leading to heart failure, liver failure, diabetes, and hypothyroidism may occur. Patients who are chronically transfused for diseases are at risk (Mazzei, Popovsky, & Kopko, 2008).

SIGNS AND SYMPTOMS

- Development of organ failure, tissue damage
- Heart failure
- Diabetes

INTERVENTIONS

- Administration of iron chelators
- Be aware that frequent infusions of RBCs can cause iron overload.

PREVENTION

The accumulation of toxic levels of iron can be reduced by use of iron chelators. Iron chelators bind iron in the body and tissues and help remove it through the urine or feces.

> EBNP A randomized phase II trial of deferasiorx (Exjade, ICL670), a once-daily, orally administered iron chelator has shown positive effects with minimal adverse effects (Piga, Galanello, Forni, et al., 2006).

Infection-Related Complications

Transfusion-Transmitted Diseases

Despite dynamic advances in blood banking and transfusion medicine, there are still risks to blood component therapy. Patients should be told of alternatives to transfusion, including risks to the patient if transfusion is not undertaken. Further, patients need to know about the blood center's autologous transfusion and patient-designated donor programs, without an implication that there is added safety to the latter.

A uniform donor history is designed to ask questions that protect the health of both the donor and the recipient. Questions asked of the donor help determine whether donating blood might endanger his or her health. If a prospective donor responds positively to any of these questions, he or she will be "deferred" or asked not to donate blood. The health history also is used to identify prospective donors who have been exposed to or who may have disease, such as human immunodeficiency virus (HIV), hepatitis, or malaria (AABB, 2008). Table 11-7 provides the incidence of transfusion-acquired infections.

Viruses

Viruses that have the potential to be transmitted include HIV types 1 and 2 (HIV-1, HIV-2), HBV, and HCV.

Human Immunodeficiency Virus

Transfusion transmission of human immunodeficiency virus (HIV) and the human T-cell lymphotropic virus (HTLV-1-11) have been almost completely eradicated since blood banks began interviewing donors about at-risk behaviors and blood tests became available in 1985. The HIV antibody tests, used on every blood donation, have undergone continuous improvement. In 1999 nucleic acid amplification testing (NAT) began to be used to directly detect the genetic material of the HIV virus in the blood (AABB, 2008). The estimated risk in Table 11-7 may be artificially low due to changes in test interpretation. The use of leukocyte reduction has reduced the risk of HTLV transmission.

Hepatitis (HBV)

Viral hepatitis, which infects the liver, accounts for only a small proportion of cases of post-transfusion hepatitis. The incidence is low owing to screening of donors for behaviors that expose them to viral hepatitis and testing of all donations of HbsAg and anti-HBc (AABB, 2008).

Hepatitis incubation period is approximately 90 days, with symptoms of dark urine, jaundice, malaise, anorexia, headache, pharyngitis, and elevated liver enzymes. Treatment is symptomatic. Seroprevalence in the U.S. population is about 5.6% and in some parts of the world greater than 50% (Fiebig & Busch, 2008). Effective blood donor screening tests and sensitive test for donors are available and their use is mandated whenever blood is collected.

Cytomegalovirus

Cytomegalovirus (CMV) is a virus belonging to the herpes group that is rarely transmitted by blood transfusion. According to the CDC about 50% to 80% of adults in the United States are infected with CMV by the age of 40. CMV infection is usually mild, but may be serious or fatal for those who are immunocompromised, for low-birthweight infants, and bone marrow and organ transplant patients. Filtered blood that decreases the number of white blood cells (the cells that carry CMV) will protect patients from getting CMV infection from a transfusion (Fiebig & Busch, 2008).

The highest risk is to immunocompromised CMV seronegative recipients. Transmission rates of up to 50% have been reported and non-leukocyte reduced cellular blood products are recommended.

West Nile Virus

West Nile virus (WNV) is spread by the bite of an infected mosquito. The virus can infect people, horses, and many types of birds. It was first detected in the United States in 1999, and the first documented cases of WNV transmission through organ transplantation and transfusion were noted in 2002. The most common symptoms of transfusion-transmitted cases of WNV are fever and headache. Screening is by blood bank interview of history of fever and headache. Blood screening with nucleic acid amplification testing (NAT) for WNV started in the summer of 2003. Blood screening has been very effective.

Bacteria

The incidence of bacterial contamination in allogeneic platelets based on culture was estimated at 1:100 to 3000 units. Screening for bacterial contamination in 2004 suggests a lower rate. Gram-positive skin saprophytes account for most of the significant organisms contaminating platelet concentrates, with the remaining attributed to gram-negative organisms. In the United States, the gram-negative bacteria *Escherichia coli*, *Providencia rettgeri*, *Klebsiella* species, and *Serratia* species account for 69% of the fatal reactions.

Detection methods for bacterial contamination were implemented in 2004. Refrigerated storage limits growth and viability of most bacteria in RBC products.

Prions

Proteinaceous infectious particles or prions are abnormally structured forms of cellular proteins that are able to convert normal protein molecules on contact into an abnormal structure. This allows prions to act like infectious agents. Prion diseases affect primarily brain tissue, causing severe, progressive dementia. The best-known prion disease in humans is Creutzfeldt–Jakob disease (CJD).

Creutzfeldt–Jakob Disease

Creutzfeldt–Jakob disease (CJD) is a rare degenerative and fatal nervous system disorder. Currently, there is no screening test for the disease, and donor leukocytes have never been shown to transmit any form of the disease. As a precaution, the FDA prohibits blood donation by individuals who may be at risk. These include potential donors who have received injections of human-derived pituitary hormone, those with a family history of CJD, or those who have had surgeries that involved transplanted dura mater.

Variant Creutzfeldt–Jakob Disease

Similar to CJD, variant CJD (vCJD), commonly known as the human form of "mad cow" disease, is a rare degenerative and fatal nervous system disorder. At this time there is no evidence that vCJD has ever been transmitted through a blood transfusion. The FDA requires donor "deferral" policies for anyone who potentially could have been exposed to the disease by eating contaminated beef products. There is no screening at this time. At this time, active efforts are underway to develop a screening test to detect prions and filters to remove them from donated blood (Cervia, Sowemimo-Coker, Ortolano, et al., 2006).

Vector-Borne Bacteria and Parasites

Parasitic Infections

A variety of parasitic infections may be transmitted through transfusions: babesiosis (transmitted by tick bites), Chagas' disease (transmitted by reduviid bugs), Lyme disease (bite of certain species of deer tick), and malaria. Blood banking facilities screen for these four parasitic infections and may "defer" the donor or permanently prohibit blood donation from those infected with these parasite infections (Fiebig & Busch, 2008).

AGE-RELATED CONSIDERATIONS

Neonatal and Pediatric Patients

Special guidelines are used for transfusion of neonates younger than 4 months of age, preterm babies weighing less than 1200 grams, and children older than 4 months. RBC transfusion support in infants older than 4 months and children is similar to that in adults. The most significant differences between this young group and adults are:

• Blood volume
• Ability to tolerate blood loss
• Age-appropriate hemoglobin and hematocrit levels.

The following are guidelines for infusion nurses to consider as part of their knowledge base:

• Blood volumes for pediatric patients vary with body weight. A full-term newborn has a blood volume of approximately 85 mL/kg, compared to 100 mL/kg in a preterm newborn. Blood banks and transfusion services must be capable of providing smaller, appropriately sized blood components to meet the needs of this population.

Transfusion Guidelines for RBCs in Infants Less than 4 Months of Age

• Hematocrit less than 20% with low reticulocyte count and symptomatic anemia
• Hematocrit less than 30% AND on 35% oxygen; or on oxygen by nasal cannula; or on continuous positive airway pressure or intermittent mandatory ventilation; or with significant tachycardia or tachypnea; or with significant apnea or bradycardia; or low weight gain (<10 g/day observed over 4 days while receiving ≥100 kcal/kg/day)
• Hematocrit less than 35% and either of the following: on greater than 35% oxygen hood; or on continuous positive airway pressure/intermittent ventilation
• Hematocrit less than 45% and either on extracorporeal membrane oxygenation or with congenital cyanotic heart disease (Wong & Luban, 2005)

Transfusion Guidelines for RBCs in Patients Older than 4 Months of Age

• Emergency surgical procedure with postoperative anemia
• Preoperative anemia when other corrective therapy is not available
• Intraoperative blood loss greater than 15% of total volume
• Hematocrit less than 24% while on chemotherapy
• Acute blood loss with hypovolemia
• Hematocrit less than 40% and with severe pulmonary disease; on extracorporeal membrane oxygenation (ECMO)
• Sickle cell disease
• Chronic transfusion programs for disorders of red cell production

Platelet Transfusion in Neonates and Older Children

With Thrombocytopenia

• Platelet count 5000 to 10,000/µL with failure of platelet production
• Platelet count less than 30,000/mL in neonate with failure of platelet production

- Platelet count less than 50,000/µL in stable premature infant with active bleeding
- Platelet count less than 100,000/µL in sick premature infant with active bleeding

Without Thrombocytopenia

- Active bleeding in association with qualitative platelet defect
- Unexplained excessive bleeding in a patient undergoing cardiopulmonary bypass
- Patient undergoing ECMO with platelet count of less than 100,000/µL

Transfusion Guidelines for Plasma Products in Neonates and Older Children

FFP

- Support during treatment of DIC
- Replacement therapy when specific factor concentrates are not available
- During therapeutic plasma exchange with FFP is indicated
- Reversal of warfarin in an emergency situation

Granulocyte Administration to Neonates and Older Children

- Neonates or children with neutropenia or granulocyte dysfunction with bacterial sepsis and lack of responsiveness to standard therapy
- Neutropenic neonates or children with fungal disease not responsive to standard therapy

(Wong & Luban, 2005).

Complications

Cytomegalovirus

The risk of transfusion-transmitted CMV infection is higher in multitransfused low-birthweight infants (<1200 grams) born to seronegative mothers. It is recommended that low birth weight infants receive CMV reduced–risk blood for transfusion. Either use blood from CMV-seronegative donors or because CMV is associated with leukocytes, leukocyte-reduced components (Josephson, 2008).

Leukocyte-Reduced Components

Neonates younger than 4 months old and infants rarely become alloimmunized to red cells or HLA antigens because of their immature immune system; therefore, transfusion reactions are infrequent.

> EBNP One study in Canada evaluated the clinical outcomes of premature infants (weighing less than 1250 grams), before and after nationwide implementation of universal leukocyte reduction, which revealed no change in mortality or rate of bacteremia. It was observed, however, that a decrease in retinopathy of prematurity and bronchopulmonary dysplasia as well as a shorter length of hospitalization occurred after implementation of the new standard.

Continued

The Older Adult

The older adult receiving transfusion therapy is at risk for transfusion-related circulatory overload. Nursing interventions include careful monitoring of intake and output, laboratory values, and daily weight and assessment of lungs and kidney function.

 Home Care Issues

Transfusing blood in a nonhospital setting requires a well-planned program that incorporates all the aspects of the hospital setting and emphasizes safety considerations. An outpatient surgery center, oncology clinic, or dialysis center are more likely settings for delivery of a transfusion yet home care might be appropriate for some patients who have difficulty getting out of the home. Transfusion services can be delivered safely and efficiently in the home setting. An advantage of home transfusion is close monitoring of the transfusion event because the personnel-to-patient ratio is one to one. The disadvantage is that there is not a trained assistant available in the event of a severe adverse reaction (Sink, 2008).

NOTE > Because of this, an important criterion for home transfusion is that the patient history includes prior transfusions without any adverse reactions.

Additional issues to consider when preparing for transfusion in the home include:
1. Availability of a competent adult in the home to assist in patient identification and summoning medical assistance if needed.
2. A mechanism to obtain immediate physician consultation
3. A telephone to contact emergency personnel and easy access for emergency services (e.g., patient does not live in rural area without rapid emergency response system).
4. The ability to properly dispose of medical waste.

Transfusions in the home setting include packed RBCs, modified RBCs, platelets, cryoprecipitate, plasma, and plasma derivatives. Whole blood is not an alternative in the home setting. Factor replacement for patients with hemophilia is often done in the home, either nurse-administered or self-infused by the patient, most often using recombinant, rather than plasma-derived products.

Home blood transfusion carries the same liability risk as hospital transfusion. During the pretransfusion visit, the informed consent and any other company-specific forms should be signed. A complete medical history and thorough physical examination is completed, along with evaluation of vascular access. An identification bracelet with the patient's full name and

Home Care Issues—cont'd

identification number is attached to the patient's wrist. The home infusion nurse also obtains blood samples for baseline chemistry.

Guidelines for Home Transfusion Therapy:

1. Ensure that a transfusion kit and protocol is available in home during the transfusion.
2. Obtain a written physician's order.
3. Evaluate the patient for:
   a. Stable cardiopulmonary status and medical condition
   b. Level of consciousness, cooperative behaviors, and ability to communicate information to the nurse
4. Evaluate the home environment for:
   a. Conducive and clean home environment
   b. Capable adult present during transfusion
   c. Telephone access available
   d. Ready access to emergency medical service and primary physician during transfusion
5. Transport blood components to the home setting using blood bank standards.
6. Procedures for blood and patient identification are in place.
7. Baseline assessments should be made according to INS Standards for monitoring the infusion.
8. An appropriate blood filter should be used.
9. Electromechanical devices may be used, but the product information should be checked to ensure that the pump is indicated for transfusion delivery and will not cause hemolysis of RBCs.
10. Use only 0.9% sodium chloride solutions to prime the administration set.
11. Administer the transfusion with constant supervision from the nurse.
12. Blood warming should not be considered for home transfusion because no more than 2 units of blood should be administered at one time in the home setting. Patients with cold agglutinins are not appropriate candidates for home transfusion.
13. A biohazard container is used to dispose of blood, and contaminated supplies and should be disposed of according to state regulations.
14. The physician must be immediately available at all times for telephone consultation.
15. Post-transfusion instructions should be left; these include but are not limited to:
    a. Emergency telephone numbers
    b. Information regarding signs and symptoms of delayed reactions
    c. Schedule of the post-transfusion assessment visit
16. Notify the physician of the transfusion completion and the patient's response to therapy.
17. Documentation must include, but not be limited to:
    a. Type of I.V. solution and time started
    b. Type of blood product
    c. Vital signs, skin condition, and appearance

Continued

Home Care Issues—cont'd

d. Any patient symptoms or complaints
e. The time blood product is discontinued
f. Volume infused
g. Reason for discontinuing the transfusion if done before completion of the infusion
h. Patient reactions to the procedure

 Patient Education

- Patients who are aware of the steps involved in a transfusion experience less anxiety.
- The nurse should explain how the transfusion will be given, how long it will take, what the expected outcome is, what symptoms to report, and that vital signs will be taken.
- The physician has the responsibility to explain the benefits and risks of transfusion therapy, as well as alternatives.
- Informed consent should be obtained.
- Instruct on the need and physiologic benefit of blood product.
- Inform on options: autologous, homologous, or directed donation.
- Instruct on current statistics of transfusion risks, if necessary

■ Nursing Process

The nursing process is a five- or six-step process for problem-solving to guide nursing action. Refer to Chapter 1 for details on the steps of the nursing process related to vascular access. The following table focuses on nursing diagnoses, nursing outcomes classification (NOC), and nursing intervention classification (NIC) for patients receiving transfusion therapy. Nursing diagnoses should be patient specific and outcomes and interventions individualized. The NOC and NIC presented here are suggested direction for development of specific outcomes and interventions.

Nursing Diagnoses Related to Transfusion Therapy	NOC: Nursing Outcomes Classification	NIC: Nursing Intervention Classification
Anxiety related to: Possibility of harm from transfusion	Anxiety level	Anxiety reduction strategies
Fatigue related to: Decreased oxygen supply to the body, increased cardiac workload	Energy conservation	Energy management (conservation and restoration)

Nursing Diagnoses Related to Transfusion Therapy	NOC: Nursing Outcomes Classification	NIC: Nursing Intervention Classification
Fear related to: Homologous blood transfusion and the transmission of disease; fear of needles	Fear control	Anxiety reduction strategies
Gas exchange impaired related to: Ventilation perfusion imbalance, decreased oxygen-carrying capacity of the blood	Gas exchange, ventilation	Acid–base management
Hypothermia related to: Exposure to cool or cold blood.	Thermoregulation	Temperature regulation
Infection risk for related to: Transfusion	Infection control	Infection control and infection protection
Knowledge deficit related to: Purpose of blood component therapy; signs and symptoms of complications	Knowledge: Treatment regimen (transfusion)	Teaching: Disease process, transfusion component risk and benefits
Protection ineffective related to: Bleeding disorder	Health-promoting behavior, blood coagulation	Bleeding precautions

Sources: Ackley & Ladwig (2008); Carpenito-Moyet (2008); McCloskey-Dochterman & Bulechek (2004); Moorhead, Johnson, & Maas (2004); NANDA-I (2007).

Chapter Highlights

- Immunohematology is the science that deals with antigens of the blood and their antibodies.
- Blood groups are based on the antigens present on the cell surface of RBCs. The two major antigen groups are the ABO and Rh systems. Every human being has two genotypes that, when paired, determine one of four blood types (A, B, AB, or O).
- The universal RBC donor is O negative; the universal plasma donor is AB.
- The majority of people (85%) have the Rh antigen D, making them Rh positive. Those without the antigen D are Rh negative.
- ABO incompatibility is the major cause of fatal transfusion reactions.
- The most common preservatives added to blood to extend the shelf life are CPDA-1 (35 days) and ADSOL (42 days).
- Blood donor collection methods include:
  - Homologous: Blood donated by someone other than the intended recipient (allogeneic)
  - Autologous: Recipient's own blood; collected in one of four ways: preoperative blood salvage, intraoperative blood salvage, ANH, postoperative blood salvage
  - Designated (directed): Blood donated from selected friends or relatives of the recipient

- Blood product transfusions are indicated for:
  - Maintenance of oxygen-carrying capacity of the blood
  - Replacement of clotting factors
  - Replacement of vascular volume
- Governmental agencies (i.e., the AABB, INS, and FDA) set standards for responsibilities of nurses in the safe administration of blood products.
- Biologic (immune) reactions include acute hemolytic transfusion reactions, delayed transfusion reactions, nonhemolytic febrile reactions, allergic reactions, and GVHD reactions.
- Nonimmune complications associated with transfusion therapy include circulatory overload, potassium toxicity, hypothermia, hypocalcemia, bacterial contamination, and infectious disease transmission.
- Key steps in the procedure to delivery of blood transfusion are:
  Step 1: Recipient consent
  Step 2: Verifying the authorized prescriber's order
  Step 3: Pretransfusion
  Step 4: Venous access; selecting and preparing the equipment
  Step 5: Assessment and education of the patient
  Step 6: Dispensing and transportation of the component
  Step 7: Initiating the transfusion
  Step 8: Monitoring the transfusion
  Step 9: Completing the transfusion.

■■ Thinking Critically: Case Study

At the beginning of your shift, you check on a unit of packed red blood cells that had been hung just prior to your shift. The unit of RBCs is infusing slowly, with approximately 200 mL left. You agitate the bag slightly and discover a pinhole at the top of the bag.

What do you do?
What legal factors are involved in this scenario?
What are the risks to the patient?
What assessments should have taken place prior to hanging this blood component?

 Media Link: Answers to the case study and more critical thinking activities are provided on the CD-ROM.

Post-Test

1. Antibodies are found in:
   a. RBCs
   b. WBCs
   c. Plasma
   d. Antigens

2. Which of the following diseases is donor blood screened for? (*Select all that apply.*)

   a. HbsAg
   b. Anti–HIV-1
   c. Anti–HTLV-1
   d. EBV (Epstein–Barr virus)

3. The initial nursing intervention for an acute hemolytic transfusion reaction would be to:

   a. Slow the transfusion and call the physician.
   b. Stop the transfusion and turn the saline side of the administration set on at a slow keep open rate.
   c. Stop the transfusion, disconnect the tubing from the I.V. catheter, and initiate new saline and tubing to keep the vein open.
   d. Stop the transfusion and turn the saline side of the administration set on at a rapid rate.

4. The component albumin 25% is hypertonic. Caution should be used by nurses when infusing 25% albumin because this product can:

   a. Cause circulatory overload
   b. Cause clotting disorders
   c. Increase RBC hemoglobin
   d. Lower the blood pressure

5. Which of the following must an RN check with another nurse before initiating a unit of blood? (*Select all that apply.*)

   a. ABO and Rh
   b. Patient name
   c. Unit number
   d. Expiration date
   e. Preservative

6. The universal recipient is a person with blood type:

   a. A-positive
   b. AB-positive
   c. O-negative
   d. AB-negative

7. Which of the following packed red blood cell preparations is considered to prevent transfusion-associated GVHD?

   a. Leukocyte-reduced RBC
   b. Washed RBCs
   c. Irradiated RBCs
   d. Frozen-washed RBCs

8. If a patient receives 2 units of packed red blood cells for a hematocrit (Hct) of 24%, what would the anticipated HCT be in 24 hours postinfusion?
   a. 26%
   b. 28%
   c. 30%
   d. 32%

9. Which of the following adverse effects of transfusion therapy has a potential for a fatal outcome for the patient?
   a. TACO
   b. Febrile reaction
   c. Citrate toxicity
   d. TA-GVHD

10. A patient with group O blood type, may receive which of the following red blood cells?
    a. Group A only
    b. Group O only
    c. Group AB and O
    d. Any blood group

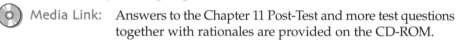 Media Link: Answers to the Chapter 11 Post-Test and more test questions together with rationales are provided on the CD-ROM.

■ References

AABB. T.H. Price (Ed.) (2008). *Standards for blood banks and transfusion services*, (25th ed.). Bethesda MD: Author.

Ackley, B.J., & Ladwig, G.B. (2008). *Nursing diagnosis handbook: An evidence-based guide to planning care* (8th ed.). St. Louis, MO: Mosby Elsevier.

Alyea, E.P., & Anderson, K.C. (2007). Transfusion-associated graft-versus-host disease. In: M.A. Popovsky (Ed.), *Transfusion reactions* (3rd ed., pp. 229–249). Bethesda, MD: AABB Press.

AuBuchon, J.P. (2008). Hemotherapy decisions and their outcomes. In: J. Roback, M. Combs, B. Grossman, & C. Hillyer (Eds.), *AABB technical manual* (16th ed., pp. 569–603). Bethesda, MD: AABB Press.

Bishton, M., & Chopra, R. (2004). The role of granulocyte transfusion in neutropenic patients. *British Journal of Haematology, 127*, 510–518.

Boucher, B.A., & Hannon, T.J. (2007). Blood management: A primer for clinicians. *Pharmacotherapy, 27*, 1394–1411.

Brecher, M.E., & Goodnough, L.T. (2001). The rise and fall of preoperative autologous blood donation. *Transfusion, 41*, 1459–1462.

Carpenito-Moyet, L.J. (2008). *Nursing diagnosis: Application to clinical practice* (12th ed.). Philadelphia: Lippincott Williams & Wilkins.

Cervia, J.S., Sowemimo-Coker, S.O., Ortolano, G.A., et al. (2006). An overview of prion biology and the role of blood filtration in reducing the risk of transfusion-transmitted variant Creutzfeldt-Jakob disease. *Transfusion Medicine Reviews, 20*, 190–206.

Cooling, L. (2008). ABO, H, and Lewis blood groups and structurally related antigens. In: J. Roback, M. Combs, B. Grossman, & C. Hillyer (Eds.), *AABB technical manual* (16th ed., pp. 361–385). Bethesda, MD: AABB Press.

Corwin, H.K. (2006). Anemia and red blood cell transfusion in the critically ill. *Seminars in Dialysis, 19*, 513–518.

Daniels, G. (2008). Other blood groups. In: J. Roback, M. Combs, B. Grossman, & C. Hillyer (Eds.), *AABB technical manual* (16th ed., pp. 411–436). Bethesda, MD: AABB Press.

Downs, K.A., & Shulman, I.A. (2008). Pretransfusion testing. In: J. Roback, M. Combs, B. Grossman, & C. Hillyer (Eds.), *AABB technical manual* (16th ed., pp. 437–460). Bethesda, MD: AABB Press.

Duff, K. (2006). You can make a difference in the administration of intravenous immunoglobulin therapy. *Journal of Infusion Nursing, 29*(3S), S5–S14.

Dutton, R.P., Hess, J.R., & Scalea, T.M. (2003). Recombinant factor VIIa for control of hemorrhage: Early experience in critically ill trauma patients. *Journal of Clinical Anesthesia, 15*, 184–188.

Dzik, W.H., Anderson, J.K., O'Neill, E.M., et al. (2002). A prospective, randomized clinical trial of universal WBC reduction. *Transfusion, 42*, 1114–1122.

Eder, A.F. (2008). Allogeneic and autologous blood donor selection. In: J. Roback, M. Combs, B. Grossman, & C. Hillyer (Eds.), *AABB technical manual* (16th ed., pp. 137–159). Bethesda, MD: AABB Press.

Fiebig, E.W., & Busch, M.P. (2008). Infectious disease screening. In: J. Roback, M. Combs, B. Grossman, & C. Hillyer (Eds.), *AABB technical manual* (16th ed., pp. 241–281). Bethesda, MD: AABB Press.

Fitzpatrick, L. (2002). Blood products: Washing away transfusion risks. *Nursing 2002, 32*(5), 36–41.

Food and Drug Administration (FDA). (2006a). Guidance: Industry consensus standard for the uniform labeling of blood and blood components using ISBT 128 version 2.0.0. Rockville, MD: CBER Office of Communication, Training and Manufacturer.

Food and Drug Administration (FDA). (2006b). Guidance for industry: Implementation of acceptable full-length donor history questionnaire and accompanying materials for use in screening donors of blood and blood components. Rockville, MD: CBER Office of Communication, Training and Manufacturer. October 2006.

Gebel, H.M., Pollack, M.S., & Bray, R.A. (2008). The HLA system. In: J. Roback, M. Combs, B. Grossman, & C. Hillyer (Eds.), *AABB technical manual* (16th ed., pp. 548–566). Bethesda, MD: AABB Press.

Giger, J.N., & Davidhizar, R.E. (2004). *Transcultural nursing: Assessment and intervention* (2nd ed., p. 140). St. Louis, MO: C.V. Mosby.

Hannon, T.J., & Paulson-Gjerde, K. (2005). Contemporary economics of transfusion. In: B. Spiess, R.K. Spence, A. Shander (Eds.), *Perioperative transfusion medicine* (pp. 46–58). Philadelphia: Lippincott Williams & Wilkins.

Harris, D.J. (2002). Immune complications associated with chronic transfusion. *Journal of Infusion Nursing, 25*(5), 316–319.

Henkel-Hank, T., & Oleck, M. (2007). Artificial oxygen carriers: A current review. *AANA Journal, 75*(3), 205–212.

Houck, D., & Whiteford, J. (2007). Improving patient outcomes: Transfusion with infusion pump for peripherally inserted central catheters and other vascular access devices. *Journal of Infusion Nursing, 30*(6), 341–344.

Infusion Nurses Society (INS). (2006). Standards of practice. *Journal of Infusion Nursing, 2* (1S).

Josephson, C.D. (2008). Neonatal and pediatric transfusion practice. In: J. Roback, M. Combs, B. Grossman, & C. Hillyer (Eds.), *AABB technical manual* (16th ed., pp. 639–663). Bethesda, MD: AABB Press.

Kakaiya, R., Aronson, C.A., & Julleis, J. (2008). Whole blood collection and component process. In: J. Roback, M. Combs, B. Grossman, & C. Hillyer (Eds.), *AABB technical manual* (16th ed., pp. 189–228). Bethesda, MD: AABB Press.

Kirmse, J. (2006). Subcutaneous administration of immunoglobulin. *Journal of Infusion Nursing, 29*(3S), S15–S20.

Kirschman, R.A. (2004). Finding alternatives to blood transfusion. *Nursing 2004, 34*(6), 58–62.

Klein, H., & Anstee, D. (2005). *Mollison's blood transfusion in clinical medicine* (11th ed.). Oxford: Blackwell.

Kopko, P.M., & Popvosky, M.A. (2007). Transfusion-related acute lung injury. In: M.A. Popovsky (Ed.), *Transfusion reactions* (3rd ed., pp. 207–228). Bethesda, MD: AABB Press.

Lockwood, W.B., Leonard, J., & Liles, S.L. (2008). Storage, monitoring, pretransfusion processing and distribution of blood components. In: J. Roback, M. Combs, B. Grossman, & C. Hillyer (Eds.), *AABB technical manual* (16th ed., pp. 248–298). Bethesda, MD: AABB Press.

Mazzei, C.A., Popovsky, M.A., & Kopko, P.M. (2008). Noninfectious complications of blood transfusion. In: J. Roback, M. Combs, B. Grossman, & C. Hillyer (Eds.), *AABB technical manual* (16th ed., pp. 715–745). Bethesda, MD: AABB Press.

McCloskey-Dochterman, J.C., & Bulechek, G.M. (2004). *Nursing interventions classification (NIC)* (4th ed.). St. Louis, MO: C.V. Mosby.

Moorhead, S., Johnson, M., & Maas, M. (2004). *Nursing outcomes classification (NOC)* (3rd ed.). St. Louis, MO: C.V. Mosby.

NANDA-I (2007). *Nursing diagnoses: Definitions and classification, 2007–2008.* Philadelphia: Author.

O'Grady, N.P., Alexander, M., Dellinger, E.P., et al. (2002). Guidelines for the prevention of intravascular catheter-related infections. *Morbidity and Mortality Weekly Report MMWR, 51*(RR-10).

Piga, A., Galanello, R., Forni, G.L., et al. (2006). Randomized phase II trial of deferasirox (Exjade, ICL670), a once-daily, orally-administered iron chelator, in comparison to deferoxamine in thalassemia patients with transfusional iron overload. *Hematologica, 91,* 873–880.

Porth, C.M., & Martin, G. (2008). *Pathophysiology: Concepts of altered health states* (8th ed.). Philadelphia: Lippincott Williams & Wilkins.

Preiksaitis, J. (2000). The cytomegalovirus –"safe" blood product: Is leukoreduction equivalent to antibody screening? *Transfusion Medicine Reviews, 14,* 112–136.

Schaefer, J. (2002). Advances and dilemmas in recombinant blood products. *Journal of Infusion Nursing, 25*(5), 305–309.

Schved, J.F. (2005). Preoperative autologous blood donation: A therapy that needs to be scientifically evaluated. *Transfusion Clinical Biology and Medicine, 12,* 365–369.

Shorr, A.F., Duh, M.S., Kelly, K.M., et al. (2004). Red blood cell transfusion and ventilator-associated pneumonia: A potential link? *Critical Care Medicine, 32,* 666–674.

Sink, B.L. (2008). Administration of blood components. In: J. Roback, M. Combs, B. Grossman, & C. Hillyer (Eds.), *AABB technical manual* (16th ed., pp. 229–238). Bethesda, MD: AABB Press.

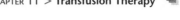

Spiess, B.D. (2004). Risks of transfusion: Outcome focus. *Transfusion 2004, 44* (S12), 4S–14S.

Stansworth, S.J., Brunskill, S.J., Hyde, C.J., et al. (2004). Is fresh frozen plasma clinically effective? A systematic review of randomized controlled trials. *British Journal of Haematology, 126,* 139–152.

Stobart, K., Iorio, A., & Wu, J.K. (2006). Clotting factor concentrates given to prevent bleeding and bleeding-related complications in people with hemophilia A or B. Cochrane Database System Reviews: 19: CD003429.

Strategic Healthcare Group (2008). What is blood management? Retrieved from www.bloodmanagment.com (Accessed August 30, 2008).

Szymanski, I.O., Teno, R.A., Lockwood W., et al. (2001). Effect of rejuvenation and frozen storage on 42–day AS-1 red cells. *Transfusion, 41,* 550–555.

Tolich, D.J. (2008). Alternative to blood transfusions. *Journal of Infusion Nursing, 31* (1), 46–50.

Vincent, J.L., Baron, J.F., Reinhart, K., et al. (2002). ABC (Anemia and blood transfusion in critical care. Investigators). Anemia and blood transfusion in critically ill patients. *JAMA, 288,* 1499–1507.

Wallis, J.P., Wells, A.W., & Chapman, C.E. (2006). Changing indications for red cell transfusion from 2000 to 2004 in the North of England. *Transfusion Medicine, 16,* 411–417.

Waters, J.H. (2008). Blood management. In: J. Roback, M. Combs, B. Grossman, & C. Hillyer (Eds.), *AABB technical manual* (16th ed., pp. 387–409). Bethesda, MD: AABB Press.

Westhoff, C.M. (2008). The Rh system. In: J. Roback, M. Combs, B. Grossman, & C. Hillyer (Eds.) *AABB technical manual* (16th ed.). Bethesda, MD: AABB Press.

Wong, C.C., & Luban, N.L.C. (2005). Intrauterine, neonatal, and pediatric transfusion. In: P.D. Mintz (Ed.), *Transfusion therapy: Clinical principles and practice* (2nd ed., pp. 159–201). Bethesda, MD: AABB Press.

Yousef, H.M., Padmore, R.F., Neurath, D.D., & Rock, G.A. (2006). The effect of patient-controlled analgesia on coadministered red blood cells. *Transfusion, 46,* 372–376.

PROCEDURES DISPLAY 11-1

Initiation of Transfusion

Equipment Needed:
0.9% sodium chloride
Blood or blood component
Blood filter
Blood administration set
Needleless infusion administration equipment
Requisition slip
0.9% sodium chloride (USP) flushes or heparin as appropriate
Blood pressure cuff, stethoscope, and thermometer

Continued

PROCEDURES DISPLAY 11-1

Initiation of Transfusion—cont'd

Delegation:
This procedure cannot be delegated. An LVN/LPN or NAP can assist by monitoring vital signs. **Note:** In California the LVN can administer blood and blood products through a peripheral line if state I.V. certified and supported by agency policy.

Procedure	Rationale
1. Verify the authorized prescriber's order, and that informed consent is signed. Order type and cross-match and order blood or blood components.	1. A written order is a legal requirement for infusion therapy. Informed consent is required for blood product administration.
2. Confirm blood is available in the blood bank.	
3. Obtain an I.V. container of 0.9% sodium chloride and Y-blood set.	3. Sodium chloride is the only solution that is compatible with blood products.
4. Introduce yourself to the patient.	4. Establishes the nurse–patient relationship
5. Verify patient identity using two forms (check ID bracelet and ask patient to state name).	5. The Joint Commission (2003) safety goal recommendation.
6. Hand hygiene: Follow standards throughout procedure.	6. Good hand hygiene is the single most important means of preventing the spread of infection.
7. Assess the patient's understanding of the procedure, then describe the procedure and provide the patient with the opportunity to ask questions and express any concerns.	7. The patient who is well-informed is better able to cope with the treatment regimen.
8. Verify that the I.V. catheter is patent before getting blood from transfusion services.	8. The blood component must be started within 30 minutes from removal from blood bank. Blood cannot be stored on the unit. The component must be infused within 4 hours.

PROCEDURES DISPLAY 11-1

Initiation of Transfusion—cont'd

Procedure	Rationale
9. Obtain baseline vital signs. Notify the physician if temperature is elevated 1° above normal. The transfusion may be held.	9. Fever can conceal the symptoms of an untoward reaction. Vital signs serve as baseline for the identification of changes that may transpire during the transfusion.
10. Prime and hand blood administration set and sodium chloride. If continuous infusion is being administered and can be discontinued during transfusion change tubing to Y-site blood tubing and sodium chloride; discard existing tubing and solution—do not save. If you cannot temporarily discontinue the existing solution, start a new I.V. for the transfusion. If intermittent access device is in place prime the Y-tubing and attach at slow rate.	10. Having all equipment at hand will save time and lessen patient anxiety. Prime the set and have equipment integrity checked and in place before obtaining the blood component from the transfusion service.
11. Obtain the component from transfusion services and record the name of the person issuing the component, as well as the date and time of issue. Inspect the component and its container for clots, hemolysis, leaks in the bag, or discoloration. If present, refuse to accept from transfusion services. Compare ABO group and Rh type on the blood label and the tag attached to it with the type	11. The correct type and crossmatch established compatibility between a donor and a recipient. The transfusion of the incompatible blood components can be serious or fatal. Most serious reactions are due to clerical errors. There is shared accountability between the nurse obtaining the component and the transfusion services.

Continued

PROCEDURES DISPLAY 11-1

Initiation of Transfusion—cont'd

Procedure	Rationale
and crossmatching information in transfusion services. Check the expiration date of the component.	
12. Return to the unit with one component (do not take more than one blood unit out of the transfusion services at a time). NEVER put a blood component in a refrigerator that is not specifically intended to store blood.	12. For safety, and integrity of blood component.
13. Reassess the patient's condition and level of consciousness. Check the component at the bedside with another nurse. Verify the following: ■ Patient name; also validate the numbers on both I.D. bands correlate with those on the laboratory form and component. ■ Physician order of the correct component ■ ABO and Rh type ■ ID number on blood bag and blood requisition slip ■ Expiration date of the component Use blood warmers only if ordered by the physician and use manufacturer recommendations for use.	13. There is less probability of error when two people verify the needed information. One person should read all of the information to the other as the second person verifies it.
14. Carry out proper hand hygiene and don gloves.	14. Gloves must be worn when handling blood components.

PROCEDURES DISPLAY 11-1

Initiation of Transfusion—cont'd

Procedure	Rationale
15. Using aseptic technique, spike the blood component bag and open the clamp to initiate the transfusion at the rate of 5 mL/min or slower. Turn off the sodium chloride. No more than 50 mL should be administered within the first 15 minutes of a transfusion. Stay with the patient for 15 minutes. Obtain a second set of vital signs. Record on the medical records.	**15.** The signs and symptoms of a severe reaction occur during the time the first 50 mL of blood are administered. The patient must be monitored throughout the course of any transfusion, but special observations should be made during the first 15 minutes.
16. Monitor and document the patient's level of consciousness, and vital signs every 30 to 60 minutes for the duration of the transfusion. (Check agency policy) Blood components must be infused within 4 hours.	**16.** Primary indicators of patient tolerance of transfusion.
17. Once the blood component has infused, flush the line with 50 mL of 0.9% sodium chloride. If another unit of blood is required, new administration set must be added. Only one administration set can be used in 4 hours.	**17.** AABB standard of practice. Flushing clears the remaining blood product that is in the tubing.
18. Discard the empty blood container and administration set in biohazard container.	**18.** OSHA standard

Continued

PROCEDURES DISPLAY 11-1

Initiation of Transfusion—cont'd

Procedure	Rationale
19. Document the time the blood component terminated and the amount infused. During the transfusion, the patient's response should also be documented, along with vital signs. **Transfusion Reaction** If a transfusion reaction occurs, notify the physician immediately; do not discard the blood container—return to transfusion services. Complete the transfusion record and place in the patient's permanent medical record. Draw post-transfusion laboratory samples as ordered. Follow agency policy on transfusion reaction. Document signs and symptoms, component administered, amount infused, time physician notified and response, time of blood bank notification, medication, and treatment ordered and administered, patient's response, and patient outcome.	19. To maintain the legal record. Immediate reactions can occur within 2 hours of completion of a transfusion. To maintain proper documentation and communicate that transfusion was administered. The remainder of the blood must be sent to the laboratory blood bank where it can be analyzed to determine the cause of the reaction. Medication and treatment will vary depending on the type of reaction.

Sources: INS (2006); Wilkinson & Van Leuven (2007).

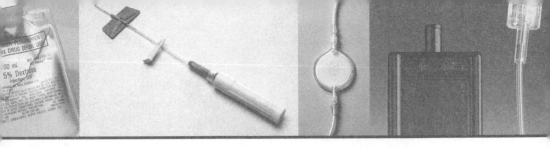

Chapter **12**

Nutritional Support

Every careful observer of the sick will agree in this that thousands of patients
are annually starved in the midst of plenty, from want of attention to the ways
which alone make it possible for them to take food.
—*Florence Nightingale, 1859*

▪ **LEARNING OBJECTIVES**

On completion of this chapter, the reader will be able to:

1. Define the glossary of terms as related to nursing care of the patient receiving nutritional support.
2. Apply the goals of parenteral nutrition to hospitalized, pediatric, and home care patients.
3. Identify the key elements of a nutritional assessment.
4. List the key points in administration of glucose, protein, and fat emulsions.
5. Describe the three major classifications of malnutrition.
6. Identify early candidates for nutritional support.
7. Identify the component used to treat essential fatty acid deficiency.
8. Describe the use of the additives heparin, insulin, and H_2 inhibitors to parenteral nutrition.
9. Describe three-in-one solutions.
10. Discuss evidence-based practice for use of cyclic therapy for the home care client.
11. Discuss the total parenteral nutrition point-of-care plan for patients with renal or liver disease.
12. Identify potential complications related to delivery of nutritional support.

⟩ GLOSSARY

Amino acid   Chief organic component of protein

Anergy   Lack of immune response to an antigen

Anthropometry measurement   Measurement of a part or whole of the body

Basal energy expenditure (BEE)   The amount of energy produced per unit of time under "basal" conditions

Cyclic therapy   Delivery of dextrose, amino acids, and fat over a regimen of reduced time frame, usually 12 to 18 hours versus a 24-hour infusion

Essential fatty acid deficiency (EFAD) Compound of carbon, hydrogen, and oxygen that combines with glycerol to form fat required in the diet. Essential fatty acids cannot be synthesized by the body, but must be obtained from the diet or intravenous infusion of lipids

Fat emulsion A combination of liquid, lipid, and an emulsifying system suitable for intravenous use because the lipid has been broken into small droplets that can be suspended in water. The solution has limited ability to be mixed with other solutions.

Kwashiorkor Malnutrition characterized by an adequate calorie intake with inadequate amount of protein

Marasmus Malnutrition characterized by decreased intake of calories with adequate amounts of protein intake

Parenteral nutrition (PN) Nutrients that are administered intravenously, comprising carbohydrates, proteins, and/or fats, and additives such as electrolytes, vitamins, and trace elements

Peripheral parenteral nutrition (PPN) Intravenous support supplied via the peripheral veins to patients whose nutritional requirements cannot be fully met via the enteral route.

Refeeding syndrome Syndrome in which the body, during its bout with starvation, adapts to nutritional deprivation and compensates by decreasing basal energy requirements

Total lymphocyte count (TLC) Integral component of the immune system

Total nutrient admixture (TNA) A three-in-one formula of amino acids, fats, and dextrose in one container

Total parenteral nutrition (TPN) The intravenous provision of dextrose, amino acids, emulsified fats, trace elements, vitamins, and minerals to patients who are unable to assimilate adequate nutrition by mouth

▪ Nutritional Support

The American Society for Parenteral and Enteral Nutrition (ASPEN) is a professional society of physicians, nurses, dietitians, pharmacists, allied health professionals, and researchers dedicated to patient's receiving optimal nutrition care and are part of the nutritional support team. Nutritional support nursing is the care of individuals with potential or known nutritional alterations. The nutrition support nurse (NSN) encompasses all nursing activities that promote optimal nutritional health. Nursing interventions are based on scientific principles. The scope of practice includes, but is not limited to, direct patient care; consultation with nurses and other healthcare professionals in a variety of clinical settings; education of patients, students, colleagues, and the public; participation in research; and administrative functions. A range of competencies that should be provided by any NSN within or outside the context of a formal nutrition support service or team are outlined in standards of practice by the American Society for Parenteral and Enteral Nutrition (ASPEN, 2007).

It is essential for nurses in all settings to respect the importance of adequate nutrition and the adverse effects of malnutrition. The goals of parenteral nutrition include:

1. To provide all essential nutrients in adequate amounts to sustain nutritional balance during periods when oral or enteral routes of feedings are not possible or are insufficient to meet the patient's caloric needs
2. To preserve or restore the body's protein metabolism and prevent the development of protein or caloric malnutrition
3. To diminish the rate of weight loss and to maintain or increase body weight
4. To promote wound healing
5. To replace nutritional deficits

 Website

American Society for Parenteral and Enteral Nutrition: www.clinnutri.org

▪ Concepts of Nutrition

Nutritional balance occurs when nutrients are provided in sufficient quantities for the maintenance of body function and renewal of these components. Nutritional balance is based on three factors: (1) intake of nutrients (quantity and quality), (2) relative need for nutrients, and (3) the ability of the body to use nutrients.

Nutritional Deficiency

When nutritional deficiency exists, the body's components are used to provide energy for essential metabolic processes. For example, body stores of carbohydrates, fats, and protein are metabolized as energy sources in nutritional deficiency states. Carbohydrates are stored in the muscle and liver as glycogen. Adipose tissue is the body's long-term energy reserve of fat. Body protein is not stored in excess of the body's needs; therefore, use of body protein without replacement adversely affects total body function (Wilson & Jordan, 2001).

Malnutrition

Malnutrition is defined as any disorder of nutrition status, including disorders resulting from deficiency of nutrient intake, impaired nutrient metabolism, or over-nutrition (ASPEN, 2002a). Malnutrition is a nutritional deficit associated with an increased risk of morbidity and mortality. Death from protein energy malnutrition and other nutritional deficiencies occurs within 60 to 70 days of total starvation in normal weight adults. After total starvation for less than 2 to 3 days in healthy adults, the losses are mainly glycogen and water. Starvation alters the distribution of carbohydrates, fats, and protein substrates. Brief starvation (24–72 hours) rapidly depletes glycogen stores and uses protein to produce glucose (gluconeogenesis) for glucose-dependent tissue. Prolonged starvation (longer than 72 hours) is associated with an increased mobilization of fat as the principal source of energy, reduction in the breakdown of protein, and increased use of ketones for central nervous tissue fuel. Stress in the form of pain, shock, injury, and sepsis intensifies the metabolic change seen in those with brief and prolonged starvation.

 NURSING FAST FACT!

> *Malnutrition is common occurrence in hospitalized patients, with an incidence of 30%–55% (Shopbell, Hopkins, & Shronts, 2001). Malnourished hospitalized patients have been shown to have increased lengths of stay, with associated increased costs of care.*

Factors indicative of malnutrition include:
- Voluntary loss or gain of 10% or greater of usual body weight over 6 months
- Loss of 5% or greater of usual body weight in 1 month
- Body weight of 20% over or under ideal body weight in the presence of chronic disease (ASPEN, 2002a)

Poor nutrition causes weight loss and generalized weakness, which affects functional ability and quality of life. Three types of malnutrition have been defined and classified by an International Classification of Diseases (ICD) diagnostic code: marasmus, kwashiorkor, and mixed malnutrition. The outcome of nutritional assessment determines the category to which an undernourished person is assigned.

Marasmus

Marasmus is caused by a decrease in the intake of calories with adequate protein–calorie ratio. In this type of malnutrition, a gradual wasting of body fat and skeletal muscle takes place with preservation of visceral proteins. The individual looks emaciated and has decreased **anthropometric** measurements and **anergy** to common skin test antigens.

 NURSING FAST FACT!

> *Marasmus may be seen in chronic illness and prolonged starvation, as well as the elderly and the patient with anorexia nervosa (McGinnis, 2002).*

Kwashiorkor

Kwashiorkor is characterized by an adequate intake of calories along with a poor protein intake. This condition causes visceral protein wasting with preservation of fat and somatic muscle. It is seen during a period of decreased protein intake as seen with liquid diets, fat diets, and long-term use of I.V. fluids containing dextrose. Loss of body protein is caused by depleted circulating proteins in the plasma. Individuals may appear obese and have adequate anthropometric measurements but decreased visceral proteins and depressed immune function.

Mixed Malnutrition

Mixed malnutrition is characterized by aspects of both marasmus and kwashiorkor. The person presents with skeletal muscle and visceral protein wasting, depleted fat stores, and immune incompetence. The affected person appears cachectic and usually is in acute catabolic stress. This mixed protein–calorie disorder is associated with the highest risk of morbidity and mortality.

Effects of Malnutrition

The hazards of malnutrition on bodily function are decreased protein stores, albumin depletion, and impaired immune status. Without protein stores in the body, a deficiency of total body protein results first in decreased strength and endurance (loss of muscle mass) and ultimately in decreased cardiac and respiratory muscle function. Skeletal muscle wasting occurs in a ratio of about 30 to 1 compared with visceral protein loss. The loss of gastrointestinal (GI) function follows skeletal muscle wasting and is associated with hypoalbuminemia. Protein–calorie malnutrition is one of the most common causes of impairment of immune function. Both B- and T-cell–mediated immune functions are impaired, causing enhanced susceptibility to infections (Porth & Martin, 2008)

The effects of malnutrition on the body include:
- Loss of muscle mass
- Impaired wound healing
- Impaired immunologic function
- Decreased appetite
- Loss of calcium and phosphate from bone
- Anovulation and amenorrhea in women
- Decreased testicular function in men

■ Nutritional Screening

Nutritional screening identifies individuals who are malnourished or who are at risk for malnutrition. The purpose of the nutrition screening is to determine if a more detailed nutrition assessment is necessary. Practice guidelines for nutrition screening include:

- A nutrition screening incorporating objective data such as height, weight, weight change, primary diagnosis, and presence of comorbidities should be a component of the initial evaluation of all patients in ambulatory, hospital, home, or alternate care settings.
- The healthcare organization should determine who will perform the screen and the elements to be included.
- A procedure for periodic nutrition re-screening should be implemented (ASPEN, 2002a).

EBNP Adult nutrition screening tools designed for use by staff nurses have been tested for validity and reproducibility and evaluated for ease of use, cost-effectiveness, validity, reliability, and sensitivity and specificity (Arrowsmith, 1999; Kovacevich, Boney, Brlaunschweig, et al., 1997).

Assessment

The nutrition assessment of overall health history provides information for identifying nutrition-related problems. It includes subjective data about the client's dietary history and related factors. The nutritional assessment also encompasses anthropometric measurements, diagnostic testing, and a complete physical examination. The nutrition assessment combines the patient history with physical and biochemical markers to define the nutritional health (Wilkinson & Van Leuven, 2007). Refer to Table 12-1.

> Table 12-1	COMPONENTS OF A NUTRITIONAL ASSESSMENT

History
- Medical
- Social
- Dietary

Anthropometric measurements
- Skinfolds
- Height and weight
- Midarm circumference
- Midarm muscle circumference

Biochemical assessment
- Serum albumin and transferrin levels
- Serum electrolytes
- Total lymphocyte count
- Urine assays (creatinine, height index)

Energy requirements

Physical examination

Other indices
- Nitrogen balance
- Indirect calorimetry
- Prognostic Nutritional Index (PNI)

The history is divided into four major components: medical, weight changes, social, and dietary. The medical history should include a specific history of weight; chronic diseases; surgical history; presence of increased losses, such as from draining wounds and fistulas; and factors such as age and drug, alcohol, and tobacco use. The social history affecting nutrient intake includes income, education, ethnic background, and environment during mealtime, along with religious considerations. The dietary history often provides clues as to the cause and degree of malnutrition. The components of a dietary history include appetite, GI disturbances, mechanical problems such as ill-fitting dentures, food allergies, medications, and food likes and dislikes (Smeltzer, Bare, Hinkle, & Cheever, 2008).

 CULTURAL AND ETHNIC CONSIDERATIONS: NUTRITION

Assess for the influence of cultural beliefs, norms, and values on the patient's nutritional knowledge. What the patient considers normal dietary practices may be based on cultural perceptions (Leininger & McFarland, 2002). Culture can determine the foods a patient eats and how they are prepared and served. Culture and religion together often determine if certain foods are prohibited and if certain foods and spices are eaten. When taking a dietary history, the nurse must be sensitive to culture and religious beliefs related to foods (Smeltzer, Bare, Hinkle, & Cheever, 2008).

Anthropometric Measurements

Anthropometry is the measurement of a part or whole of the body. It is a method of determining body composition. To estimate the size of the body fat mass, a skinfold test is done on the triceps of the nondominant arm using a caliper. Along with the skinfold measurement, a midarm circumference and midarm muscle circumference evaluation are performed. The height and weight are also part of this evaluation, with serial weights providing helpful information related to the protein–calorie status of the person. To calculate the current weight as a percentage of the usual weight, use the following calculation:

Percent ideal body weight (IBW) = (Current weight ÷ IBW) × 100

Weight loss is important because it reflects inadequate calorie intake. Weight loss indicates an increased loss of protein from the body cell mass in individuals who are malnourished. Current weight does not provide information about recent changes in weight; therefore, patients are asked about their usual body weight (UBW) (Smeltzer, Bare, Hinkle, & Cheever, 2008).

Percent of UBW = (Current body weight ÷ UBW) × 100

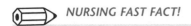 *NURSING FAST FACT!*

A loss of 10% of the usual weight or a current weight less than 90% of IBW is considered to be a risk factor of nutrition-related complications (Wilson & Jordan, 2001).

Mild malnutrition = 85% to 95% IBW

Moderate malnutrition = 75% to 84% IBW

Severe malnutrition = less than 75% IBW

In simple starvation, 20% loss of body weight is associated with marked decreases in muscle tissue and subcutaneous fat, giving the patient an emaciated appearance. Gross loss of body fat can be observed not only from appearance but also by palpating a number of skinfolds. When the dermis can be felt between the fingers on pinching the triceps and biceps skinfolds, considerable loss from body stores of fat has occurred. Protein stores can be assessed by inspection and palpation of a number of muscle groups, such as the triceps, biceps, and subscapular and infrascapular muscles. The long muscles in particular are profoundly protein depleted when the tendons are prominent to palpation.

Biochemical Assessment

Several tests are available to assess patients' biochemical nutritional status. The anergy test is recommended for assessing immunologic response and involves the intradermal injection of antigens. Proper nutrition is a key to an intact immune system, and a lack of response to antigens is considered anergic and possibly indicates malnourishment.

Biochemical assessment reflects both the tissue level of a given nutrient and any abnormality of metabolism. Studies of serum protein, albumin, globulin, transferrin, retinol-binding protein, hemoglobin, serum vitamin A, carotene, and vitamin C can reflect the utilization of nutrients. Total lymphocyte count is also measured for the body's response immunologically.

Serum Albumin and Transferrin Levels

Albumin is a major protein synthesized by the liver. Approximately 40% of protein mass is in the circulation. The serum albumin concentration is normally between 3.5 and 5.0 g/dL (DeLegge & Drake, 2007). An albumin level of 2.8 to 3.2 g/dL represents mild protein depletion, 2.1 to 2.7 g/dL reflects moderate depletion, and less than 2.1 g/dL indicates severe depletion.

Serum transferrin is a beta globulin that transports iron in the plasma and is synthesized in the liver. Transferrin is present in the serum in concentrations of 250 to 300 mg/dL. The serum levels are affected by nutritional factors and iron metabolism. Levels lower than 100 mg/dL indicate severe depletion (Smeltzer, Bare, Hinkle, & Cheever, 2008).

 NURSING FAST FACT!

> *Low serum albumin and transferrin levels are often used as measures of protein deficits in adults and many hospitals routinely screen elderly patients for these biochemicals.*

Prealbumin and Retinol-Binding Protein

Prealbumin functions in thyroxine transport and as a carrier for retinol-binding protein. Normal serum concentrations range from 15.7 to 29.6 mg/dL. Levels of 10 to 15 mg/dL reflect mild depletion, those of 5 to 9.9 mg/dL reflect moderate depletion, and a level lower than 5 mg/dL indicates severe depletion.

Total Lymphocyte Count

Immunologic testing is designed to assess nutritional deficiencies. The most commonly used test for the assessment of immunocompetence is the **total lymphocyte count (TLC)**. Reduced total lymphocyte count in people who become acutely malnourished as a result of stress and low-calorie feeding are associated with impaired cellular immunity (Dudek, 2006).

The TLC is derived from the routine complete blood count (CBC) with differential. The TLC is calculated by means of the following formula:

$$TLC = Percent\ lymph \times WBC \div 100$$

A TLC between 1200 and 2000/µL indicates mild lymphocyte depletion; a TLC between 800 and 1199/µL indicates moderate lymphocyte depletion; and a TLC lower than 800/µL indicates severe lymphocyte depletion. TLC must be interpreted with caution because many other non-nutritional factors may contribute to decreased lymphocyte counts.

Serum Electrolytes

Serum electrolyte levels provide information about fluid and electrolyte balance and kidney function. The creatinine/height index calculated over a 24-hour period assesses the metabolically active tissue and indicates the degree of protein depletion, comparing expected body mass for height and actual body cell mass (Smeltzer, Bare, Hinkle, & Cheever, 2008).

 NURSING FAST FACT!

> *Many nutrition teams have incorporated a Subjective Global Assessment into their practice. A disadvantage to the Subjective Global Assessment is that it is a subjective data collection and depends on the experience of the clinician collecting and interpreting the data.*

Energy Requirements

Energy requirements are dependent on a number of factors, which include the body surface area (derived from height and weight), age, and gender. Total daily energy expenditure has three components: (1) **basal energy expenditure** (**BEE** or BMR); (2) energy expenditure related to an activity; and (3) specific dynamic action of food. Determination of energy needs can be determined from the BEE or resting metabolic expenditure. The BEE accounts for 65% to 75% of energy expenditure and may be measured or estimated. The traditional method used to estimate BEE is the Harris–Benedict equation, which takes into consideration influence of patient's weight in kilograms, height in centimeters, age, and gender.

Physical Examination

The final phase of the nutritional assessment is a complete physical examination. Findings from a physical examination can reflect protein–calorie malnutrition along with vitamin and mineral deficiencies. The physical examination should include evaluation of the patient's hair, nails, skin, thorax and lungs, eyes, oral cavity, glands, heart, muscles, and abdomen, along with a neurologic evaluation and evaluation of delayed healing and tissue repair (Table 12-2). The physical examination should also include objective measurements of wound healing, grip strength, skeletal muscle function, and respiratory muscle function. A complete physical is not routine. Many of the body systems are selectively assessed on the basis of individuals presenting problems (Smeltzer, Bare, Hinkle, & Cheever, 2008).

> Table 12-2	PHYSICAL FINDINGS ASSOCIATED WITH DEFICIENCY STATES	
Area Assessed	**Physical Findings**	**Associated Deficiencies**
Hair	Flag sign (transverse depigmentation of hair)	Protein, copper
	Hair easily pluckable	Protein
	Hair thin, sparse	Protein, biotin, zinc
Nails	Nails, spoon shaped	Iron
	Nails, lackluster, transverse riding	Protein-calorie
Skin	Dry, scaling	Vitamin A, zinc, essential fatty acids
	Flaky paint dermatosis	Protein
	Follicular hyperkeratosis	Vitamins A, C; essential fatty acids
	Nasolabial seborrhea	Niacin, pyridoxine, riboflavin
	Petechiae, purpura	Ascorbic acid, vitamin K
	Pigmentation, desquamation (sun-exposed area)	Niacin (pellagra)
	Subcutaneous fat loss	Calorie

Continued

> Table 12-2

PHYSICAL FINDINGS ASSOCIATED WITH DEFICIENCY STATES—cont'd

Area Assessed	Physical Findings	Associated Deficiencies
Eyes	Angular blepharitis	Riboflavin
	Corneal vascularization	Riboflavin
	Dull, dry conjunctiva	Vitamin A
	Fundal capillary microaneurysms	Ascorbic acid
	Scleral icterus, mild	Pyridoxine
Perioral	Angular stomatitis	Riboflavin
	Cheilosis	Riboflavin
Oral Cavity	Atrophic lingual papillae	Niacin, iron, riboflavin, folate, vitamin B_{12}
	Glossitis (scarlet, raw)	Niacin, pyridoxine, riboflavin, vitamin B_{12}, folate
	Hypogeusesthesia (also hyposomia)	Zinc, vitamin A
	Magenta tongue	Riboflavin
	Swollen, bleeding gums (if teeth present)	Ascorbic acid
	Tongue fissuring, edema	Niacin
Glands	Parotid enlargement	Protein
	Sicca syndrome	Ascorbic acid
	Thyroid enlargement	Iodine
Heart	Enlargement, tachycardia, high output failure	Thiamine ("wet" beriberi)
	Small heart, decreased output	Calorie
	Sudden heart failure, death	Ascorbic acid
Abdomen	Hepatomegaly	Protein
Muscles, Extremities	Calf tenderness	Thiamine, ascorbic acid (hemorrhage into muscle)
	Edema	Protein, thiamine
	Muscle wastage (especially temporal area, dorsum of hand, spine)	Calorie
Bones, Joints	Bone tenderness (adult)	Vitamin D, calcium, phosphorus (osteomalacia)
Neurologic	Confabulation, disorientation (Korsakoff's psychosis)	Thiamine
	Decreased position and vibratory senses, ataxia	Vitamin B_{12}, thiamine
	Decreased tendon reflexes, slowed relaxation phase	Thiamine
	Ophthalmoplegia	Thiamine, phosphorus
	Weakness, paresthesias, decreased fine tactile sensation	Vitamin B_{12}, pyridoxine, thiamine
Other	Delayed healing and tissue repair (e.g., wound, infarct, abscess)	Ascorbic acid, zinc, protein

Other Indices

Nitrogen Balance

A sensitive indicator of the body's gain or loss of protein is its nitrogen balance. An adult is said to be in nitrogen equilibrium when the nitrogen intake from food equals the nitrogen output in urine, feces, and perspiration. The nitrogen balance is a measure of daily intake of nitrogen minus the excretion. It is used to assess protein turnover. A positive nitrogen balance indicates an anabolic state with an overall gain in body protein for the day. A negative nitrogen balance indicates a catabolic state with a net low of protein.

Negative nitrogen balance indicates that tissue is breaking down faster than it is being replaced. In absence of protein, the body converts protein to glucose for energy. This occurs with fever, starvation, surgery, burns, and debilitating diseases.

 NURSING FAST FACT!

> *Each gram of nitrogen loss in excess of intake represents the depletion of 6.25 g of protein or 25 g of muscle tissue (Smeltzer, Bare, Hinkle, & Cheever, 2008).*

Indirect Calorimetry

Indirect calorimetry is a technique used in measuring the resting energy expenditure based on oxygen consumption and carbon dioxide production.

Prognostic Nutritional Index

The prognostic nutritional index (PNI) is an assessment technique that is based on four measures selected by analysis and computer-based stepwise regression that are then incorporated into a linear predictive model. The clinically important factors as determined by this analysis include the serum albumin concentration, serum transferrin, triceps skinfold thickness, and delayed hypersensitivity. This predictive model relates the risk of morbidity to nutritional status.

■ Nutritional Requirements: Adults

Nutritional requirements are based on a basic formula that must contain all essential macro- and micronutrients for adequate energy production, support of synthesis, replacement, and repair of structural or visceral proteins; cell structure; production of hormones and enzymes; and maintenance of immune function. The basic design contains protein, and nonprotein calories: carbohydrates and fat, along with electrolytes, vitamins, trace elements, and fluid requirements.

Proteins/Amino Acids

Proteins are a body-building nutrient that function to promote tissue growth and repair and replacement of body cells. Proteins are also components in antibodies, scar tissue, and clots. **Amino acids** are the basic units of protein. There are eight essential amino acids needed by adults that must be supplied by the diet: isoleucine, leucine, lysine, methionine, phenylalanine, threonine, tryptophan, and valine.

Parenteral proteins are elemental, providing a synthetic crystalline amino acid that does not cause an antigenic reaction. These proteins are available in concentrations of 3% to 15% and come with and without electrolytes. (Some amino acid solutions are presented in Table 12-3.) An increased need for protein by the body is usually reflected by an increase in excretion of urinary nitrogen, as evidenced by laboratory values.

> Table 12-3	AMINO ACID SOLUTIONS FOR PARENTERAL NUTRITION		
Protein Solution	Concentration (%)	Nitrogen (%)	Osmolarity mOsm/L (g/100 mL)
Aminosyn	3.5	0.55	357
Aminosyn II	3.5	0.55	308
Aminosyn II	4.25	0.65	894
Aminosyn	5	0.786	500
Aminosyn II	5	0.786	438
Aminosyn	7	1.10	700
Aminosyn II	7	1.10	800
Aminosyn	8.5	1.33	850
Aminosyn II	8.5	1.3	742
Aminosyn	10	1.57	875
Aminosyn II	10	1.57	1000
Aminosyn III	15	2.3	1300
Aminosyn-HBC	7	1.12	665
BranchAmin	4	0.433	316
Clinimix (SF)	2.75	0.40	297
Clinimix E (SF) with electrolytes and calcium	2.75	0.40	297
Clinimix (SF)	4.75	0.65	480
Clinimix E (SF) with electrolytes	4.25	0.65	490
Clinimix E with electrolytes and calcium	5	0.786	550
FreAmine III	3	0.46	300
FreAmine III	8.5	1.42	810
FreAmine III	10	1.57	950
FreAmine III with electrolytes	3	0.46	405
HepatAmine	8	1.2	785
NephrAmine	5.4	1.6	718
ProcalAmine	3	0.46	736
Travasol with electrolytes	3.5	0.591	450

> Table 12-3	**AMINO ACID SOLUTIONS FOR PARENTERAL NUTRITION—cont'd**		
Protein Solution	**Concentration (%)**	**Nitrogen (%)**	**Osmolarity mOsm/L (g/100 mL)**
Travasol with electrolytes	8.5	0.924	575
Travasol with electrolytes	3.5	0.591	450
Travasol without electrolytes	5.5	0.924	575
Travasol without electrolytes	8.5	1.42	890
Travasol without electrolytes	10	1.68	970
TrophAmine	6	0.93	5.25
TrophAmine	10	1.55	875
PREMASOL Pediatric	6	0.93	525
PREMASOL Pediatric	10	1.57	950

Source: Gahart, B.L., & Nazareno, A.R. (2008). Intravenous medications (24th ed.). St. Louis, MO: C.V. Mosby.

 NURSING FAST FACT!

>   *Protein requirements for maintenance of healthy adults are 0.8–1 g/kg per day.*
>   *Catabolic patients require 1.2–2 g/kg per day*
>   *Chronic renal failure (renal replacement therapy) require 1.2–1.5 g/kg per day*
>   *Acute renal failure + catabolic patient 1.5–1.8 g/kg per day (ASPEN, 2002a)*
>   *Provisions for protein in quantities greater than 2.0 g/kg/day in PN solutions is controversial and rarely required (Jacobs, Jacobs, Kudsk, et al., 2004).*

Carbohydrates

The major nonprotein calorie sources are from carbohydrates (70%–85%) and from fat (15%–30%). This distribution may be adjusted based on tolerance. The intravenous source of carbohydrates is predominately dextrose.

 NURSING FAST FACT!

>   ■ *1 g carbohydrate = 4 kcal*
>   ■ *Dextrose increases the metabolic rate, which in turn raises ventilatory requirements.*

Glucose

The major function of carbohydrates is to provide energy. Glucose provides calories in parenteral solutions. Carbohydrates also spare body protein. When glucose is supplied as a nutrient, it is stored temporarily in the liver and muscle as glycogen. When glycogen storage capacity is reached, the carbohydrate is stored as fat. When glucose is provided parenterally, it is completely bioavailable to the body without any effects of malabsorption. When dextrose is administered rapidly, the solution acts as an osmotic diuretic and pulls interstitial fluid into the plasma for subsequent renal excretion. The nurse must be aware that when infusing 20% to 70% dextrose solutions, the rate must be kept within 10% of the prescribed order. Table 12-4 provides a list of dextrose solutions, osmolarity, and kcal/L. The pancreas secretes extra insulin to metabolize infused glucose. If 20% to 70% dextrose is discontinued suddenly, a temporary excess of insulin in the body may cause symptoms of hypoglycemia (Metheny, 2000).

Dextrose is usually administered concurrently with lipids for two reasons: (1) to prevent hyperglycemia and avert the need for extra insulin and (2) to reduce respiratory demands.

The number of dextrose calories in parenteral preparation may vary considerably, depending on the needs of the patient. The range may be from 400 to 5000 cal/day and depends on the age, weight, and clinical status of the patient along with laboratory determinations.

For peripheral infusions, a 10% or less dextrose concentration must be maintained at an isotonic or mildly hypertonic osmolarity to prevent vein irritation, damage to the vein, and thrombosis. Hypertonic concentrations of 10% and above must be administered through a central venous catheter (CVC) with tip location in the superior vena cava.

INS Standard Parenteral nutrition solutions containing final concentrations exceeding 10% dextrose and 5% protein, pH less than 5 or greater than 9, and osmolality greater than 600 mOsm/L, should be administered through a central vascular access device with tip placement in the vena cava. (INS, 2006, 69)

Fats/Lipids

Fat is a primary source of heat and energy. Fat provides twice as many energy calories per gram as either protein or carbohydrate. Fat is essential for the structural integrity of all cell membranes. Linoleic acid and linolenic

> Table 12-4   **DEXTROSE SOLUTIONS FOR TOTAL PARENTERAL NUTRITION**

Solution (%)	g/L	kcal/L	mOsm/L
5	50	170	252
10	100	340	505
20	200	680	1010
30	300	1020	1515
40	400	1360	2020
50	500	1700	2525
60	600	2040	3030
70	700	2380	3535

acid are the only fatty acids essential to humans. These two acids prevent essential fatty acid deficiency (**EFAD**). Linoleic acid is necessary as a precursor of prostaglandins. It regulates cholesterol metabolism and maintains the integrity of cell walls. Signs and symptoms of EFAD include desquamating dermatitis, alopecia, brittle nails, delayed wound healing, thrombocytopenia, decreased immunity, and increased capillary fragility.

NOTE > The majority of hospitalized adults who receive no dietary fat develop biochemical evidence of EFAD after 4 weeks of fat-free TPN (ASPEN, 2002a).

Lipid Administration

When fat or lipids is used as a calorie source in parenteral nutrition, there are fewer problems with glucose homeostasis, carbon dioxide (CO_2) production is lower, and hepatic tolerance to I.V. feedings may improve. Primarily, intravenous fats are supplied by safflower or soybean oil, with egg yolk phospholipids and glycerol to provide tonicity. Fat emulsions provide 1.1 kcal/mL (10% solution) or 2.0 kcal/mL (20% solution) (Gahart & Nazareno, 2008; Metheny, 2000). The use of 20% IVFE allows for more efficient triglyceride clearance and metabolism (ASPEN, 2004).

NOTE > A 30% fat emulsion is available but is not to be given by direct I.V. infusion.

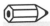 *NURSING FAST FACT!*

- *1 g of fat = 9 kcal*
- *Use of fat can help control hyperglycemia in stress states.*
- *Twenty percent (20%) fat emulsions are better utilized by the body.*

Complications associated with EFAD include impaired wound healing, platelet dysfunction, increased susceptibility to infection, and development of fatty liver. In patients with respiratory failure, the administration of fat can help decrease carbon dioxide excretion. The primary purpose of fat emulsions in patients with TPN is to prevent or treat EFAD with infusion of two or three 500-mL bottles of 10% or 20% fat emulsions per week. Table 12-5 provides a listing of lipid emulsions for TPN.

To prevent EFAD, 2% to 4% of the total calorie requirement should come from linoleic acid (25 to 100 mg/kg per day). Ten percent of calories from soy or safflower oil emulsions should provide adequate linoleic acid to prevent EFAD.

Administration sets that contain di(2-ethylhexyl) phthalate (DEHP) plasticizers extract lipids from the set. It is recommended to use a separate

> Table 12-5 | **LIPID EMULSIONS FOR TOTAL PARENTERAL NUTRITION**

Emulsion/Percentage	Available	Osmolarity (mOsm/L)
Liposyn II 10%	50/50 Safflower oil, soybean oil	10% (1.1 kcal/mL) 276
Liposyn II 20%	50/50 Safflower oil, soybean oil	20% (2.0 kcal/mL) 258
Liposyn III 10%	Soybean oil	10% (1.1 kcal/mL) 284
Liposyn III 20%	Soybean oil	20% (2.0 kcal/mL) 292
Liposyn III 30%	Soybean oil	30% (3.0 kcal/mL) 305
Intralipid 10%	Soybean oil	10% (1.1 kcal/mL) 280
Intralipid 20%	Soybean oil	20% (2.2 kcal/mL) 260
Intralipid 30%	Soybean oil	30% (3.0 kcal/mL) 310

Source: Gahart, B.L., & Nazareno, A.R. (2008). Intravenous medications (24th ed.). St. Louis, MO: C.V. Mosby.

administration set, glass infusate containers, or special non–polyvinyl chloride (non-PVC) bags. It is very important to inspect fat emulsions carefully for "breaking-out" (or "oiling out"), which is the separation of an emulsion visually. Do not use if there is an identifiable yellowish streaking or the accumulation of yellow droplets in the admixed emulsion.

 NURSING FAST FACT!

*The initial rate of **fat emulsions** should be 1 mL/min or 0.1 g of fat/min for the first 15–30 minutes of the infusion for a 10% solution; if no untoward effects, increase the rate to administer 500 mL equally distributed over 4–6 hours. For 20% solution 0.5 mL/min or 0.1 g of fat/min for the first 15–30 minutes; if no untoward effect, increase the rate to administer 250 mL equally distributed over 4–6 hours. The rate may be increased to 2 mL/min (Gahart & Nazareno, 2008).*

A 1.2-micron filter must be used when infusing total nutrient admixtures (TNAs).

INS Standard Parenteral nutrition solutions containing an intravenous fat emulsion (IVFE) should be filtered with a 1.2-micron filter during administration. (INS, 2006, 69)

Electrolytes

Electrolytes are infused either as a component already contained in the amino acid solution or as a separate additive. Standard ranges for parenteral electrolytes assume normal organ function and normal losses. Electrolytes are available in several salt forms and are added based on the patient's metabolic status. The electrolytes necessary for long-term TPN include potassium, magnesium, calcium, sodium, chloride, and phosphorus. Potassium is needed for the transport of glucose and amino acids across cell membranes. Approximately 30 to 40 mEq of potassium is necessary for each 1000 calories provided by the parenteral route. Potassium may be given as potassium chloride, potassium phosphate, or potassium acetate salt. Serum potassium levels must be closely monitored during TPN administration.

 NURSING FAST FACT!

> *Patients with impaired renal function may need decreased amount of potassium.*

Other electrolytes included in nutritional support include:
- Magnesium sulfate at 10 to 20 mEq every 24 hours
- Calcium gluceptate, gluconate, or chloride at 10 to 15 mEq in 24 hours
- Sodium chloride, acetate, lactate, or phosphate at 60 to 100 mEq in 24 hours (as needed to maintain acid–base balance)
- Phosphorous sodium or potassium at 20 to 45 mmol in 24 hours
- Chloride is provided based on acid–base status

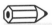 *NURSING FAST FACT!*

> *Sodium and potassium requirements for a given patient are highly variable. In general, sodium and potassium requirements in the PN formulation are 1–2 mEq/kg per day, but should be customized to meet individual needs (ASPEN, 2002a).*

Vitamins

Vitamins are necessary for growth and maintenance, as well as for multiple metabolic processes. The fat- and water-soluble vitamins are needed for patients requiring TPN. Controversy exists over the exact parenteral vitamin requirements for patients receiving TPN. Certain disease states can alter vitamin requirements, and the sequelae of vitamin deficiency can be catastrophic to very ill patients. Vitamin K is not a component of any of the vitamin mixtures formulated for adults. Maintenance requirements can be satisfied by administering vitamin K, 5 mg per week, intramuscularly (McGinnis, 2002).

 NURSING FAST FACT!

> *Sufficient vitamin K is found in lipids; if a patient receives daily lipid supplementation, vitamin K injections are not needed.*

Trace Elements

Trace elements (also called microelements) occur in the body in minute amounts. Basic requirements are very small, measured in milligrams. Each trace element is a single chemical and has an associated deficiency state. The many functions of trace elements are often synergistic (Metheny, 2000).

Zinc contributes to wound healing by increasing the tensile strength of collagen; copper assists in iron's incorporation of hemoglobin. The other trace elements (i.e., selenium, iodine, fluorine, cobalt, and nickel) all have been identified as beneficial.

NOTE > Iron is not routinely recommended for patients receiving PN therapy and is not a component of current injectable multiple trace element preparations (Krumpf, 2003).

ASPEN Standard Parenteral iron shall not be routinely supplemented in patients receiving PN therapy. It should be limited to conditions of iron deficiency when oral iron supplementation fails and followed closely in an ongoing monitoring plan. (ASPEN, 2002a)

Medication Administration with Parenteral Nutrition

Parenteral nutrition is complex and potential for physicochemical interactions exists with drug–nutrient combinations, admixture of medications with PN is not advised. Adding medications with TPN solutions depends on various factors, including the physical compatibility of the admixed components, the chemical stability of the drug, the retention of drug concentration over time, and the bioactivity of the components after admixture.

Compatibility is always an issue whenever two agents are combined. Parenteral solutions should be used immediately after mixing or else refrigerated. Stability of the admixed component dictates the appropriate length of time that the solution may be refrigerated.

INS Standard Parenteral nutrition solutions should be infused or discarded within 24 hours once the administration set is attached. (INS, 2006, 69)

 NURSING FAST FACT!

■ *Always check current information about drug compatibility with TPN solutions.*
■ *Piggybacking medications directly into TPN solutions is generally not recommended because of the guidelines that a designated port be used only for nutritional support.*
■ *Only regular insulin is appropriate for I.V. administration.*

Insulin

Insulin is commonly administered with PN. Hyperglycemia is the most common complication of TPN therapy. Hyperglycemia is caused by the high concentration of glucose in the TPN solutions. Insulin is considered to be chemically stable in parenteral nutrition. By adding regular insulin to the parenteral admixture, some patients benefit from the enhanced blood glucose levels. Insulin is responsible for adequate metabolism of carbohydrates. Insulin also has a lipolytic effect and an increased muscle uptake of amino acids.

> *EBNP Studies of medication compatibility with PN found that the compatibility differed from TNA versus 2-in-1 formulations, emphasizing that compatibility in one formulation does not predict compatibility in the other (Trissel, Gilbert, Martinez, et al., 1997, 1999).*

Parenteral Nutrition Compounding

The 1994 FDA Safety Alert highlights the serious consequences that are possible when quality-compounding practices are not in place. It is the responsibility of the dispensing pharmacist to assure that PN is prepared, labeled, controlled, stored, dispensed, and distributed properly (ASPEN, 2002a).

Automated or manual methods of PN compounding are available. Refer to Figure 12-1. Professional organizations have published guidelines for compounding and dispensing sterile products. Compounding PN formulations are classified by USP as medium-risk level given the

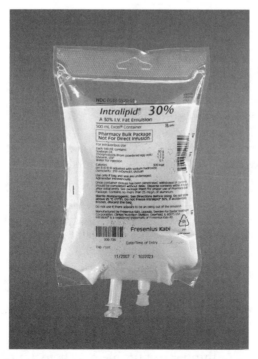

Figure 12-1 ■ Example of fat emulsion (intralipid 30%). (Courtesy of Baxter Healthcare Corp., Round Lake, IL.)

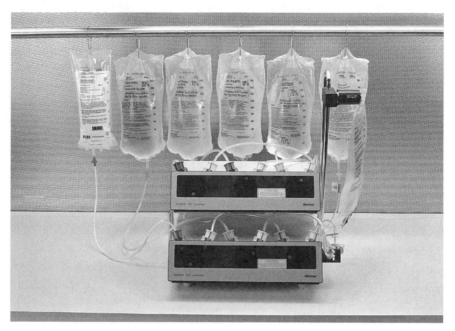

Figure 12-2 ■ Automated method of compounding parenteral nutrition. (Courtesy of Baxter Healthcare Corp., Round Lake, IL.)

multiple injections, detachments, and attachments of nutrient source products to be delivered into a final sterile container. According to the ASHP guidelines and USP standards:

- All compounded sterile preparations shall be prepared in a class 100 environment, such as a certified horizontal or vertical laminar-airflow workbench. Refer to Figure 12-2.
- Personnel are required to wear clean gowns or coveralls, as scrub attire by itself is not acceptable.
- Gloves; masks; hair covers; shoe covers; and removal of hand, finger, and wrist jewelry are recommended during the compounding process (ASPEN, 2004).

NOTE > Mishandling of these preparations has resulted in reports of septic morbidity and even death due to extrinsic contamination.

■ Delivery of Nutritional Support

Nutritional Support Candidates

Patients who are good candidates for nutritional support are those who suffer from a multiplicity of problems. Their clinical course can be complicated by malnutrition and depletion of body protein (Fig. 12-3).

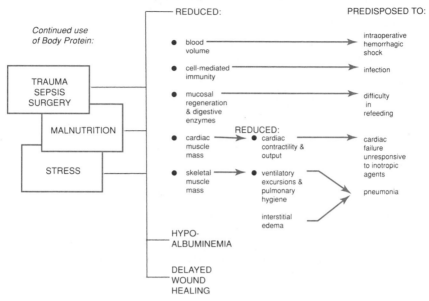

Figure 12-3 ■ Body protein depletion.

The indications for TPN in adults include a 10% deficit in pre-illness body weight; an inability to take oral food or fluids within 7 days after surgery; and hypercatabolic situations, such as major infections with fever and burns. Other conditions that have shown an efficacy for nutritional support include short gut syndrome, enterocutaneous fistulas, renal failure, and hepatic failure (Table 12-6).

> Table 12-6	CANDIDATES FOR TOTAL PARENTERAL NUTRITION

Chronic weight loss
■ Malnutrition
■ Anorexia nervosa
■ Anorexia of cancer
■ Cancer malabsorption syndrome
■ Chronic vomiting and diarrhea
■ 10% of pre-illness weight loss
Serum albumin below 3.5 g/dL
■ Bowel surgery
■ Short-bowel syndrome
■ Massive bowel resection
Conditions requiring bowel rest
■ Acute pancreatitis
■ Bowel fistulas
■ Inflammatory bowel disease
■ Obstruction

Continued

> Table 12-6	CANDIDATES FOR TOTAL PARENTERAL NUTRITION—cont'd

- Paralytic ileus
- Peritonitis
Malabsorption of enteral therapy
Excessive nitrogen loss
- Abscesses
- Fistulas
- Infections
- Wounds
Hypermetabolic states
- Burns
- Critical illness
Multiple trauma
Hepatic or renal failure
Coma

Parenteral Nutrition Orders

Life-threatening errors continue to occur in the preparation and delivery of PN admixtures to patients. A 2003 Survey of PN Practices confirmed a lack of uniformity in the ordering process from institution to institution. Research has demonstrated the benefit of standardized order writing processes in reducing prescription errors (Cerra, 1990).

Common factors associated with the majority of PN prescribing errors include:

- Inadequate knowledge regarding PN therapy
- Certain patient characteristics related to PN therapy (e.g., age, impaired renal function)
- Calculation of PN dosages
- Specialized PN dosage formulation characteristics and prescribing nomenclature

 NURSING FAST FACT!

Parenteral nutrition has been reported to be second only to anti-infective agents as a class of medications associated with errors (22% of report; Lustig, 2000).

Criteria mandatory for the PN order form is presented in Table 12-7. Figure 12-4 presents an example of PN orders.

Modalities for Delivery of Nutritional Support

Modalities for nutritional support include enteral nutrition, peripheral parenteral nutrition (PPN), total parenteral nutrition (TPN), total nutrition admixture (TNA), and cyclic therapy. There are also specialized parenteral formulas that can be used for patients in renal or liver failure or in

> Table 12-7 | COMPONENTS OF PARENTERAL NUTRITION ORDER FORM

Mandatory Components

Clarity of the form
Contact number for person writing the order
Contact number for assistance with PN ordering
Time by which orders need to be received for processing
Location of venous access device (central or peripheral)
Height, weight/dosing weight, diagnosis, PN indication
Hangtime guidelines
Institutional policy for infusion rates
Information regarding potential incompatibilities

Strongly Recommended Components

Educational tools
Guidelines to assist in nutrient/volume calculations
Recommended PN lab tests (baseline, monitoring, and special circumstances)
Guidelines for stopping/interrupting PN
Contents of multivitamin and trace element preparations
Brand names of products (e.g., amino acids, IVFE)
Guidelines for use of insulin
Guidelines for recognizing additional calorie sources.

Source: ASPEN (2004). Safe practices for parenteral nutrition. Journal of Parenteral and Enteral Nutrition, 28(S6), S44.

stress formulas. Figure 12-5 provides an algorithm for determining the choice of nutritional support.

Enteral Nutrition

Enteral nutrition is indicated for patients with functional gastrointestinal tract whose oral nutrient intake is insufficient to meet needs. The nasoenteric tube is the most common method of enteral access and is indicated for less than 4 weeks (short term). Tube enterostomies are indicated when long-term (greater than 30 days) feeding is anticipated (ASPEN, 2002b).

Advantages of enteral access include the following:

1. Maintenance of GI structure and functional integrity
2. Enhanced utilization of nutrients
3. Ease and safety of administration
4. Lower cost

Disadvantages include:

1. Contraindicated for patients with diffuse peritonitis, intestinal obstruction, intractable vomiting, paralytic ileus, or severe diarrhea that makes metabolic management difficult.
2. Not recommended during the early stages of short bowel syndrome or presence of severe malabsorption

Adult Parenteral Nutrition Orders: Orders received after 1400 will be started the next day at 2000

	Physician's Orders	

Physician: Please indicate approval of order by marking each order with a checkmark (✓). Physician must sign orders prior to initiation.

1. **Solution Order**

Patient Weight: _____ kg

☐ CENTRAL LINE FORMULA (mixed as 3 in 1)

Base Solution	Amount	Rate*		Amount	Rate*	Recommendations
Amino Acids (4 kcal/gm)	Final % _____	Total Volume/ 24 hours	OR	_____ gm/day	Total Volume/ 24 hours	1.2 gm/kg*/day Max final % is 7.5%
Dextrose (3.4 kcal/gm)	Final % _____ OR	_____ ml OR		_____ gm/day	_____ ml OR	5 gm/kg*/day Max final % is 35%
Lipids (9 kcal/gm) (2cal/ml) (2.5% ~ 40% Fat Calories in Final D20%-D25% solution)	Final % ☐ 2.5% ☐ _____	_____ ml/hr		_____ gm/day	_____ ml/hr OR ☐ Minimal vol./24 hrs	1 gm/kg*/day

*Weight is lesser of actual weight (ABW) or ideal weight (IBW) if actual is <110% of ideal. If patient is >110% of ideal weight, use the adjusted weight of IBW + 0.4(ABW − IBW).

☐ PERIPHERAL FORMULA (mixed as 3 in 1)

Final 3.5% Amino Acids, 10% Dextrose	☐ 2% Lipids ☐ No Lipids	Total Volume / 24 hrs = _____ ml or _____ ml/hour

2. **Rate:** *(Check one)   All Parenteral Nutrition bags are hung at 2000 hours daily or later if cyclic
    ☐ Administer as directed above.
    ☐ Administer over _____ hours (cyclic) (pharmacy to calculate rate)
    ☐ Rate for first 24 hours to be half of above rate or 40ml/hr (whichever is less)

3. **Electrolytes**

Additive	Per LITER		Additive	Per DAY	
Standard Lytes*	☐ Yes ☐ No		Standard Lytes*		ml
Sodium Chloride		mEq/L	Sodium Chloride		mEq
Sodium Acetate		mEq/L	Sodium Acetate		mEq
Sodium Phosphate		mM/L	Sodium Phosphate		mM
Potassium Chloride		mEq/L	Potassium Chloride		mEq
Potassium Acetate		mEq/L	Potassium Acetate		mEq
Potassium Phosphate		mM/L	Potassium Phosphate		mM
Magnesium Sulfate		mEq/L	Magnesium Sulfate		mEq
Calcium Gluconate		mEq/L	Calcium Gluconate		mEq

With "OR" between the two halves.

*Standard Lytes per 20 ml: Na$^+$ 35 mEq, K$^+$ 20 mEq, Ca^{++} 4.5 mEq, Magnesium 5 mEq, Cl$^-$ 35mEq, Acetate 30 mEq

4. **Other Additives**

Additive	Amount	Recommendation
MVI −12 10 ml	☐ Yes ☐ No	Delivered over 24hrs
Trace Elements 1ml	☐ Yes ☐ No	Delivered over 24hrs (Zinc 5 mg, Copper 1mg, Manganese 0.5 mg, Chromium 10 mcg)
Famotidine	_____ mg/day	40mg/24h unless CrCl<50ml/min then 20mg/24h
Regular Insulin	_____ Units	Consider insulin drip and sliding scales in unstable patients
Other:		

Guidelines:
→ When parenteral nutrition is discontinued, the infusion rate will be reduced by one-half for 4 hours or for the remainder of the bag.
→ If parenteral nutrition runs out before change time, begin D10W @same rate.
→ Infusion rate for the first 24 hours should be half of goal rate or 40ml/hr, whichever is less.

Physician's Signature	Date	Time

Figure 12-4 ■ Sample adult tailored parenteral nutrition order. (Courtesy of Enloe Medical Center, Chico, CA.)

3. Gastric feedings require intact gag and cough reflexes and adequate gastric emptying.
4. Gastric residuals are used to monitor safety and effectiveness of tube feedings.
5. Feeding tubes can develop mechanical complications especially clogging (ASPEN, 2002b).

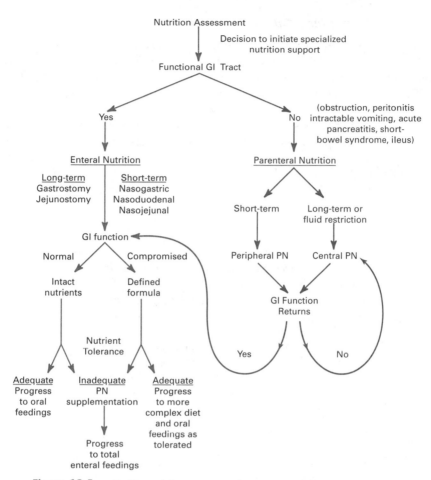

Figure 12-5 ▪ Routes to deliver nutritional support to adults: Clinical decision algorithm. This clinical decision algorithm outlines the selection process for choosing the route of nutritional support in adult patients. Major considerations for selecting the feeding route and nutritional support formula include gastrointestinal function, expected duration of nutritional therapy, aspiration risk, and the potential for or actual development of organ dysfunction.

COMPLICATIONS ASSOCIATED WITH ENTERAL NUTRITION

1. Incorrect tube placement
2. Occlusion of feeding tube
3. Pulmonary aspiration of feeding
4. Tracheoesophageal fistula
5. Acute sinusitis
6. Otitis media
7. Diarrhea
8. Metabolic imbalances: hypoglycemia, hyperglycemia, hyperosmolar nonketotic dehydration, EFAD

Peripheral Parenteral Nutrition

Peripheral parenteral nutrition (PPN) support is used to nourish patients who either are already malnourished or have the potential for developing malnutrition and who are not candidates for enteral nutrition (ASPEN, 2002a). PPN was first proposed in the early 1970s as a "nitrogen-sparing" therapy.

Prolonged infusions should be limited to solutions that are lower than 900 mOsm/L. Reports have shown that with the use of three-in-one solutions, a higher osmolality may be tolerated. No greater than 10% final concentration of dextrose should be infused peripherally (ASPEN, 2002a).

The delivery of PPN involves both advantages and disadvantages.

ADVANTAGES OF PPN

1. Avoids insertion and maintenance of a central catheter.
2. Delivers less hypertonic solutions than central venous TPN.
3. Reduces the chance of metabolic complications from that of central venous TPN.
4. Increases calorie source, along with fat emulsion.

DISADVANTAGES OF PPN

1. Cannot be used in nutritionally depleted patients.
2. Cannot be used in volume-restricted patients because higher volumes of solution are needed to provide adequate calories.
3. Does not usually increase a patient's weight.
4. May cause phlebitis owing to the osmolarity of the solution.

 NURSING FAST FACT!

> *A standardized ordering sheet is used to specify the protein, calories, and electrolyte content of each solution tailored to the client. Standard PPN includes the following basic formula:*
> - *100–150 g of dextrose with 1.0–1.5 g amino acids/kg (final concentrations of 1.75–3.5% amino acids and 5–10% dextrose), along with 500 mL of 10% or 20% lipids and electrolytes, trace elements, and vitamins.*

INS Standard Parenteral nutrition solutions in final concentrations of 10% dextrose or lower and 5% protein or lower should not be administered peripherally for longer than 7–10 days unless supplementation with oral or enteral feeding is provided concurrently to ensure adequate nutrition. (INS, 2006, 69)

 NURSING FAST FACT!

> *Assess for appropriate catheter for delivery of PPN: midline catheter should be considered for PPN. PPN is a short-term therapy for fairly stable patients whose normal GI functioning will resume within 3–4 weeks.*

Total Parenteral Nutrition (Two-in-One Admixtures)

Parenteral nutrition via central vein (**total parenteral nutrition [TPN]**) is used to provide nutrients at greater concentrations and smaller fluid volumes than is possible with PPN. Central venous access can be maintained for prolonged periods (weeks to years) with a variety of catheters that must be surgically placed and maintained. Central intravenous nutritional support is referred to as TPN. This method is also referred to as two-in-one (2-in-1) solution, which refers to combination of amino acids and dextrose solution. In 2-in-1 formulations fat solutions are delivered alone and not mixed with the dextrose and protein base solutions.

TPN reverses starvation and adequately achieves tissue synthesis, repair, and growth. TPN solutions infused through a central vein are highly concentrated and range from 1800 to 2000 mOsm/kg with final additives compared with 300 mOsm/kg in plasma. TPN is usually administered at rates of no more than 200 mL/hr.

The delivery of TPN involves both advantages and disadvantages.

ADVANTAGES

- Dextrose solution of 20% to 70% administered as a calorie source
- Beneficial for long-term use (usually longer than 3 weeks)
- Useful for patients with large caloric and nutrient needs
- Provides calories; restores nitrogen balance; and replaces essential vitamins, electrolytes, and minerals
- Promotes tissue synthesis, wound healing, and normal metabolic function
- Allows bowel rest and healing
- Improves tolerance to surgery
- Is nutritionally complete

DISADVANTAGES

- May require a minor surgical procedure for insertion of a tunneled catheter or implanted port
- May cause metabolic complications, including glucose intolerance, electrolyte imbalances, and EFAD
- Fat emulsions may not be used effectively in some severely stressed patients (especially burn patients).
- Risk of pneumothorax or hemothorax with central line insertion procedure

 NURSING FAST FACT!

Because of the high dextrose content in TPN, it is an ideal medium for microbial growth. For this reason, the CDC recommends that parenteral nutrition catheters not be used for anything other than the infusion of TPN (O'Grady, Alexander, Dellinger, et al, 2002).

PRACTICE CRITERIA FOR CENTRAL PARENTERAL ACCESS

- Parenteral nutrition should be delivered through a catheter located with its distal tip in the superior vena cava.
- Radiographic verification of catheter placement should be obtained before use of catheter.
- Full-barrier precautions should be used during the insertion of the central line

Total Nutrient Admixtures (Three-in-One Admixtures)

Total nutrient admixtures (TNAs) are systems that are combinations of dextrose, amino acids, and fat emulsions in one container. Referred to as total nutritional admixture, all-in-one solutions, three-in-one solutions (3-in-1 solutions), or trimix solutions, this product combines fat, amino acids, and dextrose in one container. The formula is provided in a large container that infuses over 24 hours. Lipids are mixed with dextrose and amino acid solution in the pharmacy. This solution is usually milky white and opaque, although a faint yellow hue may be evident with the addition of vitamins. These admixtures have been shown to be stable and well tolerated by patients via central line administration. Compounding of lipids, amino acids, and dextrose solutions raises the pH of the formula.

The TNA solutions offer a significant advantage in the ability to provide cost-effective, patient-specific nutritional support. Nursing time is saved by having only one solution container to hang each day. Pharmacy admixing is simplified by the use of computerized automixing systems, which also allow for more patient-specific formulations.

Total nutrient admixtures must be administered through a 1.2-micron filter because of the mean particle size of fat droplets (Fig. 12-6). The stability of TNA is affected by many factors, including admixture contents, storage time and conditions, addition of non-nutrient drugs, pH of the solution, and variability in temperature. The FDA strongly advises pharmacists to use care in the compounding order of nutrients, and advocates the use of a 1.2-micron filter during infusion to avoid problems with calcium and phosphate precipitation (ASPEN, 2004). There is a potential that cholestasis may develop and that long-chain triglycerides may depress the immune system. Catheter occlusion resulting from fat deposits has been reported with long-term use of this therapy.

 NURSING FAST FACT!

Most microorganisms grow rapidly in commercial 10% lipid emulsions. Infections with Malassezia furfur have been associated with administration of lipids. Use of TPN supplemented with lipids has been shown significantly to increase the risk of blood stream infection by coagulase-negative staphylococci. Candida albicans can grow in the synthetic amino acid and glucose solutions used for TPN (Maki & Mermel, 2007).

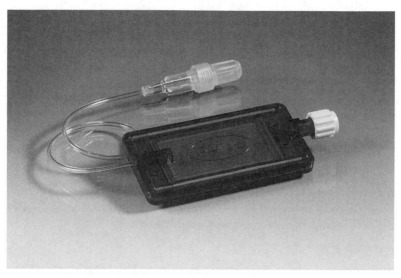

Figure 12-6 ■ Lipipor™ TNA filter set for total nutrient admixture administration with 1.2-μm air-eliminating filter. (Courtesy of Pall Corp., Ann Arbor, MI.)

Bacterial or fungal growth may be enhanced by admixture of fat emulsions with dextrose and amino acid solutions. The solutions should be observed for pink discoloration and for separation of oils in the three-in-one admixture.

 NURSING FAST FACT!

> *Examine the solution for signs of instability before hanging and periodically throughout administration*
>
> *Monitor the TNA infusion for physical or chemical phenomena which may occur with TNA solutions before administration and include:*
>
> ***a.*** *Aggregation (stratification)—rare white "streaks," which is an early stage of creaming. It is not harmful to the patient*
>
> ***b.*** *Creaming—dense white color at top of solution ("cream") layer. Reverses with gentle agitation and is not harmful. If creaming reappears in 1–2 hours it may indicate an unstable emulsion.*
>
> ***c.*** *Chemical phenomena ("oiling")—Oil globules on the surface of creamed emulsion fuse and form larger oil droplets. This is irreversible, and cannot be dispersed.*

Cyclic Therapy

For patients requiring long-term parenteral nutritional support, cyclic TPN (C-TPN) is widely used. This therapy delivers concurrent dextrose, amino acids, and fat over a regimen of reduced time frame, usually 12 to 18 hours, versus a 24-hour continuous infusion. **Cyclic therapy** is indicated for patients who have been stable on continuous TPN, and require long-term parenteral nutrition, for those receiving home TPN; for those patients who can handle total infusion volume in a shortened time period; and those who require TPN for only a portion of their nutritional needs (Wilson & Jordan, 2001).

Dehydration can occur when fluid requirements are not met. Monitoring should include pulse, orthostatic blood pressures, examination of mucous membranes, skin turgor, and laboratory tests such as blood urea nitrogen (BUN), creatinine, hematocrit, and albumin.

Symptoms of excess fluid administration should be monitored, such as weight gain resulting in edema or infusion-related shortness of breath. If too much fluid is administered during the cyclic period, the time frame should be extended. Using the C-TPN regimen requires twice the manipulations as continuous TPN; therefore, the risk of sepsis associated with central line manipulation must be considered.

ADVANTAGES

1. Prevents or treats hepatotoxicity induced by continuous TPN
2. Prevents or treats EFAD in patients on fat-free TPN
3. Improves quality of life by encouraging normal daytime activities and enhances psychological well-being

DISADVANTAGES

1. Patients must be observed for symptoms of hypoglycemia, hyperglycemia, dehydration, excessive fluid administration, and sepsis associated with central-line manipulation.
2. Hyperglycemia can develop during the peak C-TPN flow rate. Blood glucose levels should be checked whenever the patient displays symptoms of nausea, tremors, sweating, anxiety, or lethargy.

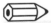 *NURSING FAST FACT!*

> The patient who is septic or metabolically stressed is not a good candidate for C-TPN
> This therapy is indicated for long-term parenteral nutrition.
> The patient's cardiovascular status must be able to accommodate large fluid volume during the cyclic phase.
> For patients without complications such as glucose intolerance or a precarious fluid balance, a 12-hour cycling regimen can be used.
> Monitor blood glucose 1 hour after tapering off C-TPN.

Specialized Parenteral Formulas

Some parenteral formulas are designed to meet the needs of patients with specific disease states such as renal and liver failure and general stress conditions such as trauma, burns, and sepsis. There are practice standards for life cycle and metabolic conditions developed by the American Society for Parenteral and Enteral Nutrition to assist the nutrition healthcare team in developing appropriate nutritional support for the patient with specific problems (ASPEN, 2002). The following are some special formulas developed for the patient with renal, liver, and special metabolic stress needs.

RENAL FORMULAS

Patients in renal failure who are in need of parenteral nutrition minimal quantities of essential amino acids enhance urea utilization and improve nephron repair. The amino acid L-histidine enhances amino acid utilization in those with uremia. Formulas used for patients in renal failure should not contain nonessential amino acids. Standard crystalline amino acid solutions contain both essential and nonessential amino acids.

Renal preparations decrease the rate of blood urea nitrogen formation and minimize deterioration of serum potassium, magnesium, and phosphorus.

Common preparations include Aminess 5.2%, Aminosyn-RF 5.2 or 5.4%, and NephrAmine. These formulas are contraindicated in the presence of severe acid–base and electrolyte imbalances or hyperammonemia.

HEPATIC FORMULAS

Protein-calorie malnutrition and nutritional deficiencies are common in liver diseases. Altered amino acid metabolism is a hallmark of liver disease, characterized by low levels of circulating branched-chain amino acid (BCAA) and elevated levels of circulating aromatic amino acids. Solutions high in branched-chain amino acids (BCAA) are designed for liver disease. Most commonly, these formulas are limited to patients with encephalopathy. The administration formulas high in BCAA would seem to be beneficial; however, as with formulas for renal failure, controversy exists (ASPEN, 2002a).

Common preparations include BranchAmin, HepatAmine, and Novamine 15%.

NOTE > These formulas are contraindicated in patients who are anuric.

Stress Formulas

Patients with infection; sepsis; and the trauma of burns, surgery, shock, and blunt or penetrating injuries often become hypercatabolic. In this situation, an increase in nitrogen excretion caused by altered protein metabolism occurs. Severely stressed patients need more protein to meet increased nutritional needs, so high metabolic stress formulas, which are similar to hepatic formulas, are available for this patient population. This group of patients has a predilection to break down BCAA in the muscles. Formulas with high BCAA replenish those depleted in the stressed patient. Examples of stress formulas include Aminosyn-HBC, BranchAmin, FreAmine HBC, and Novamine 15%.

■ Parenteral Nutrition Administration

Venous Access

The proper selection of venous access site (central vs. peripheral) depends on nutrient requirements and duration of parenteral nutrition. The hypertonic nature of total parenteral nutrition dictates that the PN be administered through a central venous access catheter (CVC) with tip placement in the superior vena cava adjacent to the right atrium (ASPEN, 2002a; CDC, 2002).

If PN is to be administered via a peripheral vein, the formulation's osmolarity along with judicious monitoring of the venous access site for signs of phlebitis and/or infiltration must be considered. The IVFE products are isotonic and can be administered via peripheral vein, or as part of a TNA when the osmolarity does not exceed 600 mOsm/L (INS, 2006, 69; Mirtallo, 2004).

NOTE > Guidelines for daily care of CVC are provided in Chapter 8.

Medical Equipment

Filters

The use of in-line filters has been recommended during the administration of intravenous products such as PN formulations (FDA, 1994). Use of a 0.22-micron filter for PN administration can remove microorganisms but this practice is limited to use with 2-in-1 formulations. The integrity of the IVFE is compromised when infused through filters less than 1.2 microns in size. A 1.2-micron filter does not remove most microorganisms from a contaminated PN formulation even though it is effective in removing particulates and microprecipitates.

 NURSING FAST FACT!

PN formulations are considered high-risk admixtures and can become contaminated during compounding or administration set up.

Administration Sets and Infusion Pumps

Specific recommendations also exist to guide the use of PN administration tubing sets. PN administration sets shall be changed using aseptic technique and standard precautions. Changes of add-on devices to the PN administration set should coincide with the changing of the PN administration set to maintain the entire PN administration system as a closed system. TNA administration sets are changed every 24 hours and immediately upon suspected contamination or if the product integrity has been compromised. Administration sets used for separate IVFE infusion are discarded after each unit is infused (CDC, 2002; INS, 2006).

Intravenous infusion pumps are an integral component of PN administration. Use of an electronic infusion device to safely administer PN is recommended (ASPEN, 2004; INS, 2006, 69). The Joint Commission (TJC) Patient Safety Goals include recommendations for infusion pumps. Free-flow protection is important to the safety of PN administration to avoid serious harm caused by rapid administration (TJC, 2004).

Practice Criteria for Administration of Parenteral Nutrition

Establish Goals

There are key monitoring concepts unique to the patient receiving PN. Considerable cost and serious complications are often associated with PN administration. Once it is determined that the individual will receive PN, goals for nutritional support should be set with specific markers and outcomes to be measured (ASPEN, 2004).

Examples of patient goals could include:

1. Replenishment of protein stores
2. Normalization of laboratory values
3. Reduction in morbidity/mortality
4. Improvement of quality of life
5. Optimization of clinical outcomes (ASPEN, 2004).

Monitoring

Monitoring individuals receiving PN is necessary to determine the efficacy of the specialized nutrition therapy; detect and prevent complications; evaluate changes in clinical condition; and document clinical outcomes.

All patients receiving PN should be monitored for:

1. Fluid and electrolyte imbalances
2. Proper blood glucose control
3. Signs and symptoms of CVC infections.

Laboratory monitoring of serum chemistries and visceral proteins is more frequent when PN is initiated, then decreases in frequency as clinically indicated. Regular assessment and meticulous care of the access device is important.

Patients may tolerate PN solutions better if the refrigerated PN is removed from the refrigerator 30 to 60 minutes before infusion. Patients have complained about discomfort while the chilled solution is infusing in the central circulation.

Reassess gastrointestinal function and readiness for oral/enteral feeding if the patient's clinical condition should change.

INS Standard Administration of Parenteral Nutrition

- Parenteral solutions should be removed from refrigeration 1 hour prior to infusion in order to reach approximate room temperature.
- Parenteral nutrition solutions not containing intravenous fat emulsion (IVFE) should be filtered with a 0.2 micron filter during administration.
- Parenteral solutions should be compounded in the pharmacy using sterile technique under a horizontal laminar flow hood.
- Parenteral nutrition administration sets, whether central or peripheral, should be dedicated to these solutions.
- Push or secondary intermittent medications should not be added to these infusion systems, with the exception of intravenous fat emulsion (IVFE), without verified compatibility.
- The nurse should monitor the patient for signs and symptoms of catheter-related complications.
- The nurse should monitor the patient for signs and symptoms of metabolic-related complications and electrolyte imbalances. (INS, 2006, 69)

NURSING POINTS-OF-CARE
ADMINISTRATION OF PARENTERAL NUTRITION

Focus Assessment
- Detailed history of weight loss
- History of disease and malnourished state
- Identify allergies and routine medications
- Vital signs, especially temperature
- Level of consciousness
- Inspect for tissue edema, and skin turgor
- Record ratios of urinary output to intake
- Inspect oral mucous membranes
- Before initiation of nutritional support obtain baseline serum blood glucose levels, serum albumin, total protein, electrolyte, and chemistry profile
- Assess vascular access for most appropriate device: TPN must be administered through central line. Midlines are appropriate for PPN.

Key Nursing Interventions
1. Assist with insertion of central line or insert PICC if competent, as appropriate for therapy.
2. Insert peripheral-short or midline catheter per agency protocol if appropriate for therapy.

3. Ascertain correct placement of CVC by radiography before beginning TPN.
4. Give strict attention to sterile technique and Standard Precautions.
5. Use appropriate hand hygiene when caring for the client with TPN.
6. Maintain central line patency and dressing per agency protocol.
7. Monitor for
   a. Infiltration and infection.
   b. Serial daily weights to track patterns of weight gain.
   c. Intake and output ratios
   d. Serum albumin, total protein, electrolyte, glucose, and chemistry profile.
   e. Vital signs every 4–6 hours initially
   f. Blood sugar every 6 hours. (As a general guideline blood glucose should be less than 200 mg/dL for patient on continuous TPN and less than 240 mg/dL for patients on cyclic TPN [Gorksi, 2005].)
8. Check the PPN or TPN solution to ensure correct nutrients are included as ordered.
9. Maintain sterile technique when preparing and hanging TPN solution.
10. Keep infusion within 10% of prescribed rate.
11. Initially TPN should be started slowly, increasing at a rate of 25 mL/hr increments until the desired rate of infusion is achieved.
12. The container of TPN must not infuse beyond a 24-hour period of time.
13. Use an electronic infusion pump for delivery of TPN solutions.
14. Change administration sets every 72 hours for 2-in-1 admixtures, every 24 hours if TNA. For IVFE administered separately, discard administration set after each infusion.
15. Avoid rapidly replacing lagging TPN solutions.
16. Administer insulin as ordered, to maintain serum glucose in the designated range as appropriate.
17. Report abnormal signs and symptoms associated with TPN to the physician and modify care accordingly.
18. Use a central line bundle for insertion and maintenance of CVC to prevent catheter-related bloodstream infection (CR-BSI).
19. Sterile dressings should be changed every 48–72 hours if nontransparent occlusive dressing is used; every 4–7 days, depending on institutional policy, if a transparent dressing is used. (See Chapter 8 for dressing management.)
20. Use of a 0.22-micron inline antimicrobial filter is recommended for TPN lines, except when lipid emulsion is added to these solutions, at which time a 1.2-micron filter should be used.
21. Observe for signs and symptoms of hypophosphatemia, hypokalemia, hypomagnesemia, and hypernatremia. (See Chapter 3 for a review of signs and symptoms.)

■ Complications Associated with Total Parenteral Nutrition

Complications associated with parenteral nutrition are divided into four groups: (1) mechanical or technical (involving catheters, pumps, and other apparatus for administration), (2) infections, (3) metabolic, and (4) nutritional (Table 12-8). The focus of this chapter is on the infection risks and metabolic and nutritional complications associated with nutritional support. Catheter-related and equipment-related complications are covered in Chapter 9.

Text continued on page 830

> Table 12-8	**COMPLICATIONS ASSOCIATED WITH NUTRITIONAL SUPPORT**		
Complication/ Etiology	**Symptoms**	**Treatment**	**Prevention**
	Mechanical/Technical Complications		
Air Embolism Cause: When line is interrupted and air is inspired while the line is open	Cyanosis, tachypnea, hypotension churning heart murmur (classic sign)	Immediately place patient on left side and lower the head of the bed; this may keep the air within the apex of the right ventricle until it is reabsorbed; administer oxygen	Line placement by appropriately trained personnel; use care in injection cap changes; do not use scissors near catheter
Vein Thrombosis Causes: Mechanical trauma to vein, TPN osmolarity, hypercoagulopathy	Swelling or pain in one or both arms, shoulders, or neck; increased anterior chest venous pattern; external jugular distension; or fluid leaking from arm May be asymptomatic	Diagnosis may be made by arm venography, contrast studies, MRI, and radionucleotide study Treatment is controversial and depends on extent of thrombus Conservative treatment without removal consists of anticoagulants Discontinuation of catheter	Tip placement in SVC not upper arm or subclavian Early recognition of symptoms
Catheter Malposition Cause: Catheter inadvertently advanced into an incorrect vein during placement Can occur spontaneously after insertion caused by coughing or vomiting	Swelling of arm or neck, pain, difficulty flushing catheter, difficulty infusing TPN Ear gurgling sound	Reposition with guidewire under fluoroscopy or remove Reposition the patient before flushing line	Not always possible to prevent Follow techniques to prevent malposition Always use radiography to confirm tip placement

> Table 12-8   **COMPLICATIONS ASSOCIATED WITH NUTRITIONAL SUPPORT—cont'd**

Complication/ Etiology	Symptoms	Treatment	Prevention
Metabolic Complications			
Altered Glucose Metabolism Hypoglycemia: Rebound Cause: Abrupt cessation of TPN	Diaphoresis, irritability, nervousness, shakiness	Administer dextrose or decrease insulin Maintain I.V. at constant rate	Maintain steady rate of infusion; wean gradually
Hyperglycemia Cause: Carbohydrate intolerance, insulin resistance, rapid TPN delivery, diabetes, sepsis, traumatic stress	Increased serum glucose, acetone breath, anxiety, confusion, dehydration, polydipsia, polyuria, malaise	Decrease dextrose TPN concentration or decrease rate administer insulin per sliding scale	Accurate glucose monitoring, gradual TPN rate, increase stable TPN infusion rate
Hyperammonemia Cause: Liver disease where ammonia is shunted past the liver and accumulates in blood	Asterixis (flapping tremor), lethargy, neurologic changes, altered ECG, vomiting, coma	Limit protein intake, enemas and antibiotics to revert growth of ammonia-producing bacteria in intestines	Accurate monitoring of serum ammonia level, monitoring of protein intake for patients with liver disease
Hypernatremia Cause: Water deprivation or loss, excessive TPN administration, profuse diaphoresis, diabetes insipidus, vomiting, diarrhea	Serum Na elevated to 145 mEq/L; urine specific gravity elevated to 1.015; thirst; elevated temperature; dry, swollen tongue; sticky mucous membrane; lethargy	Gradually decrease serum sodium levels to prevent cerebral edema Administration of water	Monitor serum electrolytes input and output, assess for insensible losses
Hypokalemia Cause: Alkalosis caused by shift of K into cells, GI losses, diuretic therapy, TPN, steroid administration, osmotic diuresis, anorexia	Serum K below 3.5 mEq/L, anorexia, fatigue, muscle weakness, decreased gastric motility, postural hypotension, ECG changes	TPN supplementation; replace GI losses	Monitor serum potassium, strict I and O, assess for digitalis toxicity
Hyperkalemia Cause: Renal impairment, iatrogenic-induced, TPN, metabolic and respiratory acidosis, tissue damage	Serum K elevated above 5.5 mEq/L ECG changes, cardiac arrest, muscular weakness, flaccid muscles, intestinal colic, diarrhea	Reduce TPN volume of K, cation exchange resins, dialysis	Accurate monitoring of K, accurate I and O

Continued

> Table 12-8   **COMPLICATIONS ASSOCIATED WITH NUTRITIONAL SUPPORT—cont'd**

Complication/ Etiology	Symptoms	Treatment	Prevention
Hypomagnesemia Cause: GI losses, refeeding after starvation, renal disease, TPN administration	Apprehension, depression, apathy, neuromuscular hyperexcitability, tremors, PVCs, tachycardia, ventricular fibrillation	Parenteral supplementation	Monitor serum Mg, assess for neuromuscular changes
Hypophosphatemia Cause: TPN supplementation without adequate phosphorus replacement, burns, malabsorptive states, and starvation	Apprehension, irritability, seizures, decreased RBCs, muscle weakness, insulin resistance	I.V. supplementation in the TPN	Monitor serum Mg levels
Hypocalcemia Cause: Vitamin D deficiency, insufficient calcium or magnesium intake, malabsorption, pancreatitis	CNS irritability, confusion, muscle cramps in extremities, muscle spasms, laryngeal spasms, seizures, tetany	Supplement TPN with calcium or I.V. calcium, correct magnesium or phosphate deficiencies	Accurate serum chemistry levels, avoid calcium-depleting medications, maintain adequate calcium intake
Infections			
Sepsis Cause: Skin contamination at insertion site, hub, and tubing junction from hands of healthcare professionals; homogeneous seeding from other sources	Chills, fever, malaise, elevated WBC count, diarrhea, tachycardia, tachypnea, flushing hypotension	Remove catheter or replace catheter over guidewire Antibiotics Administer oxygen Prepare to treat for septic shock	Maintain aseptic technique Aseptic dressing changes Use 0.22-micron filter
Nutritional Alterations			
Refeeding Syndrome Cause: Occurs during initial phase of TPN Body during its bout of starvation has adapted somewhat to nutritional deprivation: decreased basal energy requirements Causes electrolyte shift	Cardiorespiratory complications, edema, hypernatremia, hypokalemia, hypomagnesemia, hypophosphatemia	Can be averted by starting TPN gradually and gradually increasing rate	Monitor patient response to TPN

> Table 12-8	**COMPLICATIONS ASSOCIATED WITH NUTRITIONAL SUPPORT—cont'd**		
Complication/ Etiology	**Symptoms**	**Treatment**	**Prevention**
Essential Fatty Acid Deficiency Cause: Deficient intake	Minimal symptomatology until long term, soft tissue calcification, hypocalcemia, and tetany Numbness and tingling of the mouth and fingers	Fat emulsion supplementation in TPN or with intermittent infusions	Accurate calculation of protein and fat and carbohydrate ratios to maintain a positive nitrogen balance
Altered Mineral Balance Cause: Result of deficiencies caused by malnourishment or starvation	Chromium: Elevated serum lipid levels, insulin resistance, glucose tolerance Copper: hypochromic microcytic anemia, neutropenia Iron: fatigue, glossitis, hypochromic microcytic anemia Manganese: CNS changes Selenium: Cardiomyopathies Zinc: Alopecia, apathy, confusion, poor wound healing	Supply adequate supplementation in TPN	Monitor for abnormal laboratory values
Altered Vitamin Balance Cause: Disease processes can alter vitamin requirements TPN must supply the needed fat- and water-soluble vitamin supplements	Vitamin A: Dry, scaly, rough, cracked skin; decreased saliva; impaired digestion; diarrhea Vitamin D: Decreased serum calcium or phosphorus levels Vitamin E: RBC hemolysis Vitamin K: Delayed clotting Vitamin B_1: Increased serum and urine lactate or pyruvate levels, anorexia, confusion, fatigue, painful calf muscle Vitamin B_2: Glossitis, stomatitis, dermatitis, photophobia	Provide vitamin supplements in TPN	Monitor for symptoms and assess for deficits

Continued

> Table 12-8	COMPLICATIONS ASSOCIATED WITH NUTRITIONAL SUPPORT—cont'd		
Complication/ Etiology	**Symptoms**	**Treatment**	**Prevention**
	Vitamin B_3 (Niacin): Dermatitis, glossitis, diarrhea, dementia Vitamin B_{12}: Anorexia, depression dyspnea, memory lapses, delirium, hallucinations Folic acid: Macrocytic anemia, diarrhea, glossitis Vitamin C: bleeding gums, petechiae, depression		

Mechanical or Technical (Catheter-Related) Complications

Complications associated with central venous catheters (CVC) are discussed in Chapter 9. As with any CVC the main complications include pneumothorax, air embolism (during insertion and during maintenance of the device), venous thrombosis, superior vena cava (SVC) syndrome, catheter malposition, and nerve injury.

Infectious and Septic Complications

When TPN is provided by a central line, there are concerns related to the contamination of the CVC, as discussed in more detail in Chapters 2 and 9.

Local Catheter-Related Infection

Between 5% and 25% of intravascular devices are colonized by skin organisms at the time of removal. Colonized cannulas are more likely than noncolonized ones to show phlebitis or local inflammation, especially purulence at the site.

Studies have shown that use of a more effective cutaneous antiseptic, for example, chlorhexidine for antisepsis of the insertion site at the time of catheter insertion and in follow-up care of the catheter greatly reduces the risk of infusion-related BSI (Mimoz, Pieroni, Edouard, et al., 1996).

Catheter-Related Sepsis

Catheter-related bloodstream infection (CR-BSI) is a serious complication of central TPN therapy. This complication is preventable with strict aseptic techniques. Patients undergoing TPN are often immune compromised as a result of malnutrition; these patients are highly susceptible to infection. The origin of TPN catheter-related sepsis is most often the site itself; infection related to contaminated infusates is rare because of meticulous admixing protocols. CR-BSI may result from skin contaminants at the insertion site, hub, and tubing/device junction contamination; from the hands of healthcare professionals; and homogeneous seeding from other sources (e.g., lungs, urine, abdomen, wounds).

Options for management of catheter-related sepsis include exchange of the catheter over the guidewire and removal of the catheter. The decision is determined by the patient's clinical status, culture results, and the nature of the offending organism (Maki & Mermel, 2007).

Metabolic Complications

Complications associated with metabolic imbalances when administering TPN are either avoidable or controllable.

Altered Glucose Metabolism: Rebound Hypoglycemia

Rebound hypoglycemia condition is caused by abrupt cessation of TPN. Maintain a steady rate of infusion, and wean gradually when discontinuing usually prevents with condition. The patient exhibits diaphoresis, irritability, nervousness, and shaking. The infusion rate can be decreased by one half the rate for 1 to 2 hours if needed. This usually is not necessary if the patient is eating (Lyman, 2002).

Altered Glucose Metabolism: Hyperglycemia

Hyperglycemia is a common metabolic occurrence with TPN because of the high dextrose concentrations included in the admixture. Other factors that put the patient at risk for hyperglycemia are the presence of overt or latent diabetes mellitus, older age, sepsis, hypokalemia, and hypophosphatemia.

Conditions of stress result in decreased glucose tolerance and hyperglycemia in up to 25% of patients on TPN. Infusion of large amounts of glucose can also unmask latent diabetes, making hyperglycemia one of the most common complications encountered with parenteral nutrition. Other considerations when infusing formulas containing high concentrations of glucose is the potential effect of carbohydrate metabolism on respiration. Metabolism of carbohydrates results in increased production of carbon dioxide that must be compensated for by increased minute ventilation. This could precipitate respiratory failure in patients with preexisting respiratory disease or interfere with weaning from mechanical ventilation.

Factors that predispose a patient to glucose intolerance include:
- Presence of overt or latent diabetes mellitus
- Older age
- Pancreatitis
- Hypokalemia
- Hypophosphatemia
- Thiamine or B_6 deficiency
- Some antibiotics
- Steroids
- Conditions of stress, such as sepsis or surgery, result in decreased glucose tolerance and hyperglycemia in as many as 25% of TPN patients.

Essential Fatty Acid Deficiency

Lipid administration is important for delivery of essential fatty acids. If the regimen for nutritional support does not include a calorie source from fats, the patient is at risk for EFAD. Fats may be administered in amounts that supply 30% to 50% of the calories. By adding fats to the nutritional support, CO_2 production can be decreased and other metabolic complications may be avoided.

Hyperammonemia

Ammonia accumulates in the blood in those with liver disease. An elevated blood ammonia level is a common finding in infants and children receiving TPN. High protein intake may lead to elevated ammonia levels. Arginine is important in the urea cycle, and a deficiency of this amino acid may contribute to the development of hyperammonemia.

Limiting protein intake, administration of enemas, and use of antibiotics to prevent growth of ammonia-producing bacteria in the intestines may help. Monitor the serum ammonia levels and limit the essential protein in the TPN solution (Sherliker, 2000).

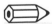 *NURSING FAST FACT!*

> *In adults, the most common laboratory finding is that of elevated transaminase levels; the most common abnormality is liver steatosis. Cholestasis and gallbladder disease are potential complications of long-term TPN (ASPEN, 2004).*

Electrolyte Imbalances

Major electrolyte imbalances associated with TPN can occur if excessive or deficient amounts of electrolytes are supplied in the daily fluid allowance. These include imbalances of sodium, potassium, magnesium, phosphate, or calcium.

- Sodium: Hypernatremia: To maintain homeostasis, the sodium ion is driven from the intracellular space into the extracellular space. This compensatory mechanism tries to combat the extracellular anion loss (Metheny, 2000). This shift can cause hypernatremia.
- Potassium: Hypokalemia: Potassium is also driven into the intracellular space during TPN. Serum potassium can become depleted with an inadequate supply of this electrolyte along with the use of insulin in the TPN solution. Insulin administration further intensifies intracellular potassium.
- Potassium: Hyperkalemia: A high potassium blood level can occur with renal impairment, iatrogenic-induced, or with metabolic and respiratory acidosis when potassium shifts out of the cells. Interventions include reducing the amount of potassium ion in the TPN solution.
- Magnesium: Hypomagnesemia: The magnesium electrolyte also is driven into the intracellular space during TPN administration. This condition is less common than hypophosphatemia or hypokalemia in patients receiving TPN (Metheny, 2000). This electrolyte should be included in TPN solution compounding. Hypomagnesemia is a common imbalance in critically ill and less acutely ill patients. This condition is often overlooked.
- Phosphate: Hypophosphatemia: Adenosine triphosphate (ATP) is required for all cell energy production. Protein synthesis begins when TPN is administered and phosphate is driven into the intracellular space as a component of ATP. Therefore, a deficiency of phosphate can occur. Include phosphate in TPN supplementation.
- Calcium: Hypocalcemia: Because of the fact that most patients receiving parenteral nutrition are malnourished and have low serum albumin levels, their total serum calcium levels are usually also below normal. The hypocalcemia is not physiologically significant and does not usually result in paresthesias or other signs of tetany. The usual TPN solution contains 5 to 10 mEq/L of calcium.

Nutrition Alterations

Refeeding Syndrome

Refeeding syndrome is a complication that can occur during the initial phases of TPN. This occurs when the body, during its bout with starvation, adapts to nutritional deprivation and compensates by decreasing basal energy requirements. This initiation of nutritional support, especially if it is undertaken too aggressively, can result in an electrolyte shift from the plasma to the intracellular fluid. Cardiorespiratory complications can occur. The result of refeeding syndrome is manifested by edema, hypernatremia, hypokalemia, hypomagnesemia, and hypophosphatemia.

Altered Mineral Balance

Mineral imbalances are usually the result of deficiencies, the cause being malnourishment or starvation and insufficient supplementation in the parenteral nutrition source. The most common deficiencies include chromium, copper, iron, manganese, selenium, and zinc.

Altered Vitamin Balance

Vitamin requirements can be altered by disease processes. The parenteral nutrition must supply the needed fat-soluble and water-soluble vitamin supplements. During illness, vitamin deficiencies can produce serious consequences for which the nurse must assess.

■ Discontinuation of Nutritional Support

Before discontinuation of parenteral or enteral nutritional support, one of the following criteria should be applicable:
- Parenteral nutrition should not be discontinued until nutrient requirements can be met by enteral or oral nutrients.
- Enteral nutrition should not be discontinued until nutrient requirements can be met by oral nutrients.
- Parenteral or enteral nutrition support should be discontinued whenever the patient's medical condition, especially complications, indicates.
- Parenteral or central nutrition support should be terminated when the physician judges that the patient no longer benefits from the therapy. The decision to discontinue support must be made according to accepted community standards of medical care and in compliance with applicable law (ASPEN, 2002b).

AGE-RELATED CONSIDERATIONS

The Pediatric Client

In the Neonatal Intensive Care Unit the most common indication for enteral nutrition is immaturity. **Parenteral nutrition (PN)** is indicated in infants and children who are unable to tolerate adequate enteral feedings to sustain their nutritional requirements. This may occur in children who suffer from chronic malnutrition (failure to thrive) or who are at high risk for developing malnutrition as a result of acute medical illness or prolonged postoperative recovery. The therapeutic goal of PN in children is both to maintain nutrition status and to achieve balanced somatic growth (American Academy of Pediatrics [AAP], 1998).

Assessment
• Nutritional assessment of pediatric patients uses standard growth curves. Calculation of the ratio of weight to height indicates wasting, and calculation of the ratio of height to age indicates stunting of growth. Anthropometric

measurements are used as gauges of somatic protein and fat stores. Visceral protein stores are evaluated by determining serum albumin, serum transferrin, prealbumin, and retinol-binding protein levels.
• Pediatric requirements for intravenous nutrition follow general guidelines and are based on protein, calorie, and fluid needs per kilogram of body weight. The nurse must monitor the child's physical status, including reporting abnormal findings of temperature spikes, inappropriate glucose spills, chills, rashes, irritability, and decreased level of consciousness. Serum level of various chemistry and hematology tests are assessed daily for the first week and then decreased to a weekly schedule for the stable hospitalized or home TPN patients.
• Another area of assessment includes psychological support. Most TPN patients are infants who are acutely ill and deprived of maternal warmth and comfort. Cuddling and holding the child should be encouraged, along with allowing the parents to participate in their child's care.
(ASPEN, 2002a)

Monitoring
Total parenteral nutrition must be monitored in the pediatric patient to meet the demands of growth and development.
• Many children require long-term support at home. Monitoring includes many of the same parameters as for adults. The monitoring during initiation of parenteral nutrition includes daily weight, strict intake and output, daily electrolytes until stable, serum glucose measurements every 8 to 12 hours, serum triglycerides and free fatty acid levels weekly, and liver function test biweekly.
• Children require evaluation of growth determinations including weight, height, head circumference, and anthropometric measurements for the duration of the therapy.
• When a child if first started on TPN, the percentage of dextrose infused is gradually increased from 5% to a maximum of 20% to 25% via a central line, according to caloric needs and tolerance of the child. Depending on caloric expenditure based on stress levels, lipids may be provided biweekly or daily.
• Children have a high basal metabolic rate per unit of body weight, an increased evaporative fluid loss, and immature kidneys. Infants and young children need additional amino acids, which are nonessential in adults. The amino acids required for infants and children include histidine, tyrosine, cystine, and taurine. Special amino acid formulas are available to meet these needs (Wilson & Jordan, 2001).
• Newborn infants require another amino acid, histidine. Premature infants also require cystine and tyrosine.
• Because of the high-risk behaviors of children, catheter sepsis rate in children may rise as high as 10% because of increased risks (e.g., teething children have been known to bite the TPN catheter).
• The use of a 2-in-1 formulation with the separate infusion of fat emulsion should be used in neonatal and infant patients (ASPEN, 2004).

Continued

- Cycling on PN formulations should be considered in select patients such as those on long-term PN or those with cholestasis (Collier, Crouch, Hendricks, Caballero, 1994).

Practice Guidelines to Prevent Complications in the Pediatric Patient
- Dextrose infusion rates in infants should not exceed 10 to 14 mg/kg per minute.
- Insulin administration by continuous infusion is safe and effective in controlling parenteral nutrition-associated hyperglycemia in infants
- PN should be tapered off over 1 to 2 hours before discontinuation in infants under age 2
- Hyponatremia in premature infants should be corrected by increasing sodium intake in order to promote tissue growth and weight gain
- Calcium and phosphate concentrations should be optimized in PN solutions to promote maximum bone mineral retention.
- Infants should receive 20% lipid emulsion to improve clearance of triglycerides and phospholipids (ASPEN, 2002a).

The Older Adult
The physiologic changes that occur with advancing age affect nutritional requirements, independent of disease or rehabilitation demands. The major physiologic changes that occur are a reduction in lean body mass, a decline in bone density and increase in total body fat with redistribution of fat stores and decrease in total body water (Flegal, Carroll, & Kuczmarski, 1998).
- It is estimated that one in four elderly people is malnourished. Elderly people who are malnourished tend to have a longer and more expensive hospital stay.
- Inadequate dietary intake in elderly people is multifaceted and includes physiologic changes in the GI tract, social and economic factors, drug interactions, disease, and excessive alcohol abuse. Poor dental health and missing teeth contribute to the malnutrition problem (Smeltzer, Bare, Hinkle, & Cheever, 2008).
- Nutritional problems of older adults are similar to adults of all ages; however, the incidence may be higher. Problems encountered by older adults related to nutrition include:
  - Loss of appetite due to diminished sense of smell and taste.
  - Unable to care for self and to obtain necessary nutrition
  - Decreased income—unable to purchase adequate nutritional meals.
  - Decreased gastric secretions occurs more frequently with older adults; therefore, medications and small frequent meals must be included in their plan of care.
  - Decreased intestinal peristalsis—older adults are more at risk of constipation.

Practice Guidelines
1. Elderly patients are at nutrition risk and should undergo nutrition screening to identify those who require formal nutrition assessment.

2. Age and lifestyle parameters should be used to assess the nutrition status of elderly persons.
3. Potential drug-nutrient interactions should be assessed in all elderly patients receiving medications.
4. Diet and specialized nutritional support for elderly persons should take into consideration altered nutrient requirements observed in this age group (ASPEN, 2002a).

 Home Care Issues

Home parenteral nutrition (HPN) has been well established and should be instituted and supervised by a multidisciplinary team with knowledge and expertise (ASPEN, 2005). Patients and their families can be taught to safely administer PN admixtures, and they can be monitored in a home setting. Hospital to home transition can be a difficult task. Keep in mind that the day of discharge is usually physically and emotionally stressful; the home care nurse should be in attendance for starting the TPN infusion at home.

Selection of Candidates
Candidates for TPN within the home care environment include patients (1) whose intake is insufficient to maintain an anabolic state; (2) whose ability to ingest food orally or by tube is impaired; (3) who are uninterested in ingesting or unwilling to ingest adequate nutrients; (4) who have underlying medical conditions that preclude their being fed orally or by tube; and (5) whose preoperative and postoperative nutritional needs are prolonged (Smeltzer, Bare, Hinkle, & Cheever, 2008). All patients identified as nutritionally-at-risk and require home PN shall have a nutrition assessment. The results of the nutrition assessment and recommendations should be shared with all patient care providers (ASPEN, 2005).

The patient must be clinically stable before going home on TPN.
• Weight maintained or increased as per goals of TPN therapy
• Stable blood chemistry levels
• Stable nutritional laboratory indicators
• No evidence of rebound hypoglycemia with discontinuation of cyclic infusions
• No adverse reactions to TPN infusion (Gorski, 2005)
Home safety must be determined before discharge from the hospital. Successful home therapy depends on several factors:
• Medical stability
• Emotional stability
• Patient's lifestyle
• Intellectual ability (client or primary caregiver)
• Visual acuity
• Manual dexterity
• Assessment of home environment
• Dry storage space for supplies

Continued

Home Care Issues—cont'd

- Refrigerator large enough to store admixtures
- Clean low-traffic area for procedure preparation
- Electronic outlets for any electronic equipment

Advantages of home treatment for nutritional support are that it involves lesser expense than treatment in the hospital; it allows the patient to remain in a familiar, comfortable surrounding, thereby decreasing the confusion associated with age-related environment changes; in many cases, it allows the patient to return to normal activities; and it is associated with a lower risk of acquiring a health-care associated infection. HPN is usually cycled or given over a 12- to 16-hour period, and most of the administration occurs during the sleeping hours. In addition, a person's control over his or her body and the self-care responsibility increase self-esteem.

Preparing for Home Parenteral Nutrition

The home education process should include but not be limited to:
- Verbal and written instructions of appropriate procedures
- Demonstration and return demonstration of procedures by the primary caregiver
  - Inspection of home parenteral nutrition containers and contents
  - Aseptic technique required for the admixture procedure and administration via an access device
  - Proper storage of formulated and admixed parenteral feeding formulations
- Evaluation and documentation of competency
- Self-monitoring instruction
- Limitations of physical activity
- Emergency intervention and problem-solving techniques
- Care of infusion equipment, solutions, and supplies
- Disposal of supplies
- Expectations of home care and medical and nursing follow-up
- State when and whom to contact when complications occur.

Home care training must be individually designed according to the individual's capabilities. Assessment of the patient's physical and emotional status before each teaching session aids in determining goals for that session. A minimum number of people should be involved with each teaching session to limit distractions and anxiety.

The TPN and related supplies are generally delivered to patient homes on a weekly basis. The TPN bags are stored in the refrigerator.

NOTE > In some cases, the home infusion pharmacy may provide a small refrigerator dedicated to TPN storage (Gorski, 2005).

Reimbursement is verified before initiation home TPN.
- Private third-party payers vary in coverage.
- Certain diagnoses and TPN infusions may be covered under the durable medical equipment benefit under Part B of the Medicare program. Patients must meet criteria that include "permanence," interpreted as requiring TPN for at least 3 months (Gorski, 2005).

Home Care Issues—cont'd

Practice criteria for delivery of TPN in the home and hospital are the same.
- Filters: 2-in-1, 0.2 micron; 3-in-1 solutions, 1.2 micron
- Change I.V. tubing every 24 hours for IVFE, 72 hours for 2-in-1 solutions, and for cyclic infusions daily.
- Use an infusion pump (ambulatory pump is preferred to assist with patient mobility).

NOTE > Ambulatory pumps have features specific for TPN administration.

- Ensure that the label on the TPN bag matches the physician's order for TPN formula.
- Inspect the TPN solution for integrity of solution.
- Verify the infusion parameters on the infusion pumps before starting the pump.
- Verify the patient's identity.
- Verify the patency of CVAD including presence of free-flowing blood return.
- Reinforce patient education as listed above. (Gorski, 2005; INS, 2006, 69 and 48)

Monitoring

The patient with home TPN must be monitored for complications related to infections, metabolic and fluid volume status, or electrolyte imbalances.
Criteria for monitoring the home TPN patient includes:
- Serum glucose, electrolyte, BUN, creatinine, magnesium, and phosphorus daily until stable.
- CBC, serum proteins, serum triglyceride every month ×3 , serum glucose, BUN, creatinine, magnesium, phosphorus, and calcium every month ×3 then every other
- Serum albumin, aspartate aminotransferase (AST), alkaline phosphatase, total bilirubin, international normalized ratio (INR), every 3 to 6 months
- Micronutrient levels as clinically necessary and/or if deficiency is suspected (ASPEN, 2002a).

Complications

Infectious complications overall is low for home TPN; risk factors for hospitalization include younger age, Crohn's disease, central vein, thrombosis and presence of a jejunostomy. Three key areas for concern in the home care setting include infectious complications and metabolic and fluid volume/electrolyte complications (Gorski, 2001).

> *EBNP A study investigated the incidence and the causative factors of complications that occur within the first 90 days after discharge from hospital to home for patient on new home PN. A complication developed in one third of the patients, and the majority required rehospitalization. Infectious complications were the most prevalent, then mechanical followed by metabolic. Trends that the authors found included (1) Patients with single-lumen catheters experienced more overall complications and (2) More complications occurred among ostomy patients (Burgoa, Seidner, Hamilton, et al., 2006).*

Continued

Home Care Issues—cont'd

Infections

As with any central line, CR-BSI is a concern. Monitoring for signs and symptoms of infection and providing patients and families with thorough education aimed at risk reduction are important aspects of home care nursing.

Metabolic Complications

Blood glucose levels should be checked during TPN infusions and compared to when the patient is off the cyclic TPN. As a general guideline include: blood glucose should be under 200 mg/dL for patient on continuous TPN and under 240 mg/dL for patient on cyclic TPN (Gorksi, 2005).

Fluid and Electrolyte Imbalances

The patient should be monitored for electrolyte imbalances as stated under monitoring home TPN. The nurse should report any signs and symptoms of fluid or electrolyte imbalances to the physician and anticipate changes in TPN formula. Refer to Chapter 3 for fluid and electrolyte imbalances.

Nutrition-Related Complications

The goals of home TPN must be kept in mind for the care plan. Assess indicators of the patient's nutritional status regularly: weight, skin integrity, elimination, behavioral changes, mucous membranes, nail bed, oral cavity (including teeth and tongue), and circulatory status. Essential fatty acid deficiency may occur in patients who do not receive lipid emulsions as part of home TPN (Gorski, 2005).

 Patient Education

The patient receiving enteral nutrition, PPN, or TPN will need education, periodic assessment, and retraining as needed. Many of the points listed in patient education for home care issues apply to patients in all settings.

- Inform the patient about the purpose and duration of the projected nutritional support.
- Instruct the patient on the product hang time of the product with the composition, intended use, and expected outcomes of the formulation.
- Educate the patient and caregiver about management of the access device.
- Instruct the patient receiving enteral feedings about clean techniques for handling the tube, maintaining the access site, and flushing the tube to maintain patency.

Patient Education—cont'd

- Inform the patient about complications associated with TPN administration, including:
  - Metabolic complications such as hypoglycemia and electrolyte imbalances (recognize and respond to these complications)
  - Mechanical or procedural problems (catheter or tube occlusion, leakage, breakage, or dislodgement)
  - Equipment malfunction or breakage
  - Infusion contamination precipitate or in homogeneity (recognize and report signs and symptoms of localized or systemic infectious process)
- Provide 24-hour phone numbers for home care agency or physician so that patient or caregiver can access professional help.

⬛ Nursing Process

The nursing process is a five- or six-step process for problem-solving to guide nursing action. Refer to Chapter 1 for details on the steps of the nursing process related to vascular access. The following table focuses on nursing diagnoses, nursing outcomes classification (NOC), and nursing intervention classification (NIC) for patients with nutritional support. Nursing diagnoses should be patient specific and outcomes and interventions individualized. The NOC and NIC presented here are suggested direction for development of specific outcomes and interventions.

Nursing Diagnoses Related to Nutritional Support	NOC: Nursing Outcomes Classification	NIC: Nursing Intervention Classification
Fluid volume excess, risk for related to: Rapid administration of TPN	Fluid balance, hydration	Fluid management
Health maintenance, ineffective related to: Poor dietary habits, with perceptual or cognitive impairment	Health beliefs: Perceived resources, health-promoting behavior, health-seeking behavior	Health education, support system enhancement
Infection, risk for, related to: Concentrated glucose solution, invasive administration of fluids; inadequate intake of calories and protein.	Infection control, risk detection	Infection control, infection protection

Continued

Nursing Diagnoses Related to Nutritional Support	NOC: Nursing Outcomes Classification	NIC: Nursing Intervention Classification
Nutrition, less than body requirements, related to: Inability to ingest or digest food or absorb nutrients as a result of biological or psychological factors	Nutritional status, nutrient intake	Feeding, nutrition management, nutrition therapy, nutrition counseling
Skin integrity, impaired or risk for, related to: Inadequate intake of protein and or vitamin A	Tissue integrity: Skin and mucous membranes	Skin care, skin surveillance, wound care

Sources: Ackley & Ladwig (2008); Carpenito-Moyet (2008); McCloskey-Dochterman & Bulechek (2004); Moorhead, Johnson, & Maas (2004); NANDA-I (2007).

Chapter Highlights

■ Candidates for nutritional support include those with:
  ■ Altered catabolic states
  ■ Chronic weight loss
  ■ Conditions requiring bowel rest
  ■ Excessive nitrogen loss
  ■ Hepatic or renal failure
  ■ Hypermetabolic states
  ■ Malabsorption states
  ■ Malnutrition
  ■ Multiple trauma
  ■ Serum albumin levels below 3.5 g/dL
■ Nutritional deficiencies fall into three categories: marasmus, kwashiorkor, and mixed malnutrition
■ Effects of malnutrition include a decrease in protein stores, albumin depletion, and impaired immune status.
■ Nutritional assessment includes:
  ■ History (medical, social, and dietary)
  ■ Anthropometric measurements (weight, skinfold tests, midarm circumference)
  ■ Biochemical assessments (serum albumin, serum transferrin, prealbumin and retinol-binding protein, total lymphocyte counts, serum electrolytes)
  ■ Energy requirements
  ■ Physical examination
  ■ Other indices (nitrogen balance, indirect calorimetry, prognostic nutritional index)
■ Parenteral nutrition is an admixture of water, carbohydrates, amino acids, lipids, electrolytes, multivitamins, and minerals formulated to meet an individual patient's needs

- Modalities for delivery of nutritional support include:
  - Enteral nutrition
  - Peripheral parenteral nutrition (PPN)
  - Total parenteral nutrition (TPN)
  - Total nutrient admixture (TNA)
  - Cyclic therapy
- Peripheral parenteral nutrition, delivered into a peripheral vein, is indicated for patients who need a complete nutrient source but are not depleted; consist of a 2% to 5% amino acid solution in combination with 5% to 10% dextrose. Fat emulsions of 10% to 20% may be combined or administered separately. This therapy is delivered for a limited time, usually 2 weeks.
- Total parenteral nutrition, delivered by central line, is the I.V. administration of hypertonic glucose (20%–70%) and amino acids (3.5%–15%), along with all additional components required for complete support.
- Nutritional support must be filtered with a 0.22-micron filter, except for when lipids are added to TNAs, which must have a 1.2-micron filter.
- Complications of parenteral nutrition include:
  - Mechanical or technical complications
  - Infectious or septic complications
  - Metabolic complications
  - Nutritional complications
- Age Related Considerations
- Home Care Issues

■■ Thinking Critically: Case Study

A 45-year-old man is admitted with severe abdominal pain. He is 6 feet 1 inches tall and weighs 132 pounds, and has experienced a 45-pound weight loss in the past 3 months (25%). He is weak and pale, has dry mucous membranes, a red beefy tongue, and cracks at the sides of his mouth. His abdomen is distended and somewhat firm. He reports decreased appetite with diminished oral intake during the past 4 months. He has been drinking 6 or more beers per day over the past 6 months. He is diagnosed with pancreatitis with pseudocyst formation. He is placed NPO and total parenteral nutrition is ordered. He is to receive a solution of 20% dextrose, 50 g of protein/L with standard electrolytes and daily multiple vitamin/ trace elements. The goal is 2 L of this solution per day. With lipids, this will provide an average of 2260 calories per day, 100 g of protein, and 2¼ L of fluid per day. The solution is initiated at 1 L/day and increases according to patient tolerance. Thiamine is added to the regimen (100 mg/day for 3 days). The TPN will be infused through a peripherally inserted central catheter.

What are the points-of-care in monitoring this patient?

Why is the patient receiving thiamine?

What potential complications related to TPN is this patient at risk for?

Media Link: Answers to the case study and more critical thinking activities are provided on the CD-ROM.

Post-Test

1. The type of malnutrition that most commonly occurs in the acutely ill hospitalized patient is:
   a. Kwashiorkor
   b. Marasmus
   c. Mixed malnutrition
   d. Anorexia nervosa

2. How many kilocalories does a 20% lipid emulsion provide?
   a. 1.0
   b. 1.1
   c. 2.0
   d. 2.2

3. Which of the following are the three essential nutrients included in parenteral nutrition required for anabolism and tissue synthesis?
   a. Trace elements, protein, and fats
   b. Protein, carbohydrates, and fats
   c. Fats, electrolytes, and carbohydrates
   d. Vitamins, electrolytes, and protein

4. Which of the following are considered anthropometric measurements? (*Select all that apply.*)
   a. Midarm muscle circumference
   b. Weight
   c. Skinfold thickness
   d. Serum transferrin

5. Which of the following filters should be used with TNA solutions?
   a. 0.22-micron filter
   b. 0.45-micron filter
   c. 1.2-micron filter
   d. 170-micron filter

6. To treat or prevent essential fatty acid deficiency which of the following should be included in parenteral nutrition?
   a. Trace elements
   b. Transferrin
   c. Crystalline amino acids
   d. Lipids

7. Which of the following visceral proteins is most useful in monitoring the effectiveness of parenteral nutritional support?

   a. Albumin
   b. Transferrin
   c. Prealbumin
   d. Total protein

8. Refeeding syndrome is associated with which of the following electrolyte abnormalities?

   a. Hyponatremia
   b. Hypercalcemia
   c. Hypophosphatemia
   d. Hypermagnesemia

9. Which of the following are common components of the nutritional assessment? (*Select all that apply.*)

   a. Social history
   b. Dietary history
   c. Physical examination
   d. Anthropometric measurements
   e. Laboratory diagnostic evaluation

10. Which of the following are points of care in delivery of PPN? (*Select all that apply.*)

    a. PPN is mildly hypertonic and should be delivered into a large peripheral vein
    b. A 20% dextrose solution can be delivered via PPN
    c. Phlebitis is a complication of PPN, the catheter site should be observed with frequent documentation of the condition of the vein and site.
    d. PPN is most commonly used for short-term therapy for fairly stable patients whose normal GI functioning will resume within 3 to 4 weeks.

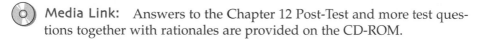 **Media Link:** Answers to the Chapter 12 Post-Test and more test questions together with rationales are provided on the CD-ROM.

▪ References

Ackley, B.J., & Ladwig, G.B. (2008). *Nursing diagnosis handbook: An evidence-based guide to planning care.* (8th ed.). St. Louis, MO: Mosby Elsevier

American Academy of Pediatrics (AAP), Committee on Nutrition (1998). *Pediatric nutrition handbook* (4th ed.). Elk Grove Village, IL: Author.

Arrowsmith, H. (1999). A critical evaluation of the use of nutrition screening tools by nurses. *British Journal of Nursing, 12,* 1483–1490.

American Society for Parenteral and Enteral Nutrition Board of Directors and Task Force (ASPEN) (2002a). Standards for specialized nutrition support: Adult hospitalized patients. *Nutrition in Clinical Practice, 20,* 103–116.

American Society for Parenteral and Enteral Nutrition Board of Directors and Task Force (ASPEN) Board of Directors and Task Force (2002b). ASPEN Guidelines: Access for administration of nutrition support. *Journal of Parenteral and Enteral Nutrition, 26S,* 36S–38S.

American Society for Parenteral and Enteral Nutrition (ASPEN) Board of Directors and Task Force. (2005a). Standards for specialized nutrition support: Hospitalized pediatric patients. *Nutrition in Clinical Practice, 20,* 103–116.

American Society for Parenteral and Enteral Nutrition (ASPEN) Board of Directors. (2005b). Standards for specialized nutrition support: Home care patients. *Nutrition in Clinical Practice, 20,* 579–589.

American Society for Parenteral and Enteral Nutrition (ASPEN) Board of Directors (2007). Standards of practice for nutrition support nurses. *Nutrition in Clinical Practice, 22,* 458–465.

American Society for Parenteral and Enteral Nutrition (ASPEN) Board of Directors and Task Force. (2004). Safe practices for parenteral nutrition. *Journal of Parenteral and Enteral Nutrition, 28*(S6), S43–S70.

Burgoa, L.J., Seidner, D., Hamilton, C., Staffor, J., & Steiger, E. (2006). Examination of factors that lead to complications for new home parenteral nutrition patients. *Journal of Infusion Nursing, 29*(2), 74–80.

Carpenito-Moyet, L.J. (2008). *Nursing diagnosis: Application to clinical practice* 12th ed. Philadelphia: Lippincott Williams & Wilkins.

Cerra, F.B. (1990). A standardized TPN order form reduces staff time and potential for error (editorial). *Nutrition, 6,* 498–499.

Collier, S., Courch, J., Hendricks, K., & Caballero, B. (1994). Use of cyclic parenteral nutrition in infants less than 6 months of age. *Nutrition in Clinical Practice, 9,* 65–68.

DeLegge, M.H., & Drake, L.M. (2007). Nutritional assessment. *Gastroenterology Clinics of North America, 36,* 1–22.

Dubek, S.G. (2006). *Nutrition essentials for nursing practice* (5th ed.). Philadelphia: Lippincott Williams & Wilkins.

Flegal, K.M., Carroll, M.D., & Kuczmarski, R.J. (1998). Overweight and obesity in the United States: Prevalence and trends 1960–1994. *International Journal of Obesity, 22,* 39–46.

Food and Drug Administration (FDA). (1994). Safety Alert: Hazardous of precipitation associated with parenteral nutrition. *American Journal of Hospital Pharmacy, 51,* 1427–1428.

Gahart, L., & Nazareno, A.R. (2008). *Intravenous medications* (24th ed.). St. Louis, MO: Mosby Elsevier.

Gorski, L.A. (2001). TPN update: making each visit count. *Home Healthcare Nurse, 19*(1), 15–21.

Gorski, L.A. (2005). *Pocket guide to home infusion therapy.* Sudbury, MA: Jones and Bartlett.

Infusion Nurses Society (INS). (2006). Infusion nursing standards of practice. *Journal of Infusion Nursing, 29*(1S), S74–S75.

Kovacevich, D.S., Boney, A.R., Braunschweig, C.L., et al. (1997). Nutrition risk classification: A reproducible and valid tool for nurses. *Nutrition in Clinical Practice, 12,* 20.

Krumpf, V.J. (2003). Update on parenteral iron therapy. *Nutrition in Clinical Practice, 18,* 318–326.

Leininger, M.M., & McFarland, M.R. (2002). *Transcultural nursing: Concepts, theories, research and practice* (3rd ed.). New York: McGraw-Hill.

Lustig, A. (2000). A medication error prevention by pharmacists. *Pharmacy & World Science, 22,* 21–25.

Lyman, B. (2002). Metabolic complications associated with parenteral nutrition. *Journal of Infusion Nursing, 25*(1), 36–44.

Maki, D., & Mermel, L.A. (2007). Infection due to infusion therapy. In: W.R. Jarvis (Ed.), *Hospital infections* (5th ed.). Philadelphia: Lippincott Williams & Wilkins.

McCloskey-Dochterman, J.C., & Bulechek, G.M. (2004). *Nursing interventions classification (NIC)* (4th ed.). St. Louis, MO: C.V. Mosby.

McGinnis, C. (2002). Parenteral nutrition focus: Nutritional assessment and formula composition. *Journal of Infusion Nursing, 25*(1), 54–64.

Metheny, N.M. (2000). *Fluid and electrolyte balance: Nursing considerations* (4th ed.). Philadelphia: Lippincott Williams & Wilkins.

Mimoz, O., Pieroni, L., Edouard, A., et al. (1996). Prospective, randomized trial of two antiseptic solutions for prevention of central venous ore arterial catheter colonization and infection in intensive care until patients. *Critical Care Medicine, 24,* 1818–1823.

Mirtallo, J.M. (2004). Complications associated with drug and nutrient interactions. *Journal of Infusion Nursing, 27*(1), 19–30.

Moorhead, S., Johnson, M., & Maas, M. (2004). *Nursing outcomes classification (NOC)* (3rd ed.). St. Louis, MO: C.V. Mosby.

NANDA-I (2007). *Nursing diagnoses: Definitions and classification, 2007–2008.* Philadelphia: Author.

O'Grady, N.P., Alexander M., Dellinger, E.P., et al. (2002). Guidelines for the prevention of intravascular catheter-related infections. *Morbidity and Mortality Weekly Report MMWR, 51*(RR-10).

Porth, C.M., & Martin, G. (2008). *Pathophysiology: Concepts of altered health states* (8th ed.). Philadelphia: Lippincott Williams & Wilkins.

Sherliker, L. (2000). Complications. In: H. Hamilton (Ed.), *Total parenteral nutrition: A practical guide for nurses.* Philadelphia: Churchill Livingstone Harcourt.

Shopbell, J.M., Hopkins, B., & Shronts, E.P. (2001). Nutrition screening and assessment. In: M.M. Gottschlich (Ed.). *The science and practice of nutrition support* (pp. 107–140). Dubuque, IA: Kendall/Hunt.

Smeltzer, S.C., Bare, B.G., Hinkle, J.L., & Cheever, K.H. (2008). *Brunner & Suddarths's textbook of medical-surgical nursing* (11th ed.). Philadelphia: Lippincott Williams & Willkins.

The Joint Commission (TJC). (2004). National patient safety goals. Retrieved from http://www.jointcommission.org/PatientSafety/National Patient Safety Goalsl/04 (Accessed September 10, 2008).

Trissel, L.A., Gilbert, D.L., Martinez, J.F., et al. (1997). Compatibility of parenteral nutrient solutions with selected drugs during simulated Y-site administration. *American Journal of Health-System Pharmacy, 54,* 1295–1300.

Trissel, L.A., Gilbert, D.L., Martinez, J.F., et al. (1999). Compatibility of medications with 3-in-1 parenteral nutrition admixtures. *JPEN, 23,* 67–74.

Wilkinson, J., & Van Leuven, K. (2007). *Fundamentals of nursing: Theory, concepts and applications.* Philadelphia: F.A. Davis.

Wilson, J.M., & Jordan, N.L. (2001). Parenteral nutrition. In: J. Hankins, R.A. Lonsway, C. Hedrick, & M. Perdue (Eds.). *Infusion therapy in clinical practice* (2nd ed., pp. 219–245). Philadelphia: W.B. Saunders.

Index

Note: Page numbers followed by f refer to figures, page numbers followed by t refer to tables.

Minimum System Requirements

PC

233 MHz processor
128 MB of RAM (256 MB of RAM recommended)
800 x 600 resolution monitor
Windows 2000/XP/Vista
8x CD-ROM drive
170 MB of available hard disk space

LICENSE AGREEMENT

1. F. A. Davis ("FAD") grants the recipient of the *Manual of I.V. Therapeutics,*
Fifth Edition, limited license for the program on the enclosed CD-ROM
"Software"). FAD retains complete copyright to the Software and associated
content.

2. Licensee has nonexclusive right to use this copy of the Software on one computer
on one screen at one location. Any other use is forbidden.

3. Licensee may physically transfer the Software from one computer to another,
provided that it is used on only one computer at any one time. Except for the
initial loading of the Software on a hard disk or for archival or backup purposes,
icensee may not copy, electronically transfer, or otherwise distribute copies.
's License Agreement automatically terminates if Licensee fails to comply
any term of this Agreement.
VARE UPDATES. Updated versions of the Software may be created or
FAD from time to time. At its sole option, FAD may make such updates
he Licensee or authorized transferees who have returned the registration
odate fee, and returned the original CD-ROM to FAD.